Personalized Medicine in Psychiatry: Challenges and Opportunities

Personalized Medicine in Psychiatry: Challenges and Opportunities

Guest Editor

Gniewko Więckiewicz

MDPI

Basel • Beijing • Wuhan • Barcelona • Belgrade • Novi Sad • Cluj • Manchester

Guest Editor
Gniewko Więckiewicz
Department of Psychiatry
Medical University of Silesia
Katowice
Poland

Editorial Office
MDPI AG
Grosspeteranlage 5
4052 Basel, Switzerland

This is a reprint of the Special Issue, published open access by the journal *Journal of Personalized Medicine* (ISSN 2075-4426), freely accessible at: https://www.mdpi.com/journal/jpm/special_issues/E4U3LF2VTQ.

For citation purposes, cite each article independently as indicated on the article page online and as indicated below:

Lastname, A.A.; Lastname, B.B. Article Title. *Journal Name* **Year**, *Volume Number*, Page Range.

ISBN 978-3-7258-7374-6 (Hbk)
ISBN 978-3-7258-7375-3 (PDF)
https://doi.org/10.3390/books978-3-7258-7375-3

Cover image courtesy of Gniewko Więckiewicz

Contents

About the Editors

Andrzej Frąckowiak

Andrzej Frąckowiak is employed as a full professor at the Institute of Thermal Energy, Poznań University of Technology. His research focuses on heat transfer and computational fluid mechanics, with a particular attention paid to the modeling of heat transfer processes through nanotube-coated surfaces and the inverse cooling of gas turbine blades using porous materials. He has conducted his research in collaboration with, and as part of research fellowships at, the University of Stuttgart, the Institute for Thermodynamics of Air and Space, the Technical University of Munich, Forschungseinheit M6, and the Free University of Berlin, Institute of Experimental Physics.

Bartosz Ciupek

Bartosz Ciupek is employed as an assistant professor at the Institute of Thermal Energy, Poznań University of Technology. His research focuses on the design and operation of heating systems and equipment, particularly boilers. He is currently conducting research on improving air quality and reducing pollutant emissions from solid fuel boilers through chemical modification of the combustion process, the use of exhaust gas cleaning systems, and alternative environmentally friendly solid fuels. He also works on improving the thermal and environmental performance of aircraft engines. He conducts his research in collaboration with, and through research fellowships with, the Cracow University of Technology, the Military University of Technology in Warsaw, the Kielce University of Technology, and the University of Kalisz. He holds a scholarship from the City of Poznań and has authored 14 patents.

Łukasz Brodzik

Łukasz Brodzik is employed as an assistant professor at the Institute of Thermal Energy, Poznań University of Technology. His research activities are focused on two fields, the first of which is space technology. In this field, he has experience solving problems with heating orbiter heat shields. His research focuses on heat transfer via thermal radiation for porous coatings in high-temperature environments, as well as their impact on structures in the event of damage. The second field is aviation. In this case, the analyses conducted concern two aspects. The first is research on miniature turbojet engines for co-combustion of aviation kerosene and hydrogen. The analyses focus on the impact of hydrogen on engine operation, primarily in terms of temperature changes in individual sections. The second aspect of our aviation sector activities is aircraft performance analysis, which involves calculating flight parameters, primarily for smaller aircraft.

Preface

This Reprint brings together selected contributions addressing contemporary issues in applied heat transfer. Its scope covers theoretical investigations, modeling, and optimization of heat transfer processes, as well as applied solutions implemented in energy devices and installations. The main purpose is to provide a comprehensive overview of innovative approaches that not only improve thermal efficiency but also support environmental protection by reducing the consumption of conventional energy sources.

The motivation for preparing this Reprint arises from the dynamic development of modern energy technologies and the growing need for sustainable practices. Heat transfer remains a central area of research with direct impact on efficiency, performance, and ecological responsibility in power engineering and related fields.

This Reprint is intended for researchers, engineers, and professionals who deal with the challenges of designing, optimizing, and implementing energy systems. It may also be of interest to graduate students and decision makers seeking insight into current research trends and technological advances in heat transfer applications.

Andrzej Frąckowiak, Bartosz Ciupek, and Łukasz Brodzik
Guest Editors

energies

MDPI

Review

Review of Thermal Calculation Methods for Boilers—Perspectives on Thermal Optimization for Improving Ecological Parameters

Bartosz Ciupek * and Andrzej Frąckowiak *

Faculty of Environmental Engineering and Energy, Institute of Thermal Energy, Poznan University of Technology, 60-965 Poznan, Poland
* Correspondence: bartosz.ciupek@put.poznan.pl (B.C.); andrzej.frackowiak@put.poznan.pl (A.F.)

Abstract: This article presents an overview of thermal calculation methods used in boilers powered by fossil fuels (solid, liquid or gas). The analysis was carried out mainly in terms of combustion chamber calculation methods. Changing standards and legal regulations regarding the use of fossil fuels in Europe and the world make it necessary to adapt calculation methods and boiler design to current requirements, and many of them are related to outdated boiler models or for fuels that are no longer so heavily used in industrial solutions. Current research and development trends implemented in the EU and in the world related to the issues of the European Green Deal, the Fit for 55 directive and other ecological trends in the energy sector make it necessary to verify and remodel the calculation methods used so far in terms of the thermal efficiency of the device, fuel consumption or the use of fuels not previously used in their wide range in a wider application. Hence, the knowledge and updating of the state of knowledge in the field of the thermal calculation of boilers in terms of their environmental performance is necessary and strongly sought after by researchers. It is undoubted that in the next few years, boilers will continue to be the main source of thermal energy, especially in the power industry or industry. A reasonable energy transition should be based on the direction of the thermal optimization of already functioning structures and adaptation of their operating parameters to the planned new ecological fuels in the sense of the intensification of energy converted from primary form to thermal energy, and in the last step, it should reorganize the energy and industrial sectors, leaving only these groups of devices treated as a stable and necessary source of energy. Therefore, it should be recognized that activities aimed at improving the thermal parameters of boilers should directly improve the thermal efficiency of the device, and this will translate into fuel savings and reduce their negative impact on the environment.

Keywords: boilers; environmental protection; thermal power; heat transfer; thermal calculations; efficiency

1. Introduction

Thermal calculations of boilers are one of the key elements of thermal engineering, especially in the context of optimizing combustion processes, energy efficiency and minimizing harmful emissions [1–3]. Boilers, used in many industrial sectors and in the energy sector, are devices whose operation must be constantly monitored and optimized to meet growing technical, environmental and economic requirements [4,5]. Increasing demands for efficient energy management and legal and regulatory requirements for exhaust emissions are driving engineers and scientists to adopt increasingly sophisticated calculation methods. Thermal calculations are the foundation of the design, operation and modernization of boilers, because they allow us to precisely determine the operating parameters of devices and predict their impact on the environment [3].

Changes in legal regulations, especially in the European Union, place increasing emphasis on energy efficiency, environmental protection and minimizing the impact of industrial activities on air quality and climate change [6]. EU directives such as the Industrial Emissions Directive (IED) and national environmental laws place a number of requirements on boiler manufacturers and industrial users regarding energy efficiency and emissions of pollutants (e.g. NO_x, SO_x, CO_2) [7,8]. Boilers based on traditional combustion methods must now be designed and modified in accordance with stringent emission standards, which forces designers and operators to carry out detailed thermal and thermodynamic calculations [3,4]. Taking the above into account, it can be concluded that as ecological parameters relating to boilers, these will be indicators assessing their impact on the natural environment, especially in the context of pollutant emissions, energy efficiency and fuel consumption. In the case of boilers, these parameters are important in assessing their compliance with environmental regulations, impact on air quality and strive for sustainable development. The key ecological parameters in the context of boilers include the following:

1. Pollutant emissions: Carbon dioxide (CO_2) as an indicator of greenhouse gas emissions, especially in fossil fuel boilers. Nitrogen oxides (NO_x) formed during high-temperature combustion affect smog and the acidification of the environment. Sulfur oxide (SO_x) emissions are associated with the use of sulfur fuels, e.g., low-quality coal leads to acid rain. Particulate matter (PM10, PM2.5) is particularly important in the case of coal or biomass-fired boilers. Carbon monoxide (CO) indicates the incomplete combustion of fuel [4].
2. Energy efficiency: The efficiency index of a boiler, i.e., the ratio of energy obtained in the form of heat to the energy contained in the fuel. Higher efficiency means lower fuel consumption and lower emissions. Condensing boilers usually have higher energy efficiency than traditional ones [2].
3. Type of fuel: Solid fuel boilers (e.g., coal, wood, biomass) are usually more emission-intensive than natural gas or fuel oil boilers. Biomass boilers can be environmentally friendly if the fuel comes from renewable sources and combustion takes place in a controlled manner [8].
4. Fuel consumption: Less fuel consumption while maintaining the same amount of heat generated is environmentally beneficial as it reduces pollutant emissions [4].
5. Flue gas temperature and heat recovery: A lower flue gas temperature indicates better energy utilization and less heat loss. The use of heat recovery techniques (e.g., in condensing boilers or economizers) reduces emissions and improves efficiency [3].
6. Flue gas filtration: The use of electrostatic precipitators, dust collectors and other technologies reduces the emission of dust and harmful gasses. Legal regulations require reduction in pollutant emissions, e.g., as part of the fight against smog [5].
7. Healthcare: Reducing dust and harmful gas emissions reduces air pollution, improving quality of life [7].
8. Economic efficiency: Higher efficiency and lower fuel consumption translate into savings for the user [4].

Therefore, it can be concluded that thermal calculation methods affect the ecological parameters of boilers by optimizing their design, the selection of operating parameters and energy efficiency. Well-conducted thermal calculations allow for minimizing energy losses and pollutant emissions, which translates into better environmental parameters of the device.

Modern thermal calculations of boilers allow for the accurate prediction of fuel consumption, the amount of heat generated in the combustion process and heat losses in various stages of boiler operation. This allows you to minimize the emission of harmful substances by optimizing the operating parameters of the devices. Legal requirements also affect the need to regularly modernize boilers in order to adapt them to standards, which requires precise thermal analyses both at the design stage and during operation [9–12].

Environmental protection is now one of the priority objectives of industrial policies, both at the national and international level. Industrial boilers, especially those of the older generation, can be a source of significant amounts of pollution if they are not properly designed and operated. One of the main problems is the emission of greenhouse gasses and harmful substances such as sulfur dioxide, nitrogen oxides and particulate matter. Thanks to precise thermal calculations, it is possible to reduce these emissions by increasing the energy efficiency of boilers and using advanced flue gas cleaning technologies [13–16].

Today's technologies, such as flue gas recirculation, condensing heat exchangers and low-emission burners, require thorough thermodynamic and thermal analyses to ensure maximum efficiency with minimum environmental impact. The professional literature, including scientific textbooks and technical articles, emphasizes the role of thermal calculations in assessing and forecasting the environmental impact of thermal installations. For example, through scientific works related to the modeling of combustion processes and the analysis of heat losses and thanks to the optimization of the combustion process, emissions can be reduced without the need to replace the entire device [17–21].

The development of technology, including the digitization of industrial processes, has contributed to a change in the approach to boiler design and operation. New-generation boilers are equipped with automatic control and monitoring systems, which allow for the ongoing adjustment of operating parameters to current needs and the optimization of energy efficiency. Modern methods of thermal calculations include computer modeling and simulations of combustion processes, which allow engineers to accurately predict the efficiency of boilers under various operating conditions. The use of numerical methods, such as finite element analysis (FEM), enables the detailed modeling of thermal and flow processes, which is necessary when designing modern boilers in order to achieve high operating parameters, such as high thermal efficiency and low emissions of harmful substances [22–24].

The scientific literature draws attention to the increase in the popularity of condensing boilers and boilers powered by alternative energy sources, such as biomass. Such devices require specialized thermal calculations that take into account the specifics of the fuel and other unique operating parameters. These boilers are highly energy efficient, but at the same time require precise design and monitoring to maximize their efficiency and minimize emissions [25–30].

The aim of this article is to analyze the existing methods of thermal calculations from the points of view of the following:

1. Available methods and tools used in the design and thermal analysis of boilers.
2. Assessment of their accuracy, merits and limitations in optimizing energy efficiency and emissions.
3. Identification of links between thermal calculations and ecological parameters.

In addition, the relationships between thermal efficiency and fuel consumption and pollutant emissions are discussed. The conclusions indicate proposals for improvements in the process of designing and operating boilers.

Thermal calculations of boilers, taking into account new legal regulations, environmental protection and the dynamic development of technology, are a key element of modern thermal engineering. They not only ensure the possibility of precise design and operation of boilers but also contribute to environmental protection and increase energy efficiency [31].

2. Method Review

2.1. Thermal Calculations of Water Tube Boilers

Water tube boilers are widely used in industrial applications due to their efficiency and ability to generate steam at high pressures. Understanding the thermal calculations involved in the operation of these boilers is essential for optimizing performance and ensuring safety. The most common methods for the thermal calculations of water and steam boilers are balance methods based on the unit heat load resulting from the fuel stream supplied to the combustion process and the assumed thermal power on the hot water or steam side. Most of the known and used methods do not take into account the stoichiometry of the fuel combustion process (they assume its complete combustion), and at the same time do not take into account the increased power demand, e.g., for flue gas cleaning. Water tube boilers operate by circulating water inside tubes that are heated by combustion gases. This design allows for a large surface area for heat transfer, which enhances efficiency. The efficiency of a water tube boiler is largely determined by its heat transfer capabilities. The primary modes of heat transfer include conduction, convection and radiation [32,33].

The basic equation in the balance sheet method is the overall heat transfer coefficient:

$$U = \frac{1}{\frac{1}{h_i} + \frac{d}{k} + \frac{1}{h_o}} \tag{1}$$

where h_i—internal heat transfer coefficient (inside the tube) [W/m^2·K]; h_o—external heat transfer coefficient (outside the tube) [W/m^2·K]; d—thickness of the tube wall [m]; and k—thermal conductivity of the tube material [W/m·K].

The thermal efficiency η of a boiler can be expressed as

$$\eta = \frac{Q_{out}}{Q_{in}} \cdot 100\% \tag{2}$$

where Q_{out}—useful heat output [W]; and Q_{in}—total energy input from fuel combustion [W].

Several factors contribute to energy losses in water tube boilers, including the following:

- Flue gas losses: heat carried away by exhaust gasses.
- Radiation losses: heat lost through the boiler casing.
- Blowdown losses: heat lost due to the removal of water to control concentration levels.

Calculating these losses is crucial for improving boiler efficiency and may be important from the point of view of improving the ecological parameters of boilers due to the reduction in harmful substance emissions through the rational management of conventional or alternative fuel resources [34,35].

Ref. [36] presents the method of the thermal conversion of radiated boilers developed by the Central Institute of Boilers and Turbines in Petersburg (CKTI), also known as the method of Gurowicz A. (1950). This method is based on scientific and experimental work carried out by the Institute, which is used in the calculations of low- and high-power boilers. In addition, the WTI method (Timofeyev B., 1934 and 1941 Moscow), the Wohlenberg method (Münzinger F., Berechnung und Verhalten von Wasserrohrkesseln, 1949), which is most widely used for the calculations of grate coal boilers, and the Ledinegg method (1952) are cited.

Ref. [37] presents thermal calculations of flame tube boilers based on the Soviet WTI method (All-Union Technical Institute in Moscow), also known as the method of Timofeyev B. (1939 and 1941), which is a standardized method, and the Wohlenberg method developed by Münzinger F. (1949). Both methods are based on calculating the heat given off by radiation in the combustion chamber bypassing the convection process, which is considered insignificant in the heat transfer of the combustion chamber. Both methods also take into account the temperature of the flue gasses leaving the combustion chamber as one of the balance conditions of the boiler, which should be assumed or calculated. The calculations are based on the classical equation for the heat of radiation resulting from the Stefan–Bolzman equation:

$$Q_{pr} = c \cdot H_{pr} \cdot \left[\left(\frac{T + 273.15}{100} \right)^4 - \left(\frac{T_{sc} + 273.15}{100} \right)^4 \right] \tag{3}$$

where T—temperature of flue gasses leaving the combustion chamber [°C]; T_{sc}—temperature of heated walls [°C]; c—total radiation coefficient (depending on the boiler design, type of fuel, etc.) [W]; and H_{pr}—radiated area [m^2].

In addition, the book presents the heat transfer coefficient (α) with the flow of flue gasses across pipes arranged in parallel and crosswise (staggered system). Both equations come from the scientific works of Antywiewa and Kozaczeński, taking into account the research of Kuznetsov and Lokrin. The equations also take into account correction factors based on Babcock–Wilcox research.

Ref. [38] present identical methods of calculating water tube boilers (flame tube boilers) as those included in [1]; however, as the most accurate measurable calculation results, they consider the CKTI method (Gurowicz A. method), taking into account the favorably calculated heat flux in individual zones of the boiler resulting directly from the WTI method (Timofeyev B., method). This method is today referred to by scientists as the zonal method. In addition, over the years, the beneficial aspects of the CKTI and WTI methods have been combined into one and established as the Soviet Steam Boiler Calculation Method.

Ref. [39] presents two Soviet methods (CKTI and WTI) as the most advantageous current methods of calculating low-, medium- and high-power boilers. In the book, both methods are considered together under the concept mentioned above. The author also presents the Wohlenberg method as a method also used in the United States (not only the German method), which has the advantage of quick and consistent calculations of the thermal parts of the boiler.

Ref. [40] presents examples of standards that allow us to define and calculate the efficiency of a boiler (German standard DIN 1942, American standard ASME PTC 4.1 and Polish standard PN–72/M–34128). In the case of the presented method of calculating thermal processes occurring in a boiler, the CKTI method is given, the description of which includes both calculations in accordance with this method, but also elements derived from the WTI method, which allows us to believe that in the scientific nomenclature, elements of the CKTI and WTI methods have been combined into one method, commonly referred to as the Soviet Method of Calculating Steam Boilers.

Ref. [41] presents, like the previous authors, a balance method of thermal calculations for boilers based on the CKTI method model.

2.2. *Thermal Calculations of Fire Tube Boilers*

Ref. [42] presents the methods of calculating thermal processes (mainly heat transfer) occurring in fire and tube boilers. The method described in this book is based mainly on the results of operational tests of operating fire and tube boilers and current scientific works on heat transfer. The described methods are based on the recommendations for determining the heat transfer coefficient (α) along the length of the fire tube and determining the temperature of the flue gas at its end, which is taken as the starting temperature for thermal calculations of the entire boiler fire tube system. Łachanin W. took this method from Dolgolenko W., who described it in the book entitled Steam Ship Devices in 1940. Another simplified method described by Łachanin W., is the determination of the velocity of flue gasses flowing in the fire tube as a determinant of the calculation of the number of tubes of the convection part of the boiler. He took this method from Barasz P., described by him in 1939 in his book entitled Fundamentals of Theory and Thermal Calculations of Steam Ship Boilers.

Ref. [43] presents methods for calculating low-temperature water heating boilers burning natural gas. It provides methods for calculating the heat given off by convection, with particular emphasis on fire tube boilers, but also flame tube boilers. The author suggests that the share of convection in the heat exchange process taking place in the combustion chamber, especially in a low-power heating boiler, is on average about 20%, although he also notes that due to the high temperature of the flue gas in the combustion chamber, the heat exchange mechanism mainly occurs by radiation, which can be considered about 80% of all energy given off by heat exchange in the combustion chamber. The author also states that in this type of construction, the heat transfer coefficient (α) can be calculated from the Sieder–Tate relation for which the Nusselt number takes the following form:

$$Nu = 1.86 \cdot \left(Re_f \cdot Pr_f \cdot \frac{d_e}{L} \right)^{1/3} \cdot \left(\frac{\nu_f}{\nu_s} \right) \tag{4}$$

where Re_f—Reynolds number of the fluid [–]; Pr_f—Prandtl number of the fluid [–]; d_e—diameter of the flue gas (internal) [m]; L—length of the flue gas [m]; ν_f—coefficient of kinematic viscosity for the mean temperature of the flue gas [m^2/s]; and ν_s—coefficient of kinematic viscosity for the flue gas for the wall temperature [m^2/s].

If the diameter of the flue gas duct (flame tube) is significantly smaller than its length and the L/d_e coefficient > 4 or more, then the equation takes the following form:

$$Nu = 6.43 \cdot \left(Re_f \cdot Pr_f \cdot \frac{d_e}{L} \right)^{1/3} \cdot \left(\frac{\nu_f}{\nu_s} \right) \tag{5}$$

The author notes that in the case of flame tubes, the condition of forced convection occurs in the laminar flow velocity range, which causes the appearance of the Grashof number in the empirical formula for the mean Nusselt number borrowed from Mikhaev (1953).

$$Nu = 0.15 \cdot {Re_f}^{0.33} \cdot {Gr_f}^{0.1} \cdot {Pr_f}^{0.43} \left(\frac{Pr_f}{Pr_s} \right)^{0.25} \varepsilon_l \tag{6}$$

where Pr_w—Prandtl number of the wall [–]; and ε_l—emissivity of the heated surface [–].

The characteristic linear dimension in this case is the inner diameter of the pipe (d_e—equivalent diameter), and the value of the physical parameters of the fluid is determined for the arithmetic mean temperature at the inlet and outlet of the tube. The author also gives the average value of the heat transfer coefficient at the flow of a single cylinder based on the work of Hilpert and Żukauskas. The equivalent thickness of the gas layer for the flow in the duct developed by Hottel is also mentioned.

Ref. [31] presents an exemplary design of thermal calculations of a fire and tube boiler based on the entapliative method, taking into account the parameters of dissociation of gasses (mainly triatomic) with the assumption of the ratio of the length of the combustion chamber to its diameter in the range of the L/d_e coefficient parameter in the range of 2–5 [–], within which the calculation of the Nusselt number value for the combustion chamber is proposed, taking into account the additional viscosity coefficient kinematic flue gas with regard to the density of flue gasses at a given point of the analyzed temperature distribution in the combustion chamber:

$$Nu = 6.43 \cdot \left(Re_f \cdot Pr_f \cdot \frac{d_e}{L} \right)^{1/3} \cdot \left(\frac{\nu_f \cdot \rho_f}{\nu_s \cdot \rho_s} \right)^{0.14} \tag{7}$$

where ρ_f—density of the fluid in the center of the stream [kg/m^3]; and ρ_s—density of the fluid on the heating surface [kg/m^3].

Within the framework of the presented method, the author divides the heat transfer processes for the combustion chamber as follows:

- Heat given by convection: about 4.5–5%;
- Heat given by flame radiation: about 75–80%;
- Heat given by flue gas radiation: about 15–20%.

2.3. Other Methods for Calculating Boiler Combustion Chambers

The method of Lobo and Evans is based on the use of the total heat transfer coefficient and radiation calculations based on the Stefan–Boltzmann equation. It has been used for systems operating in refinery–furnace design work and it is also recommended for oil- and gas-fired boilers (and also for heating natural gas-fired boilers to the max. heat power of 300–1500 kW with pipeline heat exchanger). The average deviation between the predicted and observed heat absorption for 85 tests on 19 different refinery furnaces varying widely in physical and operating characteristics was 5.3%. The max. deviation was 16%. In addition, this method is widely used in industry, especially for large furnaces [44]. According to this method, it is determined that the boiler efficiency (net) is the ratio of the amount of heat released to the heating medium circuit in a specific unit of time to the amount of heat energy generated at that time. The heat flow from the flue gas to the exchanger in the form of tubes with the circulation of the working medium takes place mainly by means of radiation and forced convection. The water or steam in the pipes receives heat energy first in the convection zone and then in the radiation zone, which increases the efficiency of heat transfer. Lobo and Evans assumed the complete mixing of the flue gasses in the radiation section, i.e., the conditions are constant throughout this zone and there are no longitudinal or transverse temperature gradients. The average radiation temperature is equal to the temperature of the gas leaving the radiation zone. Radiation to the convection zone is omitted. This method involves the use of the general heat transfer coefficient and the aforementioned Stefan–Boltzmann equation. The equation for the radiant heat flux was proposed by De Baufre [44]. It is presented below:

$$Q_R = A_{cp} \cdot E\left[\left(\frac{T_g}{100}\right)^4 - \left(\frac{T_s}{100}\right)^4\right] \tag{8}$$

where A_{cp}—a plane with an area equivalent to the exchanger area [m^2]; E—heat exchange efficiency coefficient per unit boiler volume (at the end of the sequence [W·m^2/K^4]; T_g—average temperature of the gas leaving the radiation zone [K]; and T_s—temperature of the exchanger surface (tubes) [K].

Unfortunately, this method is characterized by poor data correlation, while Lobo and Evans aimed to achieve the highest possible accuracy. The equation they determined by means of research is presented below:

$$Q_R = 0.173 \cdot F\left[\left(\frac{T_g}{100}\right)^4 - \left(\frac{T_s}{100}\right)^4\right]\alpha \cdot A_{cp} \tag{9}$$

where F—coefficient of efficiency or total heat transfer [–]; and α—coefficient decreasing A_{cp} in such a way as to obtain the effective surface of the exchanger and absorption efficiency coefficient [–].

The equation with the heat balance on the gas side is as follows:

$$Q_R = H_{in} - M \cdot c_p \cdot T_g \tag{10}$$

where H_{in}—inlet enthalpy of flue gas [W]; M—gas flow rate [kg·s]; and c_p—averaged specific heat of gas (e.g., by interpolation method) [J/kg K].

The above equation with the added convective term also takes into account the heat transfer by convection. It is presented below:

$$Q_R = 0.173 \cdot F\left[\left(\frac{T_g}{100}\right)^4 - \left(\frac{T_s}{100}\right)^4\right]\alpha \cdot A_{cp} + h_c A\left(T_g - T_s\right) \tag{11}$$

where h_c—convective transmittance coefficient [W/m^2·K]; and A—total area of the exchanger (pipes) [m^2].

The F-factor is based on Christiansen's formula and is determined as follows:

$$F = \frac{1}{\frac{1}{F_s} + \frac{1}{P_c} - 1} \tag{12}$$

where P_C—cold surface emissivity [–].

The equation of F_S, on the other hand, is determined from the following formula:

$$F_S = p_f\left[1 + \left(\frac{A_R}{\alpha A_{cp}}\right)\frac{1}{1 + \left(\frac{p_f}{1-p_f}\right)\frac{1}{F_{RC}}}\right] \tag{13}$$

where p_f—flame emissivity [–]; A_R—resistive surface [m^2]; and F_{RC}—coefficient determined empirically by Lobo and Evans [–].

The heat absorbed in the radiation zone Q_R can be determined as follows:

$$\frac{Q_R}{\alpha A_{cp} F} = 0.173\left[\left(\frac{T_g}{100}\right)^4 - \left(\frac{T_s}{100}\right)^4\right] + 7(T_g - T_s) \tag{14}$$

The Lobo and Evans method assumes constant conditions throughout the chamber and treats it as one large zone, while in reality there are temperature gradients, the degree of mixing of gasses is not complete, and the properties of the exhaust gas and the working medium are different at different points. This can result in large inaccuracies, as the model can only provide an approximate result. Nevertheless, the Lobo and Evans method works quite well for large boilers. The assumption of complete mixing of gasses is generally acceptable except in high-temperature boilers with tall, narrow furnaces, where transverse and longitudinal temperature gradients cannot be ignored. In this case, a more accurate method of estimating the temperature of the gas should be considered. To increase accuracy, the radiation zone can be divided into several sections [44].

The Wilson, Lobo and Hottel method is an empirical method that has been used in box-type furnaces powered by oils and gasses for an estimated heat load from 15,000 to 95,000 W/m^2 for the perimeter pipe area. Another limitation in the application of this method is the temperature range for the unit temperature of the pipe surface, which should not be higher than about 200 °C for the radiation parts of the boiler, taking into account the flue gas temperature. It is believed that the average length of the radiated surface should not exceed about 4.5 meters for such boilers. This method is widely used in industry and recommended for the above limitations when the accuracy of the Lobo–Evans equation is not required; therefore, it is used when the accuracy of the calculation is not strongly required (indicative method), and hence, it is considered a preliminary estimation method. The equation used to estimate the rate of heat absorption by the heat transfer surface considered in this method is given by the following equation:

$$\mu = \frac{Q}{Q_F} = \frac{1}{1 + \frac{G\sqrt{\frac{Q_F}{\alpha A_{cp}}}}{4200}} \tag{15}$$

where μ—ratio of heat absorbed to heat released in the boiler [–]; Q—net calorific value of the fuel [kJ/kg]; Q_F—heat supplied by the fuel (average calorific value or calorific value of the fuel in the operating condition) [kJ/kg]; G—ratio of air to fuel [–]; and A_{cp}—heat exchange area [m^2].

From a practical point of view, with the Wilson, Lobo and Hottel method, the heat transfer area should be properly estimated using the above equation, especially in the case of a boiler with a single and double row of fire tubes, without taking into account the surfaces washed by the flame (for the combustion chamber). This equation does not work for calculations for very low and high calorific values, because the effect of excess air on the efficiency of heat transfer by radiation is difficult to define by the ratio of excess air to fuel. This equation is used in the energy balance to calculate the amount of total radiant heat [44].

The Orrok–Hudson method, as an early empieric equation for calculating the absorbed heat in the radiating part of a water tube boiler, is used to estimate the combustion chambers on the basis of changes in and parameters of the combustion rate of the burned bed and the related air–fuel ratio (excess air coefficient). It is quite measurably used in the design of heating boilers or low-power steam boilers. It has been replaced with more precise expressions and has limited value for design work. It can be used to estimate the effects of changes in the combustion rate or air–fuel ratio for an existing coal or oil-fired boiler if the impact and degree of slag deposition on the furnace tubes is known. In such applications, it may be necessary to adjust the constant in the equation to the known operating conditions of the boiler being analyzed. The equation used in this method has the following form:

$$t_e = 20 + \frac{1000}{\frac{7.495}{\sqrt{q_i}} + \frac{1164}{h_g}} \tag{16}$$

where t_e—temperature of the exhaust gasses [°F]; q_i—one-set heat load of the combustion chamber [W/m^2 ·K]; and h_g—the amount of heat supplied per kilogram of flue gas [W].

The equation showing the dependence of the temperature of exhaust gasses to the unit heat load and the amount of heat supplied per kilogram of flue gasses, derived on the basis of the Orrok–Hudson equation at the ambient temperature of 20 °C for the boiler operating temperature range of 600–1200 °C, is characterized by a calculation error of ±20 °C (about 2–3%) [44].

The methods shown are designed to increase the precision of calculations related to heat transfer and combustion efficiency, which are critical for optimizing the efficiency of boiler combustion chambers. In conclusion, alternative methods for calculating boiler combustors are critical to meeting evolving energy efficiency and environmental compliance requirements. Their use not only improves design accuracy but also facilitates innovation in boiler technology. It is important to emphasize that it is important to choose the right method based on the type of boiler, operating requirements and available computing resources.

3. Discussion on Improving Ecological Parameters

As part of the discussion of the review of methods of thermal calculations of boilers, considering the known and used methods of thermal calculations of boilers, it can be observed that most of them derive from or refer to old methods. Most of them were developed at the beginning of the twentieth century, and therefore, due to the early principles and approaches to ecology, they do not take into account assumptions related to the optimization of the ecological parameters of boilers. The following parameters should be considered as environmental parameters of a boiler: parameters related to the emission of harmful substances into the atmosphere and greenhouse gas emissions (e.g., CO_2) [45–49]. Another environmental indicator would be the heat lost to the environment and the thermal efficiency of the boiler (on the water or steam side), which will directly affect the amount of fuel burned in the boiler, and this will affect the change in environmental parameters [50–54].

In the case of modern boiler technical solutions, flue gas treatment systems (filtration systems, catalytic converters, selective non-catalytic systems and others) are often used in their construction, and systems related to the improvement of emission parameters and efficiency, such as flue gas recirculation systems or flue gas moisture condensation systems, are used. In most cases, these systems require additional energy for their proper operation, and this energy is often associated with high flue gas temperature (e.g., selective or non-selective catalytic reactors, urea or ammonia water dosing systems or electroylters). This demand is often covered by the boiler's own energy or is supplied artificially from an additional energy source (e.g., additional burners or regenerative reactors based on other fuels or electricity). All these solutions at the stage of designing the boiler structure should be ignited and provided for as part of the boiler's energy surplus, so that the energy needed for the operation of appropriate flue gas treatment systems can be covered from the net energy produced by the boiler. In the case of boilers already in operation, another option available is the use of additional heat recovery systems; for example, with economizers, if a high chimney loss is observed on the side of high flue gas temperature and if the fuel used allows (marginal sulfur content), a possible course of action is to transform the boiler structure into a condensing system [55–67].

However, in the case of a large group of devices with an outdated design, it is necessary to modernize them or replace them with a system of modern design with the use of systems that improve the ecological parameters of the boiler. The presented analysis also shows the need to verify the currently used calculation methods and develop them in terms of taking into account the improvement of the thermal and emission parameters, especially due to the continuously strong popularity of these technical solutions and their continued use as peak or transient sources in the near future [68–72].

4. Conclusions

The most important conclusions from this review of the state of knowledge include the following:

1. Various methods of thermal calculation for boiler heating surfaces are known. Empirical methods, theoretical methods with the empirical refinement of indicators and purely theoretical formulas are used.
2. As part of the thermal calculations, both equations based only on the thermal parameters and heat transfer of the boiler are used, and there are known equations in which the parameters of the combustion process are additionally used (most often referred to as combustion stoichiometry).
3. Further activities on the thermal optimization of boilers are still carried out; attention is mainly paid to the parameters of the thermal power of the boiler and its efficiency, while issues related to the reduction in the emissions of harmful substances, including the improvement of the ecological parameters of boilers, are mainly addressed as separate issues from the construction and operation of boilers.
4. The increase in the share of biomass and alternative fuels in the construction and exploration of boilers requires the research and development of empirical coefficients for this new group within the equations for the thermal calculations of boilers in order to adapt the currently known calculation methodology to take into account these fuels (especially due to lower combustion temperatures and different stoichiometry of the combustion process compared to for conventional fuels).
5. It should be recognized that the environmental protection and ecological parameters of boilers, as a currently necessary aspect of their use, should be significantly taken into account in the process of designing new equipment or modernizing old solutions. In the case of improving the ecological parameters of boilers, the changes taking place in the scope of their operation (developed control systems) [73–76] or monitoring (carbon footprint, flue gas emission monitoring systems, drones) [77–79] should also be taken into account at the stages of design and the adaptation of the structure, so that continuous measurements of thermal and emission parameters can be carried out in a reliable manner.

The main direction of the latest research and development of boiler calculation methods is the introduction of numerical methods into boiler designs (new and those based on the formulas presented in the article). Empirical studies related to heat transfer, especially on the side of combustion chambers, take into account the processes of radiation and convection. Another important aspect is the deepening of empirical research in the field of heat transfer processes for biomass or formed, torrefied fuels or clean energy fuels, i.e., related to zero or low emissions of harmful substances, which are relatively new and still require the creation of good databases of indicators, variables or coefficients to correlate the thermal parameters of a newly built boiler or modernized in relation to the fuel intended for combustion. Hence, the direction of the development of empirical research for thermal processes and further development of numerical methods or machine learning is important from the point of view of improving the ecological parameters of boilers. However, they will still be based on well-known and refined mathematical formulas developed in the past, while of course taking into account these new aspects.

Thermal calculations for boilers involve complex interactions between heat transfer, steam generation and efficiency metrics [80–82]. By optimizing these calculations, operators can enhance performance and reduce operational costs. Understanding these principles is vital for engineers working with boiler systems in industrial settings [83–92].

Author Contributions: Conceptualization, B.C. and A.F.; methodology, B.C. and A.F.; formal analysis, B.C.; investigation, B.C.; resources, B.C.; data curation, B.C.; writing—original draft preparation, B.C. and A.F.; writing—review and editing, B.C. and A.F.; project administration, B.C. and A.F.; funding acquisition, B.C. and A.F. All authors have read and agreed to the published version of the manuscript.

Funding: This research was funded by the Poznan University of Technology's financial resources for statutory activity, grant numbers 0712/SBAD/5252 and 0712/SBAD/5280.

Data Availability Statement: Data is contained within the article.

Acknowledgments: The present work and related research were developed in the framework of the implementation of the Research Internship under contract No. 1/2024 dated 8 August 2024, under which PhD Bartosz Ciupek completed a research internship in the period of 2 September 2024 to 31 December 2024 in accordance with the Internship Program. I would like to sincerely thank the University of Kalisz, Poland, Poznan University of Technology, Poland, Andrzej Frąckowiak and Rafał Urbaniak for accepting me for a research internship and the opportunity to complete it.

Conflicts of Interest: The authors declare no conflicts of interest.

References

1. Chen, Q.; Finney, K.; Li, H.; Zhang, X.; Zhou, J.; Sharifi, V.; Swithenbank, J. Condensing boiler applications in the process industry. *Appl. Energy* **2012**, *89*, 30–36. [CrossRef]
2. Breeze, P. *Gas-Turbine Power Generation*; Academic Press: Cambridge, MA, USA, 2016; ISBN 9780128040058. (In English)
3. Incropera, F.P.; DeWitt, D.; Bergman, T.; Lavine, A. *Fundamentals of Heat and Mass Transfer*; John Wiley & Sons, Inc.: Hoboken, NJ, USA, 2007; ISBN 9780470055540. (In English)
4. Turns, S.; Haworth, D. *An Introduction to Combustion: Concepts and Applications*, 4th ed.; McGraw-Hill Book Company: New York, NY, USA, 2024; ISBN 9781260477696. (In English)
5. Wang, Y.; Pan, Z.; Zhang, W.; Borhani, T.N.; Li, R.; Zhang, Z. Life cycle assessment of combustion-based electricity generation technologies integrated with carbon capture and storage: A review. *Environ. Res.* **2022**, *207*, 112219. [CrossRef] [PubMed]
6. Schwan, L.; Hahn, J.; Barton, M.; Anders, R.; Schweigler, C. Development of Reference Buildings to Analyze the Potential for Energy-Efficient Refurbishment of Buildings. *Civ. Environ. Eng. Rep.* **2019**, *29*, 198–217. [CrossRef]
7. Calvo, V.L.V.; Giner-Santonja, G.; Alonso-Fariñas, B.; Aguado, J.M. The effect of the European Industrial Emissions Directive on the air emission limit values set by competent authorities in the permitting procedure: The case of the Spanish cement industry. *Sci. Total Environ.* **2021**, *773*, 145491. [CrossRef] [PubMed]
8. Ciupek, B. *Laboratorium Spalania Paliw Kopalnych i Biomasy*; Wydawnictwo Politechniki Poznańskiej: Poznan, Poland, 2022; ISBN 9788377756669. (In Polish)
9. Dolganov, I.; Epifanov, A.; Patsurkovskyi, P.; Lychko, B. An improved methodology for thermal calculation and design optimization of a thermosiphon waste heat boiler for CCPP. *Case Stud. Therm. Eng.* **2024**, *58*, 104402. [CrossRef]
10. Zhu, M.; Chen, L.; Zhou, L.; Jiang, L.; Su, S.; Hu, S.; Xu, K.; Wang, C.; Li, A.; Qing, H.; et al. Experimental test, numerical analysis and thermal calculation modeling of hundreds kWth-class supercritical CO_2 fossil-fired boiler system. *Energy* **2023**, *284*, 128523. [CrossRef]
11. Zima, W.; Taler, J.; Grądziel, S.; Trojan, M.; Cebula, A.; Ocłoń, P.; Dzierwa, P.; Taler, D.; Rerak, M.; Majdak, M.; et al. Thermal calculations of a natural circulation power boiler operating under a wide range of loads. *Energy* **2022**, *261*, 125357. [CrossRef]
12. Madejski, P.; Taler, D.; Taler, J. Thermal and flow calculations of platen superheater in large scale CFB boiler. *Energy* **2022**, *258*, 124841. [CrossRef]
13. Ciupek, B.; Janeba-Bartoszewicz, E.; Urbaniak, R. Effect of fineness and increased humidity of carbonaceous fuels on the chemical composition of exhaust gases. *Chem. Ind.* **2019**, *1*, 8. [CrossRef]
14. Ciupek, B. Study on hard coal combustion in heating boilers equipped with a steam-fed afterburning chamber. *Chem. Ind.* **2020**, *99*, 8. [CrossRef]
15. Ciupek, B.; Gołoś, K.; Jankowski, R.; Nadolny, Z. Effect of Hard Coal Combustion in Water Steam Environment on Chemical Composition of Exhaust Gases. *Energies* **2021**, *14*, 6530. [CrossRef]
16. Ciupek, B.; Brodzik, Ł.; Semkło, Ł.; Prokopowicz, W.; Sielicki, P.W. Analysis of the Environmental Parameters of the GTM 400 Turbojet Engine During the Co-Combustion of JET A-1 Jet Oil with Hydrogen. *J. Ecol. Eng.* **2024**, *25*, 205–211. [CrossRef]
17. Houshfar, E.; Skreiberg, Ø.; Løvås, T.; Todorovic, D.; Sorum, L. Effect of excess air ratio and temperature on NOx emission from grate combustion of biomass in the staged air combustion scenario. *Energy Fuels* **2011**, *25*, 4643–4654. [CrossRef]
18. Speth, K.; Murer, M.; Spliethoff, H. Experimental investigation of nitrogen species distribution in wood combustion and their influence on NOx reduction by combining air staging and ammonia injection. *Energy Fuels* **2016**, *30*, 5816–5824. [CrossRef]
19. Khodaei, H.; Guzzomi, F.; Yeoh, G.H.; Regueiro, A.; Pati, D. An experimental study into the effect of air staging distribution and position on emissions in a laboratory scale biomass combustor. *Energy* **2016**, *118*, 1243–1255. [CrossRef]
20. Haryanto, A.; Hong, K.S. Modeling and simulation of an oxy-fuel combustion boiler system with flue gas recirculation. *Comput. Chem. Eng.* **2011**, *35*, 25–40. [CrossRef]

21. Caposciutti, G.; Barontini, F.; Antonelli, M.; Tognotti, L.; Desideri, U. Experimental investigation on the air excess and air displacement influence on early stage and complete combustion gaseous emissions of a small scale fixed bed biomass boiler. *Appl. Energy* **2018**, *216*, 576–587. [CrossRef]
22. Yang, D.O.; Qin, C.; Qin, X.; Xie, Q.; Nian, X. The thermal response of the ignition and combustion of high-energy material projectiles under the influence of heat. *Case Stud. Therm. Eng.* **2024**, *55*, 104168. [CrossRef]
23. Yang, J.; Dong, T.; Zhou, W. Numerical investigation of the physical-thermal-chemical behaviours of particles during coal combustion and desulfurization processes in a CFB combustor. *Energy* **2024**, *308*, 132891. [CrossRef]
24. Shi, J.; Lv, J.; Behrendt, F.; Liu, Y.; Mao, M.; He, F. 3D pore-scale simulations and 1D volume-averaged calculations of the flow and thermal non-equilibrium for low-velocity filtration combustion. *Int. J. Heat Mass Transf.* **2021**, *177*, 121532. [CrossRef]
25. Judt, W.; Ciupek, B.; Urbaniak, R. Numerical study of a heat transfer process in a low power heating boiler equipped with afterburning chamber. *Energy* **2020**, *196*, 117093. [CrossRef]
26. Graham, S.; Ogunfayo, I.; Hall, M.R.; Snape, C.; Quick, W.; Weatherstone, S.; Eastwick, C. Changes in mechanical properties of wood pellets during artificial degradation in a laboratory environment. *Fuel Process. Technol.* **2016**, *148*, 395–402. [CrossRef]
27. Obernberger, I.; Brunner, T.; Bärnthaler, G. Chemical properties of solid biofuels–significance and impact. *Biomass Bioenergy* **2006**, *30*, 973–982. [CrossRef]
28. García, R.; Pizarro, C.; Lavín, A.G.; Bueno, J.L. Spanish biofuels heating value estimation. Part II: Proximate analysis data. *Fuel* **2014**, *117*, 1139–1147. [CrossRef]
29. Caracci, E.; Canale, L.; Buonanno, G.; Stabile, L. Sub-micron particle number emission from residential heating systems: A comparison between conventional and condensing boilers fueled by natural gas and liquid petroleum gas, and pellet stoves. *Sci. Total Environ.* **2022**, *827*, 154288. [CrossRef]
30. Lin, H.; Clavreul, J.; Jeandaux, C.; Crawley, J.; Butnar, I. Environmental life cycle assessment of heating systems in the UK: Comparative assessment of hybrid heat pumps vs. condensing gas boilers. *Energy Build.* **2021**, *240*, 110865. [CrossRef]
31. Ciupek, B. *Kotły Grzewcze na Paliwa Stałe. Wybrane Aspekty Budowy i Eksploatacji*; Wydawnictwo Politechniki Poznańskiej: Poznan, Poland, 2023; ISBN 9788377757215. (In Polish)
32. Babadi, K.A.; Khorasanizadeh, H.; Mirzazadeh, G.; Mirzazadeh, S. Numerical simulations and an experimental study for optimal design of a 1500 kW water-tube condensing boiler. *Energy* **2024**, *307*, 132675. [CrossRef]
33. Ranjeeth, R.; Aditya, D.; Gautam, A.; Singh, S.P.; Bhattacharya, S. Failure investigation of a water-wall tube of fossil-fuel fired boiler. *Eng. Fail. Anal.* **2024**, *155*, 107727. [CrossRef]
34. Erbas, O. Investigation of factors affecting thermal performance in a coal—Fired boiler and determination of thermal losses by energy balance method. *Case Stud. Therm. Eng.* **2021**, *26*, 101047. [CrossRef]
35. Bujak, J. Optimal control of energy losses in multi-boiler steam systems. *Energy* **2009**, *34*, 1260–1270. [CrossRef]
36. Wróblewski, T. *Kotły Parowe*; Państwowe Wydawnictwo Naukowe: Warsaw, Poland, 1954. (In Polish)
37. Tołłoczko, B. *Kotły Parowe. Tom II*; Państwowe Wydawnictwo Techniczne: Warsaw, Poland, 1956. (In Polish)
38. Wróblewski, T.; Pepłowski, A.; Górecki, H. *Urządzenia Kotłowe*; Państwowe Wydawnictwo Techniczne: Warsaw, Poland, 1960. (In Polish)
39. Orłowski, P. *Kotły Parowe. Konstrukcja i Obliczenia*; Wydawnictwo Naukowo-Techniczne: Warsaw, Poland, 1966. (In Polish)
40. Kruczek, S. *Kotły. Konstrukcja i Obliczenia*; Wydawnictwo Politechniki Wrocławskiej: Warsaw, Poland, 2001; ISBN 8370856004. (In Polish)
41. Grądziel, S. ; *Wybrane Zagadnienia z Eksploatacji Kotłów Energetycznych*; Wydawnictwo Politechniki Krakowskiej: Cracow, Poland, 2023; ISBN 9788367188432. (In Polish)
42. Łachanin, W.W. *Obliczenia Cieplne Płomienicowo-Płomieniówkowych Kotłów Okrętowych*; Wydawnictwo Komunikacyjne: Warsaw, Poland, 1952. (In Polish)
43. Kowalski, C. *Kotły Gazowe Centralnego Ogrzewania Wodne Niskotemperaturowe*; Wydawnictwo Naukowo-Techniczne: Warsaw, Poland, 1992; ISBN 8320414644. (In Polish)
44. Kern, D.Q.; Kraus, A.D. *Extended Surface Heat Transfer*; McGraw-Hill Book Company: New York, NY, USA, 1972; ISBN 9780070341951. (In English)
45. Gołoś, K.; Ciupek, B.; Judt, W.; Urbaniak, R. Impact of replacement of solid fuel heating boilers on air quality in Poland in 2000–2020. *Chem. Ind.* **2021**, *100*, 96–99. [CrossRef]
46. Ciupek, B.; Judt, W.; Gołoś, K.; Urbaniak, R. Analysis of Low-Power Boilers Work on Real Heat Loads: A Case of Poland. *Energies* **2021**, *14*, 3101. [CrossRef]
47. Ciupek, B.; Judt, W.; Urbaniak, R.; Kłosowiak, R. The emission of carbon monoxide and nitrogen oxides from boilers supplied by a pellet under the influence of changes in the air-fuel equivalence ratio. *J. Ecol. Eng.* **2019**, *20*, 34–38. [CrossRef] [PubMed]
48. Ciupek, B.; Gołoś, K. Concentration of Nitrogen Oxides When Burning Wood Pellets of Various Origins. *J. Ecol. Eng.* **2020**, *21*, 229–233. [CrossRef] [PubMed]
49. Ciupek, B.; Urbaniak, R.; Nocoń, A. Emission Models for Selected Harmful Substances Emitted During Low-Temperature Combustion of Wood Pellets. *J. Ecol. Eng.* **2024**, *25*, 267–273. [CrossRef]
50. Liu, X.; Bansal, R.C. Integrating multi-objective optimization with computational fluid dynamics to optimize boiler combustion process of a coal fired power plant. *Appl. Energy* **2014**, *130*, 658–669. [CrossRef]
51. Kačániová, M.; Vukovic, N.L.; Čmiková, N.; Galovičová, L.; Schwarzová, M.; Šimora, V.; Kowalczewski, P.Ł.; Kluz, M.I.; Puchalski, C.; Bakay, L.; et al. Salvia sclarea Essential Oil Chemical Composition and Biological Activities. *Int. J. Mol. Sci.* **2023**, *24*, 5179. [CrossRef]

52. Boman, C.; Pettersson, E.; Westerholm, R.; Boström, D.; Nordin, A. Stove performance and emission characteristic in residential wood log and pellet combustion. Part 1: Pellet stoves. *Energy Fuels* **2011**, *25*, 307–314. [CrossRef]
53. Fachinger, F.; Drewnick, F.; Gieré, R.; Borrmann, S. How the user can influence particulate emissions from residential wood and pellet stoves: Emission factors for different fuels and burning conditions. *Atmos. Environ.* **2017**, *158*, 216–226. [CrossRef]
54. Mitchell, E.J.S.; Lea-Langton, A.R.; Jones, J.M.; Williams, A.; Layden, P.; Johnson, R. The impact of fuel properties on the emissions from the combustion of biomass and other solid fuels in a fixed bed domestic stove. *Fuel Process. Technol.* **2016**, *142*, 115–123. [CrossRef]
55. Adams, D.; Oh, D.H.; Kim, D.W.; Lee, C.H.; Oh, M. Prediction of SOx–NOx emission from a coal-fired CFB power plant with machine learning: Plant data learned by deep neural network and least square support vector machine. *J. Clean. Prod.* **2020**, *270*, 122310. [CrossRef]
56. Bakhchin, D.; Ravi, R.; Douadi, O.; Faquir, M.; Essadiqi, E. Integrated catalytic systems for simultaneous NOx and PM reduction: A comprehensive evaluation of synergistic performance and combustion waste energy utilization. *Environ. Sci. Pollut. Res.* **2024**, *31*, 46840–46857. [CrossRef] [PubMed]
57. Liu, H.; Chaney, J.; Li, J.; Sun, C. Control of NOx emissions of a domestic/small-scale biomass pellet boiler by air staging. *Fuel* **2013**, *103*, 792–798. [CrossRef]
58. Bhattu, D.; Zotter, P.; Zhou, J.; Stefenelli, G.; Klein, F.; Bertrand, A.; Temime-Roussel, B.; Marchand, N.; Slowik, J.G.; Baltensperger, U. Effect of stove technology and combustion conditions on gas and particulate emissions from residential biomass combustion. *Environ. Sci. Technol.* **2019**, *53*, 2209–2219. [CrossRef] [PubMed]
59. Malico, I.; Pereira, R.N.; Gonçalves, A.C.; Sousa, A.M.O. Current status and future perspectives for energy production from solid biomass in the European industry. *Renew. Sustain. Energy Rev.* **2019**, *112*, 960–977. [CrossRef]
60. Ozgen, S.; Cernuschi, S.; Caserini, S. An overview of nitrogen oxides emissions from biomass combustion for domestic heat production. *Renew. Sustain. Energy Rev.* **2021**, *135*, 110113. [CrossRef]
61. Nussbaumer, T. Combustion and Co-combustion of Biomass: Fundamentals, Technologies, and Primary Measures for Emission Reduction. *Energy Fuels* **2003**, *17*, 1510–1521. [CrossRef]
62. Obaidullah, M.; Bram, S.; Verma, V.K.; De Ruyck, J. A Review on Particle Emissions from Small Scale Biomass Combustion. *Int. J. Renew. Energy Res.* **2012**, *2*, 147–159.
63. Ladommatos, N.; Abdelhalim, S.; Zhao, H. The effects of exhaust gas recirculation on diesel combustion and emissions. *Int. J. Engine Res.* **2000**, *1*, 107–126. [CrossRef]
64. Abd-Alla, G.H. Using exhaust gas recirculation in internal combustion engines: A review. *Energy Convers. Manag.* **2002**, *43*, 1027–1042. [CrossRef]
65. Wei, H.; Zhu, T.; Shu, G.; Tan, L.; Wang, Y. Gasoline engine exhaust gas recirculation—A review. *Appl. Energy* **2012**, *99*, 534–544. [CrossRef]
66. ElKady, A.M.; Evulet, A.; Brand, A.; Ursin, T.P.; Lynghjem, A. Application of Exhaust Gas Recirculation in a DLN F-Class Combustion System for Postcombustion Carbon Capture. *J. Eng. Gas Turbines Power* **2009**, *131*, 034505. [CrossRef]
67. Cairns, A.; Blaxill, H. *The Effects of Combined Internal and External Exhaust Gas Recirculation on Gasoline Controlled Auto-Ignition*; SAE Technical Paper; SAE International: Warrendale, PA, USA, 2005. [CrossRef]
68. Guethe, F.; de la Cruz García, M.; Burdet, A. Flue Gas Recirculation in Gas Turbine: Investigation of Combustion Reactivity and NO_X Emission. In Proceedings of the ASME Turbo Expo 2009: Power for Land, Sea, and Air. Volume 2: Combustion, Fuels and Emissions, Orlando, Florida, USA,, 8–12 June 2009; ASME: New York, NY, USA; pp. 179–191. [CrossRef]
69. Baltasar, J.; Carvalho, M.G.; Coelho, P.; Costa, M. Flue gas recirculation in a gas-fired laboratory furnace: Measurements and modelling. *Fuel* **1997**, *76*, 919–929. [CrossRef]
70. Liuzzo, G.; Verdone, N.; Bravi, M. The benefits of flue gas recirculation in waste incineration. *Waste Manag.* **2007**, *27*, 106–116. [CrossRef]
71. Andersen, V.; Solheim, I.; Gaertner, H.; Sægrov-Sorte, B.; Einarsrud, K.E.; Tranell, G. Pilot-Scale Test of Flue Gas Recirculation for The Silicon Process. *J. Sustain. Metall.* **2023**, *9*, 81–92. [CrossRef]
72. Kim, H.K.; Kim, Y.; Lee, S.M.; Ahn, K.Y. NO reduction in 0.03–0.2 MW oxy-fuel combustor using flue gas recirculation technology. *Proc. Combust. Inst.* **2007**, *31*, 3377–3384. [CrossRef]
73. Ban, D.; Li, N.; Zheng, Y.; Xue, C. CO2 Measurement under Different Pressure and Vibration Conditions Using Tunable Diode Laser Absorption Spectroscopy. *Photonics* **2024**, *11*, 146. [CrossRef]
74. Palma, A.; Gallucci, F.; Papandrea, S.; Carnevale, M.; Paris, E.; Vincenti, B.; Salerno, M.; Di Stefano, V.; Proto, A.R. Experimental Study of the Combustion of and Emissions from Olive and Citrus Pellets in a Small Boiler. *Fire* **2023**, *6*, 288. [CrossRef]
75. Tong, Y.; Gao, J.; Ma, J. Emission Characteristics, Speciation, and Potential Environmental Risks of Heavy Metals from Coal-Fired Boilers: A Review. *Sustainability* **2023**, *15*, 11653. [CrossRef]
76. Wu, C.; Sun, L.; Piao, H.; Yao, L. Adaptive fuzzy finite time integral sliding mode control of the coordinated system for 350 MW supercritical once-through boiler unit to enhance flexibility. *Energy* **2024**, *302*, 131832. [CrossRef]
77. Bayomi, N.; Fernandez, J.E. Eyes in the Sky: Drones Applications in the Built Environment under Climate Change Challenges. *Drones* **2023**, *7*, 637. [CrossRef]
78. Fosco, D.; De Molfetta, M.; Renzulli, P.; Notarnicola, B. Progress in monitoring methane emissions from landfills using drones: An overview of the last ten years. *Sci. Total Environ.* **2024**, *945*, 173981. [CrossRef] [PubMed]
79. Ho, Y.; Lin, Y. Searching for the fine particulate matter (PM 2.5) pollutant emission source using a drone. *Measurement* **2024**, *232*, 114726. [CrossRef]

80. Copik, P.; Szlęk, A.; Ditaranto, M. Simplified mathematical model of oxy-fuel combustion of municipal solid waste in the grate furnace: Effect of different flue gas recirculation rates and comparison with conventional mode. *Arch. Thermodyn.* **2024**, *45*, 13–25. [CrossRef]
81. Kijo-Kleczkowska, A.; Gnatowski, A.; Gajek, M.; Krzywanski, J.; Szumera, M.; Knaś, K.; Kwiatkowski, D. Coal-plastic waste blendings. Experimental research and prediction of the thermal process. *Arch. Thermodyn.* **2024**, *45*, 117–128. [CrossRef]
82. Demirbas, A. Potential applications of renewable energy sources, biomass combustion problems in boiler power systems and combustion related environmental issues. *Prog. Energy Combust. Sci.* **2005**, *31*, 171–192. [CrossRef]
83. Fan, X.; Wong, G.; Gan, M.; Chen, X.; Yu, Z.; Ji, Z. Establishment of refined sintering flue gas recirculation patterns for gas pollutant reduction and waste heat recycling. *J. Clean. Prod.* **2019**, *235*, 1549–6526. [CrossRef]
84. Diego, L.F.; de las Obras-Loscertales, M.; Rufas, A.; García-Labiano, F.; Gayán, P.; Abad, A.; Adánez, J. Pollutant emissions in a bubbling fluidized bed combustor working in oxy-fuel operating conditions: Effect of flue gas recirculation. *Appl. Energy* **2013**, *102*, 860–867. [CrossRef]
85. Singh, R.; Shukla, A. A review on methods of flue gas cleaning from combustion of biomass. *Renew. Sustain. Energy Rev.* **2014**, *29*, 854–864. [CrossRef]
86. Chong, P.; Zhu, X.; Li, J.; Li, X.; Deng, L. Investigation on Hydrodynamic Performance and Wall Temperature of Water-Cooled Wall in 1000 MW Boiler Under Low-Load Conditions. *Energies* **2024**, *17*, 5751. [CrossRef]
87. Han, Y.; Wang, C.; Liu, K.; Zhang, L.; Zhu, Y.; Wang, Y.; Wang, L.; Che, D. Simulation of Dynamic Characteristics of Supercritical Boiler Based on Coupling Model of Combustion and Hydrodynamics. *Energies* **2024**, *17*, 5349. [CrossRef]
88. Milovanov, O.; Klimov, D.; Kuzmin, S.; Grigoriev, S.; Mikhalev, A.; Isemin, R.; Brulé, M. Application of Torrefaction for Improved Fuel Properties of Sunflower Husks. *Energies* **2024**, *17*, 4643. [CrossRef]
89. Sołowiej, P.; Neugebauer, M.; Esmer, O. Coffee Grounds as an Additive to Wood Pellets. *Energies* **2024**, *17*, 4595. [CrossRef]
90. Puszkarek, A.; Dorobczyński, L.; Kozak, M. Main Ships Propulsion Boiler Control and Hardware-in-Loop Model Implementation. *Energies* **2024**, *17*, 4453. [CrossRef]
91. Guo, X.; Zhao, G.; Zhang, Z.; Feng, D.; Wang, Y.; Zhang, Z. A Real-Time Calculation Method to Improve Boiler Safety in Deep Peak Shaving Cases. *Energies* **2023**, *16*, 4928. [CrossRef]
92. Mojica-Cabeza, C.D.; García-Sánchez, C.E.; Silva-Rodríguez, R.; García-Sánchez, L. A review of the different boiler efficiency calculation and modeling methodologies. *Inf. Técnico* **2021**, *86*, 69–93. [CrossRef]

energies

MDPI

Review

A Review of Recent Research on Flow and Heat Transfer Analysis in Additively Manufactured Transpiration Cooling for Gas Turbines

Kirttayoth Yeranee [1] **and Yu Rao** [1,2,*]

[1] Institute of Turbomachinery, School of Mechanical Engineering, Shanghai Jiao Tong University, Shanghai 200240, China; krittayoch.y@gmail.com
[2] Shenzhen Research Institute, Shanghai Jiao Tong University, Shenzhen 518000, China
* Correspondence: yurao@sjtu.edu.cn

Abstract

Advanced gas turbine cooling technologies are required to bridge the gap between turbine inlet temperatures and component thermal limits. Transpiration cooling has emerged as a promising method, leveraging porous structures to enhance cooling effectiveness. Recent advancements in additive manufacturing (AM) enable precise fabrication of complex transpiration cooling architectures, such as triply periodic minimal surface (TPMS) and biomimetic designs. This review analyzes AM-enabled transpiration cooling for gas turbines, elucidating key parameters, heat transfer mechanisms, and flow characteristics of AM-fabricated designs through experimental and numerical studies. Previous research has concluded that well-designed transpiration cooling achieves cooling effectiveness up to five times higher than the traditional film cooling methods, minimizes jet lift-off, improves temperature uniformity, and reduces coolant requirements. Optimized coolant controls, graded porosity designs, complex topologies, and hybrid cooling architectures further enhance the flow uniformity and cooling effectiveness in AM transpiration cooling. However, challenges remain, including 4–77% porosity shrinkage in perforated transpiration cooling for 0.5–0.06 mm holes, 15% permeability loss from defects, and 10% strength reduction in AM models. Emerging solutions include experimental validations using advanced diagnostics, high-fidelity multiphysics simulations, AI-driven and topology optimizations, and novel AM techniques, which aim at revolutionizing transpiration cooling for next-generation gas turbines operating under extreme conditions.

Keywords: additive manufacturing; gas turbine cooling; heat transfer analysis; transpiration cooling

1. Introduction

1.1. Importance of Advanced Cooling Technology for Gas Turbines

Gas turbines are widely used in aviation and power generation due to their high power density, efficiency, and performance. The global market of gas turbines is projected to grow further due to technological advancements and the shift toward distributed power generation. Performance improvements are motivated by the purpose of decreasing fuel consumption, saving subsequent expenses, and reducing carbon dioxide (CO_2) emissions. According to the Brayton cycle, increasing turbine inlet temperature (TIT) is the most effective way to enhance performance [1], as shown in Figure 1a [2]. Modern combined-cycle plants with 1700 °C-class turbines achieve around 65% efficiency [3], while aero-engines will operate at TITs exceeding 1800 °C. Heavy-duty turbines, such as Mitsubishi's M701J, have reached 1600 °C, with future designs targeting 1700 °C [4].

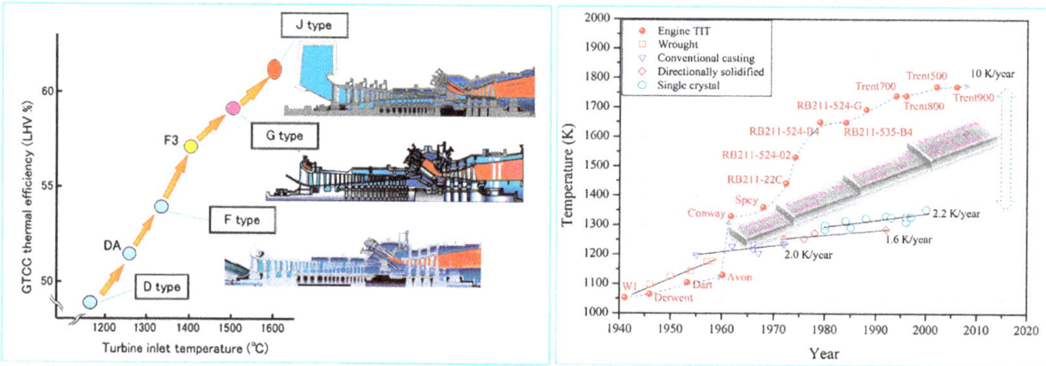

(a) (b)

Figure 1. Development in gas turbine: (**a**) TIT effects on gas turbine power and effectiveness and (**b**) Evolution of temperature capabilities of materials and thermal barrier coatings (These figures are reproduced from [2,5] under a Creative Commons Attribution (CC BY) license).

Despite these advancements, material limitations remain a critical challenge. Modern superalloys and thermal barrier coatings (TBCs) allow turbine blades to withstand temperatures around 1300 °C [6,7], as depicted in Figure 1b [5]; however, combustor temperatures are projected to exceed 1800 °C to obtain higher efficiency and power output. Furthermore, the maximum temperature for superalloys increases at a rate of only 8 °C per year, whereas the TITs are growing by up to 20 °C annually. To bridge this gap, advanced cooling technologies must be implemented to protect turbine components from thermal failure under these extreme operating conditions.

1.2. Evolution from Traditional to Transpiration Cooling

The evolution of gas turbine cooling has progressed from simple convection cooling to advanced transpiration cooling, with each stage improving cooling effectiveness, as shown in Figure 2. Early convection cooling was enhanced through various methods, including rib turbulators [8], pin fins [9], and protrusions/dimples [10]. Impingement cooling subsequently emerged as a high-performance alternative due to its superior heat transfer enhancement (Nu/Nu_0) [11,12]. However, internal cooling schemes, even combined ones, such as pin fin-dimple or rib-dimple, leave blade surfaces exposed to hot gas and cannot meet thermal protection requirements. This limitation led to the development of external cooling, i.e., film cooling, which forms a protective layer over the surface to improve cooling effectiveness. Many researchers have developed various techniques to enhance its efficiency [13]. As hole density increases, film cooling transitions to effusion cooling, which provides a full-coverage film layer to hot surfaces.

Impingement/effusion cooling, also known as double-wall cooling, has been used to improve gas turbine thermal protection since the 1980s [14,15]. This scheme combines the advantages of jet impingement and film cooling through a perforated wall with supporting structures. Studies have shown that double-wall cooling achieves higher cooling effectiveness than other conventional cooling methods, with pedestals improving heat transfer uniformity [16–19]. However, careful design is required to avoid performance degradation. The double-wall cooling system has also faced durability challenges from thermal stresses between layers. Skamniotis et al. [20–22] revealed that reducing hole ellipticity and optimizing pedestal spacing can mitigate stresses. Courtis et al. [23] showed that optimized hole spacing, particularly in the spanwise direction, can achieve film effectiveness up to 0.9, whereas increased porosity (φ) reduces mechanical strength, necessitating careful thermomechanical design trade-offs for practical implementation.

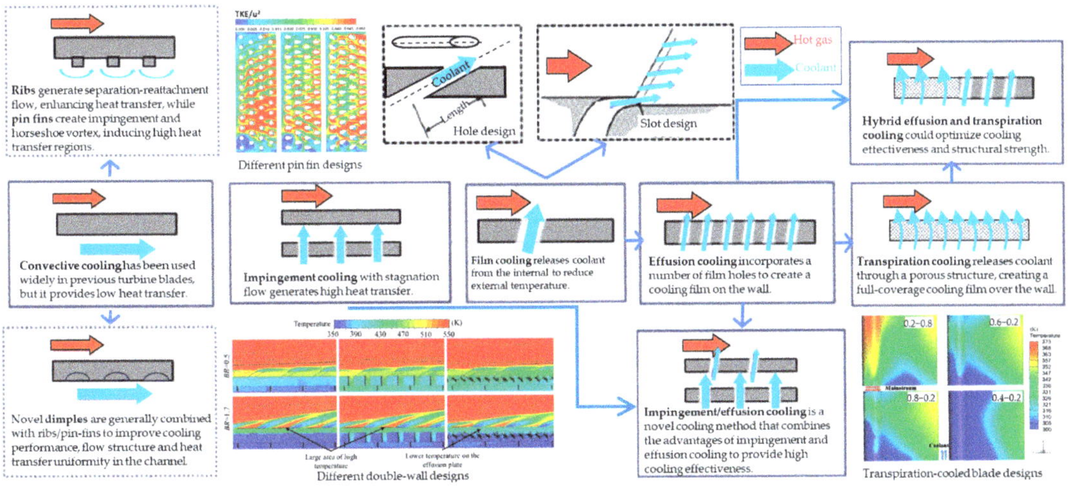

Figure 2. Overview of advanced cooling methods for gas turbine blades. Different pin fin designs, reproduced with permission from [24]. Copyright 2021 Elsevier, Different double-wall designs, reproduced with permission from [18]. Copyright 2021 Elsevier, Transpiration-cooled blade designs, reproduced with permission from [25]. Copyright 2023 Elsevier.

To balance film coverage uniformity with mechanical strength, transpiration cooling systems can be integrated with film holes [26,27]. However, conventional porous-media-based transpiration materials, such as metal foams, sintered particles, and woven meshes, lack the structural integrity required for turbine blade applications. While porous transpiration cooling has demonstrated high efficiency in rocket engines [28] and has since been adapted for gas turbines [29,30], scramjets [31], and high-speed vehicles [32], ongoing research focuses on novel materials [33], alternative coolants [34], and heat transfer enhancement techniques [35]. Additive manufacturing (AM) offers a promising solution by enabling precise and high-performance cooling designs [2]. Despite its potential, the flow and heat transfer analysis of AM-fabricated transpiration cooling remains underexplored in the existing literature [5,36–46].

1.3. Framework and Objectives

Given the urgent demand for high-performance cooling in gas turbines and the rapid advancements in AM technology, there is a critical need for a comprehensive framework that integrates both domains. This article presents a review of recent research on flow and heat transfer analysis in additively manufactured transpiration cooling systems for gas turbines, which is structured into six key sections. First, the significance and evolution of gas turbine cooling are introduced. The Section 2 summarizes the literature review of transpiration cooling, including research progress and its classification. The development of AM techniques tailored for transpiration cooling applications is then presented in the Section 3. The Section 4 analyzes flow and heat transfer characteristics in AM transpiration cooling, drawing insights from recent experimental and numerical studies, as well as optimization efforts. The Section 5 addresses challenges and future directions. Finally, the paper concludes by summarizing the main findings and their implications.

2. Literature Review of Transpiration Cooling

2.1. Research Progress and Challenges of Transpiration Cooling

The prior review articles on transpiration cooling have been widely established, mainly for aerospace and high-speed vehicles. Figure 3 summarizes the benefits, existing key challenges, and solutions, highlighting its implementation feasibility for gas turbines and high-speed vehicles. Most reviews [5,36–46] affirmed that transpiration cooling held significant promise for these applications due to high cooling performance, customizable design, and enhanced surface protection. Advances in AM technology enabled the fabrication of precision micro and transpiration cooling structures, addressing critical challenges such as particle-induced clogging, mechanical integrity, and manufacturing limitations. Additionally, research on hybrid cooling methods has been advancing, aiming to enhance thermomechanical performance under extreme conditions.

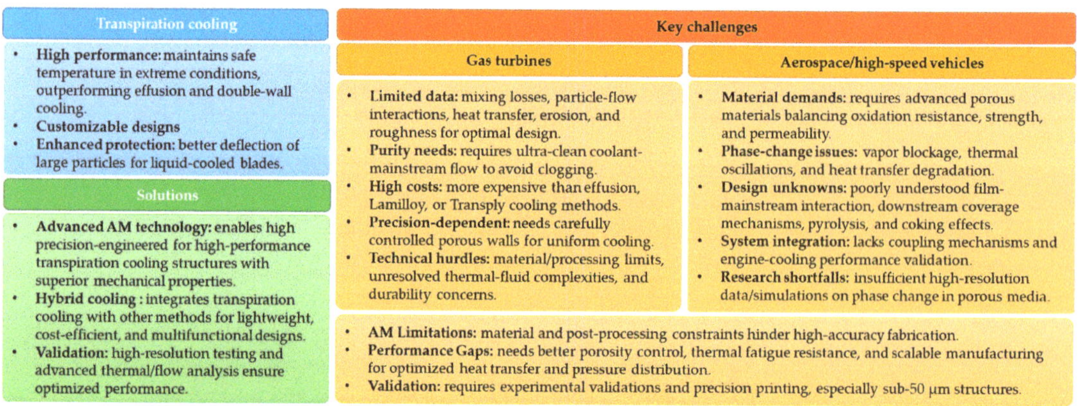

Figure 3. Summary of prior review articles on transpiration cooling techniques.

While existing reviews have thoroughly documented conventional transpiration cooling approaches, they identified critical knowledge gaps, especially in AM technology for transpiration cooling structures, experimental/numerical studies on AM-fabricated transpiration cooling systems, and detailed flow/heat transfer analysis for gas turbines. This review, therefore, addresses these gaps by evaluating recent advances in AM techniques, experimental and computational results, and optimized transpiration cooling studies, providing a comprehensive framework for implementing AM transpiration cooling in next-generation gas turbines.

2.2. Classification of Transpiration Cooling

In previous studies, transpiration cooling is also called sweat [47], effusion [48], or full-coverage film cooling [49]. Therefore, it is essential to understand the classification of transpiration cooling, as this framework defines the cooling capacity, material requirement, and manufacturing effect that guide design and performance evaluation. Transpiration cooling employs three primary mechanisms, classified based on working conditions, as summarized in Figure 4 [44]: solid cooling using phase-changing metals for passive heat absorption [50], gas cooling via forced flow through porous structures [49,51], and liquid cooling combining passive and active methods with phase-change enhancement [52–54].

The passive approach relies on material vaporization, while forced methods create protective coolant boundary layers through porous media.

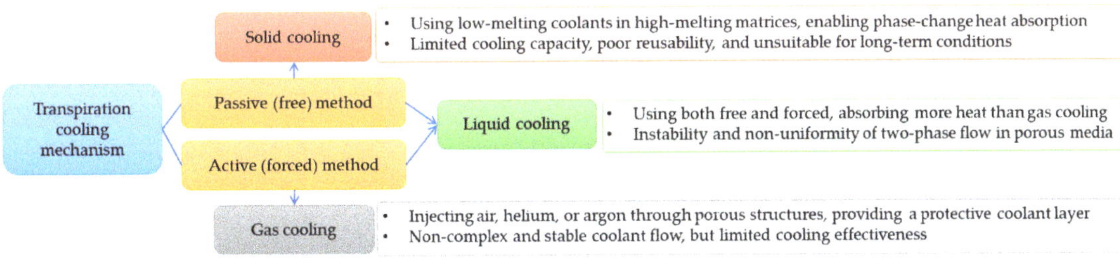

Figure 4. Classification of transpiration cooling based on working conditions.

Hypersonic vehicles and rocket engines operating above 2000 °C can achieve remarkable cooling capacities approaching 1000 MW/m^2 through liquid transpiration with phase-change enhancement [55]. Meanwhile, aero-engine turbines are limited to 50–100 MW/m^2 when using compressor bleed air through effusion or transpiration cooling, which are also constrained by the temperature limits of superalloys and ceramic matrix composites (CMCs) below 1500 °C. Moreover, liquid transpiration cooling systems, especially in gas turbines, could cause high thermal stress and pore clogging during rapid phase changes.

The current gas-phase (also known as single-phase) transpiration cooling is the most suitable for current gas turbines. The gas-phase transpiration cooling materials can be further categorized into porous media and laminated materials [38]. The porous-media transpiration materials include a metal-based type fabricated through powder sintering or advanced AM techniques and a ceramic-based type, which offers superior high-temperature performance [56]. However, sintered porous materials suffer from limited high-temperature oxidation resistance and structural strength. Meanwhile, ceramic-based transpiration faces brittleness and incompatibility with other metal structures in current technology, even though the ceramic material demonstrates excellent thermal stability and reduced coolant requirements [57].

On the other hand, laminated materials, traditionally constrained by manufacturing complexity and thermal limitations [58], have benefited from recent advances in AM technology [59–62]. Innovative approaches such as gradient laser sintering of 316 L stainless steel have enabled precise pore structure control, significantly improving anti-blockage performance and cooling efficiency [63]. Metal material with gradient φ has successfully been fabricated through the utilization of the selective laser melting (SLM) technique, in which a gradient-changing scan speed is incorporated in each SLM layer [64]. The smoothly graded pore structures are fabricated using this AM technology, resulting in optimized coolant distribution, which minimizes pore clogging and enhances cooling performance. As a result, metal-based type transpiration cooling is more viable for gas turbines when implemented in precisely engineered and non-stochastic architectures fabricated through advanced AM techniques. The following sections explore the role of AM in transpiration cooling and current flow/heat transfer analysis to address gaps identified in prior studies [5,36–46].

3. Additive Manufacturing for Transpiration Cooling

3.1. Traditional Manufacturing for Transpiration Cooling

Manufacturing developments of transpiration cooling for high-speed vehicles have been well documented in previous work [38,44,45], concluding that metal-based transpiration materials have been traditionally fabricated by powder sintering, fiber sintering, and melt casting, including bronze, stainless steel, titanium, and alloys. Powder-sintered porous metals, such as copper-based cooling systems by NASA [65], have been used in rocket engines. Recent advancements, such as metal powder injection molding (MIM), enabled precise control over pore geometry, allowing complex structures, such as inclined porous struts, for hybrid film/transpiration cooling [26]. Additionally, conventional laminated cooling fabrication involved etching or laser-cutting micro-cooling channels into thin metal sheets, followed by layer stacking and welding [66]. However, this method was time-consuming, limited to specific metals, and incapable of achieving precise complex micro-channel geometries, restricting its overall effectiveness. Therefore, the AM technique is essential to overcome the limitations of the traditional methods for efficiently fabricating advanced transpiration cooling structures for gas turbines.

3.2. Additive Manufacturing Techniques for Transpiration Cooling

Compared to conventional fabrication methods, the AM technology has offered higher precision by combining computer-aided design (CAD) with minimized material consumption and increased production efficiency. The AM allows full control over pore shape and size, making it ideal for complex designs, such as gas turbine blades with advanced cooling channels. Figure 5 shows the topology-optimized trailing edge (TE) on the scale of a gas turbine blade [67]. This study has concluded that the SLM method provided accurate printing with no micro-voids, staircase effects, or partially melted particles, and post-processing ensured a smooth external surface. Another notable example is Siemens's application of direct metal laser sintering (DMLS), developed by Electro Optical Systems (EOS), Germany, to fabricate turbine blades with optimized internal cooling structures, demonstrating the capability of the AM technology for high-performance complex cooling channels in gas turbines [68].

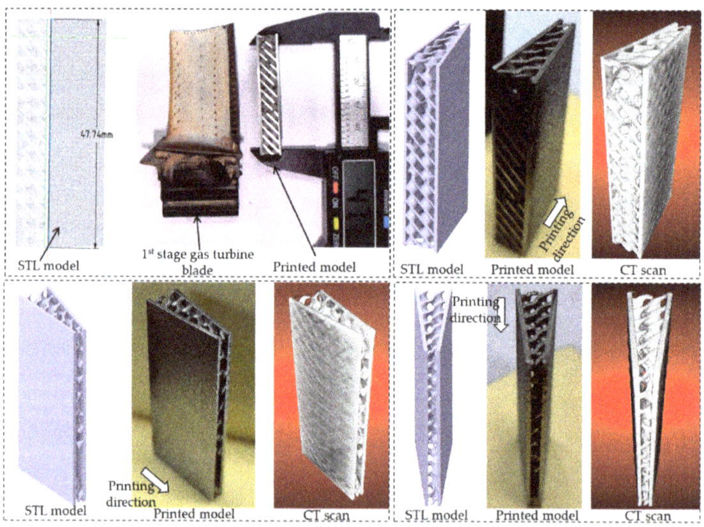

Figure 5. Complex gas turbine cooling structures fabricated using the SLM method. Reproduced with permission from [67]. Copyright 2024 Elsevier.

Three metal AM methods have emerged as key technologies for gas turbine applications, including powder bed binder jetting [69], direct laser deposition (DLD) [70], and laser powder bed fusion (LPBF) [71] for both full melt (laser melting) and partial melt (laser sintering). Each method offers distinct advantages and limitations, leading to different use cases in gas turbine component fabrication. Figure 6 summarizes the working principles, advantages, and drawbacks of these AM techniques in the context of gas turbine manufacturing [72].

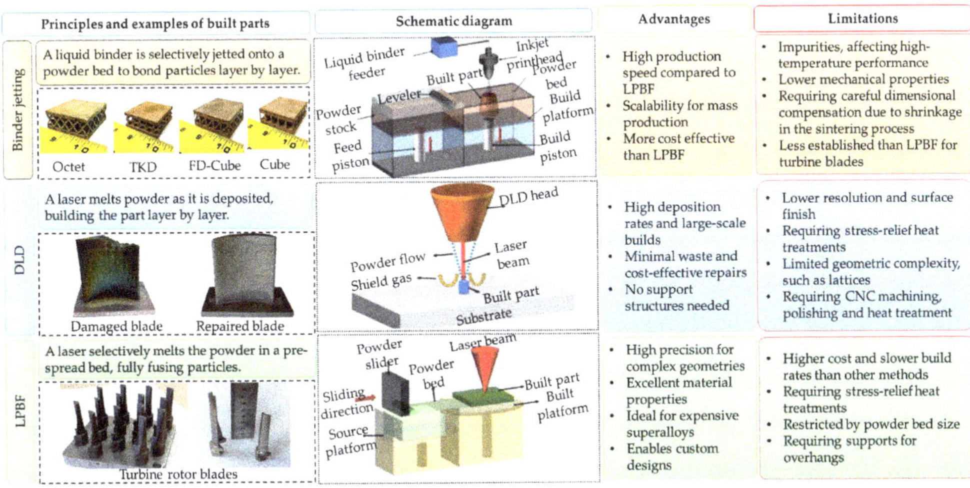

Figure 6. A summary of AM techniques for gas turbines. Lattice structures, reproduced with permission from [69]. Copyright 2022 Elsevier. Damaged and repaired blades, reproduced with permission from [70]. Copyright 2014 Elsevier. Turbine rotor blades, reproduced with permission from [71]. Copyright 2020 Elsevier. The schematic diagrams are reproduced from [72] under a Creative Commons Attribution (CC BY) license.

Most of the transpiration-cooling designs for gas turbine research have been successfully fabricated using the LPBF method, enabling detailed flow/heat transfer and structural analysis. Key studies are shown in Table 1. These studies demonstrated that the LPBF method allowed the fabrication of highly complex transpiration-cooling designs with robust mechanical properties and superior cooling performance. This represents a transformative advancement for next-generation gas turbine cooling technologies.

Table 1. Examples of metal AM-fabricated transpiration-cooling designs for gas turbine research.

Ref.	Material	Key Design/Feature	Significance
[73] [30]	Stainless steel	Porous media on a C3X single-turbine blade and cascade turbine blades	Pioneering transpiration cooling for validating the feasibility of turbine blades
[66]		0.24 mm perforated holes	Achieving a tight tolerance with only a 4% φ deviation compared to the design
[74]	Hastelloy-X	Porous-media transpiration cooling	Verifying the high-temperature material compatibility
[75]	Inconel 718	Optimized LPBF parameters for porous media	Obtaining controlled pores and accurate φ for various transpiration-cooled plates
[76]		Innovative hole topology designs	Paving the way for new research on AM-hole topology to improve cooling effectiveness and uniformity
[77]		0.2 mm perforated holes	Capable of fabricating ultra-fine holes, providing high cooling efficiencies, and desired tensile strength
[78]		Perforated holes with internal lattices	Groundbreaking research on minimizing crossflow effects in AM transpiration-cooled plates
[51]		Reinforcement for transpiration cooling	Improving mechanical integrity with a minor loss in cooling performance
[79]		Double-cavity leading edge (LE) cooling	Demonstrating advanced, complex internal and external cooling structures
[80]	Inconel 625	Gyroid TPMS-based transpiration cooling	Novel lattice design with high temperature and corrosion resistance

3.3. Additive Manufacturing-Fabricated Advanced Transpiration Cooling Structures

Advancements in AM technology have enabled the fabrication of complex and high-performance transpiration cooling structures for gas turbines, offering superior thermal management compared to conventional cooling techniques [2,46]. These structures can be categorized according to porosity control into stochastic [73–75] and deterministic structures [77,78,80–83], as shown in Figure 7. The random-pore distributions usually caused uncontrolled flow paths, limited cooling uniformity, and low mechanical strength. The non-stochastic designs also provided customizable geometry and permeability, enhanced heat transfer, predictable fluid and heat transfer characteristics, and higher mechanical strength, making them ideal for high-performance transpiration cooling in gas turbines. Notably, the mathematical equation-based designs, such as TPMS, exhibited better thermal conductivity, heat and mass transfer, and mechanical strength than the CAD-based designs [84]. In conclusion, the AM-fabricated non-stochastic structures, particularly TPMS-based designs, have demonstrated strong potential for advancing transpiration cooling in gas turbines, motivating the detailed flow and heat transfer analysis in the next section.

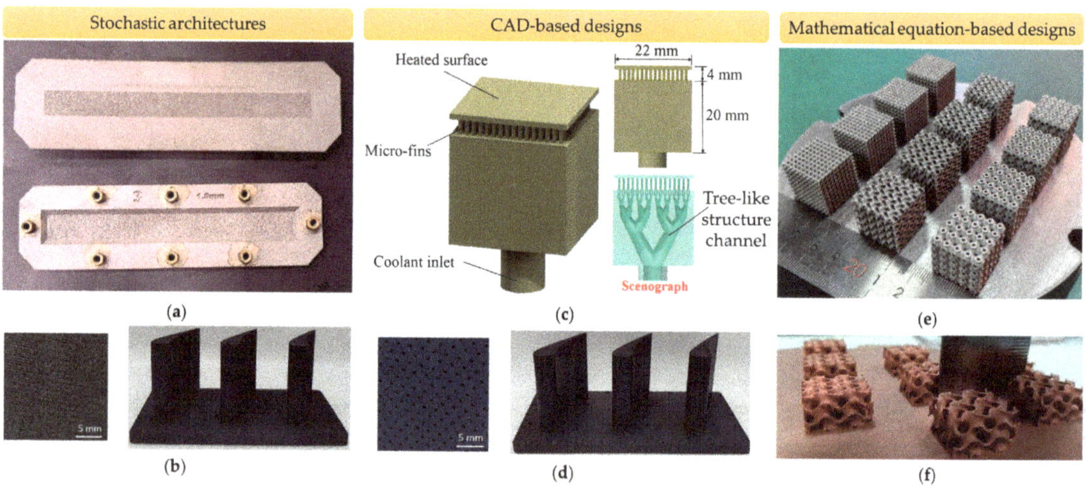

Figure 7. Advanced transpiration cooling structures in recent studies: (**a**) AM porous Hastelloy-X specimens (Reproduced with permission from [74]. Copyright 2024 Elsevier), (**b**) AM-fabricated transpiration-cooled cascade blade (Reproduced with permission from [30]. Copyright 2022 Elsevier), (**c**) Tree-like structure designs (Reproduced with permission from [83]. Copyright 2019 Elsevier), (**d**) AM-fabricated effusion-cooled cascade blade (Reproduced with permission from [30]. Copyright 2022 Elsevier), (**e**) Different TPMSs, and (**f**) Gyroid structures.

4. Flow and Heat Transfer Analysis

4.1. Heat Transfer Mechanism

The general gas-phase transpiration cooling mechanism includes forced convection within the structural matrix and a continuously developing cooling film on the hot gas side of the porous surface that protects the hot gas from attaching to the surface [85], as schematically demonstrated in Figure 8. In gas turbine applications, transpiration cooling also employs this dual-mode heat transfer mechanism to achieve enhanced thermal protection. The internal cooling process involves forced convection through the porous structures or micro holes, where coolant extracts thermal energy from the blade or combustor walls. Then, the coolant forms a film-cooling layer that interacts with the mainstream flow through convective heat transfer within the turbulent boundary layer, mass transfer-driven dilution of combustion products, and aerodynamic displacement of the stagnation line [37,86]. This combined mechanism enhances cooling effectiveness compared to discrete film cooling, primarily by eliminating jet lift-off effects.

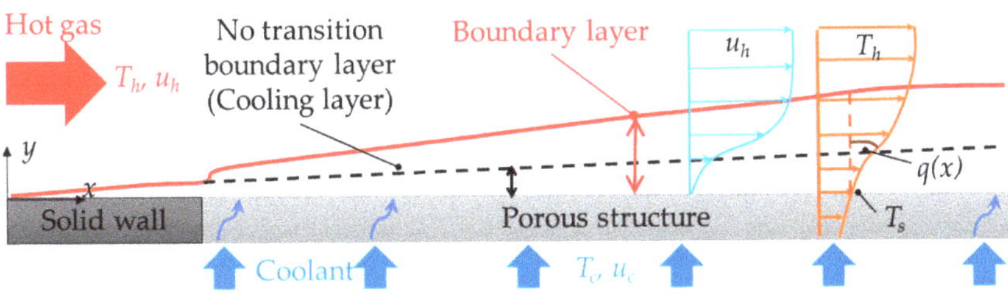

Figure 8. Schematic diagram of heat transfer mechanism of gas-phase transpiration cooling.

The particle image velocimetry (PIV) image and instantaneous velocity distribution [49] in Figure 9 show that the boundary layer remains thin in the initial cooling development region of a relatively small-diameter perforated plate. As coolant air accumulates downstream, progressive boundary layer growth is observed through the transition zone until reaching the developed cooling region. Within the developed cooling area along the wall, the boundary layer thickness stabilizes, maintaining near-constant values across the entire stabilized zone. Additionally, the boundary layer growth rate strongly depends on the cooling supplied rate, increasing linearly with coolant mass flux. Overall, this relationship closely resembles that in the sintered porous-based transpiration cooling structure [49]. Therefore, the diagram in Figure 8 could also be used to explain the flow and heat transfer phenomena of non-stochastic architectures fabricated through AM technology.

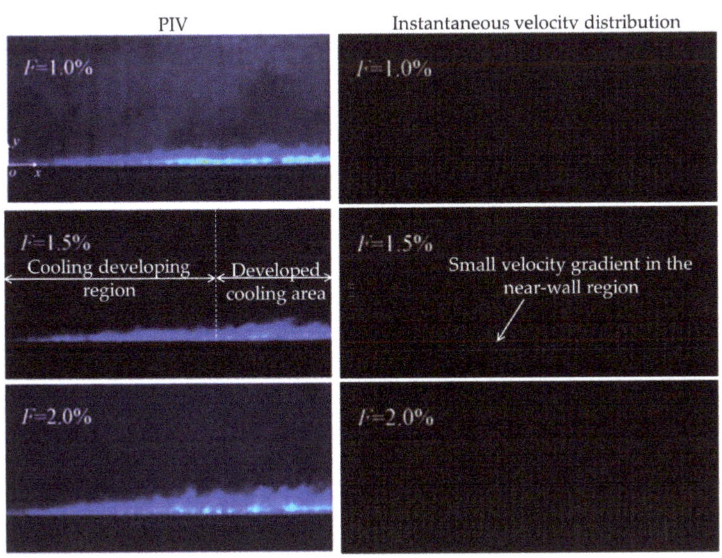

Figure 9. PIV and instantaneous velocity distributions in the near wall region of a perforated transpiration cooling plate. Reproduced with permission from [49]. Copyright 2015 Elsevier.

4.2. Related Parameters

Many pore-scale studies of transpiration cooling couple the high Reynolds number flow of the mainstream (Re_h) and the low Reynolds number flow of the coolant inside the porous matrix (Re_c) [82,87,88], defined as follows:

$$Re_h = \frac{\rho_h u_h d_h}{\mu}, d_h = 4A_h/C_h \tag{1}$$

$$Re_c = \frac{\rho_c u_D d_c}{\mu}, d_c = 4\varphi/S_V \tag{2}$$

where u_h is the mainstream flow velocity (m/s). ρ_c and ρ_h are the densities of coolant and mainstream (kg/m^3). d_h, A_h, C_h are the hydraulic diameter (m), cross-sectional area (m^2), and the circumference of the hot flow channel (m). μ signifies the dynamic viscosity of fluid (kg/(m·s)). u_D is the Darcy velocity (m/s). d_c is the hydraulic diameter of the coolant supply channel, and S_v is the specific surface area (1/m).

In transpiration cooling experiments, the mass flow ratio of coolant to mainstream (*MFR*), injection ratio (*F*), and blowing ratio (*BR*) are the key parameters for determining the coolant flow rate. The *MFR* is used in system-level cooling efficiency, such as nose cone and turbine blade cooling, to evaluate coolant supply requirements for a given cooling strategy. The *MFR* is calculated as follows:

$$MFR = \frac{\dot{m}_c}{\dot{m}_h} \tag{3}$$

where $\dot{m}_c$ and $\dot{m}_h$ are the mass flow rate of the coolant and mainstream (kg/s).

The coolant injection ratio (*F*) is used when focusing on coolant distribution per unit area, defined as follows:

$$F = \frac{\rho_c u_c}{\rho_h u_h} \tag{4}$$

$$u_c = \frac{\dot{m}_c}{\rho_c A_{eff}} \tag{5}$$

where u_c is the equivalent average cross-section coolant velocity (m/s). A_{eff} is the coolant-covered area on the hot-side surface (m^2).

In film or effusion cooling, the blowing ratio (*BR*) is the primary parameter for evaluating the coolant flow rate, focusing on momentum interaction at the injection point. Unlike the *F*, the *BR* is based on the coolant velocity defined per hole/pore rather than the total mass flow rate. The blowing ratio (*BR*) is expressed as

$$BR = \frac{\rho_c v_c}{\rho_h u_h} \tag{6}$$

where v_c is the average velocity of coolant flow in the film hole (m/s).

The v_c can be derived from the coolant flow rate and the equivalent pore diameter (d_{pore}) of the porous structure in transpiration cooling studies. Due to the significant momentum loss caused by friction within the porous medium, most studies avoid comparing micro-cooling performance using the *BR*. Instead, cooling effectiveness in various transpiration cooling studies is evaluated based on the injection ratio (*F*) or the volumetric flow rate ($\dot{V}$) of the coolant.

The convective heat transfer coefficient (h) and Nusselt number (Nu) are also important parameters to make data comparable for different transpiration cooling designs. The h

(W/m^2K) and Nu on the hot-side surface of transpiration cooling structures are defined as follows:

$$h = \frac{Q_{tot}}{A_w(T_h - T_s)} \quad (7)$$

$$Nu = \frac{hL_c}{k_f} \quad (8)$$

where Q_{tot} is the total heat transfer (W). A_w is the wetted area (m^2). T_h is the mainstream and coolant temperatures (K). T_s is the surface temperature (K). L_c is the characteristic length of the transpiration cooling designs (m). k_f is the thermal conductivity of fluid (W/m·K).

Generally, for external cooling, the heat transfer analysis quantifies cooling performance through local cooling effectiveness, calculated as

$$\eta = \frac{T_h - T_s}{T_h - T_c} \quad (9)$$

where T_c is the coolant temperature (K).

Film cooling effectiveness (η_a) is typically used in adiabatic wall studies to evaluate localized cooling performance at specific coolant injection points. In contrast, overall cooling effectiveness (η_o) is applied in conjugate heat transfer analyses, assessing the total temperature reduction in the component by accounting for external film cooling and internal cooling mechanisms, that is, the coolant flow through holes or pores.

The Biot number (Bi) is also used to analyze the thermal behavior of porous structures and the efficiency of heat transfer between the solid matrix and the coolant in transpiration cooling [89]. It can be expressed as

$$Bi = \frac{ht}{k_s} \quad (10)$$

where t is the thickness of transpiration cooling structures (m). k_s is the thermal conductivity of the solid domain (W/(m·K). In the case of porous-media structure, k_{eff}, which is effective thermal conductivity (W/(m·K), is used instead of k_s.

The flow resistance of different transpiration cooling designs is usually evaluated using the total pressure loss coefficient (ζ_{Pt}) [82,90], defined as

$$\zeta_{Pt} = \frac{p_{t,in} - p_{t,out}}{p_{t,in}} \quad (11)$$

where $p_{t,in}$ and $p_{t,out}$ are the total pressure of the coolant inlet and outlet (Pa), respectively.

The skin-friction coefficient (CF) of the transpiration cooling is employed to reveal the shear stress (τ_w) on the solid surface due to the viscous effects and show the attachment of the coolant film [91]. The CF is expressed as follows:

$$CF = \frac{\tau_w}{0.5\rho_h u_h^2} \quad (12)$$

Another parameter used to quantify the efficiency of the flow contraction through transpiration cooling structures and viscous loss due to the tortuosity of the transpiration topology is the discharge coefficient (CD). The CD is defined as the ratio of the actual mass flow rate to the theoretical mass flow rate [75,79], which can be simplified as follows:

$$CD = \frac{\dot{m}_c}{A_{pore}\sqrt{2\rho_c(p_{t,in} - p_{t,out})}} \quad (13)$$

where A_{pore} is the total cross-sectional area of transpiration cooling topology (m^2).

Due to material shrinkage, printing resolution, and post-processing, the AM structures often exhibit dimensional variations from their original designs. To assess these manufacturing tolerances, both the designed porosity (φ_{des}) and actual porosity (φ_{act}) of test specimens are quantified using

$$\varphi_{des} = \left(1 - \frac{V_{des}}{V_{sol}}\right) \times 100\% \quad (14)$$

$$\varphi_{act} = \left(1 - \frac{M_{des}}{M_{sol}}\right) \times 100\% \quad (15)$$

where V_{des} represents the designed volume of a geometry from a CAD model (m^3). V_{sol} is the volume of a solid domain with identical dimensions (m^3). M_{des} signifies the measured weight of a test specimen, while M_{sol} is the measured weight of the solid plate (kg).

Additionally, to analyze the influence of transpiration cooling design on heat transfer, the internal surface area ratio (R_{int}) and outlet area ratio (R_{out}) are usually presented [76,92], which can be calculated as

$$R_{int} = A_{int}/A_{eff} \quad (16)$$

$$R_{out} = \frac{A_{out}}{A_{eff}} \times 100\% \quad (17)$$

where A_{int} and A_{out} are the internal surfaces of the solid–fluid interface inside the specimens and the outlet area of the coolant at the outer surface (m^2), respectively. These area values are typically derived from CAD models.

4.3. *Experimental Research*

4.3.1. Experimental Setup and Measurement Method

Experiments on AM-based transpiration cooling structures are essential to address various aspects, such as the effect of geometrical designs and the influence of studied conditions, which analytical models often inadequately represent [93,94]. The experimental studies validate theoretical assumptions, reveal the interactions of porosity (φ) or topology on thermo-fluidic behavior, and quantify flow distribution in complex AM geometries. The general experimental setup for analyzing the flow and heat transfer of transpiration cooling is schematically depicted in Figure 10a.

The airflow generated by the blower or compressor passes through the inlet diffuser and enters the heater uniformly, where it is heated to the target temperature. The heated air then flows through flow stabilizers, such as honeycombs or mesh screens, to ensure a uniform mainstream flow within the test section. Maintaining consistent temperature and velocity of the mainstream inside the test section is critical. Additionally, the turbulent intensity of the airflow must be measured. For the coolant system, the coolant is supplied by the blower or compressor, and its flow rate can be adjusted using a flowmeter to vary the *MRF*, *BR*, or *F*. In flow visualization studies, techniques such as smoke-laser sheet imaging [30,73,95] or PIV [49] may be employed.

Pressure-sensitive paint (PSP) and infrared thermography (IR) methods have been widely used to acquire the cooling effectiveness of the transpiration cooling wall, as demonstrated in examples in Figure 10b,c. Meanwhile, the use of transient liquid crystal thermography (TLC) was quite limited. The PSP method measures surface pressure distributions indirectly by detecting oxygen quenching of luminescent molecules, which can then be correlated to temperature in certain applications. It provides high spatial resolution and is particularly useful for aerodynamic studies, but it requires optical access and careful calibration to separate pressure and thermal effects. In contrast, IR thermography directly captures surface temperature distributions by detecting thermal radiation emitted by the material. IR is non-invasive, works in real-time, and is well-suited for thermal analysis, but its accuracy can be affected by surface emissivity variations and environmental reflections. While PSP excels in detailed pressure mapping with temperature derivations, IR is more straightforward for pure thermal visualization, making them complementary tools depending on the experimental focus.

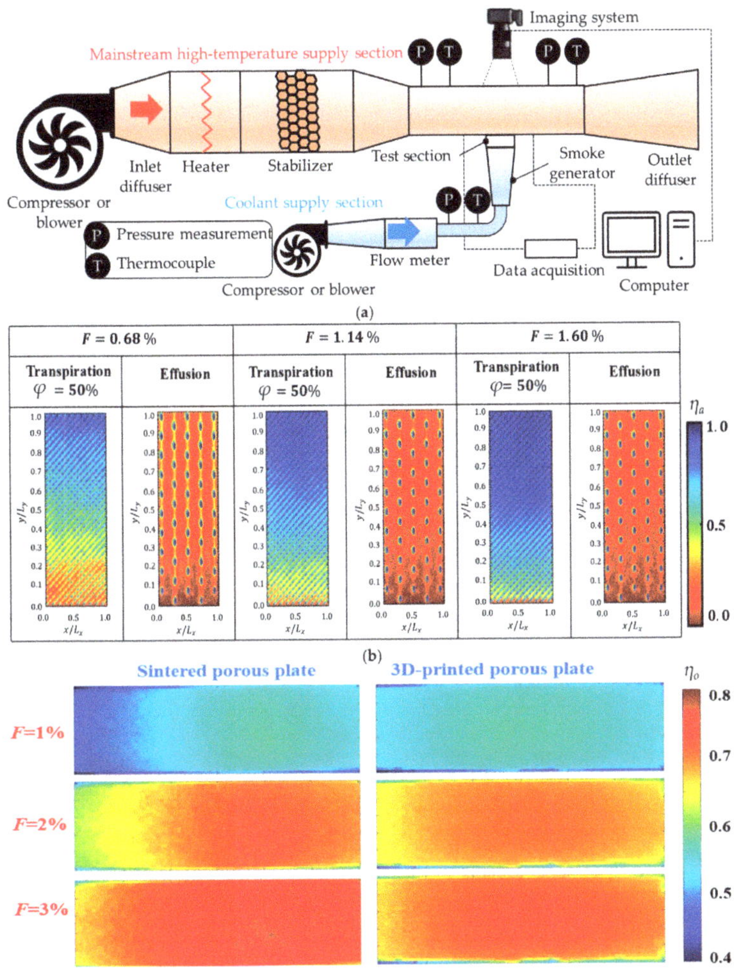

Figure 10. General experimental setup for investigation on flow and heat transfer of transpiration cooling: (**a**) Schematic diagram; (**b**) Illustration of η_a contours (Reproduced with permission from [92]. Copyright 2024 Elsevier) and (**c**) η_o distributions (Reproduced with permission from [51]. Copyright 2018 Elsevier).

Recent experimental studies on flow and heat transfer of AM transpiration cooling, suited for gas turbine applications, have been conducted, as shown in Table 2. Different measurement techniques used to acquire η, heat transfer coefficient (h), velocity (u), and discharge coefficient (CD) under various conditions are summarized. This study evaluated transpiration cooling performance across various designs, with area-averaged effectiveness (η_o and η_a) ranging from 0.05 to 0.95. Optimal configurations included sintered models with an area-averaged η_o of 0.74, staggered arrangements on an SS turbine blade with an area-averaged η_a of 0.95, and bio-inspired structures with an area-averaged η_o of 0.35–0.57. Graded porosity reduced peak temperatures by 20%, while inserting a lattice decreased area-averaged η_o by 12%. The results demonstrate that cooling efficiency was highly dependent on geometry and φ distribution.

Table 2. Overview of experimental studies on flow and heat transfer of AM transpiration cooling.

Ref.	Studied Models	Measurement Techniques (Evaluated Metric)	Studied Conditions	Significant Results
[73]	A C3X single-turbine blade with different cooling methods	IR thermography (η_o)	$T_h = 100\ ^\circ C$; $T_c = 20\ ^\circ C$; Mainstream Reynolds number (Re_h) = 100,000 ($u_h = 20$ m/s); Volumetric flow rate of coolant ($\dot{V}_c$) = 100–400 LPM	The maximum area-averaged η_o of the transpiration-cooled single turbine blade was 0.58.
[95]		Smoke-laser with a high-speed camera (u)	$T_h = T_c = 6.5\ ^\circ C$; $Re_h = 10{,}000$ ($u_h = 2$ m/s); $\dot{V}_c$ = 0–200 LPM; BR = 4.2–21.2	The coolant film on the transpiration-cooled blade was more stable.
[30]	A C3X cascade-turbine blade with different cooling strategies	IR thermography (η_o) Smoke-laser with a high-speed camera (u)	$T_h = 100\ ^\circ C$; $T_c = 20\ ^\circ C$; Re_h = 50,000–100,000 (u_h = 10–20 m/s); $\dot{V}_c$ = 50–300 LPM	The maximum area-averaged η_o of the transpiration-cooled cascade turbine blade was 0.7.
[74]	Porous-media transpiration-cooled plates	TLC (h, η_o) IR flow visualization (u)	$T_h = 70\ ^\circ C$; T_c = Ambient temperature (T_{Amb}); Re_h = 25,000 (u_h = 3.4 m/s); $BR \approx 0.4$–2.0	The highest area-averaged η_a of the transpiration-cooled plates was less than 0.4.
[75]	Porous-media transpiration-cooled specimens	Static pressure taps (CD)	The ratio of plenum stagnation and atmospheric pressures (PR) = 1.02–1.7.	The CD of the 90° laser direction was 0.02–0.07, lower than that of the 67° model.
[64]	Uniform and graded IWP TPMS plates	IR thermography (T)	T_h = 420–480 K; Mach number of mainstream (Ma_h) = 2.8; F = 0.1–0.6%.	The graded IWP reduced the maximum local temperature by around 20% compared to a uniform one.
[79]	Transpiration cooling combined with lattice structures on a leading edge	Static pressure taps (CD)	PR = 1–1.3.	The highest CD was 0.17 in the impingement sleeve.
[96]		PSP (η_a)	$T_c = T_{amb}$; Re_h = 825,313; BR = 0.03–0.15.	The area-averaged η_a was 0.11–0.34, and the maximum pressure loss was about 4.4 kPa.
[97]	Perforated transpiration-cooled turbine blade	PSP (η_a)	$T_h = T_{Amb}$; $Re_h = 1.2 \times 10^6$ ($Ma_h = 0.3$); $\dot{m}_c$ = 5–20 g/s ($BR \approx 0.1$–0.5).	The staggered arrangement on the SS turbine blade showed the highest area-averaged η_a of 0.95.
[51]	Partitional walls in transpiration-cooled plates	IR thermography (η_o)	T_h = 340 K; T_c = 296 K; u_h = 11 m/s; F = 1–3%	The maximum area-averaged η_o of the sintered and AM models was 0.74 and 0.71.
[98]		PSP (η_a)	Re_h = 395,000 (u_h = 21.6 m/s); BR = 0.1–0.7.	The highest area-averaged η_a values of the 0% and 60% blockage models were about 0.68 and 0.4.
[76]	Different transpiration topology designs	IR thermography (η_o)	T_h = 45–60 °C; T_c = 21 °C; Re_h = 98,000 (u_h = 11 m/s); BR = 1–3; F = 1.2–3.6%	The blood vessel-shaped designs showed η_o of 0.35–0.57.
[77]	Different perforated transpiration designs		T_h = 50–60 °C; T_c = 21 °C; Re_h = 98,000 (u_h = 11 m/s); F = 1.0–2.5%.	The optimal design was the 3d-pitch (d = 0.3 mm) with η_o of 0.48 and a relative UTS of 0.74.
[78]	Integrated lattice transpiration cooling structures			The area-averaged η_o was reduced by 12% when inserting a lattice in the transpiration-cooled plate. The highest area-averaged η_o was 0.67 in the pure transpiration cooling model.
[99]	Different perforated transpiration designs	IR thermography (η_a)	T_h = 50 °C; T_c = 21 °C; BR = 0.125–0.5	The spanwise-averaged η_o increased from 0.44 to 0.73 in the 2.5d-pitch (d = 0.5 mm) at BR = 0.5, higher than various multirow film hole studies.
[100]	Wire mesh porous transpiration-cooled plate	IR thermography (η_a)	T_h = 295 K; T_c = 21 °C; u_h = 18.8 m/s; F = 0.4–5.2%.	The area-averaged η_a values were within 0.05–0.36.
[101]	Different porosities and injection ratios of the Gyroid TPMS model	IR thermography (η_a)	T_c = 80 °C; $Ma_h \approx 0.27$ (u_h = 87.5 m/s); ρ_h/ρ_c = 0.83; F = 1.4–3.1%.	The area-averaged η_a values were around 0.3–0.5.
[92]	Different porosities of Diamond TPMS plates	PSP (η_a)	T_h = 50–60 °C; Re_h = 256,000 (u_h = 33 m/s); F = 0.68–1.60%.	The model with the φ of 30%, 40%, and 50% showed the highest area-averaged η_a by 0.49, 0.69, and 0.75.
[81]	Different TPMS transpiration cooling designs			The Diamond, Gyroid, and Koch models demonstrated the maximum area-averaged η_a by 0.76, 0.71, and 0.79.
[102]	Different unit cell sizes of Diamond TPMS plates			The model with the unit cell size (L) of 1.9, 2.5, and 3.1 mm provided the highest area-averaged η_a by 0.75, 0.71, and 0.66.

4.3.2. Experimental Studies on AM-Fabricated Random-Pore Porous Structures

The Korea Advanced Institute of Science and Technology pioneered innovative experimental research on state-of-the-art transpiration-cooled C3X turbine blades, showing remarkable ingenuity in advancing thermal protection for cutting-edge gas turbine cooling.

Kim et al. [73] compared internal, effusion, and 3D printed-porous transpiration cooling. The test section featured CaF_2 windows with 95% transmittance at 3–5 μm to minimize thermal interference, enabling accurate IR thermometry. The studied models included a 0.5 mm effusion-hole model fabricated by electric discharge machining and a 40 μm porous-based transpiration cooling model structure, additively manufactured within φ = 53%. The results showed that transpiration cooling demonstrated superior performance, achieving 34% and 25% higher η_o than effusion and internal cooling. The cooling effectiveness of the transpiration cooling model was more uniform, especially on the pressure side (PS).

Kim et al. [95] also used smoke-laser visualization with two diode-pumped solid-state lasers and olive oil seeding to visualize coolant flow release from the blade; then, the flow characteristics were captured by a high-speed CCD camera. It was revealed that transpiration cooling provided uniform coverage and low-momentum discharge, which prevented recirculation flow, while effusion cooling showed a large layer thickness, as shown in Figure 11a. Despite comparable coolant-to-mainstream pressure ratios, transpiration cooling required less coolant for better performance. A subsequent study [30] was conducted on a C3X cascade-turbine blade compared with different cooling methods, namely internal cooling only, effusion cooling, and transpiration cooling. They observed that in cascade blades, adjacent blades redirected and accelerated the flow along the blade chord, as shown in Figure 11b. It was obvious that the transpiration cooling showed more uniform and higher cooling effectiveness, as seen in Figure 11c. Moreover, compared to a single blade, the coolant outflow formed a thinner boundary layer in effusion and transpiration cooling. This shifted the suction-side vortex rearward, reducing mainstream/coolant mixing and stabilizing the coolant within the boundary layer. Due to these flow interactions, the cascade arrangement enhanced cooling effectiveness, as shown in Figure 11d.

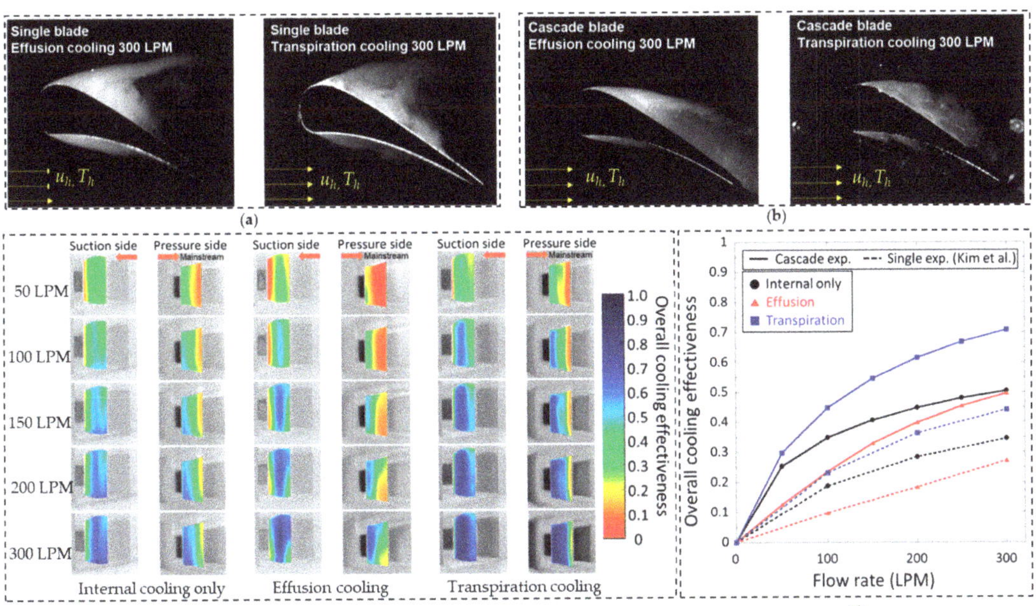

Figure 11. Transpiration-air cooled turbine blade: (**a**) visualization of coolant flow at u_h = 20 m/s and coolant volume flow rate of 300 LPM for the single blade; (**b**) for the cascade blade; (**c**) η_o distributions on the cascade blade with different cooling; and (**d**) comparisons of area-averaged cooling effectiveness between cascade and single-turbine blades from Kim et al. [73]. Reproduced with permission from [30]. Copyright 2022 Elsevier.

Researchers from Siemens Energy AB, Finspong, Sweden [74], evaluated the distributions of h and η_a of a porous Hastelloy-X transpiration-cooled plate against conventional cylindrical film holes using TLC and IR-based flow visualization with water and CO_2. Their results demonstrated that transpiration cooling enhanced lateral-averaged h and η_a compared to the cylindrical holes, owing to superior spanwise coolant coverage and reduced lift-off effects, except at a low $BR = 0.46$. The thickness (t) of the AM porous plate had a minor influence on the local and area-averaged η_a but provided more uniformity, as shown in Figure 12a. They reported that the highest area-averaged η_a was obtained at a $BR = 0.8$, and it sharply declined at the highest $BR = 2.0$ because the excessive coolant supply caused significant jet lift-off and impaired near-wall reattachment, as demonstrated in Figure 12b. To mitigate this, the research team proposed optimizing the build direction of the AM model to achieve a more favorable coolant ejection angle, thereby preserving cooling performance while minimizing flow disturbance from high discharging coolant.

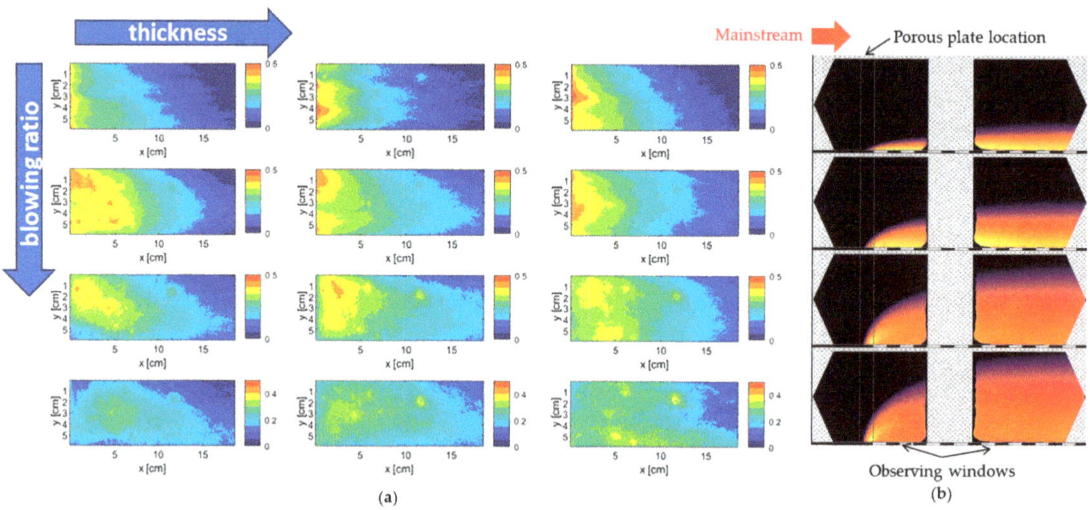

Figure 12. A porous Hastelloy-X transpiration-cooled plate: (**a**) contours of η_a at $BR = 0.5$, 0.8, 1.5, and 2.0 and $t = 0.5$, 1.0, and 2.0 mm and (**b**) IR images of concentration of ejected air at $BR = 0.5$, 0.8, 1.5, and 2.0. Reproduced with permission from [74]. Copyright 2024 Elsevier.

Fantozzi et al. [75] studied the influence of the structural parameters, including laser power, laser speed, and hatch distance of 3D-printed porous materials, on fluid flow, focusing on pore radius distribution and CD. They demonstrated that the CD increased with the pressure ratio and hatch distance but decreased nonlinearly with the thickness-to-diameter ratio. The specimens printed with a laser rotate 90° between layers, providing lower CD values than the model fabricated by a 67° rotation due to the variation in the φ. These studies demonstrated that transpiration cooling outperformed conventional methods in thermal protection, uniformity, and efficiency, with the AM method enabling optimized porous structures for enhanced gas turbine blade performance.

4.3.3. Experimental Investigations on AM-Fabricated Non-Stochastic Structures

Recent advancements in transpiration cooling for gas turbine blades have shown the superior performance of AM-fabricated deterministic structures, such as TPMS and biomimetic designs, over traditional random-pore media. Cheng et al. [64] used deionized water as a coolant for the IWP(A) TPMS-based transpiration cooling with uniform ($\varphi = 35\%$) and graded porosity ($\varphi = 25{\sim}45\%$) to enhance cooling performance. The experiments using IR thermography were conducted to observe the phase change region on the transpiration-cooled plate. Even though phase-change transpiration cooling offers high heat absorption, its complexity and instability, caused by unpredictable two-phase flow dynamics and excessive coolant use, make it impractical for gas turbine applications [103]. In contrast, single-phase transpiration cooling provides more reliable and controllable cooling performance, making it the preferred choice for gas turbines where stability and uniformity are critical.

Experiments on AM transpiration-cooled turbine blades have revealed improved film uniformity and cooling effectiveness. Ealy [79] used multiple static pressures for flow testing of the 0.5 mm perforated transpiration-cooled leading edge (LE) and revealed nearly identical discharge behavior across both internal and external cavities. This flow improved the film uniformity compared to discrete holes, even though the design yielded lower *CD* due to area calculation discrepancies. In a subsequent study, Caldero et al. [96] studied the η_o using the PSP method. They found that the effectiveness and pressure loss of the porous cavities in the LE increased at higher *BR*. The discharged coolant was uniform downstream of the porous region, and mixing became more evident with the higher *BR*.

Similarly, research by Wambersie et al. [97] showed high η_a across a 0.5 mm perforated transpiration-cooled turbine blade at a low $BR < 0.5$. They fabricated the blade using the Stereolithography (SLA) method and employed the PSP measurement that was used in their previous double-wall cooling research [104]. They found high performance on the suction-side (SS) turbine blade due to curvature and flow acceleration, enabling uniform cooling, as shown in Figure 13a,c. While the pressure side (PS) showed the lowest area-averaged η_a, large areas maintained high film effectiveness, as illustrated in Figure 13b,d. This key achievement could help justify reallocating the coolant supply. Moreover, compared to a turbine blade with impingement/effusion cooling, the transpiration cooling at the SS and PS blades provided higher area-averaged η_a and a more uniform distribution.

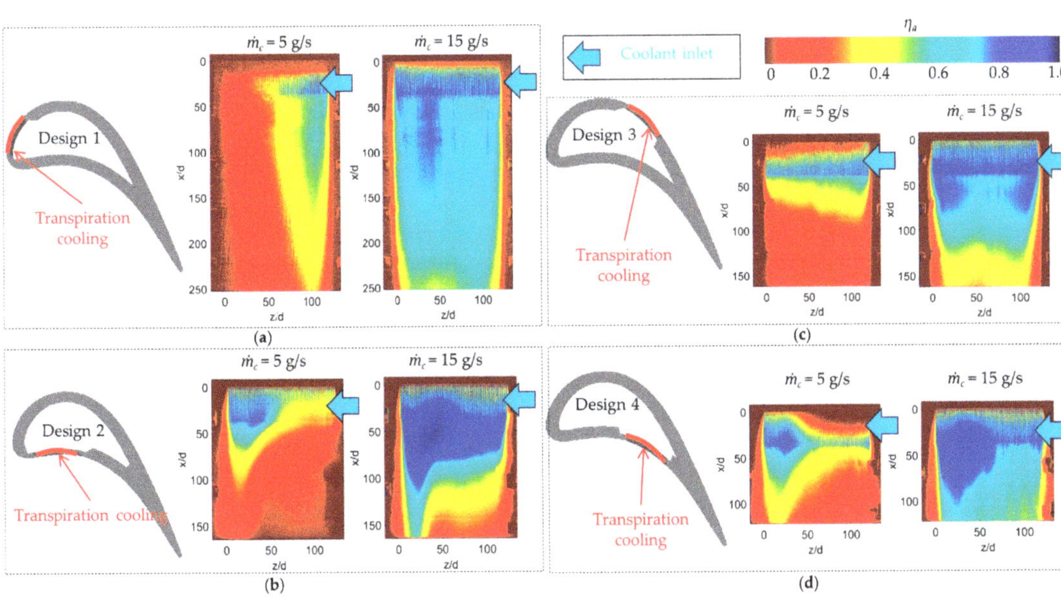

Figure 13. Distribution of η_a on transpiration-cooled blade: (**a**) SS cooling (Design 1); (**b**) PS cooling (Design 2); (**c**) SS cooling (Design 3); and (**d**) PS cooling (Design 4). This figure is reproduced from [97] under a Creative Commons Attribution (CC BY) license.

The perforated transpiration-cooled plates have been intensively studied by the research team from the National Energy Technology Laboratory, with the cooperation of the University of Pittsburgh and West Virginia University. Min et al. [77] studied various hole designs, including inline straight holes with a pitch of 1.5 *d*, 2 *d*, and 3 *d*, staggered straight holes with a pitch of 2 *d*, and 20° inclined holes with a pitch of 2 *d*. The hole diameter (*d*) also varied from 0.3 to 0.5 mm. In conclusion, as shown in Figure 14, the smaller holes (*d* = 0.3 mm) and spacing (pitch of 1.5 *d*) showed the highest and most uniform η_o but caused low mechanical strength. Chyu et al. [78] reported that integrating lattices with transpiration cooling causes a slightly lower area-averaged η_o due to partial obstruction of cooling holes by the footprint. However, the lattices mitigated η_o losses from pore blockages and offered a better alternative to pin fins for structural support due to their high surface-to-footprint ratio, addressing the inherent weakness of transpiration-only designs.

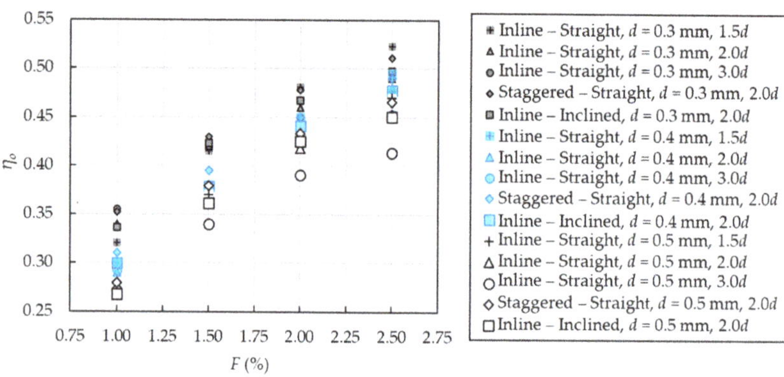

Figure 14. Area-averaged η_o comparisons at different *F*. Data collected from [77].

Heat transfer analysis on innovative hole designs of transpiration-cooled plates has been attempted by many research institutes. Huang et al. [51] compared the effects of partition walls on 0.3 mm perforated transpiration-cooled plates using IR thermography. They found that at a low *F* = 1%, the printed models with/without partition walls provided a similar area-averaged η_o value, which was higher than the sintered porous model (d_{pore} = 90 µm, φ = 32%, pore size = 33.8 µm). However, the sintered porous model was sensitive to the increase in coolant supply, generating a higher area-averaged η_o than the printed models when *F* > 2% due to increasing detached coolant on the surface of the printed model. In line with the earlier configuration, Min et al. [76] used IR thermography to investigate five topology designs for AM transpiration-cooled plates, including two perforated plates with varying hole pitches, a sphere-packing design, a wire matrix resembling woven mesh, and a biomimetic blood vessel structure. All studied *F* demonstrated a superior area-averaged η_o of all transpiration designs over shaped-hole film cooling by 10–40%. They found that the topology of the 3D-printed transpiration-cooled plate significantly influenced the η_o.

Experiments on non-metal transpiration cooling structures have been performed to assess the adiabatic film cooling effectiveness (η_a). Min et al. [99] developed a physical vapor deposition (PVD) micro-lithography technique to fabricate a surface heater for testing transpiration cooling. The IR thermography revealed that smaller coolant hole spacing and diameters improved η_a > 0.46, outperforming conventional film cooling. Aly et al. [98], employing the PSP method to study the influence of the blockage ratio on the η_a, revealed that increasing the blockage ratio reduced the area-averaged η_a, particularly at lower *BR*, due to a smaller coolant supply. Higher *BR* and blockage ratio caused non-uniform η_a

distributions within the row. Moreover, larger blockage ratios reduced lateral effectiveness, while higher BR compensated for insufficient coolant supply. In short, although the innovative partition wall designs reduced thermal efficiency, potential improvements included shaped holes, extended surfaces, vortex generators, and AM rough surfaces.

A more complex structure has been fabricated to address non-uniformity, increase cooling effectiveness, and further strengthen the structure. Fier and Bogard [100] fabricated a wire-mesh transpiration-cooled plate using a Prusa i3 3D printer based on fused deposition modeling (FDM). The proposed design demonstrated superior performance to traditional 7-7-7-shaped film-cooling holes, achieving up to 30% higher η_a at equal coolant flow rates. Brimacombe et al. [101] claimed to be the first use of the Gyroid TPMS-based transpiration cooling, 3D-printed via the SLA method at a 25 µm resolution with a 2 mm unit cell size. The IR thermography was used to measure the temperature distribution far downstream from the Gyroid-cooled plate, as shown in Figure 15a. The results showed that increasing BR and F increased the η_a, but the η_a was more sensitive to φ at a constant BR than at a fixed F, as seen in Figure 15b. The area-averaged η_a was higher than that of effusion cooling [105] but less than that of the AM wire-mesh transpiration-cooled plate with φ = 33% [100], which could be attributed to the distance of the measurement area.

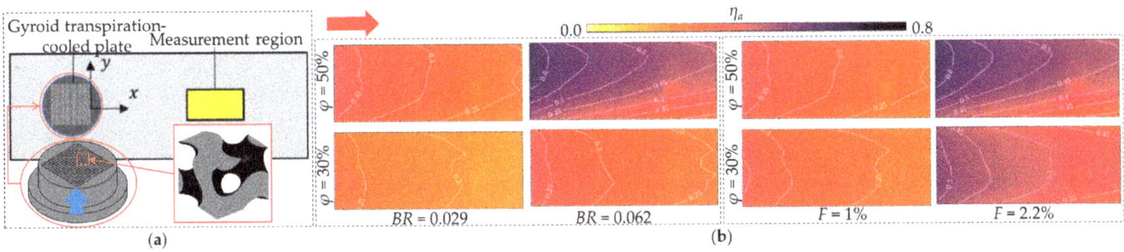

Figure 15. Gyroid TPMS-based transpiration-cooled plate: (**a**) Downstream heat transfer measurement and (**b**) the distribution of η_a at different BR, F, and φ. This figure is reproduced from [101] under a Creative Commons Attribution (CC BY) license.

The research team from the Aerospace Research Center, National Research Council of Canada has intensively conducted the heat transfer analysis of the TPMS-based transpiration cooling. Broumand et al. [92] found that the Diamond TPMS-based transpiration-cooled plate with φ = 50% outperformed conventional effusion cooling by up to five times in the area-averaged η_a using the PSP method, where the calibration and uncertainty were well-described in the report. They also revealed that the TPMS designs provided superior film coverage, reduced coolant usage, and mitigated film lift-off at high BR [106]. Using the same measurement method, Son et al. [81] found that the orientation and tortuosity of Diamond, Koch, and Gyroid TPMS topologies altered the distribution of η_a on the plate. Later, Son et al. [102] studied the variations in the unit cell size (L) of the Diamond model while maintaining φ. They found that reducing the L improved η_a. However, excessively small sizes could risk pore blockage from 3D printing or contamination, requiring optimal sizing in practical use.

4.4. Numerical Simulations

Computational modeling of transpiration cooling requires balancing accuracy and efficiency, especially when simulating phase-change effects or resolving complex porous structures. The porous-media two-phase flow model simplifies the simulation of phase-change transpiration cooling, where liquid coolant boils inside the porous structure, forming a gas–liquid mixture [107]. The phase transition absorbs significant latent heat, enhancing cooling efficiency. However, the inherent instability of boiling and non-uniform two-phase flow makes this method more complex than single-phase transpiration cooling [64]. Alternatively, Zhang et al. [80] employed the Lattice Boltzmann Method (LBM) to simulate flow through printed TPMS structures, comparing CAD and computed tomography (CT) scan geometries. They demonstrated the efficiency of the LBM in handling the complex TPMS boundaries through simple voxelized meshes, avoiding the costly unstructured meshes in conventional Navier–Stokes (NS) solvers. However, the LBM struggles with high Reynolds flows, which is the inertial regime in transpiration cooling, whereas the NS solvers with Reynolds-averaged Navier–Stokes (RANS) or large eddy simulation (LES) are more mature. Additionally, the LBM faced scalability limitations for graded or optimized complex topologies, such as the TPMS structure, requiring fine voxel resolutions. Modern NS solvers, in contrast, leverage advanced turbulence modeling to capture multiscale phenomena computationally efficiently for large-scale academic/industrial flow/heat transfer and optimization analyses.

In general, the governing equations for single-phase transpiration cooling can also be divided based on structures: deterministic and stochastic architectures. Table 3 compares the governing equations based on steady-state and non-radiation assumptions. In Table 3, ρ is the density of the fluid (kg/m^3). $\mathbf{u}$ is the velocity vector (m/s). S_m is a mass source term representing fluid injection from the wall during the cooling of porous transpiration (N/m^3). p is the pressure field, signifying the static pressure in the domain (N/m^2). $\mathbf{F}$ implies an external force, such as gravity (N/m^3). c_p is the heat capacity of the fluid (J/(kg·K)). T_{flu} and T_{sol} are the temperatures of the fluid and solid (K). S_T is the term for the energy source added/removed with the coolant (W/m^3). K and C_F are the permeability (m^2) and inertial resistance coefficient (1/m), where the empirical formula provided by Ergun and Orning [108] was mostly used.

Table 3. Governing equations of single-phase transpiration cooling in recent numerical studies.

Equation	Non-Stochastic Transpiration	Random-Pore Porous-Media Model
Mass conservation	$\nabla \cdot (\rho \mathbf{u}) = 0$	$\nabla \cdot (\rho \mathbf{u}) = S_m$
Momentum	$\rho(\mathbf{u} \cdot \nabla \mathbf{u}) = -\nabla p + \mu \nabla^2 \mathbf{u} + \mathbf{F}$	$\frac{\rho}{\varphi^2}(\mathbf{u} \cdot \nabla)\mathbf{u} = -\nabla p + \mu \nabla^2 \mathbf{u} - \left(\frac{\mu}{K} + \frac{\rho C_F}{\sqrt{K}}\lvert\mathbf{u}\rvert\right)\mathbf{u}$ $K = \frac{d_{pore}^2 \varphi^3}{150(1-\varphi^2)}; C_F = \frac{1.75}{\sqrt{150}\varphi^{3/2}}$
Energy (Fluid)	$\rho c_p(\mathbf{u} \cdot \nabla T) = \nabla \cdot \left(k_f \nabla T\right)$	$\rho c_p(\mathbf{u} \cdot \nabla T) = \nabla \cdot \left(k_{eff} \nabla T\right) + S_T$ $k_{eff} = \varphi k_f + (1-\varphi)k_s$
Energy (Solid)	$\nabla \cdot (k_s \nabla T) = 0$ (no internal heat generation)	$\nabla \cdot (k_s \nabla T) = 0$
Fluid–solid interface boundary conditions	$T_{flu} = T_{sol}$ $-k_f \nabla T \cdot \mathbf{n} = -k_s \nabla T \cdot \mathbf{n}$	

For both modes, recent numerical investigations have employed advanced computational fluid dynamics (CFD) tools to analyze various transpiration cooling configurations, utilizing different turbulence models and mesh strategies, as shown in Table 4. Major studies used STAR-CCM+ and ANSYS FLUENT with hexahedral meshes ranging from 2.3 million to 53.4 million cells, depending on the complexity of the model. The k-ω turbulence model showed the advantage of simulating the viscous sub-layer and boundary layer formation and obtained better predictability in heat transfer analysis compared to SST k-ω turbulence models in several studies [109].

Table 4. Overview of numerical analysis on flow and cooling effectiveness for AM-fabricated transpiration cooling.

Ref.	Main Study	Tool	Method	Material	Mesh Details
[95]	Flow characteristics on a transpiration-cooled single-turbine blade	STAR-CCM+	k-ω		• Hexahedral mesh = 15.3 × 10^6 cells for effusion and = 9.5 × 10^6 cells for transpiration cooling.
[30]	Flow and temperature distributions on a transpiration-cooled cascade-turbine blade	STAR-CCM+	SST k-ω	Porous media with stainless steel in the transpiration model	• Hexahedral mesh = 53.4 × 10^6 cells for effusion and = 2.3 × 10^6 cells for transpiration cooling.
[25]	Flow and overall cooling effectiveness of a non-uniform porosity transpiration-cooled blade	ANSYS FLUENT	SST k-ω		• Hexahedral mesh = 3.46 × 10^6 cells generated by FLUENT Meshing
[96]	Adiabatic cooling effectiveness and pressure loss of transpiration-cooled leading edge	STAR-CCM+	SST k-ω	Adiabatic	• Polyhedral mesh = 8.44 × 10^6
[110]	Effects of outlet angle and pattern on transpiration-cooled plates	ANSYS FLUENT	SST k-ω	Inconel 600	• Structured mesh = 1.07 × 10^6 cells
[82]	Transpiration-cooled plates with TPMS structures	ANSYS FLUENT	SST k-ω	Stainless steel	• Polygonal mesh = 5.21 × 10^6 cells generated by FLUENT Meshing
[51]	Effects of partitional walls on flow and overall cooling effectiveness in transpiration-cooled plates	ANSYS FLUENT	k-ω	Inconel 718	• Quadrilateral mesh = 2.0 × 10^6
[111,112]	Pore blockage effects on perforated transpiration-cooled plates	ANSYS CFX	SST k-ω	k_s = 1 W/(m·K)	• Hexahedral mesh = 3.1 × 10^6 cells
[113]	Pore blockage effects on tree-like transpiration-cooled plates	ANSYS FLUENT	SST k-ω	Inconel 718	• Polyhedral mesh = 5.66 × 10^6 cells, generated by FLUENT Meshing
[114]	Pore blockage effects on the oriented porous structure	ANSYS FLUENT	-	Porous media with CMC (k_s = 2 W/(m·K))	• Porous: φ = 30%, dpore = 0.1 mm, resulting in mesh = 186,500 cells
[89]	Effects of hole diameter, Biot number, and coolant distribution on perforated transpiration-cooled plates	ANSYS FLUENT	SST k-ω	Inconel 718	• Structured mesh and O-block with local refinement = 1.96 × 10^6 cells
[115]	Effects of solid thermal conductivity, wall thickness, hole spacing, and TBC on AM transpiration cooling plates with inhomogeneous porosity	ANSYS FLUENT	k-ω	Inconel 718 and ceramic (k_s = 1, 11 and 50 W/(m·K))	• Hexahedral mesh = 1.43 × 10^6 cells generated by ANSYS ICEM
[116]	Transpiration-cooled plates with varied porosity configurations and pressure gradients	ANSYS FLUENT	SST k-ω	Inconel 718 (Temperature-dependent properties)	• Hexahedral mesh = 16.38 × 10^6 cells generated by ANSYS ICEM
[117]	Swirl-chamber effusion with different inclination angles and compound angles	ANSYS FLUENT	RSM	k_s = 0.5 W/(m·K)	• Hexahedral mesh = 18.5 × 10^6 cells

However, the SST k-ω model was mostly employed to examine transpiration cooling for gas turbines due to its unique ability to accurately resolve near-wall flow physics, adverse pressure gradients, and mixing phenomena. The SST k-ω model also provided the optimal balance between accuracy and computational cost. Calderon et al. [96] found SST k-ω overpredicted the area-averaged η_a by around 25% within the $BR < 0.15$. Wang et al. [110] reported the maximum deviation in area-averaged η_o between the simulation and experimental results was 6.9%. Similarly, Yang et al. [116] and Zhou et al. [82] revealed that the maximum relative error of area-averaged η_o was less than 6%. Sun [89] observed that the SST k-ω model was more consistent with the experimental data in the literature compared to the k-ω model, and the deviation was 3%. In short, the use of turbulence models with carefully constructed meshes depended on the validation across the experimental data to balance accuracy in transpiration cooling analysis.

Many previous studies modeled transpiration cooling using the porous-media model due to lower computational costs while maintaining accuracy [118]. Kim et al. [95] revealed a series of flow results of a C3X single-turbine blade at different studied conditions. They found that transpiration cooling formed a stable boundary layer, even with increasing coolant flow, as shown in Figure 16. At high BR, the suction-side rotating flow remained near the TE. Furthermore, transpiration cooling maintained a thick, stable coolant layer on the PS, whereas effusion cooling promoted coolant-mainstream mixing due to wake recirculation. Moreover, increasing the u_h from 2 to 20 m/s while fixing the BR = 4.2 showed the same trend, as compared in Figure 16a,c. In addition, a comparative analysis of transpiration cooling simulations with experimental visualization results demonstrated excellent agreement, particularly at a low *BR*. This validation was further supported by Figure 16c, where simulation data closely matched the observed boundary layer development in overlapping visualizations. Under the tested conditions, the transpiration cooling maintained a thinner thermal boundary layer compared to effusion cooling [73].

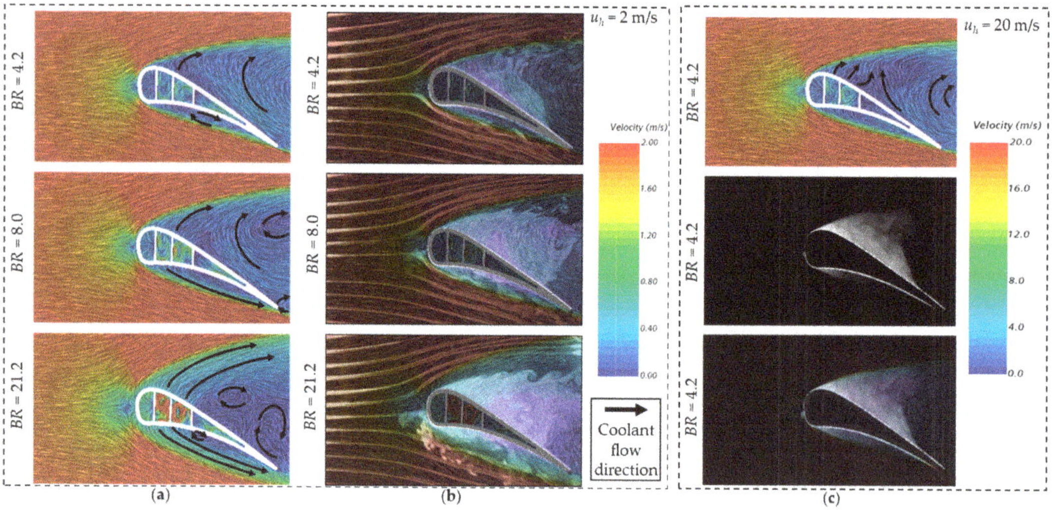

Figure 16. Flow characteristics of a C3X single-turbine transpiration-cooled blade: (**a**) Numerical results at u_h = 2 m/s; (**b**) Comparison between visualization and numerical results at u_h = 2 m/s; (**c**) Numerical results, visualized coolant flow images and comparison between visualization and numerical results at u_h = 20 m/s. Reproduced with permission from [95]. Copyright 2022 Elsevier.

Kim et al. [30] also simulated the effusion and transpiration-cooled blades. The visualization results showed that for effusion and transpiration cooling, the coolant outflow formed a thinner boundary layer compared to the single blade. This thinner layer shifted the suction-side vortex rearward, reducing mainstream/coolant mixing and stabilizing the coolant within the boundary layer. Consequently, the cascade arrangement enhanced cooling performance over a single blade due to inter-blade flow interactions. Moreover, the temperature field analysis in Figure 17 revealed that the high flow resistance of the porous-media transpiration-cooled structure significantly reduced mainstream inflow compared to effusion cooling, enabling a more stable formation of cooler internal air and thermal boundary layers. Consequently, transpiration cooling outperformed effusion cooling for both single and cascade blades.

In a related study, Ma et al. [25] focused on the effects of coolant mass flow ratio and the non-uniform φ of C3X cascade-turbine blades, validated with the experimental results of Kim et al. [30]. They concluded that increasing the coolant mass flow rate enhanced the area-averaged η_o of the blade; however, the PS caused lower values compared to the SS due to mainstream flow intrusion, particularly at a high φ = 80%. Along the coolant flow path, as pressure losses approached 100%, coolant flow stagnated, which inadequately cooled the TE. Notably, adopting a gradient φ distribution improved blade surface temperature uniformity and increased area-averaged η_o by 13.97% over conventional uniform φ designs.

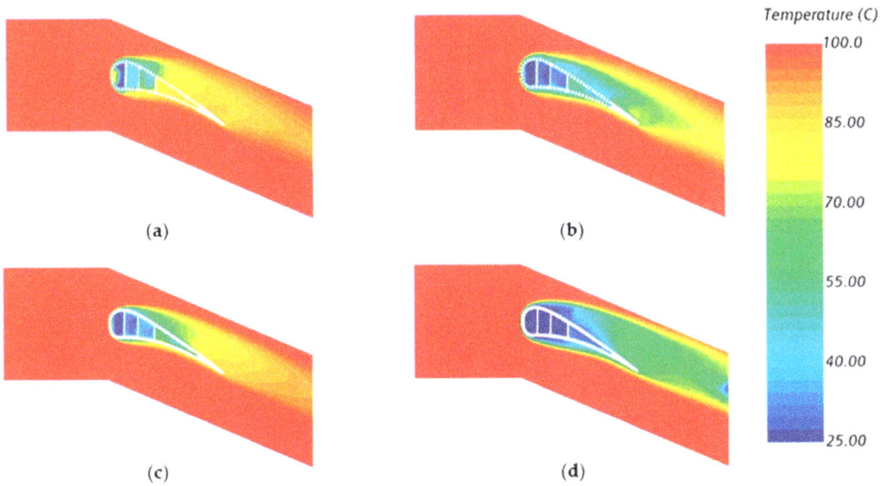

Figure 17. Temperature field of a C3X cascade-turbine transpiration-cooled blade at u_h = 20 m/s: (**a**) Effusion cooling with a volume flow rate of 100 LPM; (**b**) 300 LPM; (**c**) Transpiration cooling with a volume flow rate of 100 LPM; and (**d**) 300 LPM. Reproduced with permission from [30]. Copyright 2022 Elsevier.

Numerical studies have demonstrated the effectiveness of simplified computational methods for analyzing custom-designed transpiration cooling systems. Calderon et al. [96] adopted periodic boundary conditions to reduce the computational domain of a complex transpiration-cooled leading edge. The numerical model provided similar trends of area-averaged η_0 and pressure loss to the experiments. Similarly, Fier et al. [100] demonstrated that a 2D RANS simulation effectively captured the essential physics of the wire-mesh transpiration-cooled plate, highlighting the relative simplicity of modeling this technique.

The geometric design of the transpiration cooling shows strong influences on cooling performance. Wang et al. [110] evaluated transpiration-cooled plates with different outlet angles and patterns, revealing that while outlet angles strongly affected temperature uniformity, they only slightly affected cooling efficiency. Complementary work by Zhou et al. [82] revealed that coolant flow resistance in the TPMS-based transpiration cooling was primarily governed by pore throat geometry, though higher resistance did not require greater injection pressure due to mainstream–coolant interactions. The study also identified that counter-rotating vortex pairs (CRVPs) in the coolant film can elevate surface skin friction, but this effect can be mitigated by complex outflow angles.

Several investigations have highlighted jet lift-off challenges in transpiration cooling. Huang et al. [51] simulated the 0.25 mm perforated transpiration-cooled plates with different partitional wall designs and found major jet lift-off in the case with the largest partition walls. This phenomenon was further explored by Yang et al. [111,112], who modeled random pore blockage effects on 200 cases of transpiration cooling and confirmed that a high plugging probability (γ) caused a significant jet lift-off, decreasing cooling effectiveness, as shown in Figure 18.

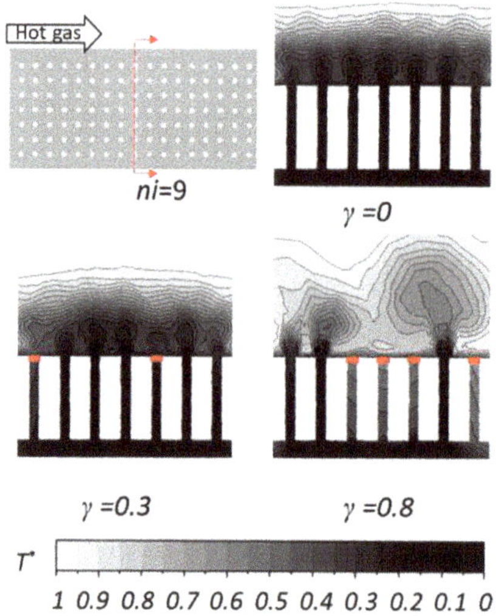

Figure 18. Simulation results showing jet lift-off of perforated transpiration-cooled plates with different pore blockage conditions. Reproduced with permission from [112]. Copyright 2018 Elsevier.

Nearly aero-engine conditions, where the T_h is above 1000 K, have also been simulated to study the impact of the φ and pressure gradient on cooling performance. Huang and He [115] used conjugate heat transfer to analyze the effect of non-uniform φ on perforated transpiration-cooled plates, where the hole diameter was varied to obtain a non-uniformity of 0–50%. Studies concluded that inhomogeneous φ had a significant influence on the cooling effects of the surface film and internal holes. Yang et al. [116] investigated transpiration cooling (d = 0.2 mm) with different φ configurations under varying mainstream pressure gradients. It was found that transpiration cooling outperforms film cooling by up to 100% in effectiveness, but non-uniform coolant distribution reduces efficiency. Li et al. [117] compared the cooling performance between 3D-printable swirl-chamber transpiration and the 30°–90° inclined film holes in a Can-type combustion chamber, considering chemical reactions. They concluded that hybrid cooling was highly effective for combustor liners, recommending smaller inclination angles and compound angles opposing the swirling flow for optimal performance. These studies demonstrated that advanced cooling designs significantly enhanced thermal performance under near-engine conditions, though coolant uniformity remained a key challenge for optimization.

4.5. Effect of Studied Conditions

Most studies agree that increasing coolant supply (*MFR*, *BR* or *F*) generally enhances cooling effectiveness, as shown in Figures 9–17. In addition, the arrangement of the perforated holes also altered the cooling effectiveness, as seen in Figure 19. However, excessive coolant flow can degrade performance. Min et al. [99] observed reduced η_a at $BR > 0.25$ due to hot gas entrainment, while Sun et al. [89] found that increasing the F from 0.2% to 1% reduced the cooling rate from 0.72 to 0.09. They solved these issues by a double coolant supply chamber, which could simultaneously improve η_o and reduce coolant consumption in perforated plate designs.

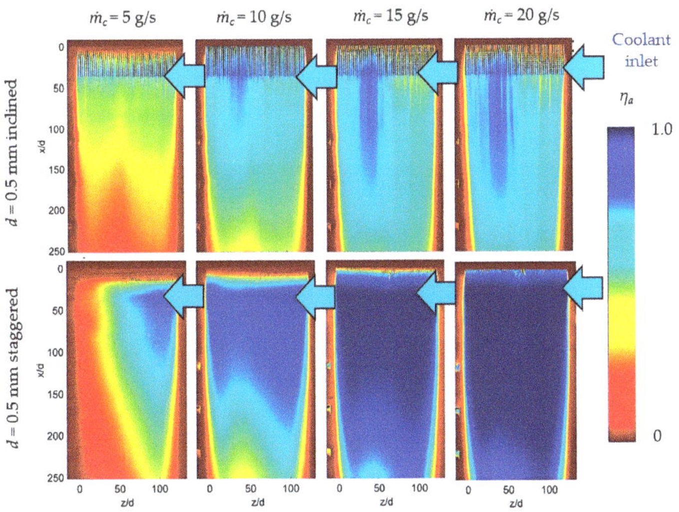

Figure 19. Influence of coolant supply and hole arrangement of transpiration cooling structures on cooling effectiveness. This figure is reproduced from [97] under a Creative Commons Attribution (CC BY) license.

Thermal resistance plays a critical role in altering the cooling effectiveness. Huang et al. [51] found that the 3D-printed transpiration-cooled plate, which was fully melted particles, enabled efficient heat conduction from the upstream to the downstream region. Therefore, it exhibited a more uniform η_0 distribution and provided a slightly higher area-averaged η_0, particularly at a low F, than the sintered porous plate. This was because the sintered model had a much lower effective thermal conductivity than its bulk material [119], leading to poorer downstream cooling performance. Sun et al. [89] showed that higher Biot numbers degraded temperature uniformity due to increased thermal resistance, particularly at low thermal conductivity.

Meanwhile, Huang and He [115] showed that higher thermal conductivity in solids significantly mitigated inhomogeneous φ effects, as compared to the variation in plate thickness and hole spacing. Also, the inhomogeneous φ strongly affected η_0 when a low-conductivity TBC was applied. The thin TBC layer introduced substantial thermal resistance, and lower conductivity worsened inhomogeneous φ effects. Yang et al. [116] further highlighted that under varying mainstream pressure gradients, the small spacing case and streamwise-decreasing φ model provided high cooling effectiveness and improved uniformity. Also, higher pressure gradients increased η_0 and uniformity.

In short, these studies showed the need for careful design balancing coolant flow, thermal conductivity, and pore geometry in the AM-fabricated transpiration cooling systems to achieve maximum performance while mitigating jet lift-off and thermal resistance.

4.6. Effect of Structural Designs

4.6.1. Influence of Porosity

Many studies have demonstrated that porosity (φ) is critical in the performance of AM-fabricated transpiration cooling systems. Fantozzi et al. [75] observed that higher-porosity AM porous media exhibited lower discharge coefficients (*CDs*), highlighting the trade-off between φ and flow efficiency. In an early study, Huang et al. [49] investigated perforated transpiration cooling with hole diameters of 0.5 mm and 1 mm, fabricated by the electric spark method, finding that smaller holes (d = 0.5 mm) with φ = 19.6%

achieved an area-averaged η_o comparable to sintered porous media with φ = 36%. However, larger holes (d = 1 mm) reduced the area-averaged η_o due to the enhanced mixing and boundary layer momentum at F > 2%. Huang et al. [51] later revealed that as the area of the reinforcing partition walls of AM transpiration-cooled plates increased (decreasing φ), the area-averaged η_o was slightly decreased within F = 2–3%.

The relationship between φ and η has been extensively studied. Broumand et al. [92] found that the Diamond TPMS transpiration-cooled plate with φ = 50% provided the highest η_a up to 0.75 at F = 1.6%, without any jet lift-off effects. Also, even a φ = 30% provided η_a = 0.36 at F = 0.68%, higher than conventional effusion cooling by 1.8 times. Smaller hole diameters (d = 0.3 mm) were shown to enhance uniformity, with staggered hole patterns providing better performance than inclined configurations [77,89]. Wambersie et al. [97] also showed that decreasing the hole spacing on a turbine blade SS (increasing φ from 20% to 30%) significantly improved film coverage, demonstrating interactions between adjacent films and mainstream flow. However, Yang et al. [116] noted that while increasing φ generally improves area-averaged η_a, reaching up to 0.83, it can lead to non-uniform coolant distribution.

Graded and non-uniform φ distributions have emerged as promising strategies for optimizing cooling performance. Cheng et al. [64] demonstrated that IWP(A)-TPMS structures with graded φ improved coolant distribution and reduced hot-spot temperatures under non-uniform heat flux. Similarly, Ma et al. [25] proposed a φ gradient from the LE to TE of turbine blades to balance coolant seepage and prevent mainstream intrusion, as shown in Figure 20. Their findings revealed that excessive φ = 80% led to uneven pressure distribution and coolant leakage, emphasizing the importance of controlled φ variation.

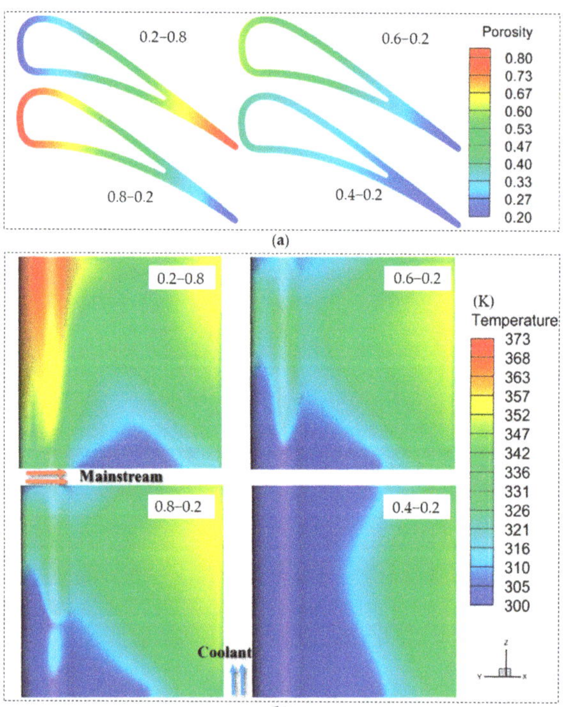

Figure 20. Non-φ distributions of the transpiration-cooled blade: (**a**) the distribution according to the dimensionless distance from the LE and (**b**) temperature contours on the blade surface. Reproduced with permission from [25]. Copyright 2023 Elsevier.

Inhomogeneous φ and manufacturing tolerances also significantly impact cooling efficiency. Huang and He [115] showed that inhomogeneous φ, which occurred during the AM process, significantly affected the surface film and internal hole cooling, causing local efficiency variations up to 41.5% and 34.5%, respectively, at a 20% non-uniformity setting. However, area-averaged and local η_o changes were minor due to heat conduction. At a non-uniformity of 50%, local impacts increased, but area-averaged η_a differences remained small. The effect of inhomogeneous φ on effusion cooling became negligible when the precision of the AM hole was maintained within a 20% variation. Overall, optimization of the φ is crucial for AM transpiration cooling systems. Graded φ designs with precise manufacturing could be a key candidate for achieving optimal coolant coverage and thermal performance in gas turbines.

4.6.2. Influence of Topology

Experimental and numerical studies have revealed that topological design critically influences the cooling effectiveness and uniformity of AM-fabricated transpiration cooling. Biomimetic approaches show particular promise, with Min et al. [76] demonstrating that blood vessel-inspired structures outperformed conventional round holes despite lower internal surface area ratios (R_{int}). This design achieved superior cooling through enhanced internal flow interaction and more uniform outlet distribution. Similarly, Sun et al. [113] reported that with the same A_{eff}, a tree-like channel achieved higher cooling efficiency than round-hole designs at equal coolant flow rates. However, Poupinha et al. [74] revealed that the unfavorable 90° ejection angle of a porous transpiration-cooled plate caused low η_a, requiring optimization of the AM build direction.

Lattice-based cooling structures exhibit significant performance variations based on their geometric configuration. Chyu et al. [78] observed that the different lattices in a transpiration-cooled plate altered the cooling performance, particularly at a $BR > 0.25$. It was observed that the η_o follows this trend: face-centered cubic > octahedral cubic ≈ body-centered cubic > Kagome. Related studies on this topic indicated that the TPMS lattices presented unique advantages for transpiration-cooling applications [46]. Zhou et al. [82] found that the IWP(B) TPMS-based transpiration cooling demonstrated an optimal balance between injection pressure and cooling performance. The Primitive(B) provided superior temperature uniformity due to reduced coolant transport along the mainstream, while the IWP(A) was the preferred choice when minimizing skin friction was critical, as it effectively suppressed CRVP formation across studied flow rates. Son et al. [81] observed that surface trough orientation and internal flow path tortuosity significantly affected the η_a. They found that the Koch model with higher tortuosity minimized orientation sensitivity, achieving uniform coolant distribution, which was only 3–5% sensitivity across flow rates, while low-tortuosity Diamond exhibited strong orientation dependence up to 15–24%. Meanwhile, the Gyroid, with moderate tortuosity, showed intermediate sensitivity of 12–17%. The Koch robustness to flow direction makes it ideal for complex surfaces with directional flows.

Findings from a similar investigation revealed that the shape of cooling holes substantially influenced thermal protection characteristics. Wang et al. [110] reported that transpiration-cooled plates (d = 0.2 mm, φ = 18.8%) with synclastic outlet angles improved cooling performance over reverse angles, while elliptical holes demonstrated an interesting trade-off between cooling efficiency and temperature uniformity based on their alignment with the mainstream flow. These findings emphasized the importance of hole geometry design for optimized transpiration cooling structures.

4.7. Optimization Studies

Recent advances in AM technologies have enabled innovative optimization approaches for transpiration cooling in gas turbines. The recent optimization studies can be categorized based on their methodologies and findings as follows:

4.7.1. Topology Optimization with Lattices

Yeranee et al. [18] showed that the topology-optimized cooling design incorporating TPMS lattices enhanced double-wall channel performance. The optimized design achieved a 9.5–12.5% enhancement in impingement heat transfer and 4.2–4.6% higher overall cooling effectiveness compared to pin fin configurations while simultaneously reducing pressure losses. They also demonstrated that TPMS-based topology optimization can address thermal challenges in advanced turbine cooling applications. This method could be used to avoid the footprint blockages on transpiration holes found in previous studies [78].

4.7.2. Machine Learning and Convolution-Based Modeling

Yang et al. [112] pioneered the use of convolution modeling to predict transpiration cooling and its associated plugging disadvantages, offering a quantitative understanding of random plugging effects and supporting optimization efforts, particularly in AM transpiration cooling, which held significant potential for mitigating plugging issues. Later, a novel convolution-based modeling approach for predicting η_o distributions was developed by treating the transpiration-cooled plates as void/solid logic functions [120]. Using conjugate CFD data from simple perforated transpiration-cooled plates for training, the high-resolution convolution model successfully reconstructed η_o for both training cases, achieving 4.04% error within 100 training steps and more complex validation geometries. They claimed that the method significantly reduced parameter space dimensionality while preserving physical interactions between coolant holes through an efficient initialization process using decoupled weight functions. In a more recent study, Yang et al. [121] developed a machine learning model using convolutional neural networks to predict the η_a in the perforated transpiration-cooled plates by integrating image conversion, convolution, and nonlinear activation processes. Training and validation used CFD data from regular and random film cooling hole arrays. Results showed that the model achieved few errors, less than 10% for training and 13% for validation. The convolution kernel revealed coolant superposition as a key factor in effusion cooling.

4.7.3. Surrogate Modeling and Evolutionary Algorithms

Several studies combined CFD with surrogate modeling and evolutionary algorithms for optimization. Wang et al. [122] used RANS simulations with the Brinkman–Forchheimer–Darcy model and a Kriging-genetic algorithm (GA) optimization framework for optimizing a transpiration-cooled C3X cascade-turbine blade with multiple porous zones of varying φ. The research revealed that the highest φ should be at the LE and PS for optimal cooling. A subsequent study [123] employed a multi-objective optimization of a transpiration-cooled C3X cascade-turbine blade using CFD modeling and a surrogate-based approach combining an artificial neural network (ANN) and a non-dominated sorting genetic algorithm-II (NSGA-II). The optimization framework treated φ distribution across different vane zones as design variables to balance cooling performance and aerodynamic efficiency. The results showed that the LE coolant discharge significantly enhanced cooling but increased porous-media pressure losses while maintaining consistent mainstream pressure losses, approximately 18% for all cases. They concluded that the optimal design required careful coolant allocation to the leading edge and adjacent SS and PS. Similarly, Lv et al. [27] showed that a porous-media plate beneath film holes improved cooling effectiveness by 30% compared to conventional double-wall cooling, with a further 8.5–8.7% improvement from the GA optimization.

4.7.4. Gradient Porosity and Response Surface Methods

Chen et al. [124] and Liu et al. [90] explored gradient φ designs using a response surface methodology and multi-objective genetic algorithms (MOGAs). Chen et al. [124] demonstrated that gradient φ plates improved temperature uniformity by 20.58–23.78% while reducing injection pressure by 84.5–86.2%. Liu et al. [90] developed an ANN-MOGA framework that increased cooling efficiency by 11.35% and reduced pressure loss by 36.23% compared to uniform φ designs. These studies emphasize the benefits of tailored φ distributions in achieving high-performance cooling.

5. Challenges and Future Directions

5.1. Additive Manufacturing Challenges and Innovations

The challenges of AM-fabricated film cooling have been well described by Dutta et al. [2]. They concluded that the AM film cooling surfaces reduced film effectiveness by disrupting jets but enhanced in-hole convection. Yeranee et al. [18] observed that the as-printed model exhibited partially fused powder particles adhering to the pedestal structures, effusion holes, and impingement cooling channels, as shown in Figure 21, attributed to non-optimized AM parameters and printing orientation. Post-processing, such as surface machining or chemical polishing, improved the external surface finish of the effusion and impingement plates, resulting in a relatively smooth exterior. However, high-resolution CT scans revealed the presence of internal micro-voids, particularly within the pedestal near the effusion plate, suggesting potential challenges in achieving fully dense structures with uncontrolled AM settings.

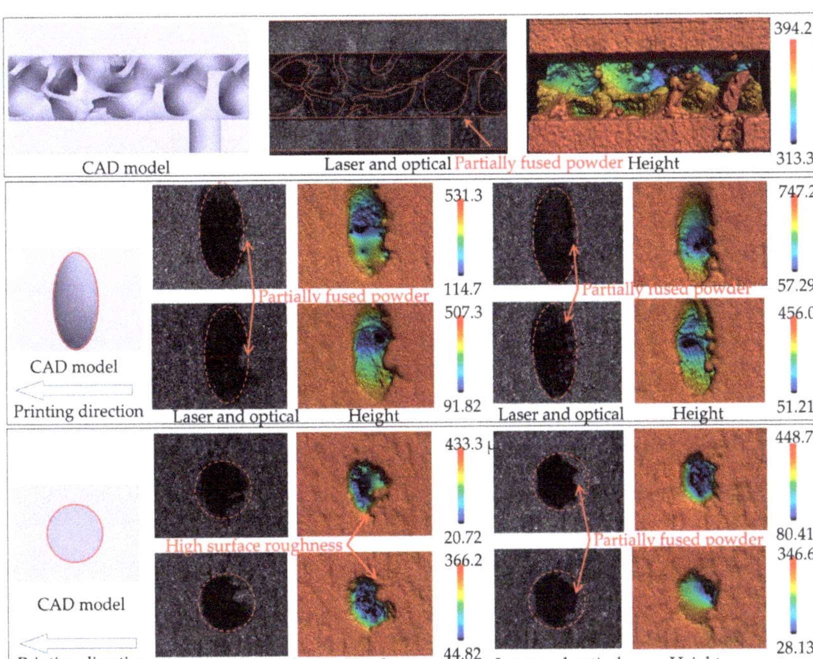

Figure 21. Deviations, defects, and surface roughness of AM-fabricated gas turbine cooling structures (unit: μm). Reproduced with permission from [18]. Copyright 2024 Elsevier.

The fabrication of transpiration cooling systems through AM technology also presents several persistent challenges that impact system performance. Dimensional accuracy issues remain prevalent, with multiple studies documenting deviations in hole sizes and φ in the AM-fabricated components. Table 5 overviews the deviations in different AM transpiration cooling designs. It can be highlighted that the etching and laser drilling obtained better accuracy than the AM methods, where most of the AM methods caused hole size and φ reduction from the designs. The SLM-produced perforations were consistently undersized compared to the design specifications, showing reductions ranging from 4% for 0.24 mm holes to 77% for 0.06 mm holes [66]. Similar findings were reported by Min et al. [76,77]. They noted that the DLMS caused φ shrinkage of about 40% for 0.3 mm holes and outlet area reduction by 27–39% for 0.5 mm holes in round-hole designs.

Table 5. Overview of deviations in different AM transpiration cooling geometries.

Ref.	Printed Geometry	Manufacturing Method (Surface Treatment)	Material	Design Values	Deviations from Designs
[66]	Oblique cylinder hole	Etching (Polish)	Stainless steel	d = 0.063 mm pitch = 0.063 mm φ = 91%	$d \approx -1\%$ to -4% pitch $\approx -1\%$ $\varphi \approx -1\%$ to -7%
	Truncated-cone hole	Laser drilling (Polish)		d = 0.06–0.24 mm pitch = 0.6–2.4 mm φ = 91%	$d \approx -8\%$ to -30% pitch $\approx -2\%$ to -5% $\varphi \approx -15\%$ to -48%
	Round hole	SLM (Laser clean)		d = 0.06–0.24 mm pitch = 0.6–2.4 mm φ = 91%	$d \approx -2\%$ to -37% pitch $\approx -33\%$ to 0.2% $\varphi \approx -4\%$ to -77%
	Quadratic-truncated-cone hole	SLA	Resin	d = 0.25 mm pitch = 2.686 mm φ = 1.0%	$d \approx -0.4\%$ to 17.2% pitch $\approx -0.6\%$ to -0.7% $\varphi \approx -29\%$ to 9%
[76]	0.3 mm-round hole (3 d-pitch) 0.3 mm-round hole (2 d-pitch) Sphere packing Wire-mesh matrix Blood vessel Film cooling	DLMS (Heat treatment, Supporting removal, De-powdering process)	Inconel 718	φ = 4.13% φ = 8.15% φ = 10.73% φ = 20.89% φ = 13.42% φ = 2.32%	$\varphi \approx -39\%$ $\varphi \approx -12\%$ $\varphi \approx -7.2\%$ $\varphi \approx -12\%$ $\varphi \approx -15\%$ $\varphi \approx -31\%$
[77]	Round hole (1.5 d-pitch) Round hole (2 d-pitch) Round hole (3 d-pitch)	DLMS (Supporting removal)	Inconel 718	A_{out} = 70,685.8 μm^2 d = 0.3 mm	$A_{out} \approx -39\%, d \approx -22\%$ $A_{out} \approx -49\%, d \approx -28\%$ $A_{out} \approx -44\%, d \approx -25\%$
	Round hole (1.5 d-pitch) Round hole hole (2 d-pitch) Round hole (3 d-pitch)			A_{out} = 125,663.7 μm^2 d = 0.4 mm	$A_{out} \approx -36\%, d \approx -20\%$ $A_{out} \approx -41\%, d \approx -17\%$ $A_{out} \approx -35\%, d \approx -19\%$
	Round hole (1.5 d-pitch) Round hole (2 d-pitch) Round hole (3 d-pitch)			A_{out} = 196,349.5 μm^2 d = 0.5 mm	$A_{out} \approx -29\%, d \approx -16\%$ $A_{out} \approx -28\%, d \approx -15\%$ $A_{out} \approx -27\%, d \approx -14\%$
[92]	Diamond TPMS lattice	SLA	Resin	φ = 30% φ = 40% φ = 50%	$\varphi = -39\%$ $\varphi = -24\%$ $\varphi = -15\%$
[80]	Gyroid TPMS lattice	LPBF	Inconel 625	φ = 61%	$\varphi = -1\%$

In addition, Huang et al. [51] reported a designed 0.3 mm hole printing at 0.25 mm due to laser beam limitations and heat diffusion, while Broumand et al. [92] noted that Diamond TPMS structures consistently achieved lower φ than designed, particularly in low-φ cases. Zhang et al. [80] found that while the LPBF-fabricated TPMS structures met φ targets, surface defects reduced permeability by around 15% compared to CAD models. Ealy et al. [79] confirmed these trends through X-ray CT analysis, showing that while 95% of surfaces met 320 μm, tolerances in the SLM Inconel 718 blades feature accuracy degraded significantly beyond 60° from the build direction. These dimensional inaccuracies directly affect pressure losses and flow distribution within the cooling structures.

Process parameter optimization presents another significant challenge, as demonstrated by Fantozzi et al. [75]. They found that increasing laser power while reducing scan speed improved geometric regularity but decreased φ, consequently increasing flow resistance. Son et al. [102] further identified critical limitations in the SLA-printed Diamond TPMS plates, where φ below 10% resulted in unprintable regions with stochastic pore clogging. Surface characteristics also significantly impact performance, with SEM analyses [51,125] confirming that as-printed channels were typically 15% smaller than designed. Huang et al. [51] noted that while adhered metal particles increased surface roughness, they enhanced heat transfer by acting as micro-fins. Min et al. [77] quantified printing accuracy through backlit imaging, finding that smaller pores (d = 0.3 mm) had >10% plugging versus 0% for 0.5 mm holes.

Future advancements in this area are focusing on several promising directions. Recent developments in AM-assisted casting of complex lattices [126,127] have shown the potential to match LPBF mechanical properties at reduced costs while achieving smoother surfaces. Emerging SLA, digital light processing, or liquid crystal display techniques [128–130] are enabling the fabrication of complex ceramic cores for transpiration channels, though challenges remain in achieving high green density post-sintering. Particularly noteworthy is the work of Min et al. [131], who developed an AM-processed oxide dispersion-strengthened coating via DMLS that demonstrated exceptional 1200 °C oxidation resistance over 2000 h while maintaining interfacial integrity. These advanced solutions could effectively mitigate the limitations of AM-fabricated transpiration cooling.

5.2. Pore Blockage and Mitigation Strategies

Pore blockage continues to be a critical reliability concern for transpiration cooling systems, with clogged holes potentially causing dangerous local temperature spikes and system failure [15]. Traditional sintered porous media are particularly susceptible to unpredictable dust-induced clogging, though AM techniques offer improved microscale control. Yang et al. [111] demonstrated the impact of increased pore blockage ratios in 0.4 mm perforated plates on cooling effectiveness, particularly in upstream regions.

Recent research has identified several promising approaches to mitigate these issues. Sun et al. [113] showed that at low F, the influence of pore blockage was minor in the tree-like channels, demonstrating their clogging resistance, while the maximum loss of the area-averaged η_o by 16.3% was found at F = 2%. Yang et al. [114] found that the proposed oriented porous structures improved cooling performance, reduced coolant consumption at equivalent cooling performance by 10–270%, and decreased the temperature gradient, eventually minimizing thermal stress and improving the reliability of the porous transpiration cooling. Sun et al. [89] introduced double coolant supply channels and found that the nonuniform coolant distribution increased area-averaged η_o by 3.27% while improving temperature uniformity.

Future work in this area will explore hybrid cooling configurations that combine the benefits of different approaches. Ding et al. [132] demonstrated that binary porous matrices could maintain 44.5% longer effective film lengths while using 20% less coolant compared to single porous matrices. Natsui et al. [133] showed synergistic effects when coupling discrete film cooling holes with transpiration cooling, effectively mitigating detrimental vortex structures. These hybrid approaches, originally developed for aerospace applications [26,134], can be adapted for gas turbine implementations with promising results.

5.3. Mechanical Integrity and Enhanced Design Approaches

The balance between mechanical strength and cooling performance remains a key challenge for AM-fabricated transpiration cooling structures. Min et al. [77] found that while 3d-pitch straight holes had the highest stress net area, staggered holes unexpectedly exhibited lower ultimate tensile strength (UTS) due to intersecting stress concentrations [135]. Huang et al. [51] provided a comparative analysis showing AM porous samples reaching 0.95 GPa UTS with 60% blockage, representing a 440% improvement over traditional sintered materials, but the samples were still 10% weaker than solid SLM specimens.

Future directions for addressing these mechanical challenges include advanced surface engineering and post-processing techniques. Ligrani et al. [136] demonstrated that abrasive flow machining methods achieved superior smoothness compared to as-built and chemically polished surfaces. Chyu et al. [125] successfully reduced surface roughness by over 40% through redesign and electrochemical processing. Arai and Suidzu [137] developed innovative plasma-sprayed porous coatings using yttria-stabilized zirconia and polyester powder that enabled active transpiration cooling under pressure gradients while maintaining low thermal conductivity. The optimized designs, advanced surface treatments, and innovative coatings significantly improve the integrity of AM transpiration cooling for next-generation gas turbines.

5.4. Experimental and Simulation Challenges with Future Methodologies

Experimental research encountered several challenges, mainly due to the current AM limitations. Firstly, most previous studies relied on simplified flat-plate models that cannot fully replicate the real applications. Since then, there has been limited high-temperature data for gas turbines due to measurement difficulties in extreme transpiration cooling flow. Meanwhile, numerical modeling of transpiration cooling faced its own set of challenges. Current approaches to single-phase cooling simulations have often oversimplified porous structures as homogeneous fluid zones with resistance terms, decreasing flow and temperature field prediction accuracy. While more detailed geometric modeling was possible, it has prohibitively high computational costs due to the number of meshes, as seen in Table 4.

Another critical challenge in AM transpiration cooling studies lies in persistent simulation–experiment discrepancies. Calderon [96] found CFD consistently over-predicted area-averaged η_a due to imperfect decay modeling. Huang et al. [51] attributed the discrepancy between simulation and experimental results to conduction heat loss apart from the roughness of the transpiration cooling samples. Unlike the simulation, the experiment involved heat conduction from the wind tunnel wall to the porous plate, which was not accounted for in the numerical model. Kim et al. [95] reported that as the *BR* increased in a transpiration-cooled C3X turbine blade, the simulated coolant film became larger than in the visualization due to resistance from the dense cooling air mixed with olive oil droplets. Yang et al. [121] found in their machine learning model that even though the method reduces computational costs and provides 2D cooling effectiveness distributions, it lacks internal cooling performance and universality for broader design applications.

Future experimental methodologies are addressing these limitations through advanced diagnostic techniques. Greifenstein et al. [76] revealed critical flame-cooling interactions in effusion-cooled combustors, where low-swirl premixed flames intensified thermal coupling. The wall temperature variations reached 150–200 K, corresponding to an area-averaged η_a = 0.45–0.62. For transpiration cooling, these findings suggested that swirl management was essential to mitigate hot spots. Also, optical diagnostics, such as hydroxyl radical, coherent anti-Stokes Raman spectroscopy, and thermographic phosphors, can validate transpiration cooling effectiveness in reacting flows. Moreover, the coolant injection strategies must account for combustion-driven thermal gradients.

High-fidelity simulations, such as LES, and rotation effect modeling are essential for the next numerical studies on transpiration cooling. Xiao et al. [138] used LES/Darcy–Forchheimer modeling to reveal Kelvin–Helmholtz jelly roll instabilities, which are critical for predicting mainstream mixing. You et al. [139] found that rotation reduced target-surface cooling efficiency, mainly due to the effects of Coriolis, buoyancy, centrifugal forces, and pressure gradient that deflected the jet impingement. For reactor conditions, Zhang et al. [140] proposed a local thermal non-equilibrium (LTNE) model for gaseous transpiration cooling, incorporating radiation via Rosseland approximation and gas expansion effects via low Mach approximation. These studies were highly relevant for gas turbine transpiration cooling, as they addressed vortex-resolved flow prediction, rotational effects, high-temperature radiation effects, coolant expansion, and pumping power optimization.

5.5. Integrated Optimization Approaches

Future advancements in transpiration cooling for gas turbine blades will increasingly rely on AI-driven optimization techniques such as ANN combined with MOGA [90,123] to design optimized non-stochastic cooling structures. Recent work shows that topology optimization combining RANS and porous-media modeling [141] effectively captures fluid-porous interactions, while meshless TPMS methods proposed by Jiang et al. [142] enable graded-φ designs with desired mechanical integrity. Though requiring improved multi-physics modeling, these approaches can revolutionize transpiration cooling by optimizing thermal protection, structural integrity, and aerodynamic efficiency simultaneously. Their integration will be key for future engines operating under extreme conditions.

6. Conclusions

Transpiration cooling, enhanced by additive manufacturing (AM), offers superior thermal management for gas turbines through complex and high-performance porous structures. This review analyzes its evolution, flow/heat transfer mechanisms, and experimental/numerical progress, demonstrating its advantages over conventional methods. However, key challenges remain, requiring advanced solutions to ensure the usability of AM transpiration cooling for practical gas turbines. The conclusions are drawn as follows:

1. AM-fabricated perforated transpiration-cooled plates achieve 10–100% higher cooling effectiveness than traditional film cooling, though dimensional inaccuracies around 4–77% porosity shrinkage in 0.06–0.5 mm holes and 10% ultimate tensile strength reductions in AM models present reliability concerns. While the integration of CAD-based lattice structures with transpiration cooling slightly reduces cooling performance, it mitigates pore blockage effects and provides superior structural support, overcoming the mechanical limitations of pure transpiration cooling.
2. Advanced AM techniques allow the precise fabrication of complex and deterministic structures, such as TPMS and biomimetic designs. These cooling models enhance adiabatic cooling effectiveness by up to five times compared to conventional film cooling. Gradient porosity/thickness of such structures balances thermal-mechanical properties, mitigates jet lift-off, and provides flow uniformity, improving temperature distributions on the surface.
3. Transpiration cooling forms a more stable boundary layer on the hot wall than effusion cooling, particularly on the blade surface, but excessive coolant supply can degrade performance due to hot gas entrainment. Precise control of the porosity and coolant supply is therefore required to avoid coolant leakages, non-uniform coolant distributions, and uneven temperature/pressure patterns.
4. Current AM technology introduces 15% hole size reductions from surface roughness and around 15% permeability deviations from CAD models, compounded by unresolved high-temperature material limitations, with only direct metal laser sintering (DMLS)-fabricated oxide coatings demonstrating reliable stability.
5. AI-driven optimization, such as artificial neural networks (ANNs) combined with multi-objective genetic algorithms (MOGAs), topology optimization, and hybrid cooling, such as discrete film holes with transpiration cooling, also offer balanced thermal-structural solutions. Nonetheless, their implementation requires advanced experimental diagnostics and high-fidelity multiphysics modeling to fully validate these innovative cooling systems for practical implementation.

Overcoming the challenges presented in this review could redefine gas turbine thermal management, enabling high-efficiency engines. Therefore, the integration of advanced AM, multiphysics validation from high-fidelity simulations and experiments, AI-driven optimization, and hybrid cooling for transpiration cooling promises revolutionary advances in gas turbine cooling technologies.

Author Contributions: Conceptualization, K.Y. and Y.R.; formal analysis, K.Y.; writing—original draft preparation, K.Y.; writing—review and editing, K.Y. and Y.R.; supervision, Y.R.; project administration, K.Y. and Y.R.; methodology, K.Y.; funding acquisition, K.Y. and Y.R. All authors have read and agreed to the published version of the manuscript.

Funding: This work received financial support through the National Science and Technology Major Project (2017-III-0009-0035) and National Natural Science Foundation of China (24Z033103800, 11972230), with additional technical support from the Chinese-German Joint Cooperation Group (GZ1577) program.

Data Availability Statement: The original contributions presented in this study are included in the article. Further inquiries can be directed to the corresponding author.

Acknowledgments: The authors would like to express their deepest gratitude to Sunanta Yeranee and Pornpana Sarawong for their encouragement throughout this research. Special thanks also go to our labmates at the Institute of Turbomachinery, School of Mechanical Engineering, Shanghai Jiao Tong University, China, for their invaluable support during the preparation of this work. Their collective strength and inspiration have been instrumental in my study.

Conflicts of Interest: The authors declare no conflicts of interest.

Nomenclature

A_{eff}	Coolant covered area on the hot-side surface (m^2)
A_h	Cross-sectional area of the mainstream channel (m^2)
A_{int}	Internal area of the solid–fluid interface inside the specimens (m^2)
A_{out}	Outlet area of the coolant at the outer surface (m^2)
A_{pore}	Total cross-sectional area of transpiration cooling topology (m^2)
Bi	Biot number (-)
BR	Blowing ratio (-)
CD, CF	Discharge and skin-friction coefficients (-)
C_F	Inertial resistance coefficient (1/m)
C_h	Circumference of the mainstream channel (m)
c_p	Heat capacity of the fluid (J/(kg·K))
d_c, d_h	Hydraulic diameter of coolant and mainstream channels (m)
d, d_{pore}	Diameter of micro hole and porous-media pore (m)
F	Injection ratio (-)
$\mathbf{F}$	External force in Navier–Stokes equation (N/m^3)
h	Convective heat transfer coefficient ($W/(m^2K)$)
k	Turbulence kinetic energy in turbulence model (m^2/s^2)
K	Permeability (m^2)
k_{eff}	Effectiveness thermal conductivity of porous media (W/(m·K))
k_f, k_s	Thermal conductivity of fluid and solid (W/(m·K))
L	Unit cell size (m)
L_c	Characteristic length of the transpiration cooling design (m)
$\dot{m}_c$, $\dot{m}_h$	Mass flow rate of coolant and mainstream (kg/s)
Ma	Mach number (-)
MFR	Mass flow ratio of coolant to mainstream (-)
Nu	Nusselt number (-)
Nu/Nu_0	Normalized Nusselt number for heat transfer enhancement evaluation (-)

p	Pressure field (Pa)
$p_{t,in}$, $p_{t,out}$	Total pressure of the coolant inlet and outlet (Pa)
$q(x)$	Heat flux (W/m^2)
Q_{tot}	Total heat transfer (W)
R_{int}, R_{out}	Internal and outlet area ratios (-)
Re_c, Re_h	Reynolds number of coolant and mainstream (-)
S_m	Mass source term (N/m^3)
S_v	Specific surface area (1/m)
t	Thickness (m)
T^*	Non-dimensional temperature (-)
T_c, T_h, T_s	Coolant, mainstream and surface temperatures (K)
T_{flu}, T_{sol}	Temperature of fluid and solid (K)
$\mathbf{u}$	Velocity vector (m/s)
u_c, u_h, u_D	Coolant, mainstream and Darcy velocities (m/s)
$\dot{V}$	Volumetric flow rate (liters per minute: LPM)
V_{des}	Design volume from CAD models (m^3)
V_{sol}	Volume of solid domain with identical dimension (m^3)
v_c	Average velocity of coolant flow in the film hole or pore (m/s)
x, y, z	Cartesian coordinate (-)
Greek letters	
γ	Plugging probability (-)
ε	Turbulent dissipation rate (m^2/s^3)
ζ_{Pt}	Total pressure loss coefficient (-)
η_a, η_o	Adiabatic and overall cooling effectiveness (-)
μ	Dynamic viscosity of fluid (kg/(m·s))
ρ_c, ρ_h	Fluid density of coolant and mainstream (kg/s)
τ_w	Shear stress (Pa)
φ	Porosity (%)
φ_{des}, φ_{act}	Design and actual porosities (%)
ω	Specific dissipation rate in turbulence model (1/s)
Abbreviations	
ANN	Artificial neural network
AM	Additive manufacturing
CAD	Computer-aided design
CCD	Charged-coupled device
CFD	Computational fluid dynamics
CMC	Ceramic matrix composite
CRVP	Counter-rotating vortex
CT	Computed tomography
DLD	Direct laser deposition
DMLS	Direct metal laser sintering
EOS	Electro Optical Systems
FDM	Fused deposit modeling
GA	Genetic algorithm
IR	Infrared thermography
IWP	I-graph and wrapped package
LES	Large eddy simulation
LBM	Lattice Boltzmann method
LTNE	Local thermal non-equilibrium
MIM	Metal powder injection molding
MOGA	Multi-objective genetic algorithms
NASA	National Aeronautics and Space Administration
NS	Navier-Stokes
NSGA-II	Non-dominated sorting genetic algorithm-II

OH-PLIF	Hydroxyl radical
PVD	Physical vapor deposit
PIV	Particle image velocimetry
PS	Pressure side of turbine blades
PSP	Pressure-sensitive paint
RANS	Reynolds-averaged Navier–Stokes
SLA	Stereolithography
SLM	Selective laser melting
SS	Suction side of turbine blades
TE	Trailing edge
TBC	Thermal barrier coating
TIT	Turbine inlet temperature
TKE	Turbulence kinetic energy
TLC	Transient liquid crystal thermography
TPMS	Triply periodic minimal surface
UTS	Ultimate tensile strength (Pa)

References

1. Perepezko, J.H. The Hotter the Engine, the Better. *Science* **2009**, *326*, 1068–1069. [CrossRef]
2. Dutta, S.; Kaur, I.; Singh, P. Review of Film Cooling in Gas Turbines with an Emphasis on Additive Manufacturing-Based Design Evolutions. *Energies* **2022**, *15*, 6968. [CrossRef]
3. Ishikawa, M.; Komori, T.; Terauchi, M.; Yasuraoka, J. Development of High Efficiency Gas Turbine Combined Cycle. *Tech. Rev. Mitsubishi Heavy Ind.* **2008**, *45*, 15–17.
4. Hada, S.; Tsukagoshi, K.; Masada, J.; Ito, E. Test Results of the World's First 1600 °C J-Series Gas Turbine. *Mitsubishi Heavy Ind. Tech. Rev.* **2012**, *49*, 18–23.
5. Wang, W.; Yan, Y.; Zhou, Y.; Cui, J. Review of Advanced Effusive Cooling for Gas Turbine Blades. *Energies* **2022**, *15*, 8568. [CrossRef]
6. Han, J.-C.; Dutta, S.; Ekkad, S. *Gas Turbine Heat Transfer and Cooling Technology*, 2nd ed.; CRC Press: Boca Raton, FL, USA, 2012, ISBN 9780429107115.
7. Clarke, D.R.; Oechsner, M.; Padture, N.P. Thermal-Barrier Coatings for More Efficient Gas-Turbine Engines. *MRS Bull.* **2012**, *37*, 891–898. [CrossRef]
8. Li, Y.; Rao, Y.; Wang, D.; Zhang, P.; Wu, X. Heat Transfer and Pressure Loss of Turbulent Flow in Channels with Miniature Structured Ribs on One Wall. *Int. J. Heat Mass Transf.* **2019**, *131*, 584–593. [CrossRef]
9. Liang, C.; Rao, Y. Computational Analysis of Rotating Effects on Heat Transfer and Pressure Loss of Turbulent Flow in Detached Pin Fin Arrays with Various Clearances. *ASME J. Heat Transf.* **2020**, *142*, 121803. [CrossRef]
10. Rao, Y.; Feng, Y.; Li, B.; Weigand, B. Experimental and Numerical Study of Heat Transfer and Flow Friction in Channels With Dimples of Different Shapes. *J. Heat Transfer* **2015**, *137*, 031901. [CrossRef]
11. YERANEE, K.; RAO, Y. A Review of Recent Studies on Rotating Internal Cooling for Gas Turbine Blades. *Chinese J. Aeronaut.* **2021**, *34*, 85–113. [CrossRef]
12. Babji, G.; Pujari, A.K. Flow and Heat Transfer Studies of Multijet Impingement Cooling for Different Configurations: A Review. *Heat Transf.* **2022**, *52*, 1604–1672. [CrossRef]
13. Ahn, J. Large Eddy Simulation of Film Cooling: A Review. *Energies* **2022**, *15*, 8876. [CrossRef]
14. Nealy, D.A.; Reider, S.B. Evaluation of Laminated Porous Wall Materials for Combustor Liner Cooling. *J. Eng. Gas Turbines Power* **1980**, *102*, 268–276. [CrossRef]
15. Wassell, A.B.; Bhangu, J.K. The Development and Application of Improved Combustor Wall Cooling Techniques. In *Turbo Expo: Power for Land, Sea, and Air*; American Society of Mechanical Engineers: New York, NY, USA, 1980; pp. 1–10.
16. Murray, A.V.; Ireland, P.T.; Romero, E. Experimental and Computational Methods for the Evaluation of Double-Wall, Effusion Cooling Systems. *J. Turbomach.* **2020**, *142*, 111003. [CrossRef]
17. Li, W.; Lu, X.; Li, X.; Ren, J.; Jiang, H. On Improving Full-Coverage Effusion Cooling Efficiency by Varying Cooling Arrangements and Wall Thickness in Double Wall Cooling Application. *J. Heat Transfer* **2019**, *141*, 042201. [CrossRef]
18. Yeranee, K.; Rao, Y.; Xu, C.; Xie, J.; Zhang, Y. Conjugate Heat Transfer and Fluid Flow Analysis on Printable Double-Wall Effusion Cooling with Internal Topology-Optimized TPMS Structures. *Therm. Sci. Eng. Prog.* **2024**, *55*, 102939. [CrossRef]

19. Rao, Y.; Liu, Y.; Wan, C. Multiple-Jet Impingement Heat Transfer in Double-Wall Cooling Structures with Pin Fins and Effusion Holes. *Int. J. Therm. Sci.* **2018**, *133*, 106–119. [CrossRef]
20. Skamniotis, C.; Cocks, A.C.F. Minimising Stresses in Double Wall Transpiration Cooled Components for High Temperature Applications. *Int. J. Mech. Sci.* **2021**, *189*, 105983. [CrossRef]
21. Skamniotis, C.; Courtis, M.; Cocks, A.C.F. Multiscale Analysis of Thermomechanical Stresses in Double Wall Transpiration Cooling Systems for Gas Turbine Blades. *Int. J. Mech. Sci.* **2021**, *207*, 106657. [CrossRef]
22. Skamniotis, C.; Cocks, A.C.F. Designing against Severe Stresses at Compound Cooling Holes of Double Wall Transpiration Cooled Engine Components. *Aerosp. Sci. Technol.* **2021**, *116*, 106856. [CrossRef]
23. Courtis, M.; Skamniotis, C.; Cocks, A.; Ireland, P. Coupled Aerothermal-Mechanical Analysis in Single Crystal Double Wall Transpiration Cooled Gas Turbine Blades with a Large Film Hole Density. *Appl. Therm. Eng.* **2023**, *219*, 119329. [CrossRef]
24. Liang, C.; Rao, Y.; Luo, J.; Luo, X. Experimental and Numerical Study of Turbulent Flow and Heat Transfer in a Wedge-Shaped Channel with Guiding Pin Fins for Turbine Blade Trailing Edge Cooling. *Int. J. Heat Mass Transf.* **2021**, *178*, 121590. [CrossRef]
25. Ma, H.; Sun, H.; Fu, H.; Luan, Y.; Sun, T.; Zunino, P. Numerical Investigation on Transpiration Cooling Performance of Turbine Blades with Non-Uniform Porosity. *Appl. Therm. Eng.* **2023**, *235*, 121394. [CrossRef]
26. Jiang, P.X.; Huang, G.; Zhu, Y.; Liao, Z.; Huang, Z. Experimental Investigation of Combined Transpiration and Film Cooling for Sintered Metal Porous Struts. *Int. J. Heat Mass Transf.* **2017**, *108*, 232–243. [CrossRef]
27. Lv, Y.; Liu, T.; Huang, X.; He, F.; Tang, L.; Zhou, J.; Wang, J. Numerical Investigation and Optimization of Flat Plate Transpiration-Film Combined Cooling Structure. *Int. J. Therm. Sci.* **2022**, *179*, 107673. [CrossRef]
28. Munk, D.J.; Selzer, M.; Seiler, H.; Ortelt, M.; Vio, G.A. Analysis of a Transpiration Cooled LOX/CH4 Rocket Thrust Chamber. *Int. J. Heat Mass Transf.* **2022**, *182*, 121986. [CrossRef]
29. Steingrimsson, A.; Marsell, B.; Mankbadi, R.; Kapat, J. Towards Prediction of Transpiration Cooling. In Proceedings of the 48th AIAA Aerospace Sciences Meeting Including the New Horizons Forum and Aerospace Exposition, Orlando, FL, USA, 4–7 January 2010. [CrossRef]
30. Kim, M.; Shin, D.H.; Lee, B.J.; Lee, J. Experimental and Numerical Investigation of Micro-Scale Effusion and Transpiration Air Cooling on Cascaded Turbine Blades. *Case Stud. Therm. Eng.* **2022**, *32*, 101892. [CrossRef]
31. Song, K.D.; Choi, S.H.; Scotti, S.J. Transpiration Cooling Experiment for Scramjet Engine Combustion Chamber by High Heat Fluxes. *J. Propuls. Power* **2006**, *22*, 96–102. [CrossRef]
32. Elnady, T.; Hassan, I.; Kadem, L.; Lucas, T. Cooling Effectiveness of Shaped Film Holes for Leading Edge. *Exp. Therm. Fluid Sci.* **2013**, *44*, 649–661. [CrossRef]
33. Reimer, T.; Kuhn, M.; Gülhan, A.; Esser, B.; Sippel, M.; Foreest, A. Van Transpiration Cooling Tests of Porous Cmc in Hypersonic Flow. In Proceedings of the 17th AIAA International Space Planes and Hypersonic Systems and Technologies Conference, San Francisco, CA, USA, 11–14 April 2011; pp. 1–13. [CrossRef]
34. Langener, T.; Von Wolfersdorf, J.; Steelant, J. Experimental Investigations on Transpiration Cooling for Scramjet Applications Using Different Coolants. *AIAA J.* **2011**, *49*, 1409–1419. [CrossRef]
35. Kumar, C.S.; Pattamatta, A. Assessment of Heat Transfer Enhancement Using Metallic Porous Foam Configurations in Laminar Slot Jet Impingement: An Experimental Study. *J. Heat Transfer* **2018**, *140*, 022202. [CrossRef]
36. Andrews, G.E.; Asere, A.A.; Mkpadi, M.C.; Tirmahi, A. Asme 1986 International Gas Turbine Conference Transpiration Cooling: Contribution of Film Cooling To the Overall Cooling Effectiveness. In Proceedings of the American Society of Mechanical Engineers (Paper), Dusseldorf, Germany, 8–12 June 1986; American Society of Mechanical Engineers: New York, NY, USA, 1986.
37. Polezhaev, J. The Transpiration Cooling for Blades of High Temperatures Gas Turbine. *Energy Convers. Manag.* **1997**, *38*, 1123–1133. [CrossRef]
38. Wang, Y.; Wang, L.; Zhou, Y.; Luo, Z.; Xie, W.; Liu, Q.; Peng, W.; Du, M. Research Progress on Transpiration Cooling Technology in Force-Thermal Concentrated Environments. *Int. J. Heat Mass Transf.* **2025**, *236*, 126262. [CrossRef]
39. Raj, R.; Moskowitz, S. *Transpiration Air Protected Turbine Blades—An Effective Concept To Achieve High Temperature and Erosion Resistance for Gas Turbines Operating in an Aggressive Environment*; American Society of Mechanical Engineers: New York, NY, USA, 1978; pp. 1–11.
40. Wadia, A.R. Advanced Combustor Linear Cooling Technology for Gas Turbines. *Def. Sci. J.* **1988**, *38*, 363–380. [CrossRef]
41. Bunker, R.S. *Gas Turbine Cooling: Moving from Macro to Micro Cooling*; American Society of Mechanical Engineers: New York, NY, USA, 2013; Volume 3C, pp. 1–17. [CrossRef]
42. Bunker, R.S. *Evolution of Turbine Cooling*; American Society of Mechanical Engineers: New York, NY, USA, 2017; Volume 1, pp. 1–26. [CrossRef]
43. Xu, L.; Sun, Z.; Ruan, Q.; Xi, L.; Gao, J.; Li, Y. Development Trend of Cooling Technology for Turbine Blades at Super-High Temperature of above 2000 K. *Energies* **2023**, *16*, 668. [CrossRef]

44. Mi, Q.; Yi, S.H.; Gang, D.D.; Lu, X.G.; Liu, X.L. Research Progress of Transpiration Cooling for Aircraft Thermal Protection. *Appl. Therm. Eng.* **2024**, *236*, 121360. [CrossRef]
45. Zhang, S.; Li, X.; Zuo, J.; Qin, J.; Cheng, K.; Feng, Y.; Bao, W. Research Progress on Active Thermal Protection for Hypersonic Vehicles. *Prog. Aerosp. Sci.* **2020**, *119*, 100646. [CrossRef]
46. Xu, R.; Cheng, Z.; Jiang, P. Fundamentals and Recent Progress of Additive Manufacturing-Assisted Porous Materials on Transpiration Cooling. *J. Glob. Power Propuls. Soc.* **2023**, *2023*, 19–48. [CrossRef]
47. Weinbaum, S.; Wheeler, H.L. Heat Transfer in Sweat-Cooled Porous Metals. *J. Appl. Phys.* **1949**, *20*, 113–122. [CrossRef]
48. Hald, H.; Ortelt, M.; Fischer, I.; Greuel, D. CMC Rocket Combustion Chamber with Effusion Cooling. In Proceedings of the 54th International Astronautical Congress of the International Astronautical Federation, the International Academy of Astronautics, and the International Institute of Space Law, Bremen, Germany, 29 September–3 October 2003; Volume 3, pp. 657–667. [CrossRef]
49. Huang, Z.; Xiong, Y.B.; Liu, Y.Q.; Jiang, P.X.; Zhu, Y.H. Experimental Investigation of Full-Coverage Effusion Cooling through Perforated Flat Plates. *Appl. Therm. Eng.* **2015**, *76*, 76–85. [CrossRef]
50. Wang, F.; Song, N.; Xia, X.; Chen, X. Experimental Investigation on Transpiration Cooling of Ammonium Carbonate in Porous Composite Structure at High-Temperature. *Appl. Therm. Eng.* **2024**, *249*, 123292. [CrossRef]
51. Huang, G.; Min, Z.; Yang, L.; Jiang, P.X.; Chyu, M. Transpiration Cooling for Additive Manufactured Porous Plates with Partition Walls. *Int. J. Heat Mass Transf.* **2018**, *124*, 1076–1087. [CrossRef]
52. Van Foreest, A.; Sippel, M.; Gülhan, A.; Esser, B.; Ambrosius, B.A.C.; Sudmeijer, K. Transpiration Cooling Using Liquid Water. *J. Thermophys. Heat Transf.* **2009**, *23*, 693–702. [CrossRef]
53. Liu, Y.; Liu, T.; Ding, R.; He, F.; Wang, J. Experimental and Numerical Investigation of Transpiration Cooling with Gradient Porosity Layout for the Thermal Protection of Nose Cone. *Aerosp. Sci. Technol.* **2024**, *149*, 109140. [CrossRef]
54. Huang, G.; Zhu, Y.; Liao, Z.; Ouyang, X.L.; Jiang, P.X. Experimental Investigation of Transpiration Cooling with Phase Change for Sintered Porous Plates. *Int. J. Heat Mass Transf.* **2017**, *114*, 1201–1213. [CrossRef]
55. Glass, D.E. Ceramic Matrix Composite (CMC) Thermal Protection Systems (TPS) and Hot Structures for Hypersonic Vehicles. In Proceedings of the 15th AIAA International Space Planes and Hypersonic Systems and Technologies Conference, Dayton, Ohio, 28 April–1 May 2008; pp. 1–36. [CrossRef]
56. Xu, G.; Liu, Y.; Luo, X.; Ma, J.; Li, H. Experimental Investigation of Transpiration Cooling for Sintered Woven Wire Mesh Structures. *Int. J. Heat Mass Transf.* **2015**, *91*, 898–907. [CrossRef]
57. Gavalda Diaz, O.; Garcia Luna, G.; Liao, Z.; Axinte, D. The New Challenges of Machining Ceramic Matrix Composites (CMCs): Review of Surface Integrity. *Int. J. Mach. Tools Manuf.* **2019**, *139*, 24–36. [CrossRef]
58. Ekkad, S.V.; Zapata, D.; Han, J.C. Film Effectiveness over a Flat Surface with Air and CO_2 Injection through Compound Angle Holes Using a Transient Liquid Crystal Image Method. In Proceedings of the ASME 1995 International Gas Turbine and Aeroengine Congress and Exposition, Houston, TX, USA, 5–8 June 1995; p. 4. [CrossRef]
59. Blakey-Milner, B.; Gradl, P.; Snedden, G.; Brooks, M.; Pitot, J.; Lopez, E.; Leary, M.; Berto, F.; du Plessis, A. Metal Additive Manufacturing in Aerospace: A Review. *Mater. Des.* **2021**, *209*, 110008. [CrossRef]
60. Kamal, M.; Rizza, G. Design for Metal Additive Manufacturing for Aerospace Applications. In *Additive Manufacturing for the Aerospace Industry*; Elsevier Inc.: Amsterdam, The Netherlands, 2019; pp. 67–86, ISBN 9780128140635.
61. Najmon, J.C.; Raeisi, S.; Tovar, A. Review of Additive Manufacturing Technologies and Applications in the Aerospace Industry. In *Additive Manufacturing for the Aerospace Industry*; Elsevier Inc.: Amsterdam, The Netherlands, 2019; pp. 7–31, ISBN 9780128140635.
62. Tian, X.; Ye, W.; Xu, L.; Yang, A.; Huang, L.; Jin, S. Optimization Research on Laminated Cooling Structure for Gas Turbines: A Review. *AIMS Energy* **2025**, *13*, 354–401. [CrossRef]
63. Li, R.; Liu, J.; Shi, Y.; Du, M.; Xie, Z. 316L Stainless Steel with Gradient Porosity Fabricated by Selective Laser Melting. *J. Mater. Eng. Perform.* **2010**, *19*, 666–671. [CrossRef]
64. Cheng, Z.; Xu, R.; Jiang, P. Transpiration Cooling with Phase Change by Functionally Graded Porous Media. *Int. J. Heat Mass Transf.* **2023**, *205*, 123862. [CrossRef]
65. Nguyentat, T.; Hayes, W.A.; Meland, T.O.; Veith, E.M.; Ellis, D.L. Fabrication of a Liquid Rocket Combustion Chamber Liner of Advanced Copper Alloy GRCop-84 via Formed Platelet Liner Technology. In Proceedings of the 42nd AIAA/ASME/SAE/ASEE Joint Propulsion Conference & Exhibit, Sacramento, CA, USA, 9–12 July 2006; Volume 10, pp. 8335–8344. [CrossRef]
66. Traub, H.; Kube, J.; Jose, S.; Prasannakumar, A.; Hühne, C. Structural and Aerodynamic Characteristics of Micro-Perforated Porous Sheets for Laminar Flow Control. In Proceedings of the ASME 2024 Aerospace Structures, Structural Dynamics, and Materials Conference, SSDM 2024, Renton, WA, USA, 29 April–1 May 2024; American Society of Mechanical Engineers: New York, NY, USA, 2024; pp. 1–10.
67. Yeranee, K.; Rao, Y.; Zuo, Q.; Xie, J. Thermal Performance Enhancement for Gas Turbine Blade Trailing Edge Cooling with Topology-Optimized Printable Diamond TPMS Lattice. *Int. J. Heat Fluid Flow* **2024**, *110*, 109649. [CrossRef]

68. Sinha, A.; Swain, B.; Behera, A.; Mallick, P.; Samal, S.K.; Vishwanatha, H.M.; Behera, A. A Review on the Processing of Aero-Turbine Blade Using 3D Print Techniques. *J. Manuf. Mater. Process.* **2022**, *6*, 16. [CrossRef]
69. Kaur, I.; Aider, Y.; Nithyanandam, K.; Singh, P. Thermal-Hydraulic Performance of Additively Manufactured Lattices for Gas Turbine Blade Trailing Edge Cooling. *Appl. Therm. Eng.* **2022**, *211*, 118461. [CrossRef]
70. Wilson, J.M.; Piya, C.; Shin, Y.C.; Zhao, F.; Ramani, K. Remanufacturing of Turbine Blades by Laser Direct Deposition with Its Energy and Environmental Impact Analysis. *J. Clean. Prod.* **2014**, *80*, 170–178. [CrossRef]
71. Kaplanskii, Y.Y.; Levashov, E.A.; Korotitskiy, A.V.; Loginov, P.A.; Sentyurina, Z.A.; Mazalov, A.B. Influence of Aging and HIP Treatment on the Structure and Properties of NiAl-Based Turbine Blades Manufactured by Laser Powder Bed Fusion. *Addit. Manuf.* **2020**, *31*, 100999. [CrossRef]
72. Yang, T.; Mazumder, S.; Jin, Y.; Squires, B.; Sofield, M.; Pantawane, M.V.; Dahotre, N.B.; Neogi, A. A Review of Diagnostics Methodologies for Metal Additive Manufacturing Processes and Products. *Materials* **2021**, *14*, 4929. [CrossRef]
73. Kim, M.; Shin, D.H.; Kim, J.S.; Lee, B.J.; Lee, J. Experimental Investigation of Effusion and Transpiration Air Cooling for Single Turbine Blade. *Appl. Therm. Eng.* **2021**, *182*, 116156. [CrossRef]
74. Poupinha, C.; Kozlowska, S.; Lluch, J.S.; Altimare, D.; Kinell, M. Experimental Study on Transpiration Cooling through Additively Manufactured Porous Structures. *Int. J. Heat Mass Transf.* **2024**, *227*, 125532. [CrossRef]
75. Fantozzi, G.; Kinell, M.; Carrera, S.R.; Nilsson, J.; Kuesters, Y. Experimental Study on Pressure Losses in Porous Materials. In Proceedings of the ASME Turbo Expo, Oslo, Norway, 11–15 June 2018; American Society of Mechanical Engineers: New York, NY, USA, 2018; Volume 5B-2018, p. V05BT21A001.
76. Min, Z.; Huang, G.; Parbat, S.N.; Yang, L.; Chyu, M.K. Experimental Investigation on Additively Manufactured Transpiration and Film Cooling Structures. *J. Turbomach.* **2019**, *141*, 1–10. [CrossRef]
77. Min, Z.; Parbat, S.N.; Yang, L.; Chyu, M.K. Thermal-Fluid and Mechanical Investigations of Additively Manufactured Geometries for Transpiration Cooling. In Proceedings of the ASME Turbo Expo 2019: Turbomachinery Technical Conference and Exposition, Phoenix, AZ, USA, 17–21 June 2019; Volume 5B-2019, pp. 1–13. [CrossRef]
78. Chyu, M.; Kang, B.; Parbat, S. *Integrated Transpiration and Lattice Cooling Systems Developed by Additive Manufacturing with Oxide-Dispersion-Strengthened (ODS) Alloys*; National Energy Technology Laboratory: Pittsburgh, PA, USA, 2022.
79. Ealy, B.; Calderon, L.; Wang, W.; Valentin, R.; Mingareev, I.; Richardson, M.; Kapat, J. Characterization of Laser Additive Manufacturing-Fabricated Porous Superalloys for Turbine Components. *J. Eng. Gas Turbines Power* **2017**, *139*, 102102. [CrossRef]
80. Zhang, K.; Hickey, J.P.; Vlasea, M. An Analysis Framework of Additively Manufactured Deterministic Porous Structures for Transpiration Cooling. *J. Mater. Eng. Perform.* **2023**, *32*, 9253–9262. [CrossRef]
81. Son, J.; Broumand, M.; Pyo, Y.; Richer, P.; Jodoin, B.; Hong, Z. Effects of Lattice Orientation Angle on Tpms-Based Transpiration Cooling. In Proceedings of the ASME Turbo Expo 2024: Turbomachinery Technical Conference and Exposition, London, UK, 24–28 June 2024; Volume 13, pp. 1–13. [CrossRef]
82. Zhou, Z.; Lv, Y.; He, F.; Liu, T.; Wang, J. Pore-Scale Investigation of Transpiration Cooling Based on Triply Periodic Minimal Surface. *Int. J. Therm. Sci.* **2024**, *201*, 109019. [CrossRef]
83. Huang, G.; Zhu, Y.; Liao, Z.; Xu, R.; Jiang, P.X. Biomimetic Self-Pumping Transpiration Cooling for Additive Manufactured Porous Module with Tree-like Micro-Channel. *Int. J. Heat Mass Transf.* **2019**, *131*, 403–410. [CrossRef]
84. Yeranee, K.; Rao, Y. A Review of Recent Investigations on Flow and Heat Transfer Enhancement in Cooling Channels Embedded with Triply Periodic Minimal Surfaces (TPMS). *Energies* **2022**, *15*, 8994. [CrossRef]
85. Nield, D.A.; Bejan, A. *Convection in Porous Media*; Springer: Cham, Switzerland, 2017; Volume 165, ISBN 978-3-319-49561-3.
86. Wolf, J.; Moskowitz, S. Development of the Transpiration Air-Cooled Turbine for High-Temperature Dirty Gas Streams. *J. Eng. Power* **1983**, *105*, 821–825. [CrossRef]
87. Cheng, Z.; Xu, R.; Jiang, P.X. Morphology, Flow and Heat Transfer in Triply Periodic Minimal Surface Based Porous Structures. *Int. J. Heat Mass Transf.* **2021**, *170*, 120902. [CrossRef]
88. Cheng, Z.; Li, X.; Xu, R.; Jiang, P. Investigations on Porous Media Customized by Triply Periodic Minimal Surface: Heat Transfer Correlations and Strength Performance. *Int. Commun. Heat Mass Transf.* **2021**, *129*, 105713. [CrossRef]
89. Sun, H.; Ma, H.; Yan, L.; Fu, H.; Luan, Y.; Zunino, P. Numerical Simulations on the Performance of Transpiration Cooling Implemented with Perforated Flat Plates. *Appl. Therm. Eng.* **2024**, *238*, 121943. [CrossRef]
90. Liu, T.; He, F.; Wu, X.; Zhou, Z.; He, Y.; Wang, J. Numerical Investigation and Multi-Objective Structure Optimization of Transpiration Cooling on the Leading Edge of Turbine Blade. In Proceedings of the ASME Turbo Expo 2024: Turbomachinery Technical Conference and Exposition, London, UK, 24–28 June 2024; Volume 7, pp. 1–11. [CrossRef]
91. Zheng, J.; Liu, X.; Zhou, W.; Bian, Y. Numerical Investigation on Directional Transpiration Cooling Performance Coupled with Regenerative Cooling. *Int. Commun. Heat Mass Transf.* **2024**, *159*, 108223. [CrossRef]
92. Broumand, M.; Son, J.; Pyo, Y.; Yun, S.; Hong, Z. TPMS-Based Transpiration Cooling for Film Cooling Enhancement. *Int. J. Heat Mass Transf.* **2024**, *231*, 125824. [CrossRef]

93. Kumar, S.; Singh, O. Thermodynamic Performance Evaluation of Gas Turbine Cycle with Transpiration Cooling of Blades Usin Air Vis-à-Vis Steam. *Proc. Inst. Mech. Eng. Part A J. Power Energy* **2010**, *224*, 1039–1047. [CrossRef]
94. Shukla, A.K.; Sharma, M.; Singh, O. Thermodynamic Investigation of Transpiration Cooled Gas Turbine Blade. In *Ergonomics fc Improved Productivity*; Springer: Singapore, 2022; Volume 2, pp. 59–69, ISBN 9789380043487.
95. Kim, M.; Shin, D.H.; Lee, B.J.; Lee, J. Flow Characterization of Microscale Effusion and Transpiration Air Cooling on Single Blad *Case Stud. Therm. Eng.* **2022**, *31*, 101863. [CrossRef]
96. Calderon, L.; Curbelo, A.; Gupta, G.; Kapat, J.S. Adiabatic Film Cooling Effectiveness of a Lam Fabricated Porous Leading Edg Segment of a Turbine Blade. In Proceedings of the ASME Turbo Expo 2018: Turbomachinery Technical Conference and Expositio Oslo, Norway, 11–15 June 2018; Volume 5B-2018, pp. 1–9. [CrossRef]
97. Wambersie, A.; Wong, H.; Ireland, P.; Mayo, I. Experiments of Transpiration Cooling Inspired Panel Cooling on a Turbine Blad Yielding Film Effectiveness Levels over 95%. *Int. J. Turbomachinery, Propuls. Power* **2021**, *6*, 16. [CrossRef]
98. Aly, O.D.; Wright, L.M.; Hassan, I. Effect of Blowing Ratio on the Film Cooling Effectiveness on a Flat Plate with Variou Blockage Ratios. In Proceedings of the ASME 2024 Heat Transfer Summer Conference; American Society of Mechanical Engineer Anaheim, CA, USA, 15 July 2024; pp. 1–11.
99. Min, Z.; Parbat, S.; Wang, Q.M.; Chyu, M.K. Surface Heater Fabrication Using Micro-Lithography for Transpiration Cooling Hea Transfer Coefficient Measurements. *J. Turbomach.* **2022**, *144*, 071003. [CrossRef]
100. Fier, N.D.; Bogard, D.G. Additively Manufactured Porous Geometries for Hybrid Turbine Cooling. In Proceedings of the ASM Turbo Expo 2021: Turbomachinery Technical Conference and Exposition, Virtual, 7–11 June 2021; Volume 5A-2021, pp. 1–1([CrossRef]
101. Brimacombe, B.J.; Scobie, J.A.; Flynn, J.M.; Sangan, C.M.; Pountney, O.J. Effect of Porosity and Injection Ratio on the Performanc of Transpiration Cooling through Gyroids. *Int. J. Turbomachinery, Propuls. Power* **2023**, *8*, 50. [CrossRef]
102. Son, J.; Pyo, Y.; Richer, P.; Jodoin, B.; Hong, Z. Impact of TPMS Structure Unit Cell Size on Transpiration Cooling. In Proceeding of the AIAA Science and Technology Forum and Exposition, AIAA SciTech Forum 2025, Orlando, FL, USA, 10 October 2024– January 2025; pp. 1–17.
103. Zhang, L.; Zhang, Y.; Sun, J.; Xu, G.; Wen, J. Model and Simulation of Two-Phase Transpiration Cooling Process for Aero-Engin Thermal Protection. In *Asia-Pacific International Symposium on Aerospace Technology*; Lecture Notes in Electrical Engineering Springer: Singapore, 2024; Volume 1051 LNEE, pp. 1047–1062, ISBN 9789819740093.
104. Ngetich, G.C.; Ireland, P.T.; Romero, E. Study of Film Cooling Effectiveness on a Double-Walled Effusion-Cooled Turbine Blade ir a High-Speed Flow Using Pressure Sensitive Paint. In Proceedings of the ASME Turbo Expo 2019: Turbomachinery Technica Conference and Exposition, Phoenix, AZ, USA, 17–21 June 2019; Volume 5B-2019, pp. 1–14. [CrossRef]
105. Meng, T.; Zhu, H.; Liu, C.; Yu, Q.; Wei, J. Accuracy of Superposition Predictions of Film Cooling Effectiveness on a Flat Plat with Double Rows of Holes. In Proceedings of the Volume 5C: Heat Transfer; American Society of Mechanical Engineers, Seou Republic of Korea, 13 June 2016; Volume 56865, pp. 1–10.
106. Son, J.; Pyo, Y.; Broumand, M.; Hong, Z.; Sarafan, S.; Wanjara, P. Advanced Transpiration Cooling Method Using Additiv Manufactured TPMS Structure. In *Proceedings of the 62nd Conference of Metallurgists, COM 2023*; Springer: Cham, Switzerland 2023; pp. 449–451, ISBN 9783031381409.
107. Chao-Yang, W.; Beckermann, C. A Two-Phase Mixture Model of Liquid-Gas Flow and Heat Transfer in Capillary Porous Media- Formulation. *Int. J. Heat Mass Transf.* **1993**, *36*, 2747–2758. [CrossRef]
108. Ergun, S.; Orning, A.A. Fluid Flow through Randomly Packed Columns and Fluidized Beds. *Ind. Eng. Chem.* **1949**, *41*, 1179–118 [CrossRef]
109. Shen, B.X.; Liu, W.Q. Effect of Hot Fuel Gas on a Combinational Opposing Jet and Platelet Transpiration Thermal Protectior System. *Appl. Therm. Eng.* **2020**, *164*, 114513. [CrossRef]
110. Wang, X.; Fan, X.; Xiong, B. Numerical Study of Transpiration Cooling at Different Outlet Angles and Hole Pattern. *Int. J. Hea Fluid Flow* **2024**, *109*, 109551. [CrossRef]
111. Yang, L.; Min, Z.; Parbat, S.N.; Chyu, M.K. Effect of Pore Blockage on Transpiration Cooling with Additive Manufacturabl Perforate Holes. In Proceedings of the ASME Turbo Expo 2018: Turbomachinery Technical Conference and Exposition, Oslo Norway, 11–15 June 2018; Volume 2D-2018, pp. 1–9. [CrossRef]
112. Yang, L.; Chen, W.; Chyu, M.K. A Convolution Modeling Method for Pore Plugging Impact on Transpiration Cooling Configura tions Perforated by Straight Holes. *Int. J. Heat Mass Transf.* **2018**, *126*, 1057–1066. [CrossRef]
113. Sun, H.; Ma, H.; Yan, L.; Fu, H.; Luan, Y.; Magagnato, F. Effect of Pore Blockage on Transpiration Cooling of Marine Turbine Blades In *International Conference on Marine Equipment & Technology and Sustainable Development*; Lecture Notes in Civil Engineering Springer: Singapore, 2023; Volume 375 LNCE, pp. 631–649, ISBN 9789819942909.
114. Yang, Y.; Zhang, B.; Fan, X.; Zhao, R. Numerical Investigation on Transpiration Cooling Performance of Oriented Porous Structure Under Local Block Conditions. *J. Thermophys. Heat Transf.* **2024**, *38*, 311–320. [CrossRef]
115. Huang, G.; He, L. Influence of Inhomogeneous Porosity on Effusion Cooling. *Int. J. Heat Mass Transf.* **2019**, *144*, 118675. [CrossRef]

116. Yang, Y.; Mao, J.; Chen, P.; Zhang, H.; Tang, H. Numerical Investigation on Transpiration Cooling Performance with Different Porosities and Mainstream Pressure Gradients. *Int. J. Therm. Sci.* **2023**, *184*, 107991. [CrossRef]
117. Li, H.; Xie, F.; Zhuang, Y.; Wang, Y.; Yan, Y.; Xu, G.; Cui, J. Numerical Investigation of Cooling Performance of 3D-Printable Cooling Structure for Aero-Engine Combustor. *Appl. Therm. Eng.* **2024**, *238*, 122196. [CrossRef]
118. Purnadiana, F.R.; Prabowo; Sasongko, H. The Performance Comparison Between Modelled and Fully Simulated Porous Media in Turbine Blade Cooling. In *International Conference on Mechanical Engineering*; Springer: Singapore, 2025; pp. 31–38; ISBN 9789819781966.
119. Nisar, F.; Rojek, J.; Nosewicz, S.; Kaszyca, K.; Chmielewski, M. Evaluation of Effective Thermal Conductivity of Sintered Porous Materials Using an Improved Discrete Element Model. *Powder Technol.* **2024**, *437*, 119546. [CrossRef]
120. Yang, L.; Min, Z.; Yue, T.; Rao, Y.; Chyu, M.K. High Resolution Cooling Effectiveness Reconstruction of Transpiration Cooling Using Convolution Modeling Method. *Int. J. Heat Mass Transf.* **2019**, *133*, 1134–1144. [CrossRef]
121. Yang, L.; Dai, W.; Rao, Y.; Chyu, M.K. A Machine Learning Approach to Quantify the Film Cooling Superposition Effect for Effusion Cooling Structures. *Int. J. Therm. Sci.* **2021**, *162*, 106774. [CrossRef]
122. Wang, W.; Tao, G.; Ke, D.; Luo, J.; Cui, J. Transpiration Cooling of High Pressure Turbine Vane with Optimized Porosity Distribution. *Appl. Therm. Eng.* **2023**, *223*, 119831. [CrossRef]
123. Wang, W.; Tao, G.; Ke, D.; Ruan, Z.; Liu, J.; Luo, J.; Cui, J. Multi-Objective Optimization of Transpiration Cooling for High Pressure Turbine Vane. *Appl. Therm. Eng.* **2024**, *246*, 122926. [CrossRef]
124. Chen, W.; Wang, K.; Wang, Y.; Tu, S.; Liu, Z.; Su, H. Numerical Investigation and Optimal Design of Transpiration Cooling Plate Structure for Gradient Porosity. *Int. J. Therm. Sci.* **2024**, *197*, 108755. [CrossRef]
125. Min, Z.; Wu, Y.; Yang, K.; Xu, J.; Parbat, S.N.; Chyu, M.K. Dimensional Characterizations Using Scanning Electron Microscope and Surface Improvement with Electrochemical Polishing of Additively Manufactured Microchannels. *J. Eng. Gas Turbines Power* **2021**, *143*, 041020. [CrossRef]
126. Carneiro, V.H.; Rawson, S.D.; Puga, H.; Meireles, J.; Withers, P.J. Additive Manufacturing Assisted Investment Casting: A Low-Cost Method to Fabricate Periodic Metallic Cellular Lattices. *Addit. Manuf.* **2020**, *33*, 101085. [CrossRef]
127. Al-Ketan, O.; Singh, A.; Karathanasopoulos, N. Strut and Sheet Metal Lattices Produced via AM-Assisted Casting and Powder Bed Fusion: A Comparative Study. *Addit. Manuf. Lett.* **2023**, *4*, 100118. [CrossRef]
128. Zocca, A.; Colombo, P.; Gomes, C.M.; Günster, J. Additive Manufacturing of Ceramics: Issues, Potentialities, and Opportunities. *J. Am. Ceram. Soc.* **2015**, *98*, 1983–2001. [CrossRef]
129. Li, H.; Liu, Y.; Liu, Y.; Zeng, Q.; Wang, J.; Hu, K.; Lu, Z.; Liang, J. Evolution of the Microstructure and Mechanical Properties of Stereolithography Formed Alumina Cores Sintered in Vacuum. *J. Eur. Ceram. Soc.* **2020**, *40*, 4825–4836. [CrossRef]
130. An, X.; Mu, Y.; Liang, J.; Li, J.; Zhou, Y.; Sun, X. Stereolithography 3D Printing of Ceramic Cores for Hollow Aeroengine Turbine Blades. *J. Mater. Sci. Technol.* **2022**, *127*, 177–182. [CrossRef]
131. Min, Z.; Parbat, S.N.; Yang, L.; Kang, B.; Chyu, M.K. Fabrication and Characterization of Additive Manufactured Nickel-Based Oxide Dispersion Strengthened Coating Layer for High-Temperature Application. *J. Eng. Gas Turbines Power* **2018**, *140*, 062101. [CrossRef]
132. Ding, R.; Wang, J.; He, F.; Dong, G.; Tang, L. Numerical Investigation on the Performances of Porous Matrix with Transpiration and Film Cooling. *Appl. Therm. Eng.* **2019**, *146*, 422–431. [CrossRef]
133. Natsui, G.; Johnson, P.L.; Torrance, M.C.; Ricklick, M.A.; Kapat, J.S. The Effect of Transpiration on Discrete Injection for Film Cooling. In Proceedings of the ASME Turbo Expo, ASMEDC, Vancouver, BC, Canada, 1 January 2011; Volume 5, pp. 509–520.
134. Lv, Y.; Liu, L.; Ma, Y.; Dou, Y.; He, F.; Wang, J. Experimental Investigation on Cooling Characteristic of Transpiration-Film Combined Cooling Structure Using Liquid Coolant. *Int. Commun. Heat Mass Transf.* **2024**, *158*, 107964. [CrossRef]
135. Supar, K.; Ahmad, H. Stress Distribution Study on Multi-Holes Configurations in Woven Fabric Kenaf Composite Plates. *IOP Conf. Ser. Mater. Sci. Eng.* **2017**, *271*, 012005. [CrossRef]
136. Ligrani, P.M.; Bueschges, C.; Tatge, M.; Weigand, B.; Subramanian, C.; Collopy, H.L.; Taylor, Z.; Sheth, J.; Gradl, P. Heat Transfer and Aerodynamic Losses of Additively Manufactured Turbine Alloy Blades with Different Surface Enhancement Post-Processing. *Int. J. Therm. Sci.* **2025**, *214*, 109914. [CrossRef]
137. Arai, M.; Suidzu, T. Porous Ceramic Coating for Transpiration Cooling of Gas Turbine Blade. *J. Therm. Spray Technol.* **2013**, *22*, 690–698. [CrossRef]
138. Xiao, X.; Zhao, G.; Zhou, W.; Martynenko, S. Large-Eddy Simulation of Transpiration Cooling in Turbulent Channel with Porous Wall. *Appl. Therm. Eng.* **2018**, *145*, 618–629. [CrossRef]
139. You, R.; Liu, Z.; Wang, Q.; Li, H. Study on the Flow and Heat Transfer Characteristics of a Double-Wall Structure with Multiple-Jet Impingement Cooling under Rotating Conditions. *Int. Commun. Heat Mass Transf.* **2025**, *161*, 108299. [CrossRef]
140. Zhang, W.; Yi, Y.; Bai, X.; Nakayama, A. A Local Thermal Non-Equilibrium Analysis for Convective and Radiative Heat Transfer in Gaseous Transpiration Cooling through a Porous Wall. *Int. J. Heat Mass Transf.* **2020**, *162*, 120389. [CrossRef]

141. Munk, D.J.; Selzer, M.; Steven, G.P.; Vio, G.A. Topology Optimization Applied to Transpiration Cooling. *AIAA J.* **2019**, *57*, 297–312. [CrossRef]
142. Jiang, Y.; Hu, J.; Wang, S.; Lei, N.; Luo, Z.; Liu, L. Meshless Optimization of Triply Periodic Minimal Surface Based Two-Fluid Heat Exchanger. *CAD Comput. Aided Des.* **2023**, *162*, 103554. [CrossRef]

energies

MDPI

Review

Surface Air-Cooled Oil Coolers (SACOCs) in Turbofan Engines: A Comprehensive Review of Design, Performance, and Optimization

Wiktor Hoffmann * and Magda Joachimiak

Faculty of Environmental Engineering and Energy, Institute of Thermal Energy, Poznan University of Technology, 60-965 Poznań, Poland; magda.joachimiak@put.poznan.pl
* Correspondence: wiktor.hoffmann@put.poznan.pl

Abstract

Surface Air-Cooled Oil Coolers (SACOCs) can become a critical component in managing the increasing thermal loads of modern turbofan engines. Installed within the bypass duct, SACOCs utilize high-mass flow bypass air for convective heat rejection, reducing reliance on traditional Fuel-Oil Heat Exchangers. This review explores SACOC design principles, integration challenges, aerodynamic impacts, and performance trade-offs. Emphasis is placed on the balance between thermal efficiency and aerodynamic penalties such as pressure drop and flow distortion. Experimental techniques, including wind tunnel testing, are discussed alongside numerical methods, and Conjugate Heat Transfer modeling. Presented studies mostly demonstrate the impact of fin geometry and placement on both heat transfer and drag. Optimization strategies and Additive Manufacturing techniques are also covered. SACOCs are positioned to play a central role in future propulsion systems, especially in ultra-high bypass ratio and hybrid-electric architectures, where traditional cooling strategies are insufficient. This review highlights current advancements, identifies limitations, and outlines research directions to enhance SACOC efficiency in aerospace applications.

Keywords: SACOC; heat-exchangers; geared turbofan engines; thermal management; aerodynamics

1. Introduction

Surface Air-Cooled Oil Coolers (SACOCs), also known as surface air-oil heat exchangers (SAOHE), can become an essential part of the thermal management of turbofan engines, which are increasingly experiencing increased thermal loads due to advances. Sources of additional heat can be gearboxes in geared fan engines like Rolls-Royce UltraFan [1] or increased electrical systems requirements. In the first case, increasing the bypass ratio requires the use of a gearbox that adjusts the rotation speed of the fan, which is limited by its increased outer diameter with the rotation speed of the turbine. In the other case, replacing mechanical controllers as well as hydraulic actuators with fly-by-wire systems, as well as a general increase in the number of electrical systems that replace the work of the pilots, results in more heat being dissipated. This causes the capabilities of conventional heat sinks to be insufficient.

SACOCs can be located on the wall of the turbofan engine bypass duct, where they use the high-mass flow stream of air as an effective heat dissipation medium. The potential integration of SACOCs in modern aeroengine designs is based on their ability to simplify

https://doi.org/10.3390/en18154052

oil cooling under rigorous operational conditions, which supports improved lubrication, thermal management, and overall engine reliability. It is important to mention that their implementation introduces aerodynamic challenges like pressure drop and flow distortion, which can affect engine performance. Therefore, a complex aerodynamic and thermal analysis is necessary to optimize their design and integration.

Engine oil serves the dual function of lubricating and cooling, by transferring heat absorbed from bearings and gears to the fuel through Fuel-Oil Heat Exchangers (FOHEs). This method uses the ability of the fuel to act as a heat sink before combustion, which increases the thermal efficiency. However, this method has limitations. The mass flow of the fuel changes during flight, resulting in an irregular heat absorption capacity. Furthermore, accurate regulation of fuel temperature is required to avoid issues such as coking, which can cause damage to engine components or lead to unstable work of fuel injectors. In addition, the increasing application of composite materials in aircraft structures, characterized by lower thermal conductivity compared to traditional alloys, undermines the efficacy of the airframe in dissipating heat [2,3].

Surface Air-Cooled Oil Coolers (SACOCs) represent an innovative approach to dealing with high thermal loads. These devices are conventionally positioned within the engine's bypass duct, where they use bypass flow as an effective heat sink, making it easier to transfer heat from the engine oil. This configuration reduces the dependence on fuel as the primary heat sink while simultaneously using existing airflow, thus reducing the need for additional cooling systems. However, integration of SACOCs poses aerodynamic challenges, including potential pressure drops and flow distortions, which can affect engine efficiency. Consequently, the accurate design and optimization of the SACOC geometry is mandatory to achieve a balance between efficient thermal management and minimal aerodynamic losses [2,4,5].

2. Function and Integration of SACOCs in Turbofan Engines

2.1. SACOC Working Principle and Structure

Surface Air-Cooled Oil Coolers (SACOCs) are based on convective heat transfer. Hot oil flows internally through channels in a finned block while the cooler bypass air flows around the external surface, absorbing thermal energy. SACOCs can be installed along the inner wall of the bypass duct (Figure 1), thus taking advantage of the high mass flow and relatively low temperature of the bypass air, even under high thrust conditions [2].

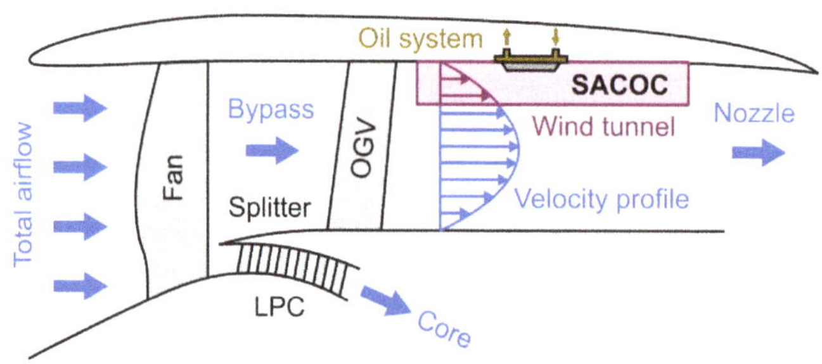

Figure 1. SACOC localization in the bypass duct, assumed for the experiment by Broatch et al. [2].

In the further examples discussed below, SACOCs are proposed to take the shape of an array of fins, pin fins, strip fins, or microchannel structures, having oil tubes inside, which serve to increase the surface area and thus increase the rate of heat transfer [6,7]. These solutions require an equilibrium between thermal effectiveness and aerodynamic performance to prevent significant pressure drop or flow distortion [2,5]. Given the high-velocity characteristics of the external air flow, often high Mach number, proper fin geometry design, surface roughness, and material selection are required. [8].

2.2. Placement in the Bypass Duct

The placement of SACOCs within the bypass duct in the bypass duct provides a continuous high-mass flow of relatively cool air, which is ideal for convective heat rejection. Unlike the core flow, which is highly energetic and contains combustion products, the bypass flow remains cleaner and more thermally stable, making it more suitable as a heat sink for sensitive cooling applications [4]. Additionally, the geometry of the bypass duct geometry allows for the installation of heat exchangers without increasing the frontal area of the engine or requiring additional ducting [5], which is possible due to the low height and compact geometry. The curved inner wall of the bypass duct provides a large surface area for SACOC integration, and its proximity to the fan and low-pressure compressor stages ensures airflow in all operating conditions, including low-speed ground operations and take-off [9].

2.3. Integration Challenges: Aerodynamic Penalties and Thermal Efficiency Trade-Offs

Maximizing the heat transfer rate requires increasing the wetted surface area, which leads to higher viscous drag and pressure drop in the bypass stream [10]. Such pressure losses can affect engine efficiency, especially in high-speed flows where Mach numbers in the bypass duct approach 0.5 or higher [8]. Furthermore, inappropriate and incompatible with flow parameters, SACOC geometries can introduce flow separation, shock wave interaction, or secondary vortices that distort bypass flow, potentially affecting downstream components and reducing engine performance [11]. To mitigate these aerodynamic losses, designers must carefully tune the density, orientation, and surface roughness of the fin to balance heat dissipation with acceptable drag levels. This is challenging because improvements in thermal performance, such as more aggressive fin profiles, often worsen pressure loss, requiring iterative design and optimization informed by both Computational Fluid Dynamics (CFD) and wind tunnel testing [6,12]. When reducing pressure losses and flow distortion, it should not be forgotten that for turbulent flow, heat transfer coefficient h depends on the velocity v and air density ρ as follows:

$$h \propto (\rho \cdot v)^{0.8}. \tag{1}$$

This means that pressure losses and distortion of the velocity profile are detrimental to both engine efficiency and the efficiency of SACOCs themselves.

2.4. The Meredith Effect and Performance Recovery

Broatcch et al. [13] suggest that SACOCs can benefit energy conversion through the phenomenon called the Meredith effect, where heated bypass air expands and produces additional thrust in the secondary nozzle. This can make the bypass duct not only a practical location from a thermal point of view but also a contributor to overall propulsive efficiency, which will be analyzed in a later section.

This effect was first described in 1936, by British engineer Frederick William Meredith in his "Cooling of Aircraft Engines. With Special Reference To Ethylene Glycol Radiators Enclosed In Ducts" report [14]. Meredith's work demonstrated that by designing the cooling ducts to allow heated air from the radiator to exit at high velocity, it was possible to generate forward thrust, partially offsetting the drag caused by the radiator itself. More specifically, increasing the air enthalpy before it exits through the secondary nozzle can lead to partial compensation for the drag introduced by the heat exchanger.

The effectiveness of this mechanism depends on multiple factors, including the placement of the heat exchanger, the air pressure and velocity in the bypass duct, and the degree of increase in temperature imparted to the air [11]. Although the Meredith effect was originally exploited in piston-engine aircraft of the WWII era, its relevance in turbofan applications has grown with the increasing thermal loads and compact engine architectures that demand localized heat rejection solutions [15]. Modern SACOC designs can be optimized not only for minimal pressure drop and maximum heat dissipation, but also to maximize the thrust benefit derived from bypass air heating, effectively turning a cooling requirement into a performance enhancement opportunity [6].

However, due to the lack of reliable data, it is difficult to calculate the level of thrust recovered from heat for a real engine. Anyway, based on the known Rolls-Royce UltraFan 800 geared turbofan engine, with a bypass ratio 14:1, 360 kN of thrust, and 64 MW of fan power, and adding assumptions such as bypass mass flow $\dot{m}_b$ = 882 kg/s (hypothetical, ideal, based on thust and bypass ratio), almost exactly 1 N of thrust will be received. Such a low propulsion efficiency of such a system is obviously due to insufficient compression for optimal Brayton Cycle usage.

3. Aerothermal Characterization of SACOCs

3.1. Experimental Techniques for SACOC Testing

Experimental evaluation plays a crucial role in the development and validation of SACOC designs, especially given the complexity of flow and thermal interactions within the bypass duct environment. Due to the costs and logistical difficulty of full-scale engine testing, scaled-down SACOC prototypes are mostly used in transonic wind tunnels that can replicate the flow conditions found in engine bypass ducts. The test section used in the study by Broatch et al. [2] replicates a part of the bypass duct, as shown in Figure 1. These facilities allow researchers to analyze heat transfer rates, pressure drop, and flow distortion under controlled and repeatable conditions.

To look deeper into flow velocity field and aerodynamic losses, non-intrusive optical diagnostics, such as Particle Image Velocimetry (PIV) and Schlieren imaging, can be used, offering high-resolution visualization and shock interactions near the SACOC surfaces [13]. Advances in Additive Manufacturing make possible complex SACOC geometries, including internal fin structures and conformal duct surfaces that would be difficult or impossible to fabricate using traditional machining methods. This leads to the acceleration of the design iteration cycles and allows researchers to explore new shapes of the heat exchangers and internal channel topologies [16].

3.2. Numerical Simulations and Validation Approaches

Numerical simulation has become an important tool in the aerothermal development of SACOCs, enabling the detailed exploration of complex flow and heat transfer phenomena that are difficult, too expensive, or impossible to capture experimentally. Computational Fluid Dynamics (CFD) allows for the visualization of local temperature gradients, flow separation zones, and turbulent structures around and inside the SACOC geometry, providing an overview of performance limiting factors such as hot spots or excessive pressure drops, especially those that are impossible to measure directly during an experiment [7]. Reynolds-Averaged Navier–Stokes (RANS) [17] and Large Eddy Simulation (LES) [18] models are used depending on the desired level of detail and computational cost. Conjugate Heat Transfer (CHT) [19] simulations are often used to capture the simultaneous interaction between solid fins and fluids, typically oil inside and air outside, allowing for accurate heat flux predictions [6]. The validation of numerical results should be carried out via comparison with experimental data, using surface temperature distributions, outlet air temperatures, and pressure profiles [5]. Recent studies have combined CFD with parametric optimization algorithms to explore the effect of fin geometry, pitch, and orientation on both thermal and aerodynamic performance, improving design based on multiple design variables [12].

3.3. Representative Studies

The biggest impact on understanding SACOC performance was achieved by integrating experimental, numerical, and optimization methodologies. The studies mentioned above, performed by Broatch et al. [2], conducted experimental investigations in transonic wind tunnels to characterize the aerodynamic and thermal performance of SACOCs under realistic bypass conditions, where the SACOCs were placed in a tunnel channel in which the velocity field corresponding to the actual bypass flow was created by the distorting screen (Figure 2). Based on this, the same authors examined the effect of rounded fin geometries [12], highlighting how minor changes in cross-sectional curvature could improve heat transfer efficiency and decrease aerodynamic drag. Then, in 2024, the same research group introduced the use of optical measurement techniques and Additive Manufacturing to improve prototyping and achieve high-resolution flow diagnostics, allowing for rapid iteration in early design phases [13]. Parallel to these investigations, Chávez-Modena et al. [6] developed a numerical framework for fin shape optimization using CHT simulations, allowing for detailed sensitivity analyses of geometric parameters. Their work also lead to experimental experimental validation in 2023, confirming its precision and suitability to guide the design of the SACOC [5], where the CFD error relative to the experiment did not exceed 3.1% for pressure drop and 1.2% for heat transfer. Together, these studies form a set of work that addresses both fundamental mechanisms and practical design trade-offs in the integration of SACOCs. More case-specific studies will be presented in the following sections about optimization and high-speed flows.

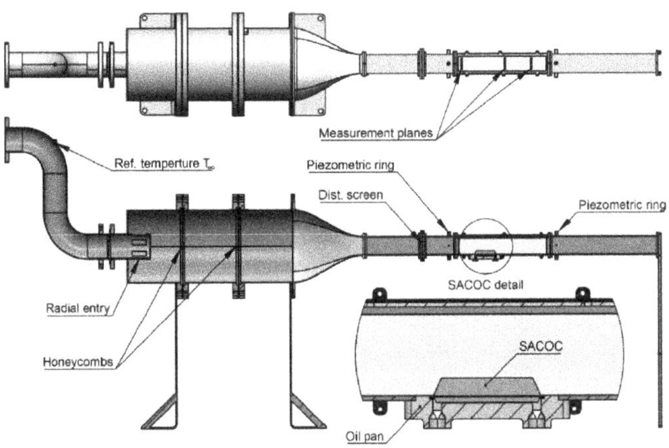

Figure 2. Drawing of the wind tunnel detailing the installation of the SACOCs [2].

4. Fin Geometry and Design Optimization

4.1. Influence of Fin Geometry on Pressure Drop, Heat Transfer, and Flow Uniformity

The performance of SACOCs has critically influenced how pin geometries affect pressure drop, heat transfer rates, and flow uniformity across the heat exchanger surface. High-performance fins promote turbulence and disrupt boundary layers, increasing convective heat transfer. However, these same features often result in increased friction losses and non-uniform velocity distributions, leading to higher-pressure drop penalties. Jeng and

Tzeng [20] showed that staggered pin-fin arrays provide better heat transfer performance than in-line configurations but at the cost of significantly greater pressure loss. For example, for Reynolds Number 12,500, a staggered array of square pin-fins can reach 20% better heat transfer than in-line circular fins but also 25% greater losses.

Similarly, Jonsson and Moshfegh [21] demonstrated that bypass of the flow that outflows the finned core can reduce both the thermal effectiveness and the predictability of flow patterns in plate-fin and pin-fin heat sinks. Importantly, the authors point out that diversities in temperature and velocity fields also increase local thermal stresses on fins, which can impact mechanical durability over time. Experiments and calculations are carried out for different pin shapes (Figure 3) and for Reynolds Numbers in the range 2500 to 15,000. Numerical simulation has become an important tool in the aerothermal development of SACOCs, enabling the detailed exploration of complex flow and heat transfer that are difficult, too expensive, or impossible to capture experimentally.

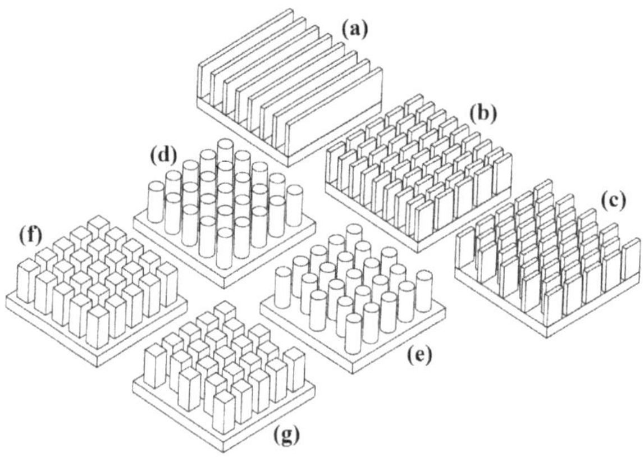

Figure 3. Type of geometries studied by Jonsson and Moshfegh [21]: (**a**) plate fins, (**b**) in-line strip fins, (**c**) staggered strip fins, (**d**) array of in-line circular pin fins, (**e**) array of staggered circular pin fins, (**f**) array of in-line square pin fins, and (**g**) array of staggered pin fins.

The study by M.Kim et al. [7,10] explored the aerothermal behavior of the slanted pin fin arrangements, such as the plate fin and the slanted fins for four different angles (Figure 4), as well as different fin heights and Reynolds Numbers, for their ability to enhance convective heat transfer while minimizing aerodynamic losses. The first flat plate fin and pin fin comparison showed an increase in pressure losses of 27% and an increase of 12.5% in heat transfer for square pin fins in Reynolds Number 12,000 (graph in Figure 5).

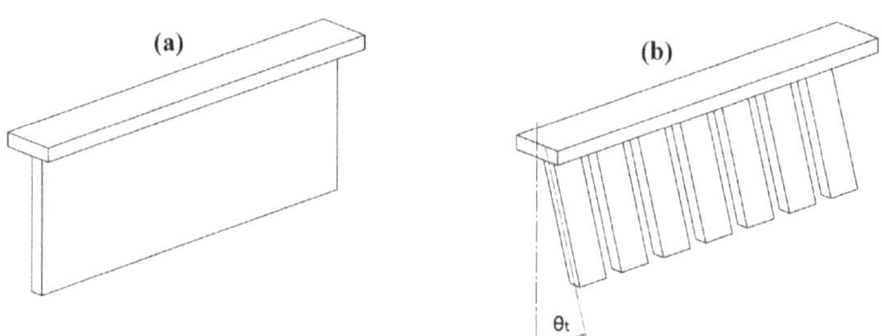

Figure 4. Plate fin (**a**) and cross-cut slanted pins (**b**) [10].

The slant angle influences flow, resulting in certain increases in heat transfer as well as in an increase in pressure losses, but the studies are confusing because the results for different slant angles do not show clear patterns, as well as results in diagrams (b) and (c) in Figure 5 show fewer differences than declared accuracy (3.2% for pressure drop). In addition, the inaccuracy between CFD and experiment is 9% for aerodynamics and 7.5% for heat transfer. In addition, the results are shown for different Reynolds numbers, where the fin height is given as the characteristic dimension, which varies from case to case. Moreover, the Reynolds Numbers chosen for the study appear to be too low for the bypass channel of the turbofan engine. Additionally, S.Kim et al. [4] showed that the interaction between bypass flow and SACOC geometry is related not only to the drag profile but also the internal oil-side temperature distribution, affecting the uniformity and predictability of thermal performance. These findings emphasize that SACOC performance cannot be evaluated under low-speed assumptions and must instead account for the complex aero thermal coupling that arises in high-speed bypass conditions.

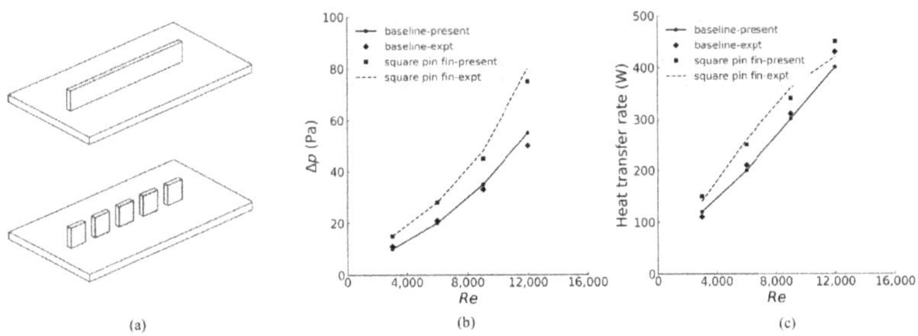

Figure 5. Comparison of calculation results with experimental data for fins in channel: (**a**) geometry, (**b**) pressure drop, and (**c**) thermal resistance [10].

4.2. Optimization Techniques and Design Trade-Offs

Designing SACOC fins involves a multi-objective optimization process that balances heat transfer enhancement and aerodynamic performance. Traditional trial-and-error methods, as mentioned above in research, have been increasingly replaced by computational optimization techniques, including genetic algorithms [22], response surface models, and adjoint-based solvers [23]. These methods allow designers to evaluate large parametric spaces efficiently, identifying optimal configurations. Guo et al. [24] demonstrated an example of using a structured optimization for the geometry of counterflow plate-fin heat exchangers, achieving notable improvements. Similarly, as mentioned above, Chávez-Modena et al. [6] applied a simulation-based Conjugate Heat Transfer (CHT) approach to optimize fin geometry and spacing under bypass duct conditions. These optimizations often reveal nonintuitive design choices, such as asymmetrical fin layouts or nonuniform spacing, that can be better than traditional symmetric configurations. The example of results can be seen in Figure 6, which shows a noticeable decrease in turbulent kinetic energy for optimized fin shape. The new geometry results in a significant decrease in pressure drop of 10.6%, while the change in heat transfer is minimal (around 0.3 %). However, performance gains must be carefully weighed against complexity and manufacturing constraints, especially if they are related to internal oil pipes.

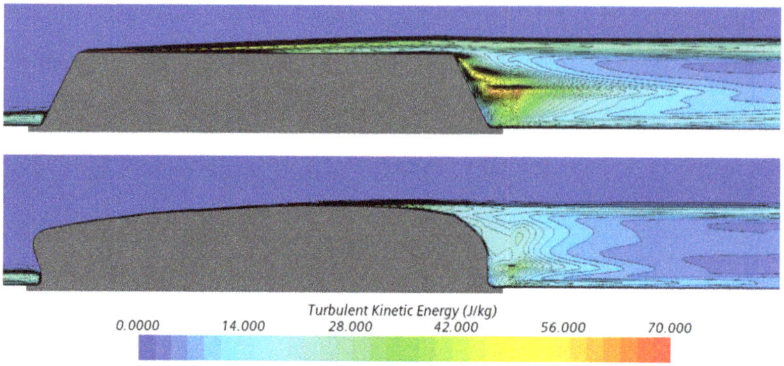

Figure 6. Turbulent kinetic energie field for original and optimized fin shapes [6].

5. High-Speed Flow Effects and Aerodynamic Interactions

5.1. Impact of Transonic and High Bypass Flows on SACOC Performance

In modern engines, bypass Mach Number can exceed 0.5 during cruise and take-off, placing SACOCs in a transonic or even locally supersonic regime. These conditions fundamentally alter the flow structure on the heat exchanger surface, increasing the complexity of pressure recovery, turbulence generation, and boundary layer behavior. Sousa et al. [11] demonstrated that transonic effects lead to localized shock formation and unsteady flow separation on the fin surfaces, which can significantly impact thermal effectiveness and introduce dynamic loads that degrade structural integrity over time. These studies were also one of the best representations of the actual geometries of the bypass channel and flow conditions. The cooling demands are indicated to be the highest in take-off conditions and a heat exchanger sensitivity less than 10% for the flight envelope. Continuing research in similar channel geometry and Mach Number 0.8, Villafañe and Paniagua [8] performed tests for "continuous fins" and "interrupted fins", which are smilar geometries to Plate fin and square Pin-Fins tested by M.Kim et al. [7]. It was noted that interrupted fins generate greater flow distortion than perturbations in the case of continuous fins.

5.2. Flow Distortion, Pressure Losses, and Mitigation Strategies

The bypass air interacts with the SACOC surfaces and densely packed or high-profile fins, which can lead to flow separation, vortex shedding, turbulence intensification, and non-uniform outlet velocity profiles. These effects are even more important when approaching transonic flow. Rebassa et al. [25] quantified these distortions using a high-speed wind tunnel, for Mach Number 0.3 to compare with previous studies and Mach Number 0.5 as closer to bypass duct conditions. The tests were performed for finned geometries, similar to those designed by Modena et al. [6] (Figure 6). Unfortunately, the article lacks numerical results for Mach 0.5, making a comparative evaluation impossible.

In parallel, studies mentioned above by Villafañe and Paniagua [8] showed a transonic wind tunnel experiment for Mach Number of approximately 0.8. In this case, the geometries tested were similar to those tested by M. Kim et al. [10]. Again, it is difficult to make a comparison, since both the flow parameters and geometric dimensions were completely different. However, it should be mentioned that these were the first tests in which the wind tunnel channel reproduced the actual curvature of the bypass duct wall.

6. Advanced Heat Exchanger Concepts for Aero Engines

6.1. Cooled Cooling Air (CCA) and Precooled Engine Technologies

Advanced cooling strategies such as Cooled Cooling Air (CCA) systems and pre-cooled engine cycles are gaining prominence. CCA technology involves preconditioning the cooling air, typically by expanding or cooling it before it reaches heat exchangers, thus enhancing its capacity to absorb heat from lubricating oil or other thermal sources. C. Kim et al. [26] developed and experimentally validated a compact CCA heat exchanger, demonstrating significant improvements in heat transfer performance and structural durability under representative engine conditions. Similarly, Zhuang et al. [27] conducted an analysis of CCA for low bypass ratio engines, showing it to be an alternative to conventional oil or fuel-based heat sinks. In parallel, pre-cooled engine concepts, borrowed from hypersonic propulsion, use regenerative heat exchangers to cool the air that enters before compression. Wang et al. [28] modeled the performance of such systems for intake precooling in hypersonic engines, revealing potential thrust and fuel efficiency.

6.2. New Materials and Manufacturing Methods (e.g., SLM)

Advancements in materials and manufacturing technologies enable novel geometries, improved thermal performance, and enhanced mechanical resilience. One of the most transformative developments is the use of Selective Laser Melting (SLM), also known as Selective Laser Sintering (SLS), and other Additive Manufacturing (AM) techniques, which allow for the fabrication of intricate, high-performance heat exchanger structures that were previously unachievable using traditional subtractive methods. Wong et al. [16] demonstrated that SLM-produced heat sinks could achieve complex internal geometries with high dimensional accuracy, resulting in both improved convective heat transfer and reduced pressure losses compared to their conventionally machined counterparts. Another paper by Silva et al. [29] presents an interesting analysis of various heat sinks, one of which, shown in Figure 7, is a great example of a geometry that is impossible to mill or cast (due to thin walls) but is an excellent demonstrator of SLM technology.

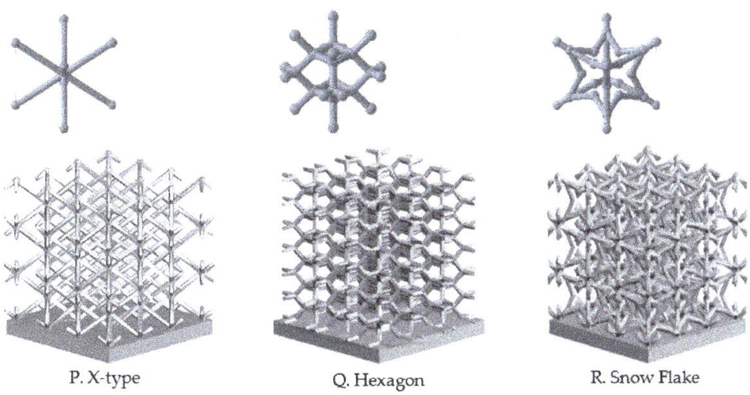

Figure 7. Example of SLM-fabricated heat sinks [29].

Furthermore, AM supports the integration of graded materials and controlled porosity, which can be used to locally optimize thermal conductivity and mechanical strength [30]. In parallel, new high-temperature alloys and composite–metal hybrids are being investigated to withstand thermo-mechanical environments inside bypass ducts.

7. Future Challenges and Research Directions

7.1. Integration with Next-Gen Propulsion (Hybrid-Electric, Ultra-High Bypass)

The integration of SACOCs into future propulsion systems creates new challenges and opportunities, particularly in the context of hybrid-electric architectures and ultra-high bypass ratio (UHBR) engines like Rolls-Royce UltraFan or Pratt and Whitney PW1000G (Figure 8). These next-generation systems introduce increased thermal loads (even up to 100 MW of fan power) and reduced availability of traditional heat sinks (especially when fuel consumption is decreased). In hybrid-electric configurations, power electronics, batteries, and electric motors all contribute significant waste heat, which must be managed by a highly integrated thermal management system. SACOCs, with their advantages, are well positioned to support this function but must be adapted to operate effectively under different mission profiles and variable engine operating conditions [31]. In UHBR engines, the increased fan diameter and reduced core flow limit the effectiveness of core-mounted cooling strategies, creating a greater dependence on the bypass stream for heat rejection. As a result, SACOCs must be designed to conform to increasingly constrained aerodynamic and structural envelopes, often within curved duct geometries or composite casings. This requires enhanced flexibility in SACOC architecture and integration with structural components, which could lead to multifunctional heat exchanger designs that simultaneously provide load-bearing, acoustic, and thermal management functions.

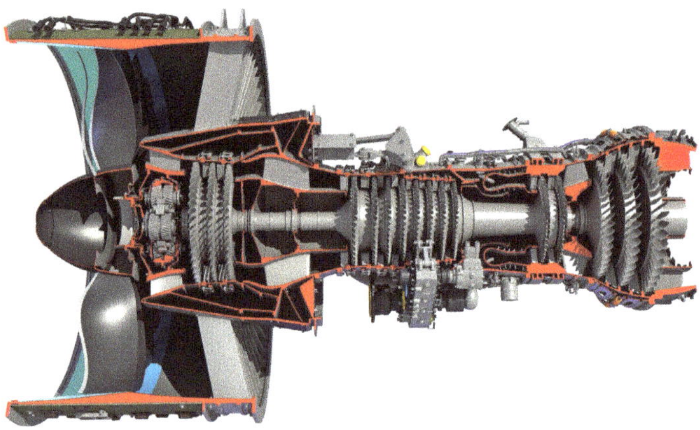

Figure 8. Cut-away of geared turbo fan engine Pratt and Whitney PW1000G [32].

7.2. Smart SACOCs (Adaptive Fins, Real-Time Monitoring)

Emerging trends in aerospace thermal management point toward the development of "smart" SACOCs that incorporate adaptive features and real-time sensing to respond dynamically to changing flight and engine conditions. Unlike conventional passive designs, smart SACOCs could integrate shape-memory alloys, piezoelectric actuators, or thermally responsive materials to alter fin geometry or flow pathways during operation, optimizing performance across a wider operating envelope [33]. For example, variable-geometry fins could minimize drag during cruise while expanding surface area during high thermal load events such as takeoff or climb. In parallel, embedded sensors capable of measuring oil temperature, pressure, vibration, or local heat flux would enable condition-based monitoring and predictive maintenance, reducing the risk of thermal failure and improving reliability. Lumped-parameter and reduced-order models linked to real-time data streams could provide onboard diagnostic tools to adapt thermal strategies in response to flight mission profiles. Although still in early research phases, these smart SACOC systems align with broader trends in "more-electric" and "intelligent" engine systems, where adaptability and autonomy are becoming core performance attributes.

7.3. Sustainability and Fuel Efficiency Impact

SACOCs also play an increasingly strategic role in the broader goals of aviation sustainability and fuel efficiency. As regulatory pressures and industry commitments push towards lower CO_2 and NO_x emissions, improving the thermal efficiency of propulsion systems becomes essential. Effective oil cooling directly contributes to reduced mechanical losses, extended engine life, and higher component reliability, all of which support lower specific fuel consumption throughout the engine's lifecycle. More critically, optimized SACOC designs can enable higher overall engine pressure ratios and bypass ratios by alleviating thermal bottlenecks, indirectly improving thermodynamic efficiency. Studies such as those by Liu et al. [34] have highlighted the link between thermal system management and engine failure modes, suggesting that proactive cooling strategies can mitigate hot-spot-induced degradation. Furthermore, integrating SACOCs with advanced fuel-saving engine cycles or hybrid-electric systems requires high adaptability and compactness to maintain overall system efficiency. As part of a holistic thermal management architecture, SACOCs contribute not only to engine-level improvements but also to fleet-wide reductions in fuel burn and emissions, aligning with the industry's long-term decarbonization strategies.

8. Conclusions

Surface Air-Cooled Oil Coolers (SACOCs) have become a critical component in the thermal management strategies of modern and future turbofan engines. As engine architectures evolve toward higher bypass ratios, increased electrification, and compact integrated systems, SACOCs offer a viable and efficient means of dissipating thermal loads using the bypass airstream. This review has outlined the fundamental working principles of SACOCs; their challenges in aerodynamic and thermal integration; and the significant role they play in optimizing engine reliability, fuel efficiency, and performance.

A wide range of experimental and numerical studies have been conducted to evaluate and enhance the performance of SACOCs. These efforts have included the characterization of fin geometries, mitigation of pressure loss, and heat transfer optimization through conventional and advanced techniques such as Additive Manufacturing. Furthermore, this article has highlighted the adoption of high-fidelity CFD tools, transonic wind tunnel testing, and smart materials as emerging enablers for next-generation SACOC designs.

In the future, SACOCs are expected to play a central role in the thermal architecture of hybrid electric propulsion, ultra-high bypass engines, and intelligent aerospace systems. Their integration into multifunctional structures, adaptive designs in real time, and engine cycles driven by sustainability underscores the need for continued innovation in both modeling and experimental validation. Addressing these challenges will not only support the development of efficient propulsion systems but will also contribute to the broader decarbonization and performance goals of the aviation industry.

Unfortunately, some of the studies described raised confusion, especially in the context of studies with relatively low Reynolds Numbers. Also, the Meretith effect is more of a curiosity than a meaningful phenomenon.

All presented studies lack an analysis of the effect of ambient temperature on the efficiency of SACOCs. For example, in hot climates, assuming an air temperature above the runway of 320 Kelvins and 16% lower air density than standard atmosphere, we can easily reach above 400 Kelvins just before SACOCs.

Funding: This research received no external funding

Conflicts of Interest: The authors declare no conflicts of interest.

Abbreviations

The following abbreviations are used in this manuscript:

AM	Additive Manufacturing
CCA	Cooled Cooling Air
CFD	Computational Fluid Dynamics
CHT	Conjugate Heat Transfer
FOHEs	Fuel-Oil Heat Exchangers
LES	Large Eddy Simulation
RANS	Reynolds Averaged Navier–Stokes
SACOCs	Surface Air-Cooled Oil Coolers
SAOHE	Surface Air–Oil Heat Exchangers
SLS	Selective Laser Sintering
SLM	Selective Laser Melting

References

1. Rolls-Royce Plc. UltraFan—Demonstrator Aero Engine. 2025. Available online: https://www.rolls-royce.com/innovation/ultrafan.aspx (accessed on 20 July 2025).
2. Broatch, A.; Olmeda, P.; García-Tíscar, J.; Felgueroso, A.; Chávez-Modena, M.; González, L.; Gelain, M.; Couilleaux, A. Experimental aerothermal characterization of surface air-cooled oil coolers for turbofan engines. *Int. J. Heat Mass Transf.* **2022**, *190*, 122775. [CrossRef]
3. Ryemill, M.; Bewick, C.; Min, J.K. The Rolls-Royce PLC UltraFan Heat Management Challenge. In Proceedings of the 30th Congress of the International Council of the Aeronautical Sciences (ICAS), Daejeon, Republic of Korea, 25–30 September 2016.
4. Kim, S.; Min, J.K.; Ha, M.Y.; Son, C. Investigation of high-speed bypass effect on the performance of the surface air–oil heat exchanger for an aero engine. *Int. J. Heat Mass Transf.* **2014**, *77*, 321–334. [CrossRef]
5. Chávez-Modena, M.; González, L.M.; Valero, E.; Broatch, A.; García-Tíscar, J.; Felgueroso, A. Experimental and numerical methodology for the aero-thermal analysis of a SACOC heat exchanger. *Appl. Therm. Eng.* **2023**, *219*, 119409. [CrossRef]
6. Chávez-Modena, M.; González, L.M.; Valero, E. Numerical optimization of the fin shape experiments of a heat conjugate problem surface air/oil heat exchanger (SACOC). *Int. J. Heat Mass Transfer* **2022**, *182*, 121971. [CrossRef]
7. Kim, M.; Ha, M.Y.; Min, J.K. A numerical study on various pin–fin shaped surface air–oil heat exchangers for an aero gas-turbine engine. *Int. J. Heat Mass Transf.* **2016**, *93*, 637–652. [CrossRef]
8. Villafañe, L.; Paniagua, G. Aerodynamic impact of finned heat exchangers on transonic flows. *Exp. Therm. Fluid Sci.* **2018**, *97*, 223–236. [CrossRef]
9. Gelain, M. Aerothermal Characterisation of a Surface Heat Exchanger Implemented in a Turbofan By-pass Duct. In Proceedings of the 33rd Congress of the International Council of the Aeronautical Sciences (ICAS), Stockholm, Sweden, 4–9 September 2022.
10. Kim, M.; Ha, M.Y.; Min, J.K. A numerical study on the aero-thermal performance of a slanted-pin-fin cooler under a high-speed-bypass condition. *Int. J. Heat Mass Transf.* **2018**, *119*, 791–812. [CrossRef]
11. Sousa, J.; Villafañe, L.; Paniagua, G. Thermal analysis and modeling of surface heat exchangers operating in the transonic regime. *Energy* **2014**, *64*, 961–969. [CrossRef]
12. Broatch, A.; García-Tíscar, J.; Felgueroso, A.; Chávez-Modena, M.; González, L.; Valero, E. Numerical and experimental analysis of rounded fins for high speed air-cooled heat exchangers. *Int. J. Heat Mass Transf.* **2023**, *201*, 123575. [CrossRef]
13. Broatch, A.; García-Tíscar, J.; Quintero, P.; Felgueroso, A. Rapid aerodynamic characterization of surface heat exchangers for turbofan aeroengines through optical techniques and additive manufacturing. *Therm. Sci. Eng. Prog.* **2024**, *55*, 102966. [CrossRef]
14. Meredith, F.W. *Cooling of Aircraft Engines with Special Reference to Ethylene Glycol Radiators Enclosed in Ducts*; Technical Report R&M No. 1683; Aeronautical Research Committee: London, UK, 1935.
15. Murray, J.J.; Guha, A.; Bond, A. Overview of the development of heat exchangers for use in air-breathing propulsion pre-coolers. *Acta Astronaut.* **1997**, *41*, 723–729. [CrossRef]
16. Wong, M.; Owen, I.; Sutcliffe, C.; Puri, A. Convective heat transfer and pressure losses across novel heat sinks fabricated by Selective Laser Melting. *Int. J. Heat Mass Transf.* **2009**, *52*, 281–288. [CrossRef]
17. Reynolds, O. On the Dynamical Theory of Incompressible Viscous Fluids and the Determination of the Criterion. *Philos. Trans. R. Soc. Lond. A* **1895**, *186*, 123–164.

18. Smagorinsky, J. General Circulation Experiments with the Primitive Equations. I. The Basic Experiment. *Mon. Weather. Rev.* **1963**, *91*, 99–164. [CrossRef]
19. Perelman, T.L. On Conjugated Problems of Heat Transfer. *Int. J. Heat Mass Transf.* **1961**, *4*, 273–281. [CrossRef]
20. Jeng, T.M.; Tzeng, S.C. Pressure drop and heat transfer of square pin-fin arrays in in-line and staggered arrangements. *Int. J. Heat Mass Transf.* **2007**, *50*, 2364–2375. [CrossRef]
21. Jonsson, H.; Moshfegh, B. Modeling of the Thermal and Hydraulic Performance of Plate Fin, Strip Fin, and Pin Fin Heat Sinks—Influence of Flow Bypass. *IEEE Trans. Components Packag. Technol.* **2001**, *24*, 142–149. [CrossRef]
22. Peng, H.; Ling, X. Optimal design approach for the plate-fin heat exchangers using neural networks cooperated with genetic algorithms. *Appl. Therm. Eng.* **2008**, *28*, 642–650. [CrossRef]
23. Burghardt, O. The Discrete Adjoint Solver in SU2 and Its Application to Aeroelastic Optimization. In Proceedings of the 2024 SU2 Conference, SU2 Foundation, Accessible via NASA Aeronautics Meeting Summaries, Villa Monastero in Varenna, Italy, 9–12 September 2024. Available online: https://www.nas.nasa.gov/assets/nas/pdf/ams/2024/AMS_20240912_Burghardt.pdf (accessed on 20 July 2025).
24. Guo, K.; Zhang, N.; Smith, R. Optimisation of fin selection and thermal design of counter-current plate-fin heat exchangers. *Appl. Therm. Eng.* **2015**, *78*, 491–499. [CrossRef]
25. Rebassa, A.; Rahbari, I.; Paulson, J.; Paniagua, G. Aerothermal characterization of finned surfaces in high-speed flows. *Appl. Therm. Eng.* **2023**, *227*, 120331. [CrossRef]
26. Kim, C.; Kim, H.; Cho, J.; Park, S.; Ha, M. Manufacturing and mechanical evaluation of cooled cooling air (CCA) heat exchanger for aero engine. *Int. J. Precis. Eng. Manuf.* **2016**, *17*, 1195–1200. [CrossRef]
27. Zhuang, L.; Xu, G.; Liu, Q.; Li, M.; Dong, B.; Wen, J. Superiority analysis of the cooled cooling air technology for low bypass ratio aero-engine under typical flight mission. *Energy Convers. Manag.* **2022**, *259*, 115510. [CrossRef]
28. Wang, C.; Eri, Q.; Wang, Y.; Ding, W. Flow and heat transfer characteristics of intake-precooler system for hypersonic precooled aero-engine. *Appl. Therm. Eng.* **2023**, *229*, 120596. [CrossRef]
29. Silva, E.C.; Álvaro M. Sampaio.; Pontes, A.J. Evaluation of Active Heat Sinks Design under Forced Convection—Effect of Geometric and Boundary Parameters. *Materials* **2021**, *14*, 2041. [CrossRef] [PubMed]
30. Gu, X.; Wang, J.; Wang, H.; Liu, X.; Wang, Y. Hybrid optimization for structure of printed circuit heat exchanger with airfoil fins. *Int. J. Therm. Sci.* **2025**, *212*, 109803. [CrossRef]
31. Van Heerden, A.S.; Judt, D.M.; Lawson, C.P.; Jafari, S.; Nikolaidis, T.; Bosak, D. Framework for integrated dynamic thermal simulation of future civil transport aircraft. In Proceedings of the AIAA Scitech 2020 Forum, Orlando, FL, USA, 6–10 January 2020. [CrossRef]
32. Iemoto, K. Pratt & Whitney PW1000G Cutaway (Geared Turbofan). 2010 . Available online: https://commons.wikimedia.org/wiki/File:Pratt_%26_Whitney_PW1000G_(4339944349).jpg (accessed on 20 July 2025).
33. Kholi, F.K.; Son, H.J.; Park, J.; Ha, M.Y.; Klingsporn, M.; Chetwynd-Chatwin, J.; Yang, J.S.; Min, J.K. Enhanced prediction of the decongealing performance of aero-engine oil coolers with various fin types and operating conditions using lumped model. *Case Stud. Therm. Eng.* **2023**, *51*, 103530. [CrossRef]
34. Liu, Y.; Xu, G.; Fu, Y.; Wen, J.; Huang, H. Thermal dynamic and failure research on an air-fuel heat exchanger for aero-engine cooling. *Case Stud. Therm. Eng.* **2023**, *42*, 102715. [CrossRef]

energies

MDPI

Article

Particle Image Velocimetry Flow Characterisation of High-Convection Slot Nozzle Systems for Impingement Heat Transfer

Eileen Trampe *, Ida Daube *, Dominik Büschgens, Herbert Pfeifer and Christian Wuppermann

Department for Industrial Furnaces and Heat Engineering, RWTH Aachen University, 52074 Aachen, Germany; bueschgens@iob.rwth-aachen.de (D.B.); pfeifer@iob.rwth-aachen.de (H.P.); wuppermann@iob.rwth-aachen.de (C.W.)

* Correspondence: trampe@iob.rwth-aachen.de (E.T.); ida.daube@rwth-aachen.de (I.D.); Tel.: +49-241-80-26051 (E.T.)

Abstract: Impingement jets are used in many applications for high convective heat transfer. In order to optimise specialised nozzle systems, a comprehensive understanding of the gas flow is essential. The aim of this work is to investigate high-convective flows at Re = 10,000 to Re = 50,000 for a single slot nozzle (slot width W = 5 mm) and a slot nozzle array (distance between nozzle slots s = 70 mm) consisting of five nozzles. Particle image velocimetry measurements are taken for a distance between strip and nozzle exit of H = 50 mm and are compared to verify if the results from a single slot nozzle are transferable to a nozzle array. The presence of an array of nozzles not only creates a distinct zone where the individual jets interact but also changes the flow characteristics of the respective free jets. The potential core length in the nozzle field is significantly reduced compared to the single nozzle. It is therefore not possible to make a direct transfer of the results. Direct transferability of the results is therefore not possible. This means that further studies on whole arrays are needed to optimise nozzle arrays.

Keywords: impingement jets; convective heat transfer; thermal process technology; potential core length; turbulent flow; PIV visualisation; turbulent kinetic energy

1. Introduction

Energy-intensive industries like metal, glass, or paper manufacturers use impingements jets to efficiently heat or cool products, where highly efficient nozzle systems are essential to minimise energy consumption [1]. Climate protection and resource efficiency are key issues in society and politics. Innovative and resource-efficient lightweight construction solutions are needed to reduce emissions and achieve our climate, sustainability, and electromobility goals [2]. High-strength aluminium and steel alloys are important factors for lightweight automotive construction. An amount of 100 kg less weight reduces the fuel consumption of a car by 0.7 l per 100 km. For electric vehicles a weight reduction is reflected in increased range. [3]. The materials optimised for these properties are characterised by demanding production routes, especially in terms of heat treatment. The complex requirements for the material properties place high demands on the nozzle systems. It is therefore imperative to continuously improve highly efficient nozzle systems for various applications across all industries.

Despite many studies [4] that have been carried out on impingement jets, further research is needed to optimise nozzle systems for specific applications with high Reynolds numbers $Re > 10{,}000$ due to the complex flow characteristics of impingement jets when striking a surface (see Figure 1). In this work, an industrial nozzle system used in the heat treatment of metal strips is analysed. The original nozzle array can be analysed without simplifications. An impingement jet can be divided into three zones: free jet zone, stagnation zone, and wall jet zone. For nozzle arrays an additional mixing zone is taken into consideration [5,6].

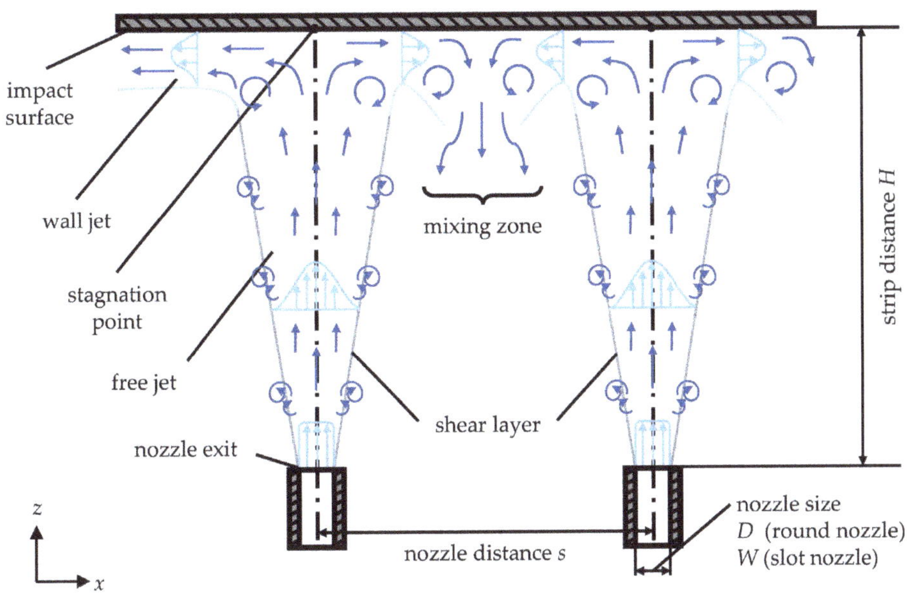

Figure 1. Schematic illustration of the flow of an impingement jet.

Starting from the nozzle, a free jet is formed which continuously expands and mixes with the surrounding medium (shear layer). As a result, the vertical velocity component decreases continuously until it is reduced to zero at the stagnation point. At the same time, the horizontal velocity component increases and a wall jet zone is formed. The area between individual nozzles in a nozzle field is referred to as a mixing zone. The characteristics of this flow depend on the nozzle geometry (round nozzle: nozzle diameter D, slot nozzle: slot width W), the distance between the nozzle outlet and the impact surface (strip distance H), the nozzle exit velocity u, and, in the case of a nozzle array, the distance between the individual nozzles s. In addition, the flow and therefore the heat transfer is very sensitive to the nozzle arrangement. A low ratio of strip distance to nozzle size is aimed for to maximise heat transfer but is not always technically feasible.

Within the free jet, the potential core jet is of importance for heat transfer. Here, the velocity remains constant and is equal to the nozzle exit velocity. The length of the core jet depends on the degree of turbulence of the nozzle flow and the nozzle exit velocity. The potential core jet length is defined as the position where the mean flow dynamic pressure (proportional to speed squared) reaches 95% of the initial value at the nozzle exit. For slot nozzles, the core jet length is between 4.7 and 7.7 times the nozzle width [7,8].

The basis for optimising nozzle systems is a sufficient understanding of the flow. The challenge is to visualise the real flows and their properties such as velocity and direction. One way to build up this understanding is through experiments supported by particle-based optical measurement techniques for describing velocities in flows. These include Laser Doppler Anemometry (LDA), Particle Image Velocimetry (PIV), Doppler Global

Velocimetry (DGV), and Laser Transit Velocimetry (LTV) [9]. PIV's ability to capture the flow velocity of a large number of points in an area simultaneously, the possibility for quantitative visualisation of flow structures, and gradient-based variables such as vorticity have led PIV to be used in various nozzle systems before [10]. Due to the wide range of applications of impingement jets, various optical flow investigations which have been carried out are summarised in Table 1.

Table 1. Optical flow studies on nozzle systems by other authors.

Author (Year)	Method	Nozzle System	Reynolds Number *Re*
Buchlin (2002) [11,12]	PIV/CFD	Slot nozzle array	11,000
Geers (2004) [13]	PIV/LDA	Single round nozzle (D = 36 mm) Round nozzle array (D = 12 mm)	23,000
Angioletti (2005) [14]	PIV	Single round nozzle	1000–4000
Wang (2016) [15]	PIV	Double slot nozzle (W = 5.8 mm)	9100
Khayrullina (2017) [16]	PIV/LDA	Single slot nozzle (W = 8; 16 mm)	7200–13,500
Nguyen (2019) [17]	PIV	Single square nozzle with round edges (W = 12.7 mm)	Re > 450,000
Berthold (2020) [18]	PIV	Round nozzle array (D = 12 mm)	7200
Barbosa (2022) [19]	PIV	Round nozzle array (D = 5 mm, X_{Nozzle} = 5)	5000
Barbosa (2023) [20]	PIV	Round nozzle array (D = 5 mm, X_{Nozzle} = 3)	5000

Different types of nozzles and settings have been studied, including single nozzles and nozzle arrays with different shapes. The focus of the studies is also varied, e.g., Barbosa et al. [19,20] investigate the influence of the impact plate shape. Only a few studies deal with flows Re > 10,000, resulting in a specific field of research for highly convective heat transfer, which is characterised by very high flow velocities and special nozzle systems. In addition, often only individual nozzles are investigated, leaving the transferability of results to entire nozzle arrays limited. Especially for slot nozzle arrays, there is little data availability.

The aim of this study is to fill this research gap by investigating highly convective air flows at Re = 10,000 to Re = 50,000 using PIV. The experiments are carried out on a single slot nozzle and on an array of slot nozzles. In particular, the visualisation of the flow in entire slot nozzle arrays on an industrial scale in thermal process technology is unique.

2. Experimental Setup and Data Processing

2.1. Experimental Test Rig

The test rig for concluding the heat transfer of industrial nozzle systems by determining both the heat transfer coefficient and the flow visualisation is shown in Figure 2. The test rig is based on a radial fan with a power of 90 kW_{el} and a maximum volume flow rate of 10,800 m^3/h.

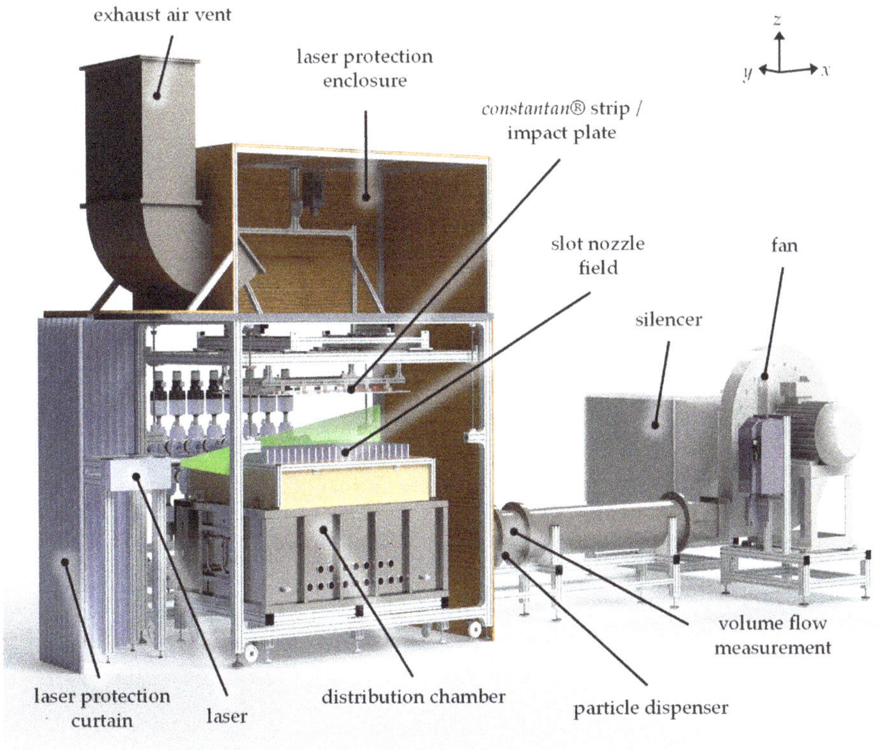

Figure 2. Test rig for optical flow measurements and heat transfer characterisation; dimensions: 8 m × 5 m × 4 m.

The fan draws in ambient air and accelerates it through an inlet section equipped with a flow meter into a distribution chamber. Particles are injected via the particle dispenser into the inlet section for visual observation of the flow. Various nozzle arrays up to industrial size (1480 × 1560 mm^2) can be mounted on the distribution chamber. The heat transfer coefficient was calculated based on measurements taken from an IR camera directed at an electrically heated constantan® strip. For further technical details please refer to the detailed description which is included by Trampe and Rademacher in [21].

This test rig was extended by laser measurement technology including a Nd:YAG laser, a camera system, a particle dispenser, and laser protection to carry out optical investigations of the flows within various nozzle systems. In order to investigate the flow of the impinging jets using laser-optical measurement techniques, the heated strip is replaced by a steep plate. This provides an accurate and straight edge for alignment of the PIV camera system and protects the sensitive electrical connections from contamination by the tracer particles. In addition, the test rig was equipped with a full laser protection system.

The presented results are derived by an investigation of a single slot nozzle with a slot width of W = 5 mm and length of L = 100 mm. The slot nozzle array consists of five single slot nozzles (W = 5 mm, L = 100 mm). According to Holger [22] heat transfer reaches its maximum when Equation (1) is satisfied.

$$s_{op} = \frac{7}{5}H \tag{1}$$

Since the strip distance is kept constant at H = 50 mm, a nozzle spacing of s = 70 mm results. Accordingly, a flow-optimised slot nozzle array is assumed in this work. The geometric data of the investigated nozzle systems are summarised in Figure 3. The hydraulic diameter D_h is given for the dimensionless relations. For a slot nozzle, this is $D_h = 2W$.

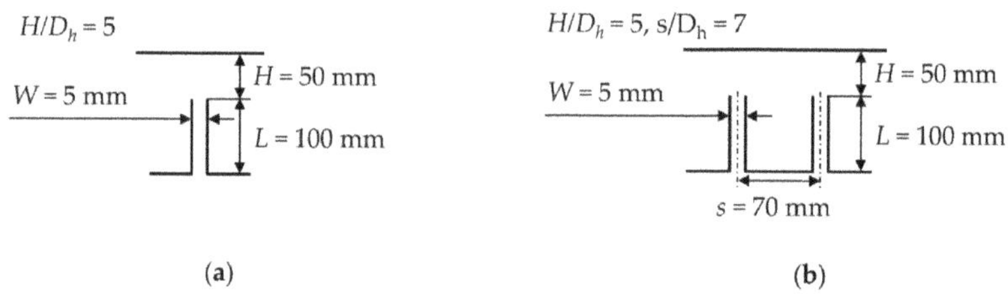

Figure 3. Schematic of the investigated (**a**) single nozzle and the (**b**) slot nozzle array.

The experiment utilised air as the test medium, with a temperature of T_{Air} = 30 °C, resulting in a fluid density ρ = 1.161 kg/m^3 and the dynamic viscosity η =17.1 µPa·s. The nozzle outlet velocity was determined through the usage of Equation (2) and the measurement of the dynamic pressure p at the nozzle outlet. Prior to each measurement, a pitot tube was installed and subsequently removed to avoid influencing the flow. The corresponding Reynolds numbers Re were calculated from the determined nozzle exit velocities using Equation (3).

$$u = \sqrt{\frac{2 \cdot p}{\rho}} \quad (2)$$

$$Re = \frac{\rho \cdot u \cdot 2W}{\eta} \quad (3)$$

For both nozzle systems three different nozzle exit velocities are investigated representing the range of different Reynolds numbers. Table 2 provides an overview of all tests carried out.

Table 2. Overview of the analysed nozzle exit velocities.

Nozzle System	Nozzle Exit Velocity u	Reynolds Number Re
Single slot nozzle	19.3 m/s	10,670
Single slot nozzle	48.7 m/s	33,750
Single slot nozzle	70.1 m/s	48,600
Slot nozzle array	15.4 m/s	13,360
Slot nozzle array	48.4 m/s	33,570
Slot nozzle array	70.8 m/s	49,080

As part of the experimental investigation, a comparison of the outlet velocities of the single slot nozzle and the slot nozzle array was ensured, with a comparable value being recorded in each case. The nozzle outlet velocity that could be stably set for the single slot nozzle was labelled u = 19.3 m/s, which is 4 m/s higher than that of the slot nozzle array. It was not possible to set a lower volume flow with the fan. Opening the nozzle box could have caused cross-flow.

2.2. Measurement Setup

The measurement setup for carrying out PIV measurements includes a laser, a high-resolution camera, and a computer for recording and processing the data. A double-pulsed Nd:YAG laser (wavelength 532 nm) from Litro Lasers Ltd. is used. The maximum pulse energy is 200 mJ with a pulse length of 6–9 ns. The repetition rate can be adjusted between 0–15 Hz. The light sheet of the laser has a width of 2 mm. The liquid di-ethyl-hexyl sebacate (DEHS) is used as tracer particles for applications in air. This odourless and colourless liquid has a density of ρ_p = 0.912 g/cm^3 and, using a seeding device from LaVision, has an average particle size of d_p < 1 µm [23].

The high-resolution Imager digital camera CX2-16 from LaVision is integrated into the test rig. The camera is aligned at 90° to the laser sheet with a distance of approximately 880 mm. The maximum resolution of the camera is 5312 × 3024 pixels. The image dimensions are 241.5 × 137.5 mm, obtaining a resolution of 22 pixels/mm. LaVision's DaVis 11 software is used for the processing of the measurement data. The local velocity vectors are calculated by cross-correlation, which is the basis for evaluating the PIV method [24]. For this purpose, the two recorded images are divided into frames of 64 × 64 pixels. An overlap factor of these frames is set on 75%. Further processing is used to reduce reflections and background noise. The background is deducted over a spatial length of 4 and a filter is used to remove or insert any outliers. In the following measurements, all outliers above 0.5 are removed and those below 3.0 are reinserted. Due to the processing parameters 20 vectors per orifice width are counted.

3. Results

The velocity and the turbulent kinetic energy (TKE) k distributions are determined for each case from the vector fields of the PIV measurements. While the velocity is derived directly from the vector displacement of the particle motion, the turbulent kinetic energy is calculated based on the Reynolds stress R_{xx} and R_{yy} according to Equation (4).

$$k = \frac{3}{4}\left(R_{xx} + R_{yy}\right) \tag{4}$$

Since a 2D planar PIV system is used in the present study, the turbulent kinetic energy can only be calculated in the laser slice plane with the vector components V_x and V_y. It is assumed that the turbulent kinetic energy in the third not-measured dimension V_z has the same dimension as V_x and V_y [25]. Turbulent kinetic energy characterises the energy in the fluctuating velocity field and can therefore be understood as a measure of the energy content of the turbulent motion in a flow. Since it is well known that heat transfer increases with increasing turbulence, knowledge of the distribution of turbulent kinetic energy is an important contribution for the optimisation of nozzle systems [26].

The singe-slot nozzle was measured within a range from x = ± 40 mm. The measurement of the slot nozzle array focused on the middle three nozzles (x = ± 90 mm). This allows the influence of increasing nozzle exit velocities on the formation of flow structures to be analysed. In addition, for the slot nozzle array, the interaction between the nozzles can be evaluated. To ensure a visual comparison of the data between the results of the single slot nozzle and the slot nozzle array, the scales per nozzle exit velocity have been kept the same. However, it should be noted that the TKE values of the slot nozzle array exceed the maximum value of the scale. Adjusting the scales to present the results of the single slot nozzle would result in a significant loss of information. This also applies to standardised scaling over the velocities.

3.1. Single Slot Nozzle

Initially, the flow through a single slot nozzle with a strip distance of H = 50 mm is analysed at different nozzle exit velocities. Figure 4a shows the velocity distributions for the three different exit velocities, while Figure 4b illustrates the corresponding distributions of turbulent kinetic energy. Note that the scales had to be adapted to the increasing exit velocity. A uniform scaling across all velocities leads to reduced contrast, resulting in reduced readability of the measured data.

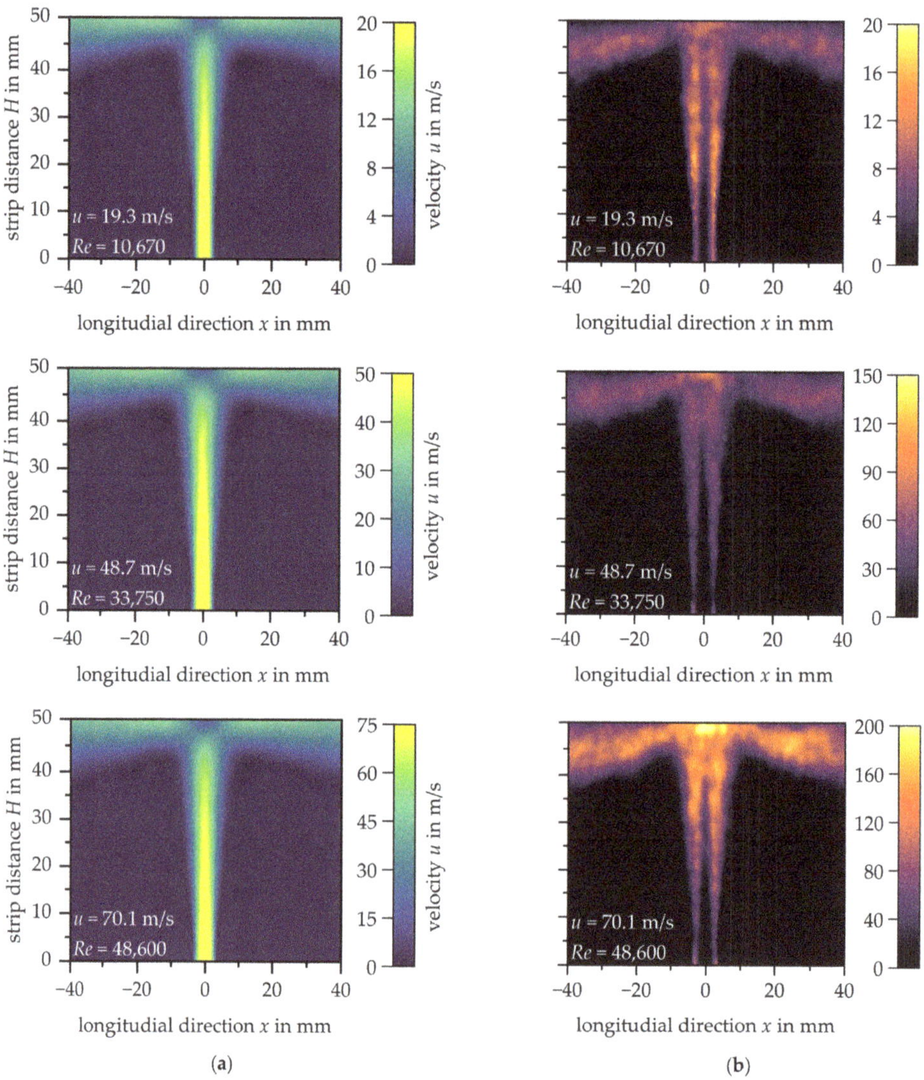

Figure 4. Representation of (**a**) the velocity and (**b**) the turbulent kinetic energy distribution for an impingement jet with three different nozzle exit velocities with H = 50 mm.

The influence of the nozzle exit velocity u on the flow is limited since only higher velocities in both the free jet and the wall jet can be observed. The dimension of the stagnation zone remains unaffected, as does the expansion of the shear layer.

The distribution of turbulent kinetic energy (TKE) throughout the impingement jet changes with increasing nozzle exit velocity. Turbulent kinetic energy is generally lowest in the centre of the free jet and wall region and highest in the shear layers of the free jet and the wall jet. The formation of the impingement jet is symmetrical.

For the lowest nozzle exit velocity of u = 19.3 m/s (Re = 10,670), the highest turbulent kinetic energy of k = 15 m^2/s^2 is reached in the shear layer of the free jet. The turbulent kinetic energy increases with increasing nozzle exit velocity at u = 48.7 m/s and reaches its maximum at the stagnation point at k = 95 m^2/s^2. The wall jet reaches a turbulent kinetic energy value up to k = 65 m^2/s^2. In the shear layer of the free jet a turbulent kinetic energy of k = 40 m^2/s^2 is reached.

At the maximum investigated nozzle exit velocity u = 70.1 m/s, the turbulent kinetic energy reaches up to k = 200 m^2/s^2 at the stagnation point. It is noticeable that the zone of increased turbulent kinetic energy in the area of the stagnation point expands as the nozzle exit velocity increases. Analogous to the doubling of the turbulent kinetic energy at the stagnation point of the impingement jet by increasing the nozzle exit velocity from u = 48.7 m/s to u = 70.1 m/s, the turbulent kinetic energy in the wall jet (k = 134 m^2/s^2) and in the shear zone (k = 89 m^2/s^2) also doubles.

3.2. Slot Nozzle Array

Single nozzles are not commonly used in an industrial setting; therefore, a slot nozzle array consisting of five single slot nozzles is considered. The flow from the three centre nozzles is evaluated as it is anticipated that the flow formation will repeat symmetrically. The left nozzle appears to be slightly displaced inwards. This, however, does not affect the key findings of the study. Figure 5a shows the velocity distribution of the slot nozzle array at a nozzle exit velocity of u = 15.4 m/s.

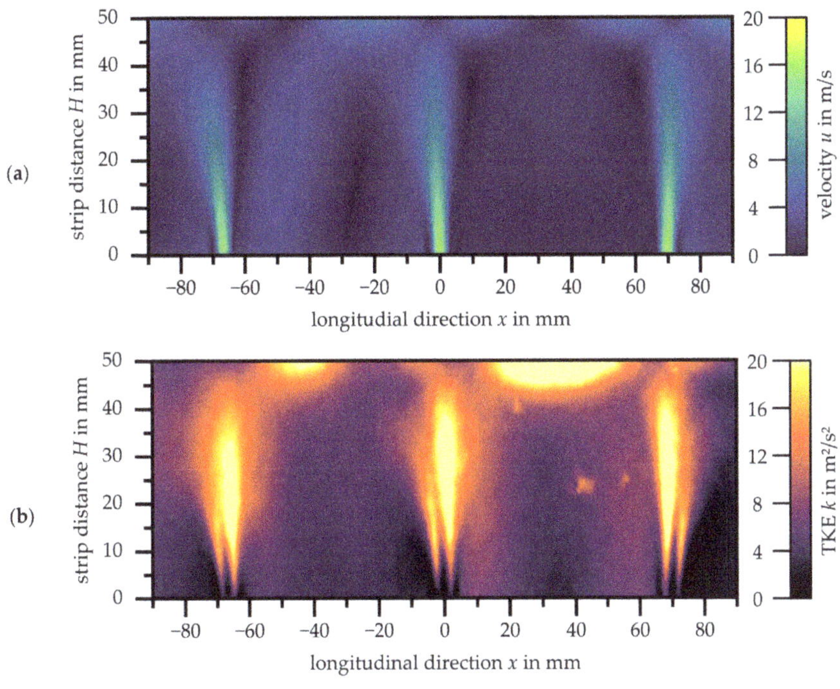

Figure 5. Representation of (**a**) the velocity and (**b**) the turbulent kinetic energy distribution for an impact jet array with a nozzle exit velocity of u = 15.4 m/s with H = 50 mm.

The impingement jets from each of the three nozzles are clearly visible. The mixing zone between the left and middle nozzle is more pronounced than the mixing zone between the middle and right nozzles. This is also apparent in the distribution of turbulent kinetic energy in Figure 5b. There are local maxima of $k = 20\ m^2/s^2$ both in the shear layer of the individual free jets and in the area of the mixing zone where two wall jets meet. The distribution of the turbulent kinetic energy in the individual impingement jet is not symmetrical.

Figure 6 provides in (a) the velocity distribution and in (b) the turbulent kinetic energy distribution of the slot nozzle array with a nozzle exit velocity of $u = 48.7$ m/s. Due to the increased nozzle exit velocity, the velocity in the wall jets also increases, resulting in a clearer formation of the wall jet flow and the flow in the mixing zone.

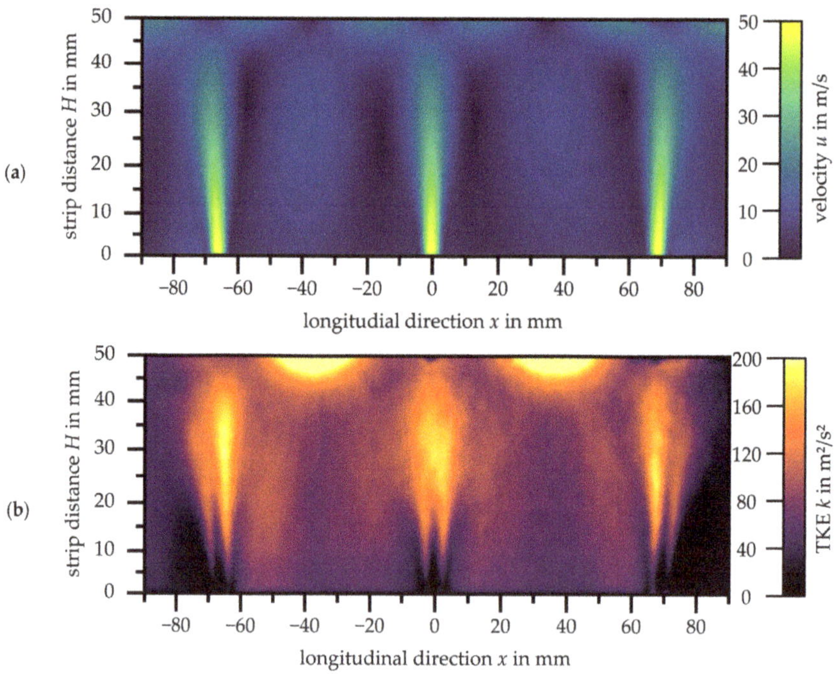

Figure 6. Representation of (**a**) the velocity and (**b**) the turbulent kinetic energy distribution for an impact jet array with a nozzle exit velocity of $u = 48.4$ m/s with $H = 50$ mm.

The areas with high turbulent kinetic energy have increased significantly in proportion. After just one third of the free jet, a turbulent kinetic energy of $k = 170\ m^2/s^2$ is reached in the entire impingement jet. The zone around the interaction between two wall jets has also increased and reaches a turbulent kinetic energy of $k = 200\ m^2/s^2$. It is now noticeable that the mixing zone extends between the nozzles. There is no change in the flow characteristics when the nozzle exit velocity is increased up to $u = 70.1$ m/s in the slot nozzle array (see Figure 7).

(a)

(b)

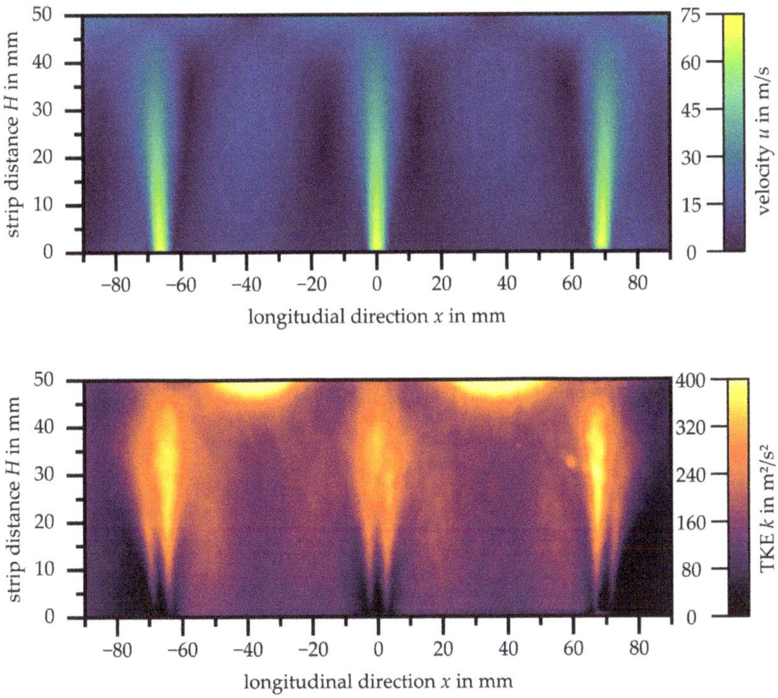

Figure 7. Representation of (**a**) the velocity and (**b**) the turbulent kinetic energy distribution for an impact jet array with a nozzle exit velocity of u = 70.8 m/s with H = 50 mm.

3.3. Uncertainty

The most important criterion for PIV measurements is that the tracer particles follow the flow for any velocity u without delay. The Stokes number, as shown in Equation (5), is used to verify this criterion. For $Stk << 1$ the particles follow the flow closely [9].

$$Stk = \frac{\tau_\mathrm{p}}{\tau_\mathrm{f}} \tag{5}$$

Therefore, τ_p describes the response time as defined in Equation (6) and τ_f is the characteristic time scale of the flow (see Equation (7)) [24].

$$\tau_p = d_p^2 \cdot \frac{\rho_\mathrm{p}}{18 \cdot \mu} \tag{6}$$

$$\tau_\mathrm{f} = \frac{L}{u} \tag{7}$$

The response time formula is valid for $Re < 1$. For the velocity range studied, Re is in the interval of Re = 10,000 to 50,000 (see Table 2). Due to the high Reynolds numbers, an additional factor, a standard drag correlation C_D, must be added [27]. The material data of the DEHS tracer particles (particle diameter d_p, particle density ρ_p) were mentioned in Section 2.2; the dynamic viscosity of the air is specified as $\mu = 1.185 \cdot 10^{-5}$ Pa·s. With the characteristic length of the slot nozzle $L = D_h = 2W$ and the additional factor C_D, this results in τ_p being between $1.86 \cdot 10^{-6}$ s–$1.98 \cdot 10^{-6}$ s. This leads to Stokes numbers between Stk = 0.00353–0.01384. Due to the small Stokes numbers for all velocities, the tracing error can be estimated to be less than 1% [9].

The overall measurement uncertainty is also analysed directly in the software DaVis based on the uncertainty of standard deviation [25]. According to Wieneke [28], a value of 0.01 pixels is considered 'excellent' and 0.3 pixels 'poor'. As an example, the measurement uncertainty is illustrated by the single slot nozzle with a nozzle exit velocity of u = 48.7 m/s in Figure 8. The measurement uncertainty of the velocity distribution u_u is shown in pixels in Figure 8a and in m/s in Figure 8b. At this point, both units are selected in order to show the accuracies of the PIV measurement carried out in pixels but also the more comprehensible deviation of the velocity distribution in m/s.

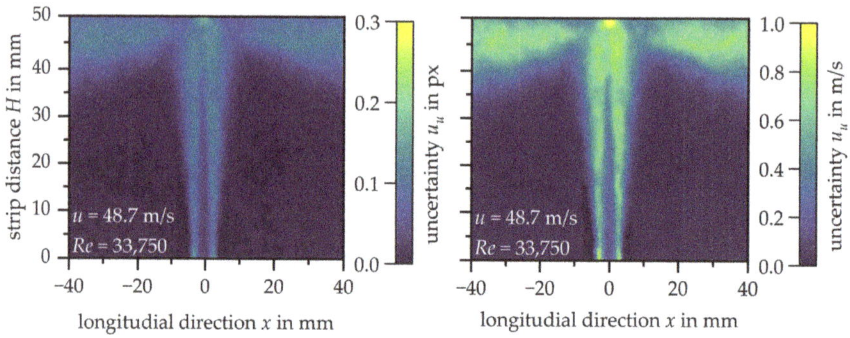

(**a**) (**b**)

Figure 8. Measurement uncertainty of the single slot nozzle at u = 48.7 m/s to be specified in (**a**) u_u in px and (**b**) u_u in m/s with H = 50 mm.

The measurement uncertainty of the PIV measurements is on average less than u_u < 0.1 px, except for the stagnation point, where the measurement uncertainty reaches its maximum deviation at u_u = 0.16 px. The illustration in Figure 8b shows that the corresponding measurement uncertainty is u_u = 0.5 m/s on average and the increased measurement uncertainty at the stagnation point is u_u = 1 m/s.

Figure 9 presents the measurement uncertainty u_u of the velocity distribution of the slot nozzle array with a nozzle exit velocity of u = 48.7 m/s, given in m/s. As with the single nozzle, the accuracy of the PIV in pixels is less than 0.1 px.

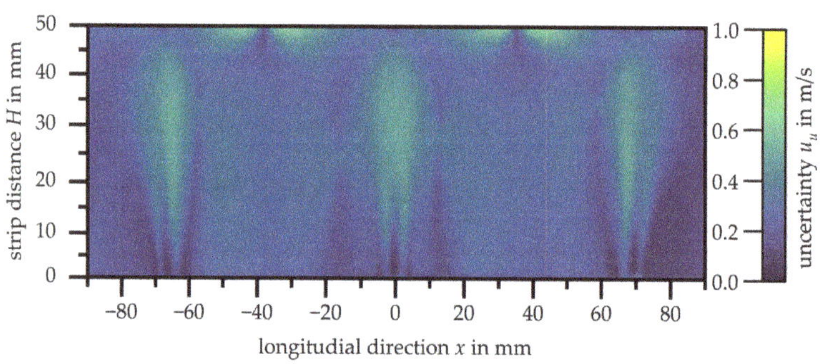

Figure 9. Measurement uncertainty of the slot nozzle array at u = 48.4 m/s to be specified in u_u in m/s with H = 50 mm.

The measurement uncertainty of the other investigated nozzle exit velocities are within the shown range and can be considered overall as 'good' according to Wieneke [28]. Higher accuracies, especially in the area near the stagnation point, have to be accepted at this point, as the focus is on a comprehensive flow investigation of the impingement jets. A high-resolution analysis of the boundary layer is beyond the scope of this study.

4. Conclusions

The highly convective flow of an impingement jet generated by a single slot nozzle (W = 5 mm) and a slot nozzle array consisting of five single slot nozzles with a nozzle spacing of s = 70 mm have been investigated for three different nozzle exit velocities. The nozzle exit velocities correspond to Reynolds numbers from approximately Re = 10,000 to 50,000. The resulting flow profiles of the single slot nozzle and the slot nozzle array are subsequently compared and evaluated.

The results for the single slot nozzle show that the formation of the characteristic flow pattern is independent from the nozzle exit velocity leading to an increase in the mean velocity of the impingement jet. The same applies to the turbulent kinetic energy distribution. The turbulent kinetic energy increases reciprocal to the increase in velocity. The same was observed when analysing the slot nozzle array. Furthermore, it can be seen that the velocity in the mixing zone increases with increasing nozzle exit velocity, which leads to a higher turbulent kinetic energy. Figure 10 compares the results of the single slot nozzle and the slot nozzle array at a nozzle exit velocity of $u \approx 48.5$ m/s. The central slot nozzle of the slot nozzle array has been selected for this comparison.

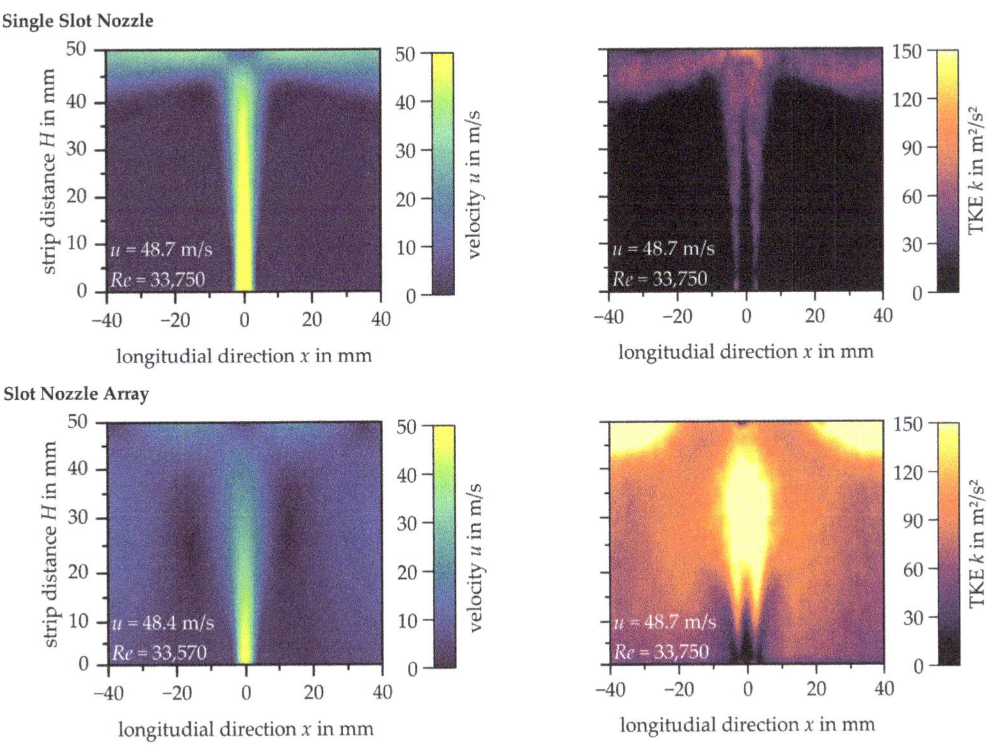

(a) (b)

Figure 10. Comparison of the (**a**) velocity and (**b**) turbulent kinetic energy distribution of the flow from a single slot nozzle and a slot nozzle array (centre nozzle) at a nozzle exit velocity of $u \approx 48.5$ m/s with H = 50 mm.

Comparison of the velocity profiles at the same nozzle exit velocity shows that the potential core jet length in the free jet of the impingement jet is about one third shorter for the centre nozzle of the slot nozzle array and therefore has a significantly lower velocity. Table 3 shows the theoretical velocities according to Livingood and Hrycak [7] for the associated nozzle exit velocities of the single slot nozzle as well as the centre nozzle in the slot nozzle array. The corresponding absolute core jet length and the core jet length as a function of the nozzle width W from the PIV measurement are also given in the table.

Table 3. Comparison of core jet lengths between single slot nozzle and slot nozzle array with $W = 5$ mm.

Nozzle System	Nozzle Exit Velocity	Velocity Potential Core Jet End	Core Length	Core Length W Related
Single slot nozzle	19.3 m/s	18.8 m/s	31.8 mm	6.4
Single slot nozzle	48.7 m/s	47.2 m/s	24.3 mm	6.9
Single slot nozzle	70.1 m/s	69.0 m/s	34.0 mm	6.8
Slot nozzle array	15.4 m/s	15.0 m/s	6.5 mm	1.3
Slot nozzle array	48.4 m/s	47.5 m/s	8.2 mm	1.6
Slot nozzle array	70.8 m/s	78.3 m/s	13.9 mm	2.8

With a relative core jet length of between 6.4 and 6.9, the core jet length of the single slot nozzle is within the range predicted by Zuckermann [8]. The reduced relative core jet length of 1.3 to 2.8 in the centre nozzle of the slot nozzle array deviates significantly from this specification. In the area between the core jet and the impact surface, a substantial reduction in the velocity of the impingement jet can be recognised.

In the mixing region of the impingement jet a higher velocity is observed due to the interaction with the adjacent jets for the slot nozzle array. The turbulent kinetic energy in the shear layer and in the area of the wall jet where the jets meet is three times higher compared to the single slot nozzle. Even between the nozzles, away from the shear layer, the turbulent kinetic energy is significantly higher. The reverse is observed at the stagnation point. Due to the reduced velocity in the stagnation zone of the slot nozzle array, no local maximum of the turbulent kinetic energy is reached here.

This finding leads to the conclusion that interference between multiple impinging jets is not limited to the mixing zone near the wall. The mixing zone partially extends along the length of the jet, resulting in further interaction with the jet. This leads to a significant reduction in the velocity of each individual impingement jet, but also to a disproportionate increase in turbulent kinetic energy. Geers [13] made similar observations when analysing single round nozzles and a round nozzle array. The flow in round nozzles is rotationally symmetrical, which is not the case with slot nozzles. Therefore, the results cannot be directly compared to each other. Nevertheless, this work confirms that it is not possible to extrapolate the results of flow investigations on individual nozzles to entire nozzle fields, without compensating for the observed interaction. Further investigations with other nozzle arrangements are essential to confirm the observations of both studies. Larger nozzle spacings are expected to reduce the interaction between the impinging jets, but the effect on the core jet length is still largely unknown.

Due to the limited database for impingement flows from slot nozzle systems, there is a need for further research. Most of the work has been carried out on single nozzles, and the present work raises questions about the applicability of the flow results to nozzle arrays. For this reason, experimental and numerical investigations on impinging heat transfer problems, especially for industrial applications, must examine more nozzle arrays. Otherwise, the extrapolated results from single slot nozzles will not be sufficient for the efficient design of nozzle systems.

Author Contributions: E.T., I.D., D.B., H.P. and C.W. Conceptualization, methodology, software, validation, and formal analysis, investigation, resources, data curation, writing—original draft preparation, writing—review and editing, visualization, supervision, project administration, funding acquisition. All authors have read and agreed to the published version of the manuscript.

Funding: This research received no external funding.

Data Availability Statement: Data are contained within the article.

Acknowledgments: The presented experimental data were generated during trials within the IGF project ("Impingement jets—Development and experimental validation of numerical heat transfer models for impingement jets"; IGF no. 22751 N) funded by the Federal Ministry for Economic Affairs and Climate Action based on a resolution of the German Bundestag.

Conflicts of Interest: The authors declare no conflict of interest.

Nomenclature

The following abbreviations are used in this manuscript:

C_D	Standard drag correlation	
D	Diameter (round nozzle)	mm
d_p	Particle diameter	µm
H	Strip distance	mm
k	Turbulent kinetic energy	m^2/s^2
L	Nozzle length	mm
s_{op}	Optimised nozzle distance	mm
Re	Reynolds number	
R_{xx}, R_{yy}	Reynolds stress	
s	Nozzle distance	mm
Stk	Stokes number	
u	Nozzle exit velocity	m/s
u_u	Uncertainty of the velocity distribution	m/s, px
V_x, V_y, V_z	Vector components	
W	Width	mm
X	Number of nozzles	
μ	Dynamic viscosity	Pa·s
ρ_p	Particle density	g/cm^3
ρ_{Fluid}	Fluid density	g/cm^3
τ_f	Response time	s
τ_p	Characteristic time scale	s

References

1. Fleiter, T.; Rehfeldt, M.; Hirzel, S.; Neusel, L.; Aydemir, A.; Schwotzer, C.; Kaiser, F.; Gondorf, C.; Hauch, J.; Hof, J.; et al. *CO_2-Neutrale Prozesswärmeerzeugung*; UBA: New York, NY, USA, 2023.
2. European Parliament. Resolution of 15 January 2020 on the European Green Deal (2019/2956(RSP)). Available online: https://www.europarl.europa.eu/doceo/document/TA-9-2020-0005_EN.html (accessed on 4 March 2025).
3. Umweltbundesamt. Ökosteuer—Sparen Oder Zahlen?: Sprit Sparen und Mobil Sein. 2009. Available online: https://www.umweltbundesamt.de/sites/default/files/medien/publikation/long/3705.pdf (accessed on 4 March 2025).
4. Plant, R.D.; Friedman, J.; Saghir, M.Z. A review of jet impingement cooling. *Int. J. Thermofluids* **2023**, *17*, 100312. [CrossRef]
5. Bergman, T.L.; Lavine, A.S.; Incropera, F.P.; Dewitt, D.P. *Fundamentals of Heat and Mass Transfer*; John Wiley & Sons: Hoboken, NJ, USA, 2011; ISBN 978-0470-50197-9.
6. Hofmann, H.M. *Wärmeübergang Beim Pulsierenden Prallstrahl*; KIT Scientific Publishing: Karlsruhe, Germany, 2005; ISBN 3-937300-57-0.
7. Livingood, J.N.B.; Hrycak, P. Impingement Heat Transfer from Turbulent Air Jets to Flat Plates: A Literature Survey. NASA-TM-X-2778. 1973. Available online: https://ntrs.nasa.gov/citations/19730016200 (accessed on 4 March 2025).

8. Zuckerman, N.; Lior, N. *Jet Impingement Heat Transfer: Physics, Correlations, and Numerical Modeling*; Elsevier: Amsterdam, The Netherlands, 2006; pp. 565–631. ISBN 9780120200399.
9. *Springer Handbook of Experimental Fluid Mechanics*; Tropea, C., Ed.; Springer: Berlin/Heidelberg, Germany, 2007; ISBN 9783540302995.
10. Scharnowski, S.; Kähler, C.J. Particle image velocimetry—Classical operating rules from today's perspective. *Opt. Lasers Eng.* **2020**, *135*, 106185. [CrossRef]
11. Buchlin, J. Convective Heat Transfer in Impinging-Gas-Jet Arrangements. *JAFM* **2011**, *4*, 137–149. [CrossRef]
12. Buchlin, J.-M.; Gouriet, J.-B.; Planquart, P.; van Beeck, J.; Renard, M. Experimental and Numerical Study of Convective Heat Transfer in an Array of Slot Jets. In Proceedings of the 2002 ASME Joint U.S.-European Fluids Engineering Conference, Montreal, QC, Canada, 14–18 July 2002; pp. 13–19, ISBN 0-7918-3616-9.
13. Geers, L.F.G.; Tummers, M.J.; Hanjalic, K. Experimental investigation of impinging jet arrays. *Exp. Fluids* **2004**, *36*, 946–958. [CrossRef]
14. Angioletti, M.; Nino, E.; Ruocco, G. CFD turbulent modelling of jet impingement and Its validation by particle image velocimetry and mass transfer measurements. *Int. J. Therm. Sci.* **2005**, *44*, 349–356. [CrossRef]
15. Wang, H.; Lee, S.; Hassan, Y.A. Particle image velocimetry measurements of the flow in the converging region of two parallel jets. *Nucl. Eng. Des.* **2016**, *306*, 89–97. [CrossRef]
16. Khayrullina, A.; van Hooff, T.; Blocken, B.; van Heijst, G.J.F. PIV measurements of isothermal plane turbulent impinging jets at moderate Reynolds numbers. *Exp. Fluids* **2017**, *58*, 31. [CrossRef]
17. Nguyen, D.T.; Maher, B.; Hassan, Y. Effects of Nozzle Pressure Ratio and Nozzle-to-Plate Distance to Flowfield Characteristics of an Under-Expanded Jet Impinging on a Flat Surface. *Aerospace* **2019**, *6*, 4. [CrossRef]
18. Berthold, A.; Haucke, F.; Weiss, J. Flow Field Analysis of a Dynamically Forced Impingement Jet Array. In Proceedings of the AIAA Scitech 2020 Forum, Orlando, FL, USA, 6–10 January 2020; American Institute of Aeronautics and Astronautics: Reston, VA, USA, 2020; p. 1062020, ISBN 978-1-62410-595-1.
19. Barbosa, F.V.; Teixiera, S.F.; Teixeira, J.C. 2D PIV analysis of the flow dynamics of multiple jets impinging on a complex moving plate. *Int. J. Heat Mass Transf.* **2022**, *188*, 122600. [CrossRef]
20. Barbosa, F.V.; Teixeira, S.F.C.F.; Teixeira, J.C.F. Flow dynamics and heat transfer characterization of confined multiple jets impinging on a complex surface. *Exp. Fluids* **2023**, *64*, 153. [CrossRef]
21. Trampe, E.; Rademacher, N.; Wulfmeier, M.; Büschgens, D.; Pfeifer, H. A High-Resolution Method for the Experimental Determination of the Heat Transfer Coefficients of Industrial Nozzle Systems in Heat Treatment Plants. *Appl. Sci.* **2024**, *14*, 3024. [CrossRef]
22. Martin, H. Heat and Mass Transfer between Impinging Gas Jets and Solid Surfaces. In *Advances in Heat Transfer*; Elsevier: Amsterdam, The Netherlands, 1977; Volume 13, pp. 1–60. ISBN 9780120200139.
23. LaVision GmbH. Seeding Particles: DEHS. Available online: https://shop.lavision.de/en/seeding-particles/1/dehs (accessed on 4 March 2025).
24. Raffel, M. *Particle Image Velocimetry: A Practical Guide*, 3rd ed.; Springer International Publishing AG: Cham, Switzerland, 2018; ISBN 9783319688527.
25. LaVision GmbH. *Product Manual for DaVis 11.0*; LaVision GmbH: Göttingen, Germany, 2023.
26. Pope, S.B. *Turbulent Flows*; 1. Publ., 12. Print; Cambridge University Press: Cambridge, UK, 2015; ISBN 9780521591256.
27. COMSOL Multiphysics®. *Users Guide 5.6: Theory for the Particle Tracing for Fluid Flow Interface*; COMSOL: Stockholm, Sweden, 2020.
28. Wieneke, B. PIV uncertainty quantification from correlation statistics. *Meas. Sci. Technol.* **2015**, *26*, 74002. [CrossRef]

energies

MDPI

Article

Application of Neural Network Models for Analyzing the Impact of Flight Speed and Angle of Attack on Flow Parameter Non-Uniformity in a Turbofan Engine Inlet Duct

Adam Kozakiewicz, Maciej Adamczyk * and Rafał Kieszek

Institute of Aviation Technology, Faculty of Mechatronics, Armament and Aerospace, Military University of Technology, 00-908 Warszawa, Poland; adam.kozakiewicz@wat.edu.pl (A.K.); rafal.kieszek@wat.edu.pl (R.K.)

* Correspondence: maciej.adamczyk01@wat.edu.pl; Tel.: +48-510-146-332

Abstract: This study investigates the aerodynamic performance of a fourth-generation normal shockwave inlet system, with a primary focus on minimizing pressure losses and ensuring uniform airflow distribution. A computational model was developed, incorporating a section of the fuselage along with the complete inlet duct. The model was discretized using a hybrid mesh approach to enhance numerical accuracy. The analysis was conducted at a flight altitude of 8000 m, encompassing 370 distinct cases defined by varying angles of attack and Mach numbers. This comprehensive parametric study yielded a dataset of 10,800 total pressure measurements across predefined sampling locations. Based on the obtained results, flow distortion coefficients in both circumferential (CDI) and radial directions (RDI) were systematically determined for each test case. The interdependencies between CDI, RDI, Mach number, and angle of attack (α) were analyzed and presented in a consolidated manner. In the second phase of the study, an artificial neural network (ANN) utilizing a Feed-Forward architecture was implemented to predict pressure distributions for intermediate flight conditions. The ANN was trained using the CFG algorithm, and the predictive accuracy was assessed through the determination coefficients computed by comparing ANN-based estimates with numerical simulation results. The findings demonstrate the efficacy of ANN-based modeling in enhancing the predictive capabilities of inlet flow dynamics, offering valuable insights for optimizing next-generation supersonic air intake systems.

Keywords: turbofan engine; inlet system; AIP; circumferential pressure distortion index; radial pressure distortion index; neural network

1. Introduction

The task of individual aircraft components and systems is to ensure their integrity and optimization for the changing nature of the missions performed by the aircraft. As a result of the evolution of these requirements, further concepts have emerged and developed in the design of individual components and systems, including the propulsion systems and their components. All aviation turbine engines are turbomachines that require the air supply necessary for their operation, up to 1200 kg/s. The basic task of the inlet system is to pre-compress and, above all, to supply a sufficient, stable, uniform airflow to the engine compressor. Given the complexity of the problem, determining the appropriate design criterion for the inlet system design and the inlet system control solution must consider the following basis:

- flight speed and altitude;
- angles at which the flight is performed;
- shape of the inlet cross-section;
- inlet location in the fuselage;
- length of flow duct;
- mechanization system;
- stealth technology.

The final compromise in the design of the inlet system is based on the criterion between the parameters determining pressure loss and the aerodynamic drag. The pressure loss coefficient relates to the internal efficiency of the inlet duct and significantly affects the engine thrust through the mass flow rate. It is estimated that for every 1% increase in pressure loss, the engine thrust decreases by the same or greater amount. The phenomenon is intensifying and is non-linear, especially for high Mach numbers, where for example, for Mach number = 2.0 with a pressure loss of 8%, the engine thrust decreases by 13% while fuel consumption increases by 5% [1]. The design, and the operation of the inlet system, which is a simple component, involves many decisions that affect not only the performance of the engine but also the overall functionality of the entire aircraft.

In the area of turbine engine inlet systems, some studies are being conducted on the criteria mentioned. The analysis of inlet operation at high angles of attack [2–5] is of great interest. For example, the study [2] examined the inlet of an F/A-18A supersonic aircraft. The calculations dealt with pressure field distribution and inlet vortices. Static pressure distributions on the front part of the fuselage surface were studied. The results from the flight tests were comparable to the numerical results. The problem of vortex migration was presented. It has been proved that vortices generated along the inlet edge can be less intense. The effects of the inlet edge were found to have a significant impact on the development of the secondary flow field in the inlet duct.

Another problem may be the shape of the inlet duct [3,6]. A study of the flow in an S-type duct was performed in the article [3]. Reference aerodynamic data for compressible flow through the S-type duct were presented. The results of measurements of the three-dimensional velocity field, total pressure, and static pressure were presented. Thin turbulent boundary layers were achieved at the inlet. The results present that an area of flow separation occurred in the duct. Measurements indicate that the curvature of the duct induced strong secondary flows, which may be amplified by pressure. The analyses performed showed that these vortices moved low-momentum fluid from the boundary layer toward the center of the duct, degrading both the uniformity and magnitude of the overall pressure profile.

The issue of the pressure loss coefficient and the distortion of the total inlet pressure as a function of flight maneuverability is included in the article [7]. A study of the recovery (pressure loss coefficient) of the inlet pressure and distortion effects observed under varying maneuverability conditions of the F-16 aircraft was conducted. The maneuverability of the F-16 was defined using three parameters: Mach number, angle of attack, and angle of bank. Pressure recovery and distortion values were measured at the aerodynamic interface plane (AIP). Two simulations were performed: one to compare flight conditions at sea level and 10 km altitude. The results of the flight level comparison showed a slightly higher pressure loss coefficient of 0.985 at 10 km altitude compared to a value of 0.983 at sea level. The obtained values of the distortion coefficient of the impact pressure fields for both conditions were similar and amounted to 0.120.

Analyses of the performance of the fuselage-integrated Diverterless Supersonic Inlet (DSI) are being carried out for the most maneuverable aircraft. The study [8] presents the results of an experimental study to investigate the effect of the angle of attack on the performance of the DSI. Experiments were conducted using a typical front part of the fuselage, including an elliptical nose, to consider the effect of fuselage geometry on the incoming flow. Tests were conducted at a constant Mach number of free stream, $M\infty = 1.65$, zero bank angle, and various angles of attack ranging from −2 to 6 degrees. Consequently, for a positive angle of attack, the DSI yield point moves towards subcritical conditions, and for a negative angle, it deviates towards supercritical conditions.

The use of neural networks in this area is proving to be an important element of modern aircraft engine research. The application of ANN in the aviation industry is rapidly evolving and plays a significant role in engineering research. Dong et al. [9] present a review of current studies in this field. Five deep learning methods are introduced, and their applications in aviation are discussed. The authors observed that the current use of artificial neural networks is expanding in the areas of aircraft design, dynamics and control, and aircraft operations monitoring. Examples of this kind of work can be found in the articles [10–16]. These studies focus on optimizing the structure of the components [10,11], diagnosing the powerplant system [12,13], and investigating detailed aerodynamic behaviors under various flight conditions [14]. The application of ANN is also widely utilized in operational aspects, such as fuel consumption prediction [15] and the improvement of radionavigation systems [16]. Published studies have not examined the potential use of ANN for detailed aerodynamic analyses of flow disturbances in the inlet systems of combat aircraft. The introduction of ANN in this area could enable significantly faster and more efficient analyses of fuselage–intake interactions, as well as the patterns and distributions of disturbances under various flight conditions. This is particularly relevant in cases where analysis requires the consideration of a large number of computational scenarios, such as varying flight speeds, angles, and altitudes. The application of more efficient and faster methods for characterizing the performance of inlet systems could also potentially be utilized in aircraft or engine control systems.

The authors of this article discuss issues related to the study of inlet systems in terms of flow issues regarding the influence of various factors on vortex formation and the stability of the operation of this component. The accumulated experience and development of numerical models for individual intake systems are discussed in articles [17–19]. The new tool of neural networks is also used in the analyses [20,21].

This study combines two areas of scientific activity. As a first stage, the analysis was performed and thus, the effects of changes in the angle of attack and Mach number on the distributions of flow non-uniformity expressed by dimensionless pressure coefficients were presented. In the second stage, using the obtained database, calculations were performed based on neural networks.

This study investigates the impact of flight speed and angle of attack on flow parameter non-uniformity in a turbofan engine inlet duct, focusing on flow distortion and pressure loss. By integrating numerical simulations with artificial neural networks (ANN), the research enhances predictive capabilities for aerodynamic performance assessment. The first stage involves high-fidelity numerical simulations analyzing circumferential and radial distortion indices (CDI and RDI) under 370 flight conditions, covering the Mach number and angle of attack variations. This yields a dataset of 10,800 total pressure measurements. The study examines how these parameters influence inlet flow stability and uniformity, which are critical for efficient engine operation. In the second stage, a Feed-Forward ANN trained with the CFG algorithm predicts pressure distributions for intermediate flight conditions, reducing computational costs compared to traditional simulations. The ANN model's accuracy is evaluated through determination coefficients comparing predicted CDI and RDI values with numerical results. This research contributes to optimizing turbofan inlet design by demonstrating the effectiveness of ANN-based modeling in aerodynamic flow analysis. The findings support future advancements in supersonic and highly maneuverable aircraft propulsion systems, improving efficiency and performance under diverse operational conditions.

2. Computational Fluid Dynamics (CFD) Modeling Approach

A so-called fourth-generation normal shockwave inlet system was used for the study. This type of inlet is characterized by a cross-sectional, ellipse-type shape and a relatively short inlet duct. The requirements for this construction solution are high efficiency (performance) over a wide range of mean Mach numbers (0.60 ÷ 1.20) and a simple design with no changing geometries, which also ensures a lower mass. Therefore, this type of inlet has been referred to as a 'normal shockwave' and is placed centrally under the fuselage, which is the optimum solution for a high-maneuverability aircraft. As for the disadvantages of this type of inlet, these include increased aerodynamic drag and greater distortion generated at high flight speeds. In addition, there is an increased risk associated with the FOD phenomenon when the engine is running on the ground.

A hybrid mesh, which is a combination of structured and unstructured elements, was used to digitize the inlet system model. Hybrid mesh allowed us to accurately reproduce the complex geometry of the aircraft fuselage. In principle, the fluid domain consists of tetrahedral cells. Five layers of prismatic mesh were applied to the structural mesh on the fuselage and in the inlet duct to increase the accuracy of the results in the near-wall layer body. The final dimensions of the computational domain were 40.0 [m] × 22.0 [m] × 22.0 [m]. To improve the calculation results, a Body of Influence was added around the object. By applying this approach, it is possible to maintain a high accuracy of results in an area where changes in fluid parameters are expected to be large, while at the same time having a smaller total number of elements. The dimensions of the BOI are 7.16 [m] × 4.0 [m] × 3.746 [m]. The final mesh consisted of over 8 million elements, with an average skewness of 0.22649 and an average orthogonality of 0.77254. The lowest mesh quality was observed at the sharp upper edge of the inlet, which caused significant stretching of the triangular surface mesh, resulting in elements with skewness higher than average. Prior to conducting the main computations, a mesh dependency analysis was performed using three different grid resolutions: 6 million, 8 million, and 10 million elements with and without BOI. The criterion selected for this analysis was the average outlet pressure of the inlet system. The final mesh was chosen based on the best trade-off between computational cost and result quality, given the available hardware resources. The applied mesh has been presented in Figure 1.

A pressure far-field boundary condition was used for the external surfaces, which corresponds to the undisturbed flow under flight conditions. The plane located at the end of the inlet duct, downstream of which the engine fan is located, is assigned a pressure outlet boundary condition with atmospheric pressure value that allows the vacuum at the outlet of the fluid domain to be altered to match the natural operating conditions of the inlet system. Calculations were conducted with the k-ω SST turbulence model due to its effective representation of flows in both wall-adjacent areas and free-stream regions.

The analysis was performed for a flight altitude of 8000 m. The atmospheric parameters at the analyzed altitude were assumed according to the ISA model. A distribution of measuring points was introduced for further analysis and determination of coefficients (Figure 2). The Ansys Fluent software (2023 R2) allows the definition of fixed points or lines (Rake/Line function), which can be used to read parameter values or visualizations. The function allows a specified number of points to be positioned at fixed distances relative to defined geometric parameters. This resulted in a consistent distribution of points, irrespective of the changing shape of the channel (transition from an ellipse section to a circular section).

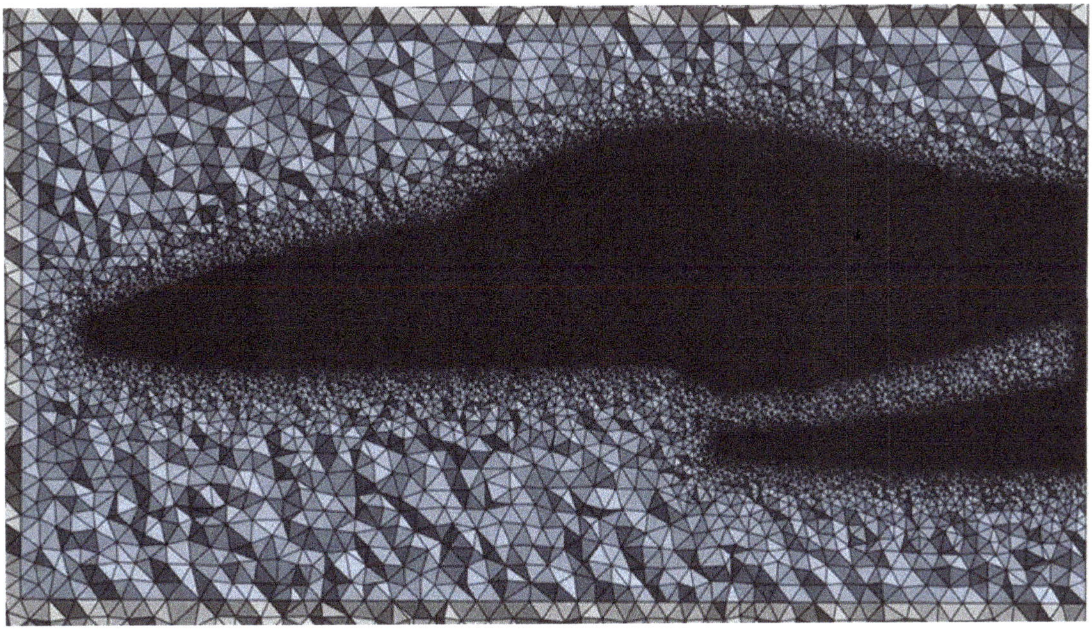

Figure 1. Mesh in the plane of symmetry of the intake duct.

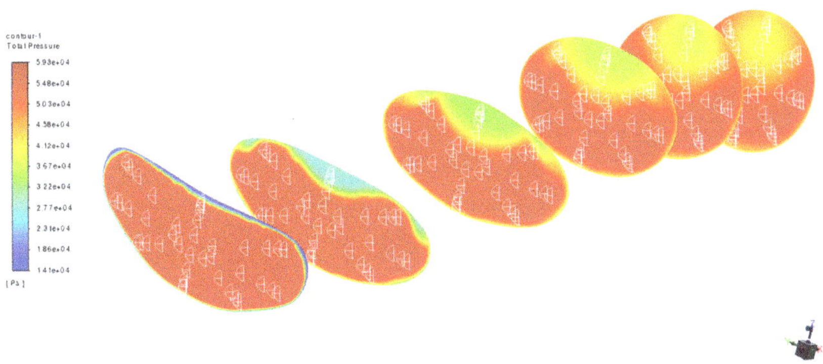

Figure 2. Applied distribution of measuring points in the inlet duct.

Figure 3 shows the distribution of design points on the final cross-section (AIP) of the inlet duct. The points were distributed in five rings, every 45°, using a slight density towards the inlet duct wall. Determining the coefficients based on the selected points allows a quantitative description of the uniformity of the pressure field at the outlet of the inlet system. Total pressure values were taken from the designated points, and the cross-sectional area-weighted average total pressure was determined. This resulted in 40 total pressure values for each of the ten angles of attack cases. In total, 370 cases (combinations of angle of attack and Mach number) were analyzed, resulting in a total of read 10,800 total pressure values for the adopted number of measuring points.

For the operation of the inlet system, the most critical factor is the uniformity of the pressure distribution. In the literature, two coefficients are commonly used to describe the intensity of disturbances along the circumferential and radial directions of the inlet cross-section. Based on the obtained results, two coefficients describing the intensity of the flow distortion in the inlet system were determined:

- Circumferential distortion index CDI, presents the relative value of the deviation, minimum pressure to the mean value in a given circle:

$$CDI = \frac{p_{i_r} - p_{i_{min}}}{p_{i_r}}, \quad (1)$$

where
p_{i_r}—average pressure for the *i*-th ring [Pa],
$p_{i_{min}}$—minimal average pressure for the *i*-th ring [Pa].

- Radial distortion index (RDI) presents the relative value of the pressure deviation for a given circle relative to the average pressure of the entire cross-section:

$$RDI = \frac{p_{0_r} - p_{i_r}}{p_{0_r}}, \quad (2)$$

where
p_{i_r}—average pressure for the *i*-th ring [Pa],
p_{0_r}—average pressure for the entire cross-section [Pa].

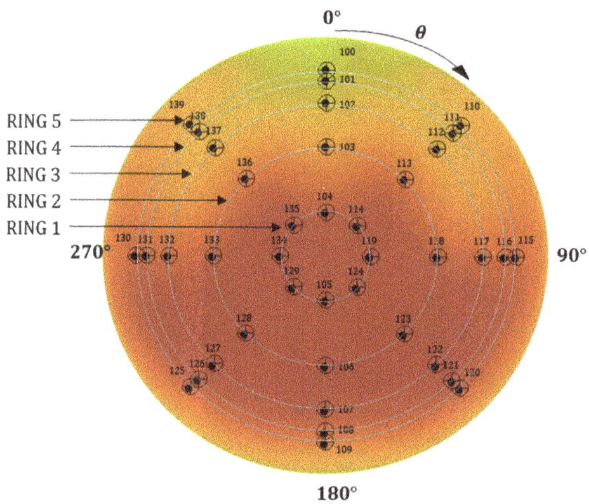

Figure 3. Applied distribution of design points in the AIP cross-section of the inlet duct.

The characteristics of the CDI and RDI coefficients as a function of flight speed and angle of attack for the inlet system are presented in Figure 4. The determined values for specific Mach numbers and angles of attack were presented as points for which approximation curves were then determined for each angle of attack using a third-degree polynomial. The curve highlighted in red, according to the mean values, comes from the entire range of angles of attack. As the observed distortion has an obvious single-lobe pattern, the RDI coefficient values are an order of magnitude smaller than CDI. An increased angle of attack does not result in an increased distortion of the total pressure field at the AIP cross-section in every case. Some combinations of flight speed and angle of attack will cause the area of reduced pressure to shift toward the center of the duct cross-section. As a general rule, however, the distortion of the inlet flow increases as the Mach number increases. The intensity of the distortion generated in the circumferential direction is several times greater than the radial element for all the angles of attack that are being studied in this article. For low Mach numbers, in the range Ma = 0.30 ÷ 0.65, there are strong dependencies of the observed distortion as a function of the angle of attack. The spread of coefficient values is significant in this respect. Higher flight speeds result in greater stability of the distortion against changes in the angle of attack, even though the distortion itself generally increases as the Mach number increases.

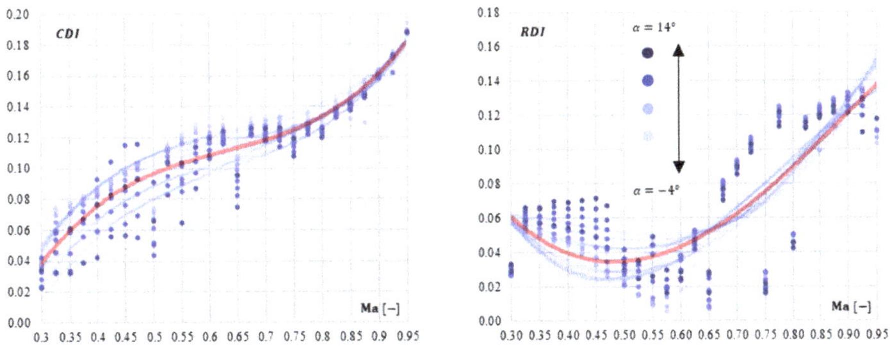

(**a**) (**b**)

Figure 4. Characteristics regarding the effect of Mach number and angle of attack (α) on the variation of: (**a**) CDI; and (**b**) RDI coefficients.

Figure 5 presents a generalization of the CDI coefficient as a function of the Mach number and angle of attack α. Regarding the circumferential distortion generated by the inlet system, there is a strong relationship concerning flight speed and thus Mach number. As such, it should be regarded as the most significant parameter affecting the distortion, in contrast to the angle of attack, which does not affect the obtained values of the CDI parameter to such a significant extent. Nevertheless, the distortion values for negative angles of attack are higher than for positive angles of attack. The underlying cause of this phenomenon is mainly the nature of the shockwave entering the inlet, which naturally increases in strength with the increasing flight speed.

Figure 6 presents an analogous generalization of the RDI coefficient in terms of the Mach number and angle of attack α. The radial distortion presents the lowest values for all angles of attack in the range of numbers Ma = 0.55 ÷ 0.60. Thus, for low Mach numbers, below Ma = 0.50, the occurring radial distortions are several times higher for positive angles of attack than for negative angles of attack, with a completely inverse relationship occurring for high Mach numbers above Ma = 0.65. Nevertheless, again, the main factor on which RDI values depend is the Mach number. It is important to note the cyclic operation of the inlet system concerning the decreasing value of the RDI coefficient for the areas in the range Ma = 0.60, through Ma = 0.70, 0.78, and 0.85. In these fields, there are large gradients of change in the RDI coefficient, reaching up to six times the value. Analyzing the behavior of the CDI coefficient value from this angle (Figure 5), no such large changes were obtained in the circumferential direction. For the inlet system being studied, the intensity of both the radial and circumferential distortion, it is to be believed, will depend mainly on the wave phenomena occurring in the inlet duct. For high flight speeds, and therefore high Mach numbers, the non-uniformity of the pressure field will be significant, due to the occurrence of a separation zone in the upper part and center of the fan inlet cross-section.

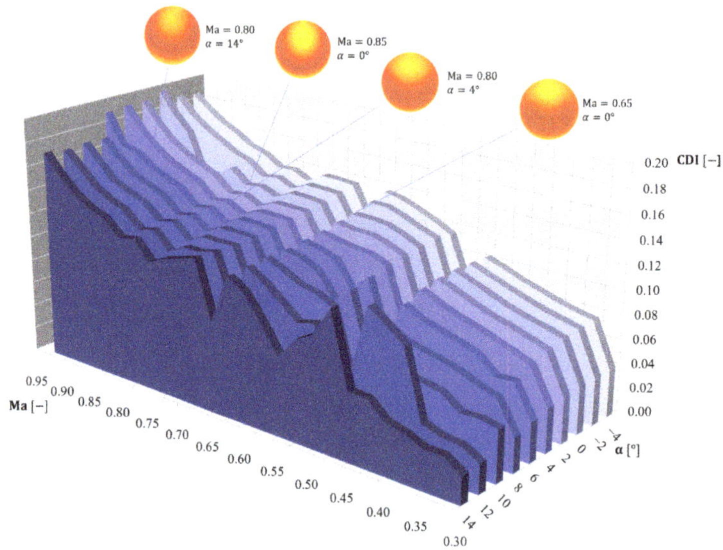

Figure 5. Characteristics of the CDI coefficient as a function of Mach number and angle of attack.

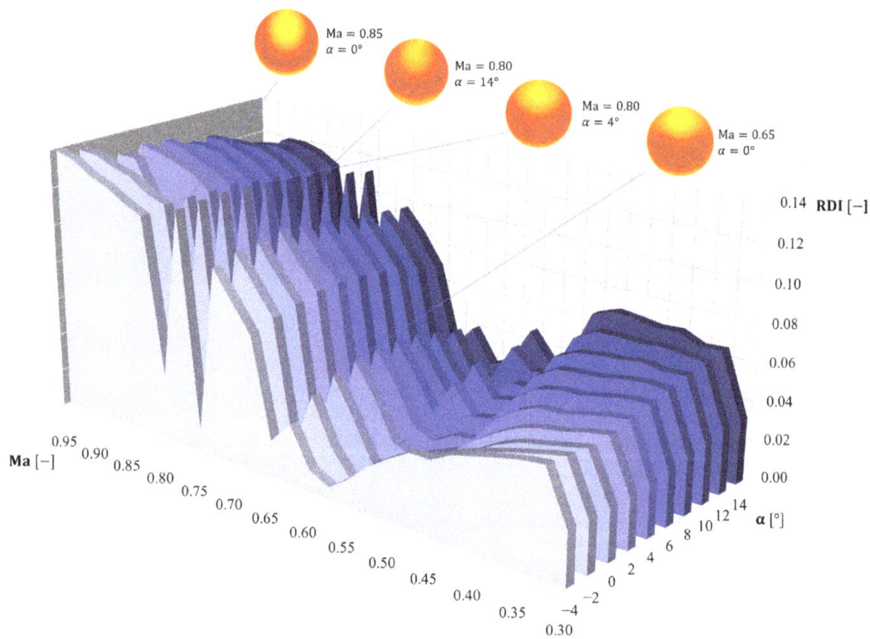

Figure 6. Characteristics of the RDI coefficient as a function of Mach number and angle of attack.

The geometry of the investigated inlet duct results in a characteristic single-lobe distortion pattern in the upper part of the initial cross-section. The separation occurs as a result of the curvature of the channel and originates at the edge of the diverter. An increase in the angle of attack of the aircraft for a given Mach number increases the separation zone observed on the last cross-section of the inlet duct (AIP). The increase in Mach number also increases the intensity of distortion generated in the inlet system, with the increases being much greater than when the angle of attack is increased. The most intense distortions occur for flights and maneuvers performed with a Mach number of Ma = 0.95.

3. Artificial Neural Network

The second part of the study used a Feed-Forward neural network to predict the pressure distribution in the inlet for intermediate values of angles of attack (α) and Mach numbers (Ma_H). The input parameters required to train the ANN are the angle of attack of the selected aircraft $\alpha \in \langle -10; 16 \rangle^{\circ}$, i.e., 2°, and the Mach number $Ma_H \in \langle 0.3; 0.925 \rangle$, i.e., 0.025. The output parameters from the network are the total pressure p^* [Pa]. The same six sections as in the first part were used for the study. Forty landmarks, numbered according to the scheme on each cross-section, have been identified in Figure 7.

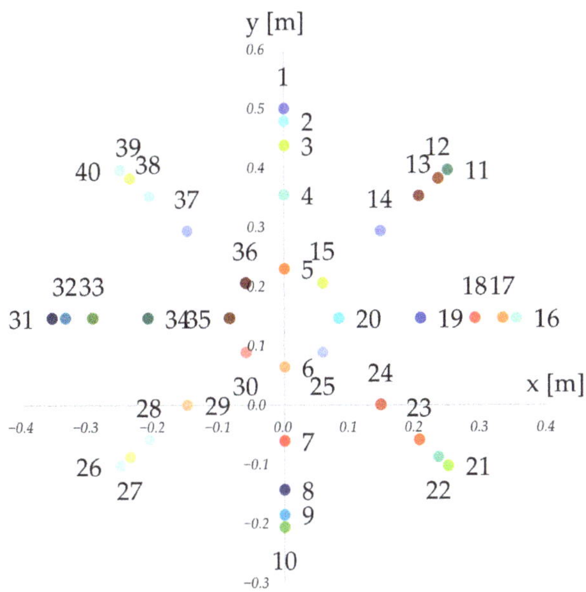

Figure 7. Example of the applied distribution of measuring points for cross-section six.

The distribution of points was normalized along lines defined at angles of 45° from the angle 0°, corresponding to the positive part of the y-axis. Using the Ansys Fluent solver, 10,400 combinations of input data were analyzed to obtain the pressures necessary to teach the neural networks at the standardized 240 points. The 10,400 cases are the values of pressure readings for individual points in selected sections for all possible combinations of Reynolds number Re and angle of attack α in the range: $Re = 0.3 : 0.025 : 0.925$ and $\alpha = -4 : 2 : 14$. The learning data were divided into training, validation, and testing sets according to a $20 : 3 : 3$ ratio.

240 Artificial Neural Networks (ANNs) were prepared, 40 for each cross-section. A single neural network predicted the dynamic pressure for a single, selected point. The MATLAB (MATLAB 2024a, Deep Learning Toolbox) Neural Network Toolbox was used as the environment for the neural networks. The ANN architecture was defined as a Feed-Forward neural network (2-50-20-2-1), and they were trained using the CFG algorithm (Conjugate gradient backpropagation with Fletcher–Reeves update). The structure of the neural networks stems from an earlier, unsuccessful attempt to predict RDI and CDI coefficients in between selected characteristic points. The analysis started with a network with more hidden layers, which was not able to learn with sufficient accuracy. The network

learned quickly and accurately enough, so the process of optimizing its structure was abandoned. In future publications, where the authors will try to use ANN to predict the pressure distribution between selected points, the optimization of the network's hyperparameters will be carried out. However, our experience shows that the applied activation functions (linear for output layer and sigmoidal for rest of them) and learning rate equal 0.01 are working correctly.

The training aimed to minimize the mean squared error (MSE) of the data fitting. The training was repeated until the maximum relative error of the impact pressure prediction was no greater than 4%. Of the 240 networks, 71 had an error greater than 1%, with 31 greater than 2% and 17 greater than 3%. The training error histogram of all 240 networks is shown in Figure 8. The error histogram and MSE for one of each randomly chosen neural network are shown in Figure 9. The high value of errors (absolute error) is not a major problem, because relatively speaking, most of these errors do not exceed 5%.

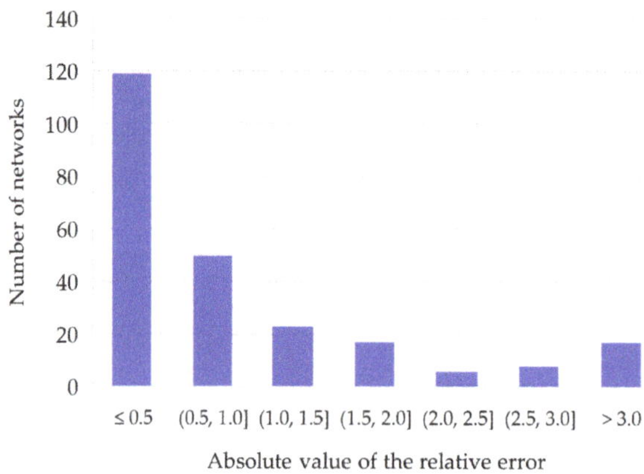

Figure 8. Histogram of ANN relative training error.

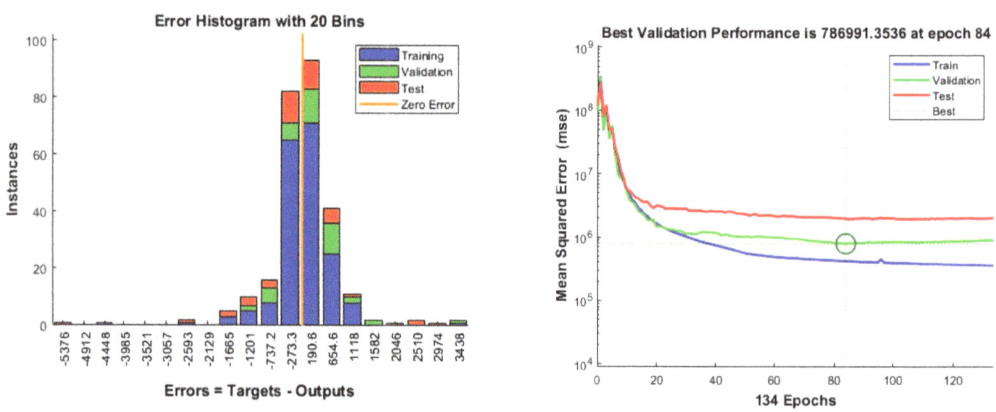

(a) (b)

Figure 9. Error histogram (**a**) and MSE (**b**) for one of each randomly chosen neural network. Where green circle is point of best performance.

Figure 10 presents the R^2 coefficient of determination of the artificial neural networks used, trained for all angles of attack α and Ma numbers about the data achieved based on hard calculations (CFD), is presented.

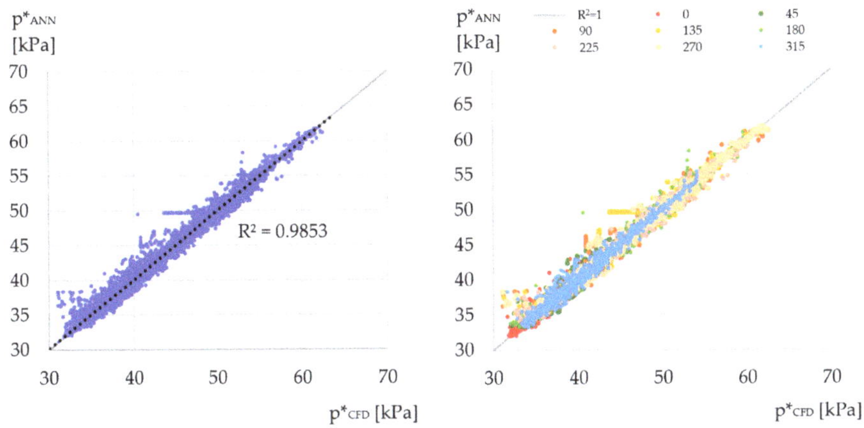

(a) (b)

Figure 10. The R^2 coefficient of determination for impact pressure, achieved by numerical studies (p^*_{CFD}) and ANN (p^*_{ANN}) (**a**), and divided into angles, which is consistent with Figure 7 (**b**).

The resulting data fitting distribution and the coefficient of determination was 0.9854. This demonstrates that the neural networks are well-trained for pressure distribution prediction. Figure 11 presents the R^2 coefficient of determination for the impact pressure achieved by numerical studies (p^*_{CFD}) and ANN (p^*_{ANN}) for individual position vectors, which is consistent with Figure 7.

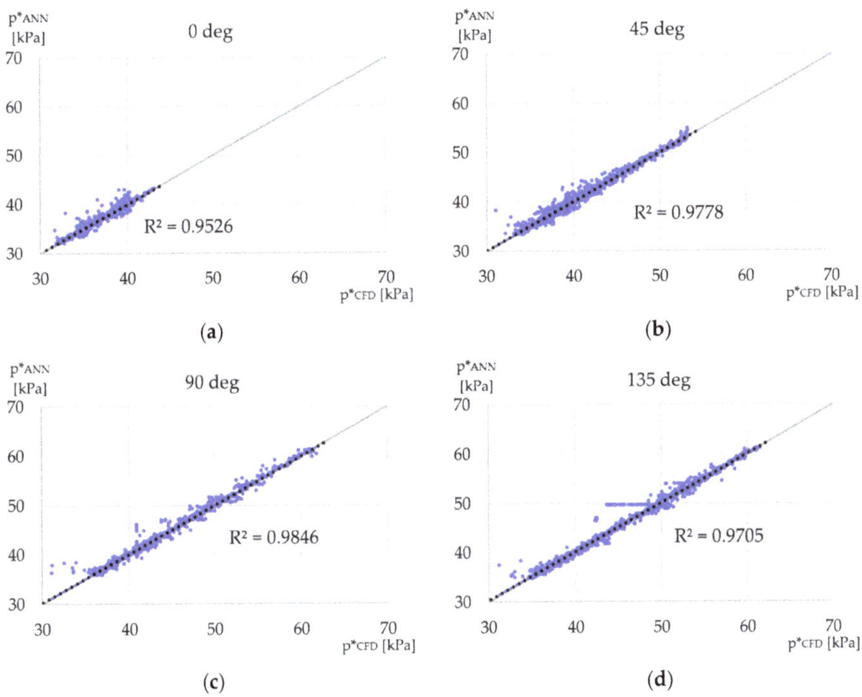

(a) (b) (c) (d)

Figure 11. *Cont.*

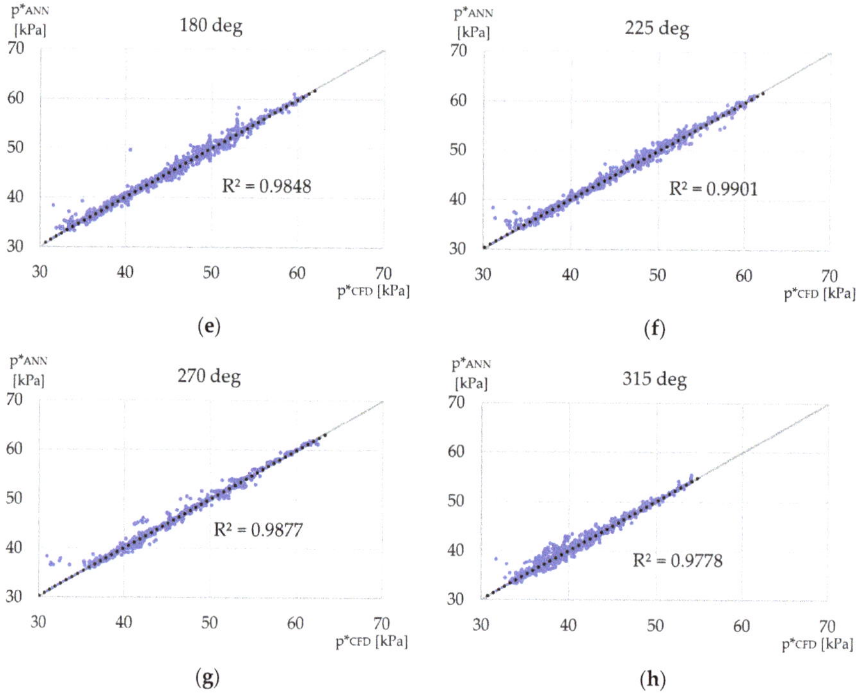

Figure 11. The R^2 coefficient of determination for the impact pressure achieved by numerical studies (p^*_{CFD}) and ANN (p^*_{ANN}) for individual position vectors. The division was made by Figure 7.

The network achieved the worst coefficient of determination on the vertical line from the axis of rotation (0°), which was equal to $R^2 = 0.9526$. The higher coefficient of determination corresponds to the angular position for which, according to Figure 11, there is a lower pressure gradient.

Figure 12 presents the R^2 coefficients of determination for the CDI and RDI coefficients calculated based on the prediction of ANN pressures and numerical calculations.

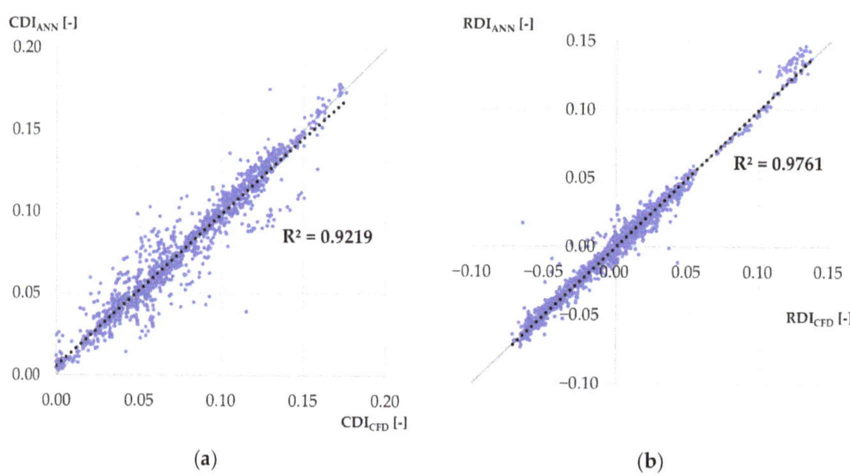

Figure 12. R^2 coefficient of determination for CDI (**a**) and RDI (**b**) coefficients were determined by numerical analyses and ANN.

As presented in Figure 12, the R^2 coefficients of determination for the CDI and RDI coefficients are, respectively, $R^2_{CDI} = 0.9219$ and $R^2_{RDI} = 0.9761$. The prediction accuracy of the CDI and RDI coefficients is sufficiently high to conclude that the developed neural metamodel enables the prediction of the aforementioned coefficients for predicting the nature of the pressure variations in the inlet duct to the turbine engine.

4. Conclusions

The analysis of the fourth-generation inlet system highlights its critical role in ensuring both propulsion efficiency and overall aircraft performance. Through a comprehensive evaluation of flow distortion indices, it was determined that the radial distortion index (RDI) is an order of magnitude smaller than the circumferential distortion index (CDI). Notably, an increase in the angle of attack does not consistently lead to higher total pressure distortion at the aerodynamic interface plane (AIP).

For low Mach numbers (Ma = 0.30–0.65), a strong dependence between flow distortion and angle of attack was observed. The CDI coefficient exhibited higher distortion values for negative angles of attack compared to positive angles, primarily due to the influence of shockwave behavior. A similar trend was noted for RDI at higher Mach numbers, whereas at lower Mach numbers, the relationship was reversed. Additionally, cyclic behavior in inlet flow was identified, with RDI coefficients exhibiting significant gradients—up to sixfold variations—across specific Mach number ranges.

The application of artificial neural networks (ANN) demonstrated high predictive accuracy in modeling CDI and RDI coefficients. The trained ANN exhibited strong data fitting capabilities, with determination coefficients indicating robust predictive performance. These results confirm the viability of neural networks as an effective tool for analyzing turbine engine inlet dynamics, providing a computationally efficient approach to predicting pressure distribution patterns.

The proposed method enables its application in various aspects related to turbine engines as well as other turbomachines. The first area of application concerns the design of new intake systems, while the second focuses on the improvement of existing designs. The potential utilization of neural networks in this context can be of significant importance in turbine engine control systems due to their speed and accuracy. This is particularly relevant for engines installed on highly maneuverable aircraft as well as those used for commercial or transport applications.

A disturbance in the system induces an off-design operating state for the subsequent component, the fan or compressor. Exceeding critical thresholds under such conditions introduces the risk of surge phenomena, potentially leading to engine shutdown. The ability to determine instability ranges using neural networks and subsequently convert these into control signals for stabilizing components, including variable guide vanes, handling bleed systems, and rotor speed adjustments, can effectively protect the engine from thrust or power loss.

Control systems based on such solutions can address various challenges arising from flight operations in turbulent atmospheric conditions under different flight parameters (e.g., speed, altitude, and angles). This is achieved by generating predictive models of possible behavior for individual components, including the intake system.

This study enhances the understanding of fourth-generation inlet system behavior under varying flight conditions, contributing to improved engine control strategies for mitigating stall and surge risks. The findings support ongoing advancements in turbine engine inlet system research, reinforcing the importance of data-driven modeling in modern aerospace engineering.

Author Contributions: Conceptualization, A.K.; methodology, A.K., M.A. and R.K.; software, M.A., R.K.; validation, A.K., M.A. and R.K.; formal analysis, A.K., M.A. and R.K.; investigation, A.K., M.A. and R.K.; resources, A.K., M.A. and R.K.; data curation, A.K., M.A. and R.K.; writing—original draft preparation, M.A. and R.K.; writing—review and editing, A.K., M.A. and R.K.; visualization, M.A. and R.K.; supervision, A.K.; project administration, A.K. and R.K.; funding acquisition, A.K. All authors have read and agreed to the published version of the manuscript.

Funding: This research was funded by the Military University of Technology, Warsaw, Poland, under research project No. UGB Nr 531-000039-W200-22 dated 28 January 2025.

Data Availability Statement: Data is contained within the article.

Conflicts of Interest: The authors declare no conflicts of interest.

References

1. Whitford, R. *Design for Air Combat*; Jane's: London, UK, 1987.
2. Smith, F.C.; Podleskit, S.D. Installed F/A-18A Inlet Flow Calculations: A Grid Study. *J. Propuls. Power* **1995**, *11*, 1250–1256. [CrossRef]
3. Wellborn, S.R.; Reichertt, B.A.; Okiishiij, T.H. Study of the Compressible Flow in a Diffusing S-Duct. *J. Propuls. Power* **1994**, *10*, 668–675. [CrossRef]
4. Bruns, J.E.; Smitht, F.C. Installed F/A-18 Inlet Flow Calculations at a High Angle of Attack. *J. Propuls. Power* **1994**, *10*, 110–115. [CrossRef]
5. Mohankumar, B.; Hall, C.A.; Wilson, M.J. Fan Aerodynamics With a Short Intake at High Angle of Attack. *J. Turbomach.* **2021**, *143*, 051003. [CrossRef]
6. Sudasinghe, A.; Rajakareyar, P.; Matida, E.; Abo El Ella, H.; El Sayed, M.S.A. Aerodynamic Shape Optimization of an Aircraft Propulsor Air Intake with Boundary Layer Ingestion. *Appl. Mech.* **2022**, *3*, 1123–1144. [CrossRef]
7. Ibrahim, I.H.; Ng, E.Y.K.; Wong, K. Flight Maneuverability Characteristics of the F-16 CFD and Correlation with its Intake Total Pressure Recovery and Distortion. *Eng. Appl. Comput. Fluid Mech.* **2011**, *5*, 223–234. [CrossRef]
8. Askari, R.; Soltani, M.R.; Mostoufi, K.; Khajeh Fard, A.; Abedi, M. Angle of Attack Investigations on the Performance of a Diverterless Supersonic Inlet. *J. Appl. Fluid Mech.* **2019**, *12*, 2017–2030. [CrossRef]
9. Dong, Y.; Tao, J.; Zhang, Y.; Lin, W.; Ai, J. Deep Learning in Aircraft Design, Dynamics, and Control: Review and Prospects. *IEEE Trans. Aerosp. Electron. Syst.* **2021**, *57*, 2346–2368. [CrossRef]
10. Li, Z.; Chen, C.; Pei, H.; Kong, B. Structural Optimization of the Aircraft NACA Inlet Based on BP Neural Networks and Genetic Algorithms. *Int. J. Aerosp. Eng.* **2020**, *2020*, 8857821. [CrossRef]
11. Rai, M.M.; Madavan, N.K. Application of Articial Neural Networks to the Design of Turbomachinery Airfoils. *J. Propuls. Power* **2001**, *17*, 176–183. [CrossRef]
12. Lu, P.J.; Zhang, M.C.; Hsu, T.C.; Zhang, J. An Evaluation of Engine Faults Diagnostics Using Artificial Neural Networks. *J. Eng. Gas Turbines Power* **2001**, *2001*, 340–346. [CrossRef]
13. Kobayashi, T.; Simon, D.L. Hybrid Neural-Network Genetic-Algorithm Technique for Aircraft Engine Performance Diagnostics. *J. Propuls. Power* **2005**, *21*, 751–758. [CrossRef]
14. Mirmohammadi, A.; Taheri, A.; Mohammadi-Amin, M. Numerical Framework to Investigate Intake Aerodynamics Behavior in Icing Conditions, World Academy of Science. *Eng. Technol. Int. J. Mech. Mechatron. Eng.* **2009**, *3*, 717–722. Available online: https://zenodo.org/record/1084598/files/15208.pdf (accessed on 1 March 2025).
15. Baklacioglu, T. Predicting the fuel flow rate of commercial aircraft via multilayer perceptron, radial basis function and ANFIS artificial neural networks. *Aeronaut. J.* **2020**, *125*, 453–471. [CrossRef]
16. Julian, K.D.; Kochenderfer, M.J.; Owen, M.P. Deep Neural Network Compression for Aircraft Collision Avoidance Systems. *J. Guid. Control. Dyn.* **2018**, *42*, 598–608. [CrossRef]
17. Kozakiewicz, A.; Kachel, S.; Frant, M.; Majcher, M. Intake-System-Performance Stability as a Function of Flow Throttling. *Energies* **2022**, *15*, 6291. [CrossRef]
18. Kozakiewicz, A.; Adamczyk, M.; Wróblewski, M. Areas of Investigation into Air Intake Systems for the Impact on Compressor Performance Stability in Aircraft Turbine Engines. *Adv. Sci. Technol. Res. J.* **2022**, *16*, 62–64. [CrossRef]
19. Kozakiewicz, A.; Frant, M.; Majcher, M.; Adamczyk, M. Analysis of the Impact of Aircraft Manoeuvring on Intake Disturbance. *Int. Rev. Aerosp. Eng. (IREASE)* **2023**, *1*, 159–168. [CrossRef]

20. Kieszek, R.; Kachel, S.; Kozakiewicz, A. Modification of Genetic Algorithm Based on Extinction Events and Migration. *Appl. Sci.* **2023**, *13*, 5584. [CrossRef]
21. Kozakiewicz, A.; Kieszek, R. Artificial Neural Network Structure Optimisation in the Pareto Approach on the Example of Stress Prediction in the Disk-Drum Structure of an Axial Compressor. *Materials* **2022**, *15*, 4451. [CrossRef] [PubMed]

energies

MDPI

Article

Evaluating the Thermohydraulic Performance of Microchannel Gas Coolers: A Machine Learning Approach

Shehryar Ishaque [1], Naveed Ullah [2], Sanghun Choi [1,2] and Man-Hoe Kim [1,*]

[1] KNU Institute of Engineering Design Technology (IEDT), Kyungpook National University, Daegu 41566, Republic of Korea; shehryarbangash1@gmail.com (S.I.); s-choi@knu.ac.kr (S.C.)

[2] School of Mechanical Engineering, College of Engineering, Kyungpook National University, Daegu 41566, Republic of Korea; naveedullah@knu.ac.kr

* Correspondence: manhoe.kim@knu.ac.kr

Abstract: In this study, a numerical model of a microchannel gas cooler was developed using a segment-by-segment approach for thermohydraulic performance evaluation. State-of-the-art heat transfer and pressure drop correlations were used to determine the air and refrigerant side heat transfer coefficients and friction factors. The developed model was validated against a wide range of experimental data and was found to accurately predict the gas cooler capacity (Q) and pressure drop (ΔP) within an acceptable margin of error. Furthermore, advanced machine learning algorithms such as extreme gradient boosting (XGB), random forest (RF), support vector regression (SVR), k-nearest neighbors (KNNs), and artificial neural networks (ANNs) were employed to analyze their predictive capability. Over 11,000 data points from the numerical model were used, with 80% of the data for training and 20% for testing. The evaluation metrics, such as the coefficient of determination (R^2, 0.99841–0.99836) and mean squared error values (0.09918–0.10639), demonstrated high predictive efficacy and accuracy, with only slight variations among the models. All models accurately predict the Q, with the XGB and ANN models showing superior performance in ΔP prediction. Notably, the ANN model emerges as the most accurate method for refrigerant and air outlet temperatures predictions. These findings highlight the potential of machine learning as a robust tool for optimizing thermal system performance and guiding the design of energy-efficient heat exchange technologies.

Keywords: thermohydraulic performance; gas cooler; machine learning; ANN; KNN; SVR

1. Introduction

In recent years, the global adoption of new energy vehicles (NEVs), particularly electric vehicles (EVs), has surged due to increasing environmental concerns and the transition toward sustainable transportation. Governments and manufacturers worldwide are promoting EV technologies to reduce greenhouse gas emissions and urban noise. Among these vehicles, battery electric vehicles (BEVs) dominate the market [1]. As a result, the efficiency of vehicle thermal management systems, especially for cabin air conditioning, has become a critical factor affecting overall energy consumption and driving range.

With the growing global demand for EVs, energy-efficient and eco-friendly cooling strategies must be developed for these vehicles. Transcritical CO_2 microchannel gas coolers (MCGCs) are one of the promising solutions, offering compactness, high thermal efficiency, and reduced environmental impact compared to conventional cooling systems that employ refrigerants with high global warming potential. The unique feature of CO_2 is its low critical temperature (31.1 °C), which differentiates it considerably from other refrigerants.

Above this critical point, the heat transfer capacity of the condenser becomes ineffective which subsequently replaces the condenser with a specialized heat rejection device (gas cooler). In a gas cooler, the conventional condensation process is replaced with a unique gas cooling process in which the temperature of the refrigerant decreases significantly, while pressure changes remain minimal. The gas cooling process operates within the supercritical region, where temperature and pressure are decoupled. This unique process determines the enthalpy of CO_2 at the outlet of a gas cooler, influenced by both temperature and pressure [2]. The performance of these gas coolers is important for the overall efficiency and effectiveness of the EV's air conditioning system [3]. Strategies for improving the performance of transcritical CO_2 systems primarily focus on two key aspects: optimizing system components and improving system design. In terms of system component optimization, this approach mainly involves optimizing the performance of the gas cooler, evaporator, or compressor [4,5].

Accurate prediction of the thermohydraulic performance of MCGCs for EV applications is essential for their design and optimization. Conventional methods such as empirical correlations and numerical simulations have been extensively used in the field of heat transfer for evaluating the performance of MCGCs. These well-established techniques rely on physical principles and consider specific system details, including geometry, materials, and working fluid properties. Empirical correlations are basically derived from experimental data and are often tailored to specific geometries and flow regimes. Although these correlations offer a quick and straightforward solution, their accuracy may be limited, especially when applied to novel designs or nonstandard operating conditions. In contrast, numerical simulations offer a more comprehensive evaluation of the MCGC performance. Computational fluid dynamics (CFD) techniques such as finite element and finite volume methods are utilized to numerically solve the governing equations of fluid flow and heat transfer. These methods consider the intricate geometry of microchannels, the properties and behavior of the working fluid. By discretizing the domain and iteratively solving the equations, CFD simulations can provide insights into the thermohydraulic performance of MCGCs under various operating conditions. Both empirical correlations and numerical simulations have their advantages and limitations. Empirical correlations are relatively simple and can provide quick estimates; however, they may lack accuracy for complex designs or under unconventional operating conditions. Conversely, numerical simulations offer a more detailed understanding of the underlying physical processes but require significant computational resources and expertise. Both approaches have been widely used considering the specific details of the system being modeled. In addition, emerging techniques such as neural networks offer promising options for more accurate, cost effective, and quick estimation of MCGC performance [6–8]. Neural networks can learn complex relationships between input parameters (e.g., geometrical and operational variables) and the corresponding thermohydraulic performance. By training the neural network with a diverse dataset generated from experimental or simulation data, MCGC performance can be accurately predicted under various operating conditions. ML algorithms are faster than numerical simulations, allowing for more rapid optimization of air conditioning system design. In addition, they are more flexible than numerical simulations, enabling performance prediction under a wider range of operating conditions and cooler designs. ML techniques have been extensively studied in heat transfer and fluid mechanics [9,10].

Saeed et al. [11] performed 3D-Reynolds-averaged Navier–Stokes simulations to calculate the heat sink performances with various fin configurations. Subsequently, this data was employed to train six ML regression techniques to identify the most accurate method for predicting heat transfer coefficients and ΔP values. The selected ML model was combined with a multi-objective genetic algorithm to determine the ideal heat sink geometry. The multilayer perceptron method, adapted into a deep neural network model, effectively predicted the heat transfer coefficients and ΔP using the available data. The performance of the optimized channel geometry increased 2.1 times compared to that of the best existing channel configuration, with a 14% higher heat transfer coefficient and five times lower ΔP. Arman et al. employed a committee neural network (CNN) to estimate the ΔP in microchannels under varying conditions and demonstrated that incorporating multiple techniques into the CNN increased the accuracy of the results, suggesting its strong predictive potential across diverse fields [12]. Kim et al. developed general ML models using power law regression and a database comprising 906 data points from 15 different sources. The ML models were found to have mean absolute errors of 7.5–10.9%, an approximately fivefold improvement in prediction accuracy compared with existing regression correlations [13]. Yu et al. performed numerical simulations of the flow and heat transfer process in an elliptical pin-fin microchannel heat sink, and ANNs were used to predict the average temperature, temperature nonuniformity, and ΔP of the microchannel [14]. Sikirica et al. introduced a framework using CFD, ML-based surrogate modeling, and multi-objective optimization to optimize microchannel heat sink designs. The optimized designs showed enhanced performance while reducing the computational time compared with traditional methods. The designs generated achieved temperatures more than 10% lower than that of a typical microchannel design under the same pressure limits. When limited by temperature, ΔP decreased by more than 25% [15].

Recent advancements underscore the growing role of machine learning (ML) and deep learning (DL) in optimizing thermal system performance, particularly in complex geometries and multiphase flow conditions. For example, Zohora et al. [16] applied multilayer perceptron and XGBoost models to CFD data from pin-fin microchannel heat sinks, achieving over 95% accuracy in thermal and fluid flow predictions. Efatinasab et al. [17] developed ANN and CNN models trained on a large experimental dataset to predict heat transfer and ΔP in micro-finned tube heat exchangers, achieving mean absolute errors under 4.5% and leveraging SHAP analysis for interpretability. Similar trends are evident in vortex generator optimization [18], multimodal data fusion for boiling heat sinks [19], and hybrid physics-informed frameworks for pool boiling on structured surfaces [20]. Other works demonstrate the effectiveness of LSTM and Transformer-based models in capturing complex flow dynamics in plate heat exchangers [21,22], while XGBoost and SGBoost models have proven to be reliable surrogates for CFD in nanofluid systems [23,24]. Collectively, these studies highlight the current shift toward data-driven modeling strategies in thermal engineering, emphasizing high accuracy, physical interpretability, and substantial reductions in computational cost.

To meet the growing demand for compact, energy-efficient, and eco-friendly thermal systems in electric vehicles, transcritical CO_2 microchannel gas coolers (MCGCs) have emerged as a promising solution due to their high heat transfer efficiency and low environmental impact. However, their design and operation involve significant challenges, such as complex two-phase flow, maldistribution, high-pressure conditions, and performance sensitivity to varying parameters. While experimental and CFD-based approaches have been used to investigate these systems, they often have high computational and resource costs, particularly when analyzing a wide range of conditions. In this context, machine learning (ML) offers a powerful and efficient alternative for predicting thermohydraulic performance by capturing nonlinear interactions among design and operating variables. This study aims to develop and validate ML-based models to provide fast and accurate predictions for MCGCs, supporting advanced design and optimization efforts.

In this work, we aim to investigate and compare the ability of ML algorithms in predicting the thermohydraulic performance of an MCGC for mobile air conditioning applications. Utilizing over 11,000 data points from an experimentally validated numerical model, we developed and optimized predictive models using five ML techniques: XGB, RF, SVR, KNNs, and ANNs. By carefully tuning hyperparameters and evaluating performance metrics such as coefficient of determination (R^2) and mean squared error (MSE), our study provides insights into the unique abilities of each model, offering enhancement of the energy efficiency and design optimization of complex thermal systems in automotive applications.

2. Numerical Model Development of MCHX

2.1. Geometric and Operating Conditions

In this study, a numerical model was developed using MATLAB R2024b code for single-slab MCHX. The baseline geometry consists of 34 tubes arranged in three passes (13-11-10), each tube with 11 circular ports as illustrated in Figure 1. CO_2 refrigerant flows through microchannel tubes and air across louvered fins. The geometric specifications and operating conditions are provided in Tables 1 and 2, respectively.

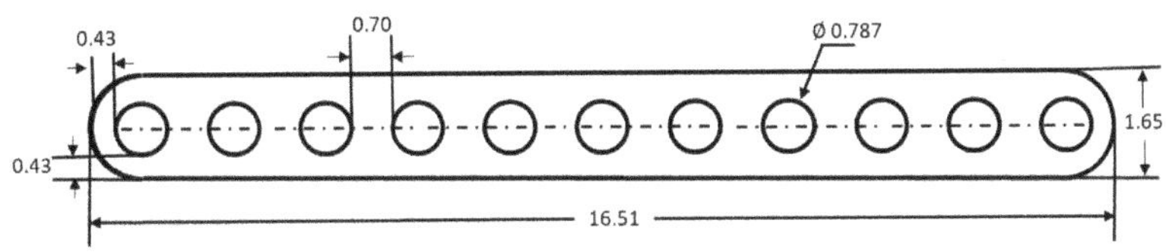

Figure 1. Microchannel tube cross-section.

Table 1. Geometric specifications.

Number of Tubes	34
Tube length (mm)	545
Number of ports	11
Ports diameter (mm)	0.79
Fin type	Louvered fins
Fin height (mm)	8.89
Fin pitch (mm)	2.5
Fin width (mm)	16

Table 2. Operating conditions.

S.No	T_{ri} [°C]	P_{ri} [kPa]	T_{ai} [°C]	$\dot{m}_r$ [g/s]	$\dot{m}_a$ [g/s]
I17-1	106.8	9833	43.6	20.78	451
I17-2	111.7	10,355	43.6	19.8	451
I17-3	115.8	10,888	43.6	19.02	452
I17-4	119.7	11,388	43.6	18.45	452
I17-5	123	11,854	43.6	17.96	452
I6-1	115.8	12,464	55.1	26.39	457
I6-2	118	12,672	55	25.91	457
I6-3	119.2	12,855	55	25.61	457
I6-4	120.5	12,960	54.9	25.26	0.456
I6-5	125	13,335	54.9	24.47	456
I6-6	126.6	13,592	54.9	23.94	456
M03-1	124.7	10,937	42.7	37.84	537
M03-2	124.3	10,950	42.8	38.05	537
M03-3	125	10,974	42.9	37.75	537
M03-4	124.7	10,975	42.9	37.93	537

Table 2. *Cont.*

S.No	T_{ri} [°C]	P_{ri} [kPa]	T_{ai} [°C]	$\dot{m}_r$ [g/s]	$\dot{m}_a$ [g/s]
H03-1	129.3	10,338	43.6	56.39	701
H03-2	129.5	10,351	43.9	56.39	700
H03-3	138.6	10,792	43.5	56.36	701
H03-4	142.6	11,025	43.7	54.83	700
H03-5	148.9	11,756	43.5	50.13	700

2.2. Modeling Approach

A segment-by-segment modeling approach was used due to the strong sensitivity of CO_2 properties near the critical point. Each tube was divided into five segments, each modeled as an independent crossflow heat exchanger. Heat transfer and ΔP were calculated using the ε-NTU method. Properties of CO_2 and air were calculated using REFPROP (v10.0). The model assumes steady-state, one-dimensional flow, and uses empirical correlations for heat transfer and ΔP, which may introduce deviations under highly transient conditions or at the extremes of operating parameters (e.g., extremely low or high mass flow rates, very large channel aspect ratios, or non-uniform refrigerant distribution). The schematic flow chart of the numerical methodology is shown in Figure 2.

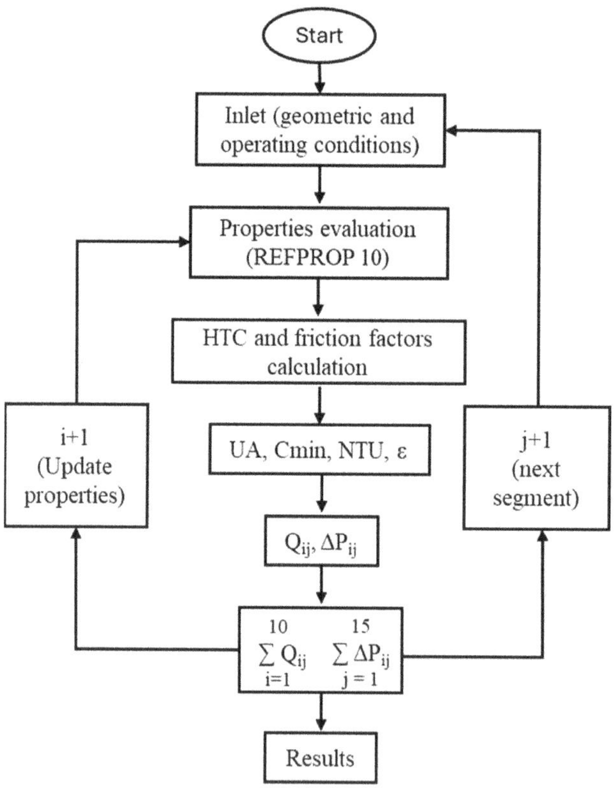

Figure 2. Flow chart of a numerical model for transcritical CO_2 gas cooler.

2.3. Heat Transfer and Pressure Drop Correlations

Appropriate correlations for heat transfer and ΔP are essential for model accuracy. The convective heat transfer coefficient on the air side is selected based on the fin configuration.

In the present model, the Colburn j factor and friction f factor correlations for louvered fins, as developed by Kim and Bullard [25], were employed. These correlations are widely used for flat-tube heat exchangers with louvered fins and have been validated in the literature under comparable operating conditions, making them well-suited for the geometry and application considered in this study.

$$j = Re_{Lp}^{-0.487}\left(\frac{L_\alpha}{90}\right)^{0.257}\left(\frac{F_p}{L_p}\right)^{-0.13}\left(\frac{H}{L_p}\right)^{-0.29}\left(\frac{F_d}{L_p}\right)^{-0.235}\left(\frac{L_l}{L_p}\right)^{0.68}\left(\frac{T_p}{L_p}\right)^{-0.279}\left(\frac{\delta_f}{L_p}\right)^{-0.05} \quad (1)$$

$$f = Re_{Lp}^{-0.781}\left(\frac{L_\alpha}{90}\right)^{0.444}\left(\frac{F_p}{L_p}\right)^{-1.682}\left(\frac{H}{L_p}\right)^{-1.22}\left(\frac{F_d}{L_p}\right)^{0.818}\left(\frac{L_l}{L_p}\right)^{1.97} \quad (2)$$

The refrigerant side heat transfer coefficient is calculated by Gnielinski correlation [26], valid in the range of $3000 \lesssim Re \lesssim 5 \times 10^6$ and $0.5 \lesssim Pr \lesssim 2000$. The Darcy friction factor f_D is obtained from Equation (4) developed by Petukhov [26], a single correlation that spans a wide range of Reynold numbers, $3000 \lesssim Re \lesssim 5 \times 10^6$.

$$Nu = \frac{(f_D/8) \times (Re - 1000) \times Pr}{1 + 12.7(f_D/8)^{\frac{1}{2}}\left(Pr^{\frac{2}{3}} - 1\right)} \quad (3)$$

$$f_D = (0.79ln(Re) - 1.64)^{-2} \quad (4)$$

The ΔP is calculated from friction along ports as follows:

$$\Delta P = \frac{L_t}{D_{port}} \times \frac{f_D \times G_r^2}{2\rho_r} \quad (5)$$

2.4. Numerical Model Validation

The numerical model for Q and ΔP is validated against experimental data from Yin and Bullard [27]. Results showed strong agreement, with maximum errors within ±3.79% for capacity and ±10.24% for ΔP, respectively, which is within the acceptable range as shown in Figure 3.

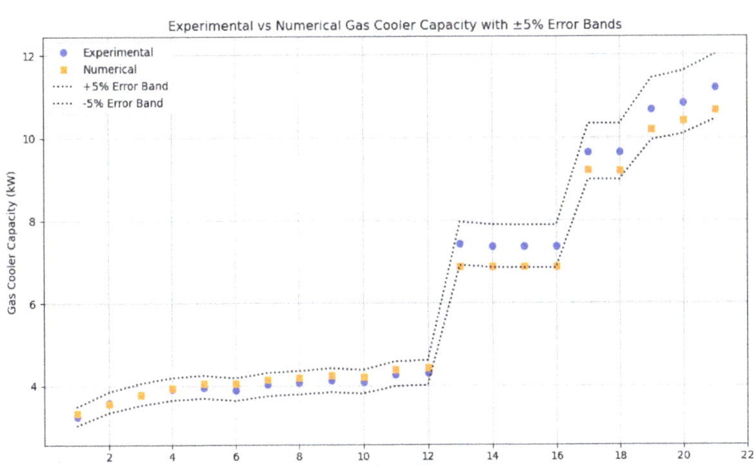

(a)

Figure 3. *Cont.*

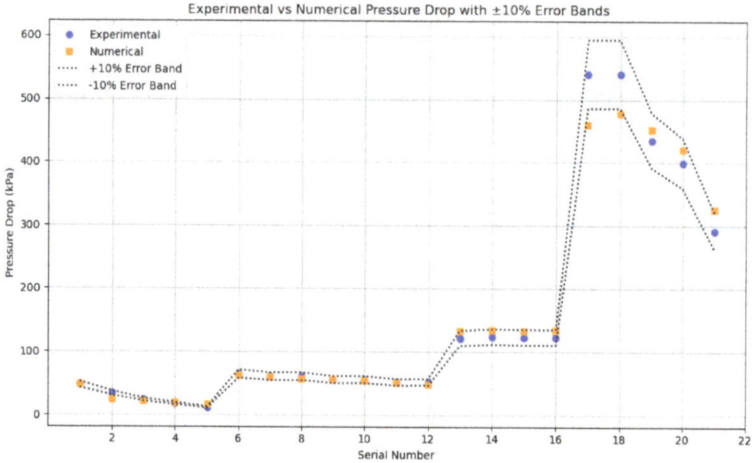

(b)

Figure 3. (**a**) Comparison of experimental vs. simulated Q. (**b**) Comparison of experimental vs. simulated gas cooler ΔP.

3. Predictive Modeling of MCGC Using Machine Learning Approach

The methodology for predicting MCGC performance in mobile air conditioning systems (MACSs) is built upon a robust machine learning (ML) framework that incorporates five advanced algorithms: XGB, RF, SVR, KNN, and ANNs. Each algorithm was selected to represent a diverse range of modeling approaches, ensuring a comprehensive evaluation of their individual capabilities, from XGB's robustness in handling tabular data to RF's resilience against overfitting, SVR's efficiency in capturing non-linear patterns, KNN's interpretability for local relationships, and ANN's capacity to learn intricate, non-linear interactions. By comparing their performance on the same dataset, the framework facilitates a comparative analysis of their performance, highlighting both their general-purpose utility and scenario-specific strengths. All algorithms were implemented using the scikit-learn library, with configurations tailored to optimize predictive accuracy while minimizing the risk of overfitting. This systematic and well-rounded approach provides valuable insights into the strengths and limitations of each algorithm, enabling informed decision-making for performance prediction in MACSs.

3.1. Problem Formulation

The task of performance prediction is framed as a supervised learning problem. Given a dataset containing input features $X = \{x_1, x_2, \ldots, x_n\} \in \mathbb{R}^n$, where n is the number of features, representing geometric and operational parameters, and output variables $Y = \{y_1, y_2, \ldots, y_m\} \in \mathbb{R}^m$, where m is the number of output variables, representing system performance metrics, the objective is to learn the functional relationship:

$$Y = f(X) + \varepsilon \tag{6}$$

where $f(X)$ is the true mapping function and ε is the error. Each algorithm separately models this relationship, predicting the outputs $\hat{Y}$. To evaluate model performance, two metrics were used: mean squared error (MSE) and the coefficient of determination (R^2). The MSE is defined as follows:

$$MSE = \frac{1}{N}\sum_{i=1}^{N} (y_i - \hat{y}_i)^2 \tag{7}$$

which quantifies the average squared difference between predicted $\hat{y}_i$ and true y_i values. The R^2 metric is defined as follows:

$$R^2 = 1 - \frac{\sum_{i=1}^{N}(y_i - \hat{y}_i)}{\sum_{i=1}^{N}(y_i - y_i)} \tag{8}$$

measures the proportion of variance in the dependent variable that is predictable from the independent variables.

The overall workflow of the system is depicted in Figure 4, providing a clear representation of the sequential processes involved. Each component of the workflow is meticulously detailed in the subsequent sections, offering an in-depth explanation of their roles and functionality within the system.

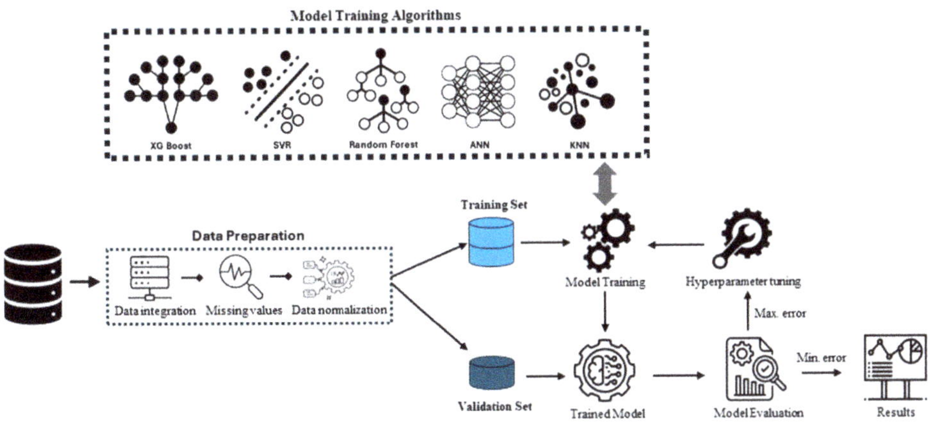

Figure 4. Schematic flow chart of the proposed framework.

3.2. Data Preparation

The dataset used for machine learning model development was generated from a validated numerical model of the MCGC [27,28]. By systematically varying key geometric and operational parameters such as number of passes (3–5), number of tubes (18–60), number of circular ports (9–21), ambient temperature (42–56 °C), inlet air flow rate (0.45–0.70 kg/s), and refrigerant flow rate (0.018–0.057 kg/s), a total of approximately 13,000 datasets were generated. Each data point includes twenty-three input parameters and four output performance indicators. While the numerical model exhibits some errors relative to experimental data, our ML framework will be trained and tested exclusively on those same simulated outputs, so this bias will not affect the reported ML accuracy.

The dataset was thoroughly examined for missing, constant, and duplicate values, followed by necessary preprocessing steps to ensure its integrity and readiness for analysis. A rigorous approach was also applied for outlier removal to maintain the quality of the regression modeling. To enhance predictive accuracy and model efficiency, a systematic feature selection process was carried out on the preprocessed dataset. Statistical techniques and correlation analysis were used to identify the most influential variables affecting the target outputs, thereby reducing the original 27 features to an optimized set of 13 (nine input features and four output features). Features with constant values such as heat exchanger volume, tube pitches, fin pitch, tube thickness, and fin height were removed due to their lack of variance. Redundant features were excluded based on high correlation and engineering relevance. For example, among airflow-related parameters (velocity, mass flow rate, and volume rate), only the air mass flow rate was retained. Similarly, the number of tubes and number of ports were chosen over the more dependent geometric dimensions like height and width. A single categorical feature "passes" was used to represent the variation in refrigerant flow configurations. This refined feature set not only reduces model complexity and the risk of overfitting but also ensures better interpretability and relevance to the thermal and hydraulic behavior of CO_2 gas coolers.

The input features include air flow rate ($\dot{m}_{ca}$), air inlet temperature (T_{cai}), refrigerant flow rate ($\dot{m}_r$), refrigerant inlet pressure (P_{cri}), refrigerant inlet temperature (T_{cri}), heat exchanger length, number of tubes, ports, and passes. Output variables are Q, ΔP, and air and refrigerant outlet temperatures (T_{ao} and T_{ro}). Ranges of geometric and operating conditions for machine learning models are given in Table 3.

Table 3. Ranges of geometric and operating conditions used for machine learning models.

Parameter	Range/Values
Passes	3–5
Tube Numbers	18–60
Number of Circular Ports	9–21
MCGC Dimensions	Length: 545 mm, Depth: 16.51 mm, Height: 1.65 mm
Ambient Temperature	42–56 °C
Inlet Air Flow Rate	0.45–0.70 kg/s
Refrigerant Flow Rate	0.018–0.057 kg/s

The dataset was preprocessed to ensure compatibility with the ML algorithms. Input features were standardized using the StandardScaler function to achieve zero mean and unit variance.

3.3. *Train Test Split Technique*

In ML, evaluating a model's performance on unseen data is crucial for the assessment of its generalizability. To achieve this, the dataset is commonly divided into two subsets: a training set and a testing set. The training set is used to train the model, enabling it to learn the underlying patterns and relationships between the input features and output values. On the other hand, the testing set is employed to assess the model's performance on new, unseen data, which helps determine how effectively the model can generalize its predictions to novel data points. In this study, the testing set size was defined as 0.2, indicating that 20% of the dataset was dedicated to testing, while the remaining 80% was allocated for the training set. Moreover, the random state parameter was set to 1, ensuring that the data split was reproducible across multiple runs. By setting this parameter, we obtained consistent results when evaluating the models. Consequently, the resulting training set, represented as X_{train} (input features) and y_{train} (output values), was employed to train various models, and the testing set, denoted as X_{test} (input features) and y_{test} (output values), was used to evaluate the performances of these models. Using this systematic approach, we effectively determined the capabilities and limitations of the different models under consideration.

3.4. *Model Training*

As described earlier, five different machine learning algorithms, i.e., XGB, RF, SVR, KNN, and ANNs, were independently used to train multiple models. Each algorithm was optimized using hyperparameter tuning to ensure accurate predictions and robust performance across the dataset. To prevent overfitting, early stopping techniques were employed during model training.

3.4.1. Algorithms for MCGC Performance Predictions

These algorithms were implemented using Python 3.11, and utilized a suite of powerful open-source libraries. For seamless data handling and preprocessing, pandas enabled efficient loading and manipulation of tabular datasets, while NumPy facilitated complex mathematical computations. To visualize insights and trends, matplotlib provided dynamic and intuitive plotting capabilities. Key machine learning operations, including data transformation, model implementation, and evaluation, were powered by scikit-learn. Specifically, sklearn.linear_model supported the implementation of various regression models, sklearn.preprocessing ensured the data was appropriately transformed, sklearn.model_selection streamlined data splitting and cross-validation, and sklearn.metrics allowed for comprehensive performance evaluation using diverse metrics. Together, these tools not only enabled precise coding of the models but also ensured their performance could be rigorously assessed. Each algorithm's underlying principles were carefully considered to match the dataset's complexity and diversity, creating a framework that combines analytical rigor with computational efficiency.

The Extreme Gradient Boosting Algorithm

XGB, introduced by Chen [29], is a powerful ML algorithm that belongs to the class of ensemble methods. It builds an ensemble of weak learners (decision trees) in a sequential, additive manner while minimizing a given loss function to form a strong predictive model. XGB employs regularization techniques to control model complexity and reduce overfitting. The objective function of XGB can be expressed as follows:

$$Obj(\theta) = \sum_{i=1}^{n} l\left(y_{\mathrm{i}}, \hat{y}_{\mathrm{i}}^{(t-1)} + f_{\mathrm{t}}(x_{\mathrm{i}})\right) + \Omega(f_{\mathrm{t}}), \tag{9}$$

where θ is the model parameters, l is the loss function, y_{i} is the true label of the ith observation, $\hat{y}_{\mathrm{i}}^{(t-1)}$ is the predicted label of the ith observation at the (t − 1)th iteration, $f_{\mathrm{t}}(x_{\mathrm{i}})$ is the tth weak learner (i.e., decision tree) that maps the features (x_{i}) to a predicted label, and Ω is a regularization term that penalizes complex models. The objective function comprises two parts: the loss function and the regularization term. The loss function measures the difference between the predicted and true labels, whereas the regularization term penalizes complex models to avoid overfitting. Figure 5 shows the schematic of the XGB model.

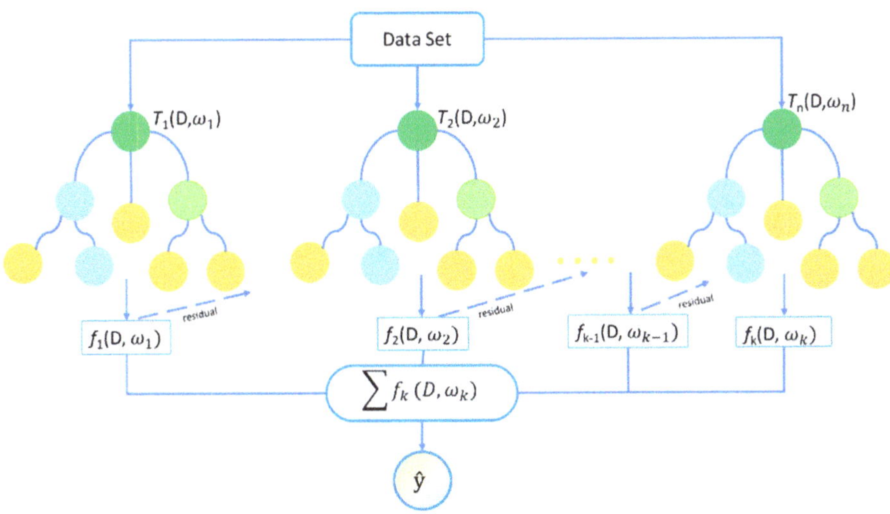

Figure 5. Schematic of the XGB model.

Random Forest Algorithm

RF is an ensemble learning algorithm developed by Breiman and Leo [30]. It combines multiple decision trees to improve the accuracy and robustness of the model. The mathematical equation for the RF model is expressed in Equation (10) as follows:

$$f(x) = \Sigma(b_j * I(x \in R_j)), \tag{10}$$

where $f(x)$ is the predicted value for a new observation with the feature vector x. The decision tree comprises a set of regions R_j that divide the feature space into mutually exclusive and exhaustive regions. Each region R_j is associated with the predicted value b_j. The equation $I(x \in R_j)$ is an indicator function that takes the value 1 if the new observation x belongs to region R_j and takes the value 0 otherwise. Therefore, $\Sigma(b_j * I(x \in R_j))$ computes the predicted value by summing the predicted values b_j of all regions to which the new observation x belongs:

$$\hat{y} = mode(f_1(x), f_2(x), \ldots, f_n(x)). \tag{11}$$

In Equation (11), $\hat{y}$ is the predicted value for the new observation with the feature vector x. It comprises n decision trees trained on the randomly selected subsets of the training data and the randomly selected subsets of the features. Each decision tree produces the predicted value $f_i(x)$ for the new observation x. The function mode returns the most common value among its arguments, which are the predicted values of all the decision trees. Therefore, the equation $\hat{y} = mode(f_1(x), f_2(x), \ldots, f_n(x))$ computes the predicted value by taking the majority vote of the predicted values of all decision trees in the RF. The schematic of the RF model is shown in Figure 6.

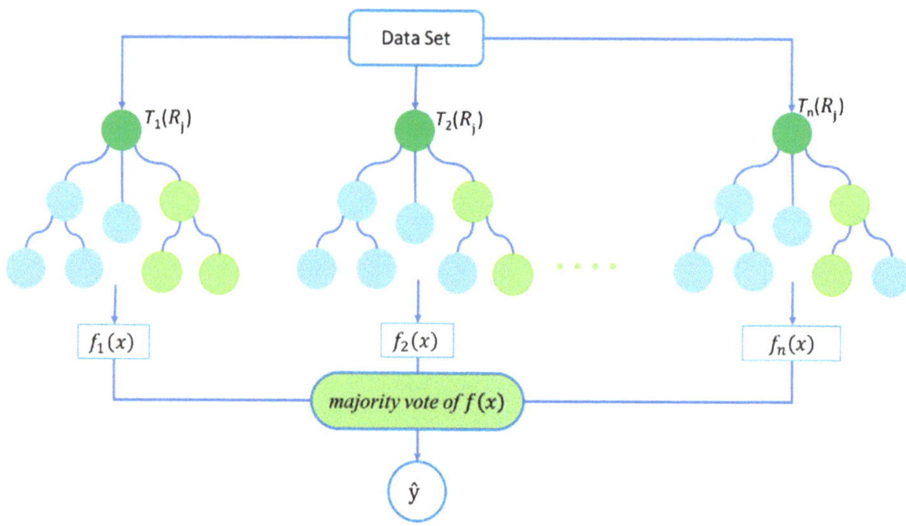

Figure 6. Schematic of the RF model.

Support Vector Regression Algorithm

SVR is an ML algorithm developed by Vapnik and fellows [31] for regression tasks. It is a variant of support vector machine (SVM) and is particularly useful when dealing with nonlinear and complex data using different kernel functions. SVR aims to find the best-fitting hyperplane that maximizes the margin while minimizing the prediction error. SVR can be expressed as follows:

$$y = b + \sum(\alpha_{\mathrm{i}} \cdot K(x_{\mathrm{i}},\ x)), \tag{12}$$

where y is the target variable, b is the bias term, and α_{i} are the Lagrange multipliers or support vector weights associated with each data point. $K(x_{\mathrm{i}},\ x)$ is the kernel function that calculates the distance between the input data points x_{i} and x in a higher-dimensional feature space.

k-Nearest Neighbors Algorithm

In ML, a KNN is a nonparametric algorithm that predicts the value of a target variable by considering the k-nearest training examples in the feature space. To determine the nearest neighbors, the KNN algorithm uses a distance metric to measure the distance between each pair of observations in the feature space. The most used distance metric is the Euclidean distance, which can be described by Equation (13):

$$d(x_{\mathrm{i}},\ x_{\mathrm{j}}) = \sqrt{\sum\left(x_{ik} - x_{jk}\right)^2}, \tag{13}$$

where x_{ik} is the kth feature of observation i, and x_{jk} is the kth feature of observation j.

Once the distance between each pair of observations is calculated, the algorithm selects the KNNs for the new observation. The value of k is a hyperparameter set before training the algorithm. Then, the KNN algorithm assigns the label of the new observation based on the majority class of its KNNs, as described by Equation (14):

$$\hat{y} = argmax(\sum(I(y_{\mathrm{i}} = y))), \tag{14}$$

where $\hat{y}$ is the predicted label for the new observation, y_{i} is the label of the ith nearest neighbor, and $I(y_i = y)$ is an indicator function that equals 1 if $y_{\mathrm{i}} = y$ and 0 otherwise. The function argmax returns the value of the argument that maximizes the function inside the parentheses. In other words, argmax returns the label y that has the highest frequency among the KNNs.

Artificial Neural Networks Model

ANNs are computational models inspired by biological neural networks and are used in various ML applications. They comprise interconnected layers of neurons, including the input, hidden, and output layers as shown in Figure 7. ANNs learn through back-propagation, adjusting their weights to minimize the error between the predicted and actual outputs. Activation functions introduce nonlinearity, enabling the network to learn complex relationships, as described by Equation (15):

$$Y_i^h = \sum_{j=1}^{n_{h-1}} W_{ij}^h * a_j^{h-1} + b_i^h, \tag{15}$$

where Y_i^h represents the preactivation value of neuron i in the hidden layer h, W_{ij}^h denotes the weight connecting neuron j in layer $(h-1)$ to neuron i in layer h, a_j^{h-1} represents the activation value of neuron j in layer $(h-1)$, and b_i^h represents the bias term associated with neuron i in layer h. n_{h-1} is the number of neurons in layer $(h-1)$.

The topology of the ANN employed in predicting the performance of an MCGC comprised an input layer, three hidden layers, and an output layer. In total, 9 features were considered, with model outputs including Tao, Tro, Q, and ΔP.

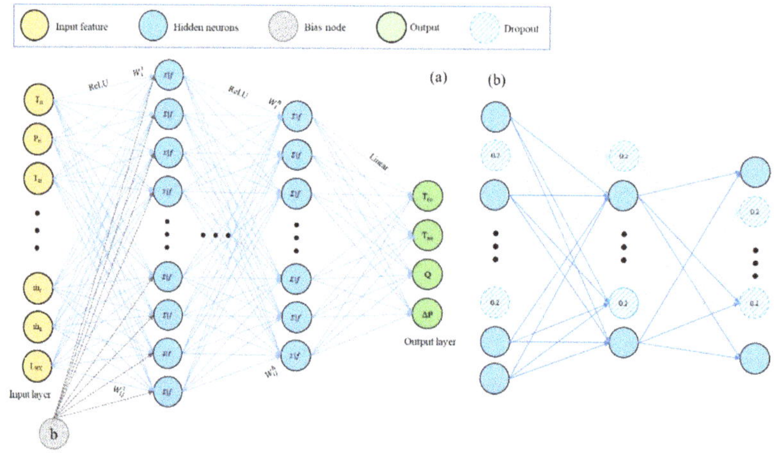

Figure 7. (**a**,**b**) Schematic of the ANN model.

To prevent overfitting and enhance generalization, the dropout technique is utilized in neural networks. This technique selectively deactivates neurons in hidden layers during training, thus improving the network's ability to generalize unseen data. Through dropout regularization, the architecture of the neural network is adjusted, contributing to more robust model performance.

3.5. Hyperparameter Tuning

The predictive capability of an ML model heavily relies on fine-tuning its hyperparameters. Hyperparameters are configuration settings that are not directly learned from the data but influence the learning process. Optimizing these hyperparameters is crucial to achieve the best model performance. In ML, various methods are commonly employed to fine-tune a model's hyperparameters. The manual search involves manually tweaking the hyperparameters based on prior knowledge and intuition. The grid search systematically explores a predefined grid of hyperparameter combinations and evaluates the model's performance for each configuration. Moreover, the random search employs a randomized search strategy by sampling hyperparameters from predefined distributions. In this study, the RandomizedSearchCV method is used for parameter tuning. RandomizedSearchCV combines the benefits of random search and cross-validation. It randomly samples hyperparameters from the defined distributions and evaluates the model's performance using cross-validation techniques. This approach allows for a more efficient exploration of the hyperparameter space, enabling the identification of promising combinations that yield improved model performance. Once the hyperparameters are fine-tuned using RandomizedSearchCV, the model is deemed ready for training, testing, and prediction. With the optimized hyperparameters, the model can be trained on the training data, allowing it to learn the underlying patterns and relationships. Subsequently, the model's performance is assessed on the testing set to evaluate its ability to make accurate predictions on unseen data. Finally, with the trained and evaluated model, predictions can be made on new, unseen data to facilitate decision-making and inference tasks.

4. Results and Discussion

4.1. Feature Importance

The SHAP analysis provides a detailed interpretation of feature contributions to the machine learning model's predictions for both Q and ΔP in the gas cooler system. As shown in Figure 8a, for the output variable Q, the $\dot{m}_r$ emerges as the most influential parameter, as indicated by consistently high SHAP values. This reflects the direct thermodynamic relationship between increased refrigerant flow and higher heat capacity. The $\dot{m}_{ca}$ also contributes positively to Q, although with slightly less variability than $\dot{m}_r$. A higher air flow rate enhances the convective heat transfer on the air side, thereby increasing overall heat transfer. The T_{cri} shows a positive impact on Q at higher values, indicating that warmer T_{cri} improves the energy transfer potential. In contrast, the T_{cai} displays a negative relationship with Q, meaning lower T_{cai} values result in larger temperature differentials between air and refrigerant, enhancing heat transfer and increasing Q. The P_{cri} has a minimal effect, as evidenced by SHAP values clustered near zero, suggesting a negligible marginal contribution under the modeled conditions.

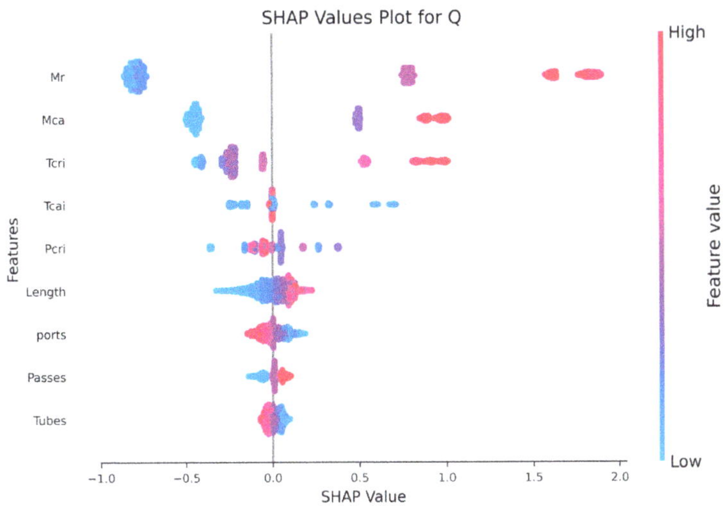

(a)

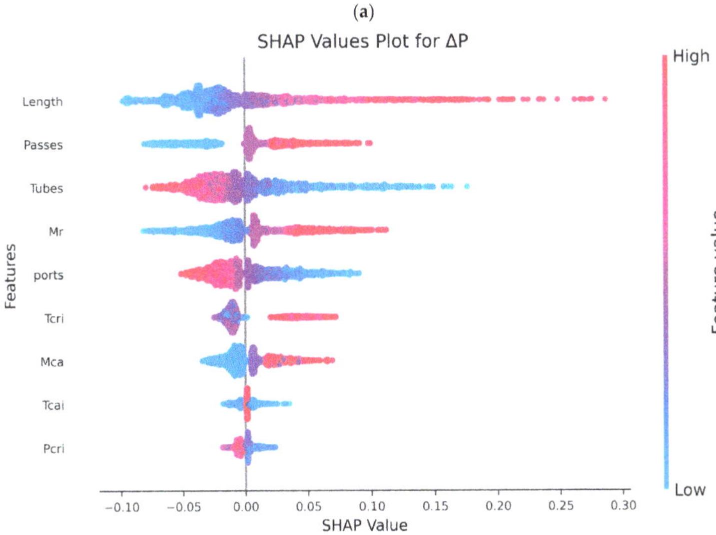

(b)

Figure 8. Impacts of various input parameters on (**a**) SHAP feature impact on output Q, and (**b**) SHAP feature impact on ΔP.

Regarding the geometrical parameters, tube length demonstrates a significant positive influence on Q. A longer tube provides an extended heat transfer surface area and contact time, enhancing thermal exchange. The number of passes also positively affects Q, as it increases the effective refrigerant path length. However, the number of tubes and ports shows a negative impact on Q. This may be attributed to the division of flow among a higher number of channels, potentially reducing the velocity and convective heat transfer effectiveness in individual tubes or ports. Overall, the operating conditions exert a more dominant influence on Q than the geometrical features.

In contrast, the SHAP analysis for ΔP, as illustrated in Figure 8b, reveals a shift in the dominant contributing features. Tube length again shows the highest impact, with longer lengths correlating with increased ΔP due to higher frictional losses over a longer path. Similarly, an increased number of passes leads to higher ΔP, as the flow is redirected more frequently, increasing turbulence and head loss. The number of tubes has a negative contribution; more tubes reduce ΔP by allowing a greater number of parallel flow paths, thereby reducing the velocity and associated frictional losses per tube. The $\dot{m}_r$ has a strong positive impact on ΔP, as higher flow rates increase velocity and, consequently, the pressure loss due to friction. The number of ports shows a negative influence, possibly due to more distribution and reduced local velocities. Notably, the SHAP values for operating conditions such as T_{cri}, $\dot{m}_{ca}$, T_{cai}, and P_{cri} are relatively low, indicating minimal effect on ΔP compared to geometrical parameters. Overall geometrical features dominate the contributions to ΔP while operating parameters have less impact.

These findings highlight the importance of distinguishing the roles of thermodynamic and geometric parameters in influencing different aspects of gas cooler performance. The SHAP analysis not only quantifies each feature's impact but also aligns with engineering principles, offering interpretable and physically consistent insights into the model's decision-making process.

4.2. *Gas Cooler Capacity Predictions*

In Figure 9a–e, the predicted Q of an MCGC is visually represented using advanced ML models such as (a) XGB, (b) RF, (c) SVR, (d) KNNs, and (e) ANNs. Two key metrics, the coefficient of determination (R^2) and the mean squared error (MSE), were used to evaluate the performance and accuracy of each model. The R^2 values, which reflect the proportions of predictable variance, showcase excellent predictive performance across all models, with XGB at 0.99841, RF at 0.99818, SVR at 0.99844, KNNs at 0.99825, and ANNs at 0.99836. Simultaneously, the MSE values, which indicate the average squared differences between the predicted and actual values, exhibit noteworthy accuracy, with XGB at 0.09945, RF at 0.10639, SVR at 0.09858, KNNs at 0.10536, and ANNs at 0.09918.

Possible reasons for obtaining these results are attributed to the inherent strengths of each algorithm. XGB, known for its ensemble learning and boosting techniques, reveals high accuracy and efficiency in capturing complex patterns in the data. RF utilizes multiple decision trees, provides robustness in handling diverse features and reducing overfitting. SVR, which is based on the identification of optimal hyperplanes, excels in handling nonlinear relationships in the data. KNNs rely on proximity and are effective in capturing local patterns and dependencies. Lastly, ANNs, inspired by human brain functioning, showcase significant performance in capturing intricate relationships in large datasets. The combined use of these models allows for a comprehensive evaluation, providing valuable insights into Q predictions and aiding in the selection of the most suitable model for practical applications.

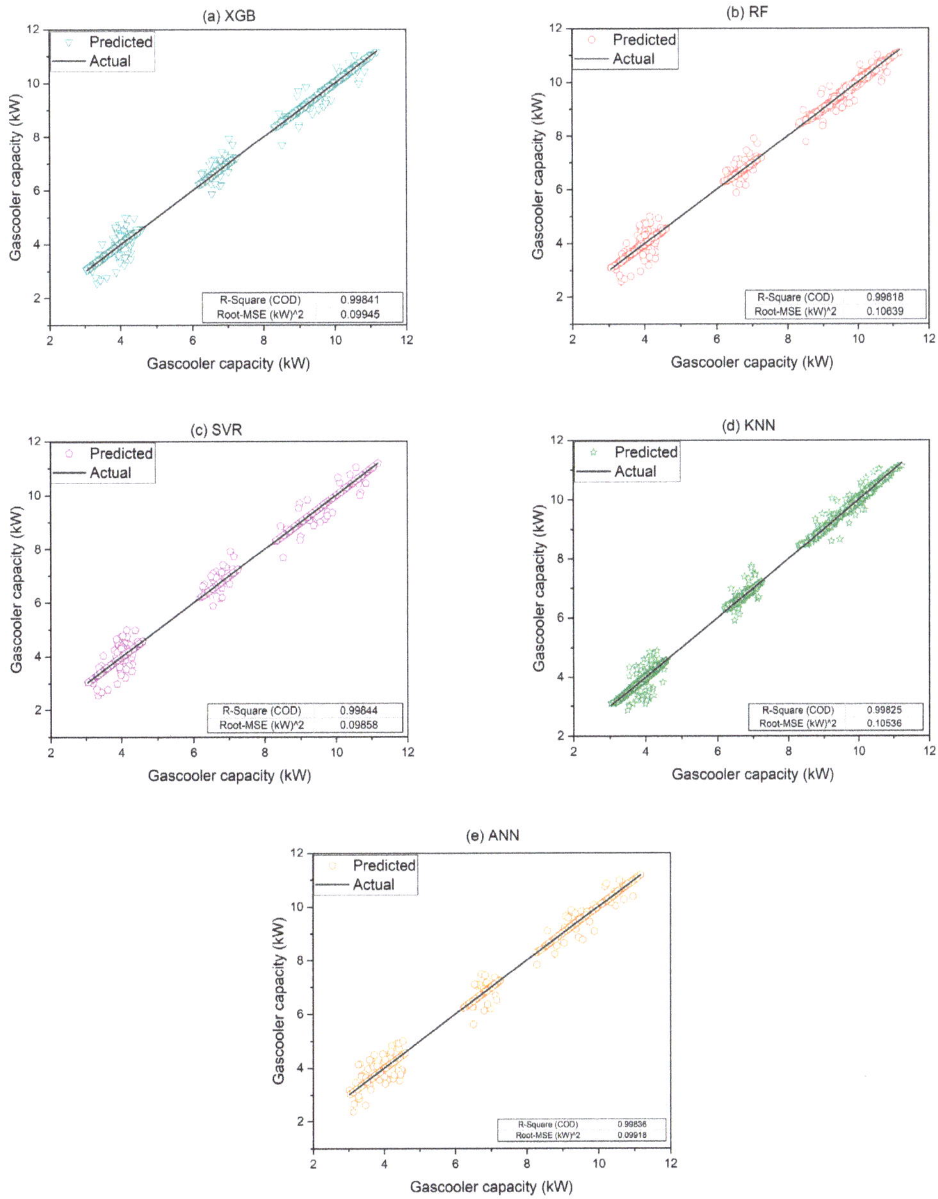

Figure 9. Comparison of the actual and predicted gas cooler capacities using (**a**) XGB, (**b**) RF, (**c**) SVR, (**d**) KNNs, and (**e**) ANNs.

4.3. Gas Cooler Pressure Drop Predictions

The graphical results shown in Figure 10a–e represent ΔP predictions using XGB, RF, SVR, KNNs, and ANNs. As with the capacity prediction, R^2 and MSE were used to assess model reliability, showing consistently high accuracy across all approaches. Notably, XGB stands out with an exceptional R^2 value of 0.99398, highlighting its robust capability in predicting ΔP. SVR and ANNs also exhibit significant R^2 values of 0.99166 and 0.98954, respectively, emphasizing their accuracy. RF maintains a notable R^2 value of 0.96809, whereas the KNN model, with its focus on proximity-based predictions, displays a somewhat lower R^2 value of 0.86713. This is primarily due to the local nature of KNN, which performs well in dense regions but lacks a global modeling structure, making it less suitable for capturing complex ΔP patterns. In contrast, ANN excels by modeling intricate non-linear dependencies, while XGB and SVR effectively manage high variance through boosting and margin optimization, respectively.

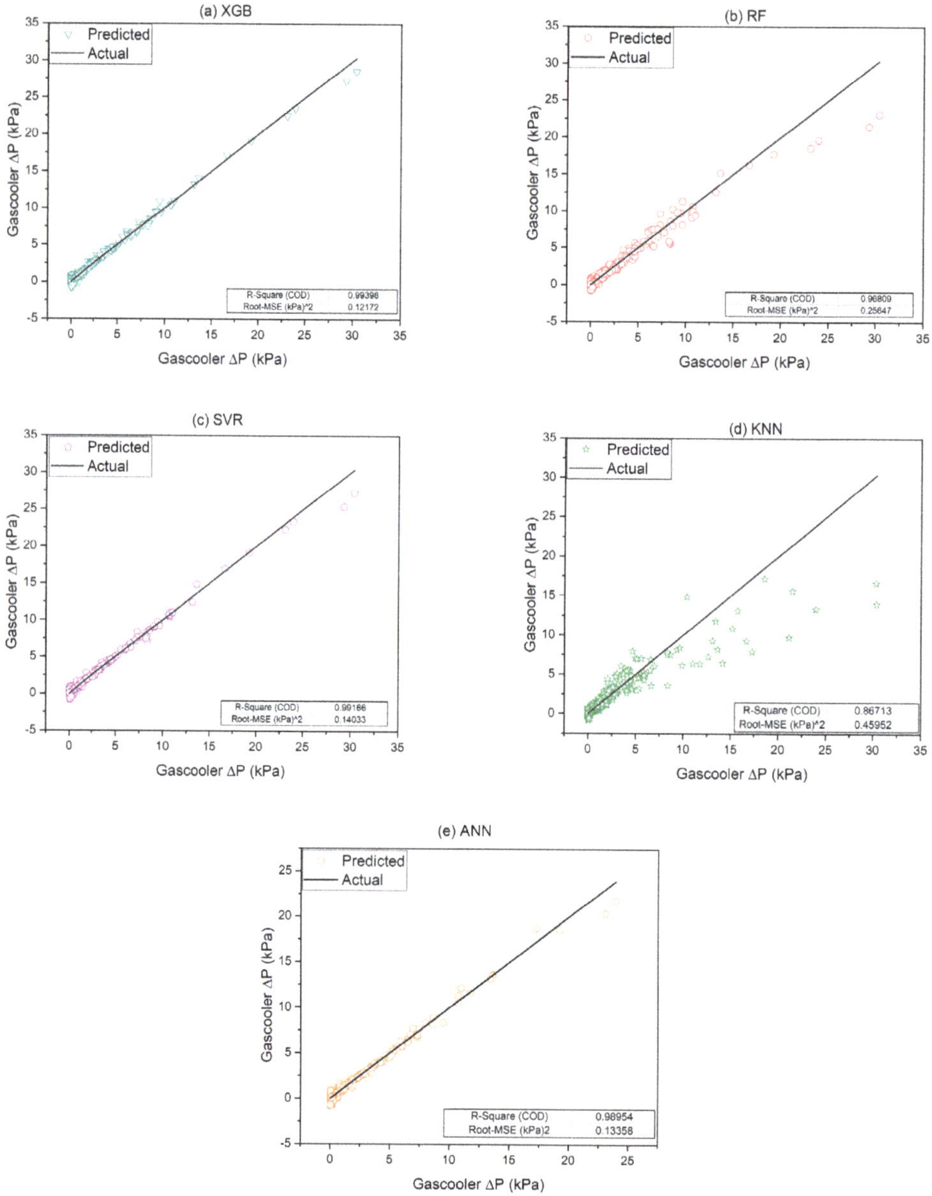

Figure 10. Comparison of the actual and predicted gas cooler ΔPs using (**a**) XGB, (**b**) RF, (**c**) SVR, (**d**) KNNs, and (**e**) ANNs.

At the same time, the MSE values, which offer insights into the average squared differences between the predicted and actual values, confirm the accuracy of the models. XGB demonstrates exceptional precision with a low MSE of 0.12172, indicating minimal discrepancies in its ΔP predictions. SVR and ANN exhibit reliability with MSE values of 0.14033 and 0.13358, respectively. However, RF, despite its robust R^2 value, presents a higher MSE of 0.25647, indicating some variability in prediction accuracy. The KNN model, which relies on local patterns, demonstrates a higher MSE of 0.45952, indicating potential challenges in capturing complex relationships within the data. The small variations in the performances of the models emphasize the importance of selecting suitable algorithms based on specific data characteristics and the complexities of the prediction task. Among all the models, XGB stands out as an effective predictor, producing impressive and reliable ΔP predictions. The RF model exhibits slight dispersion in its predictions. The SVR model presents more detailed behavior, providing dispersed predictions for lower ΔP while exhibiting enhanced accuracy for higher ΔP. This intriguing distinction shows the SVR model's sensitivity to ΔP ranges and its potential applicability in scenarios with high ΔPs. In contrast, the KNN model shows considerable inconsistency, delivering highly dispersed predictions that deviate significantly from the acceptable range. Such divergence raises concerns about the suitability of the KNN model for ΔP analysis. On the other hand, the ANN model emerges as the best predictive model for ΔP prediction. The results highlight exceptional performance, surpassing the performance of other models. This superiority can be attributed to the ANN's unique approach based on deep learning principles, enabling it to effectively capture complex patterns and dependencies in the ΔP data. XGB shows robust predictive capabilities, RF exhibits promise with slight fluctuation, and SVR reveals distinct behavior across ΔP ranges. While KNN's highly dispersed predictions raise concerns about its reliability, the ANN model stands out as a dominant model due to its precision and accuracy in ΔP predictions, substantiating the power of deep learning techniques.

4.4. Refrigerant (CO_2) Outlet Temperature Predictions

Figure 11 illustrates that all models reveal remarkable accuracy in their predictions of refrigerant (CO_2) outlet temperature. Among the models, the ANN demonstrates superior performance, providing the most accurate predictions of outlet temperature. This high level of precision can be attributed to its deep learning architecture, which effectively captures complex patterns and dependencies within the data, resulting in highly reliable outcomes. Furthermore, the SVR model notably avoids overfitting in this specific case. This indicates that SVR's margin-based learning is well-tuned for smooth continuous outputs like temperature, though its performance may still be constrained in the presence of high-dimensional feature interactions, where ANN has a natural advantage.

4.5. Air Outlet Temperature Predictions

Our detailed assessment of predictive models for outlet air temperature forecasting revealed the notable potential of all models to achieve accurate predictions. Among them, the ANN model exhibits the highest precision and reliability in its predictions, as shown in Figure 12. Its superior performance can be attributed to its utilization of sophisticated DL techniques, which enables it to discern intricate patterns and dependencies within the data. The XGB and SVR models closely follow the ANN model in proficiency, demonstrating commendable predictive capabilities. Their competitive performance attests to their capacity to capture meaningful insights from the data, although they fall short of the exceptional results achieved using the ANN model. Moreover, the RF and KNN models offer noteworthy outcomes, though RF may have oversmoothed predictions due to averaging across trees, and KNN's instance-based learning is more sensitive to local variations, limiting its generalization across broader operating conditions.

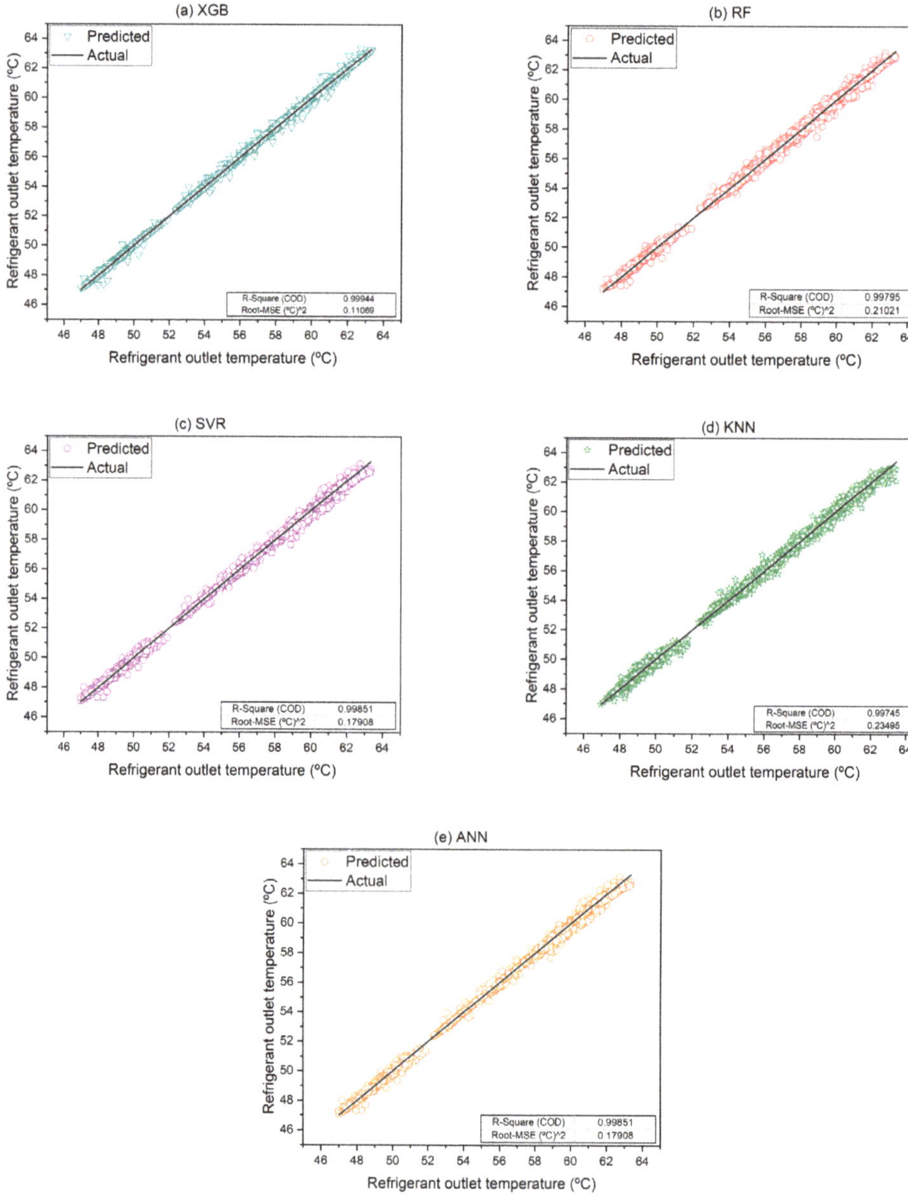

Figure 11. Comparison of the actual and predicted refrigerant outlet temperatures using (**a**) XGB, (**b**) RF, (**c**) SVR, (**d**) KNNs, and (**e**) ANNs.

4.6. Comparitive Analysis of Numerical Model and ANN

Figure 13a evaluates the percentage error in predicting Q by comparing experimental data with numerical simulation results, and numerical results with ANN predictions. The error between experimental and numerical results averages 3.63%, indicating that the numerical model effectively captures the thermal behavior of the gas cooler. This level of agreement suggests that the numerical model accurately incorporates the key thermo-physical properties of the working fluid, heat transfer mechanisms, and flow distribution effects. On the other hand, the ANN model, trained on numerical data, demonstrates a slightly higher average error of 4.14%. This reflects the ANN's capacity to generalize from training data and estimate thermal capacity under varying input conditions with reasonable accuracy. Despite the black-box nature of ANNs, their predictive reliability in this context highlights their suitability for quick performance estimation, especially when rapid analysis is needed in parametric studies or optimization routines.

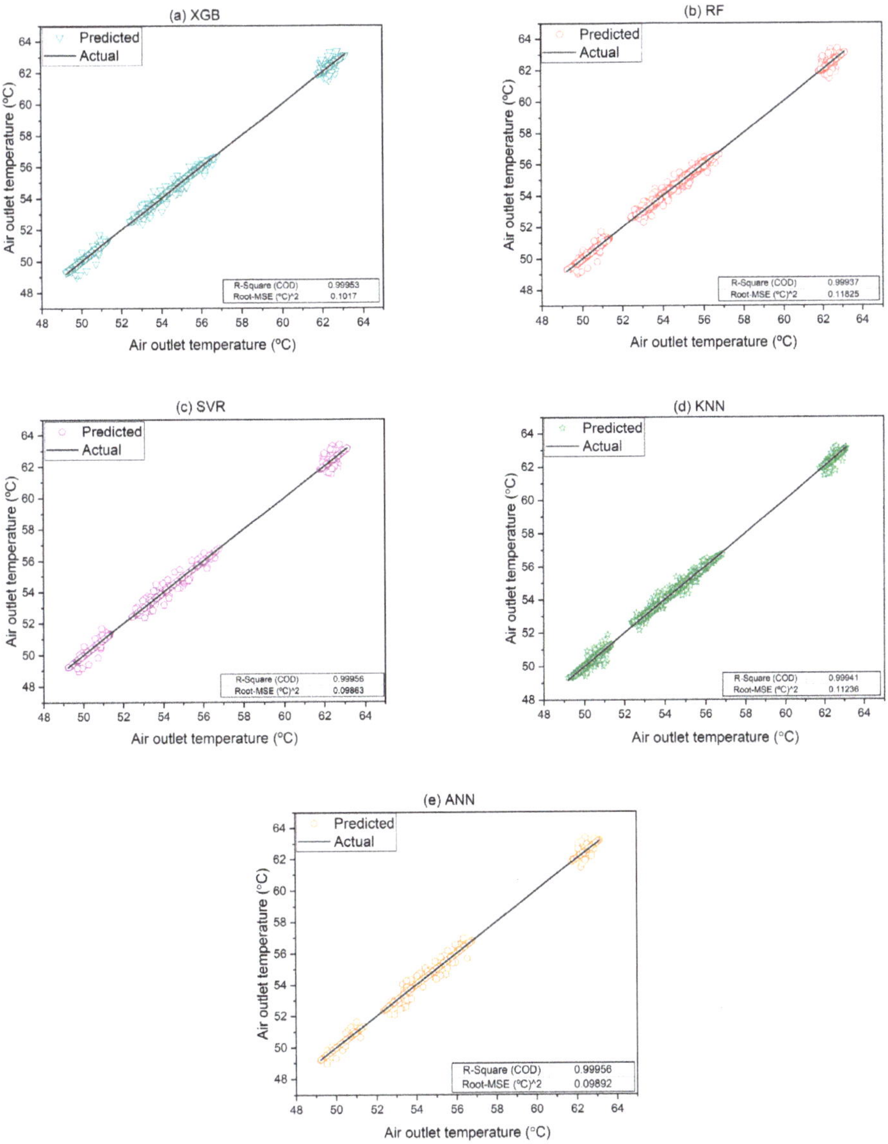

Figure 12. Comparison of the actual and predicted air outlet temperatures using (**a**) XGB, (**b**) RF, (**c**) SVR, (**d**) KNNs, and (**e**) ANNs.

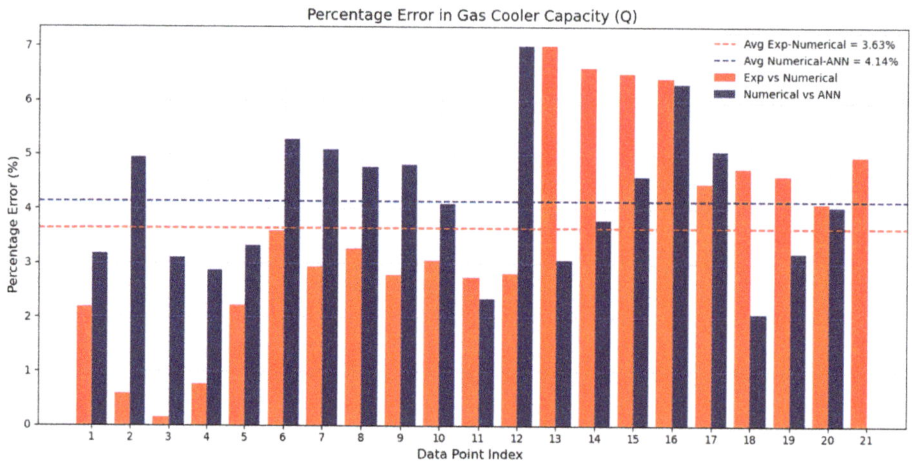

(**a**)

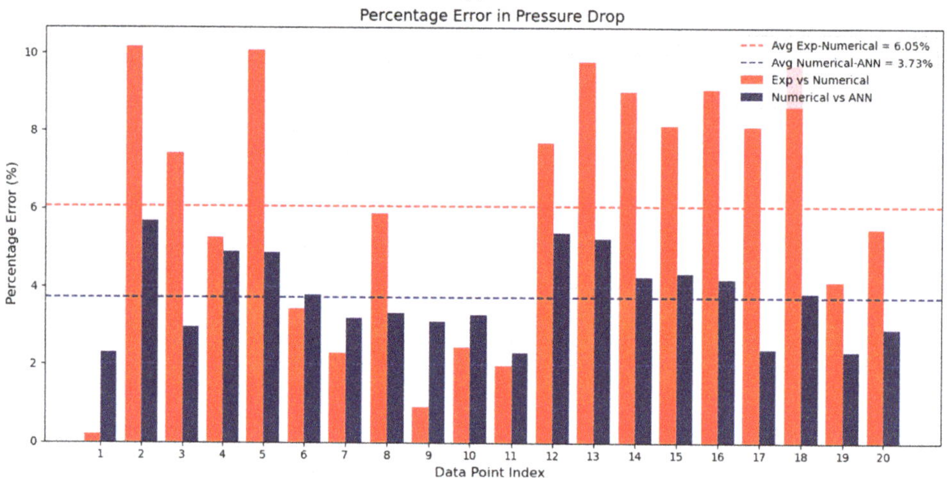

(**b**)

Figure 13. (**a**) Comparison of percentage difference in Q predictions (experimental vs. numerical) and (numerical vs. ANN). (**b**) Comparison of percentage difference in gas cooler ΔP predictions (experimental vs. numerical) and (numerical vs. ANN).

Figure 13b analyzes the percentage error in predicting gas cooler ΔP, again comparing experimental data with numerical results, and numerical data with ANN predictions. ΔP prediction typically involves more sensitivity to geometric features, flow regime transitions, and localized effects such as entrance losses or maldistribution. The numerical model shows an average error of 6.05% when compared to experimental values, suggesting that while it captures the general trend, it may have limitations in modeling detailed flow resistance or minor losses. In contrast, the ANN model achieves a lower average error of 3.73% compared to the numerical results, indicating effective learning of the complex nonlinear mapping between inputs (e.g., geometric and operating conditions) and output (ΔP). Moreover, once the ANN model is trained, it can produce predictions in nanoseconds, offering a significant computational advantage over simulation-based methods, which are typically resource-intensive and time-consuming. This speed advantage makes ANN particularly attractive for real-time control, iterative design, and optimization applications.

5. Conclusions

This study employed various machine learning algorithms (XGB, RF, SVR, KNN, and ANN) to predict the thermohydraulic performance of a microchannel gas cooler (MCGC). The models were trained on high-fidelity data generated from a validated numerical model, and their hyperparameters were carefully optimized to ensure robust performance. SHAP plots were used to interpret models and identify the influence of key operational and geometric parameters.

Among the tested models, ANN consistently delivered the highest accuracy across all performance metrics, including Q, ΔP, and outlet temperatures. XGB and SVR also performed well in certain cases, while KNN showed limitations in consistency. SHAP-based interpretability helped uncover important trends, such as the significant effect of flow rates and air-side temperatures.

This work adds novelty by focusing specifically on transcritical CO_2 MCGCs, a relatively less-explored application in ML-based thermal system modeling. The integration of explainable ML techniques (e.g., SHAP) further enhances its practical relevance, offering insights that can support the design and optimization of advanced cooling systems, particularly in automotive and energy applications.

From a comparative standpoint, the findings highlight the importance of aligning model choice with data characteristics. ANN's deep learning framework excels at capturing intricate nonlinear relationships in complex thermofluidic data, while XGB's ensemble boosting effectively reduces bias and variance. SVR demonstrates strength in handling smooth trends without overfitting, and RF provides stability through averaging, albeit sometimes at the cost of precision. KNN, despite being intuitive and easy to implement, is more sensitive to local noise and less suited for capturing global patterns. These distinctions offer guidance for model selection in future applications of ML in heat exchanger performance prediction.

6. Practical Implications and Design Recommendations

The findings of this study offer practical guidance for the design and optimization of CO_2 gas coolers in electric vehicle (EV) thermal management systems. The integration of machine learning (ML) models with SHAP-based interpretability highlights the most influential operating and geometric parameters affecting thermal performance. Specifically, refrigerant and air mass flow rates, as well as refrigerant inlet temperature, emerged as key factors influencing cooling capacity. This indicates that strategies such as adjusting refrigerant flow rates, enhancing air-side heat transfer via fan speed or duct design, and managing inlet conditions can yield significant improvements. Additionally, geometric factors such as tube length, number of passes, and number of ports should be carefully balanced to maximize heat transfer while avoiding flow maldistribution. The developed ML models, coupled with SHAP insights, not only support accurate performance prediction but also offer a robust framework for real-time control, early-stage design, and integration into digital twins, thereby translating data-driven methods into actionable engineering solutions.

Author Contributions: Conceptualization, S.I. and N.U.; Methodology, S.I. and N.U.; Validation, S.I. and N.U.; Formal analysis, S.I. and N.U.; Investigation, S.I. and N.U.; Data curation, S.I., N.U. and S.C.; Writing—original draft, S.I. and N.U.; Writing—review & editing, S.I., N.U., S.C. and M.-H.K.; Supervision, S.C. and M.-H.K.; Project administration, M.-H.K.; Funding acquisition, M.-H.K. All authors have read and agreed to the published version of the manuscript.

Funding: This research received no external funding.

Data Availability Statement: The original contributions presented in the study are included in the article, further inquiries can be directed to the corresponding author.

Acknowledgments: This work was partly supported by the Korea Institute of Energy Technology Evaluation and Planning (KETEP) grant funded by the Korea government (MOTIE) (Project number: RS-2025-02313376).

Conflicts of Interest: The authors declare no conflict of interest.

Nomenclature

$\dot{m}_{ca}$	Air flow rate, kg/s
ΔP	Gas cooler pressure drop, kPa
$\dot{m}_r$	Refrigerant mass flow rate, kg/s
P_{cri}	Refrigerant inlet pressure, kPa
Q	Gas cooler capacity, kW
T_{cai}	Air inlet temperature, °C
T_{ao}	Air outlet temperature, °C
T_{cri}	Refrigerant inlet temperature, °C
T_{ro}	Refrigerant outlet temperature, °C
Abbreviations	
CFD	Computational fluid dynamics
DL	Deep learning
EVs	Electric vehicles
ML	Machine learning
MCGC	Microchannel gascooler
MACS	Mobile air-conditioning system
SHAP	Shapley additive explanations
XGB	XGBoost
RF	Random Forest
SVR	Support Vector Regression
KNNs	k-Nearest Neighbors
ANNs	Artificial Neural Networks
R^2	Coefficient of determination
MSE	Mean squared error

References

1. The Number of New-Energy Vehicles in China Reached at 7.84 Million by the End of 2021. Available online: http://www.gov.cn/xinwen/2022-01/12/content_5667734.htm (accessed on 3 May 2023).
2. Ji, H.; Pei, J.; Niu, J.; Ding, C.; Guo, F.; Wang, Y. Hybrid offline and online strategy for optimal high pressure seeking of the transcritical CO_2 heat pump system in an electric vehicle. *Appl. Therm. Eng.* **2023**, *228*, 120514. [CrossRef]
3. Wang, H.; Song, Y.; Qiao, Y.; Li, S.; Cao, F. Rational assessment and selection of air source heat pump system operating with CO_2 and R407C for electric bus. *Renew. Energy* **2022**, *182*, 86–101. [CrossRef]
4. Okasha, A.; Müller, N.; Deb, K. Bi-objective optimization of transcritical CO_2 heat pump systems. *Energy* **2022**, *247*, 123469. [CrossRef]
5. Qin, X.; Zhang, D.; Zhang, F.; Gao, Z.; Wei, X. Experimental and numerical study on heat transfer of gas cooler under the optimal discharge pressure. *Int. J. Refrig.* **2020**, *112*, 229–239. [CrossRef]
6. Song, X.; Yuan, H.; Zhang, Y.; Yu, B.; Wang, D.; Shi, J.; Chen, J. Experimental study on improved performance of an automotive CO_2 air conditioning system with an evaporative gas cooler. *Int. J. Refrig.* **2022**, *140*, 39–48. [CrossRef]
7. Wang, D.; Yu, B.; Shi, J.; Chen, J. Experimental and theoretical study on the cooling performance of a CO_2 mobile air conditioning system. *Energies* **2018**, *11*, 1927. [CrossRef]
8. Na, S.I.; Kim, M.; Kim, M.S. Performance simulation of CO_2 transcritical cooling system with mechanical subcooling cycle for automobile air conditioning. *J. Mech. Sci. Technol.* **2022**, *36*, 4797–4807. [CrossRef]
9. Nie, F.; Wang, H.; Zhao, Y.; Song, Q.; Yan, S.; Gong, M. A universal correlation for flow condensation heat transfer in horizontal tubes based on machine learning. *Int. J. Therm. Sci.* **2023**, *184*, 107994. [CrossRef]

10. Saeed, M.; Berrouk, A.S.; Al Wahedi, Y.F.; Singh, M.P.; Dagga, I.A.; Afgan, I. Performance enhancement of a C-shaped printed circuit heat exchanger in supercritical CO_2 Brayton cycle: A machine learning-based optimization study. *Case Stud. Therm. Eng.* **2022**, *38*, 102276. [CrossRef]
11. Saeed, M.; Kalule, R.S.; Berrouk, A.S.; Alshehhi, M.; Almatrafi, E. Machine Learning-Based Optimization of a Mini-Channel Heatsink Geometry. *Arab. J. Sci. Eng.* **2023**, *48*, 12107–12124. [CrossRef]
12. Haghighi, A.; Shadloo, M.S.; Maleki, A.; Abdollahzadeh Jamalabadi, M.Y. Using committee neural network for prediction of pressure drop in two-phase microchannels. *Appl. Sci.* **2020**, *10*, 5384. [CrossRef]
13. Kim, K.; Lee, H.; Kang, M.; Lee, G.; Jung, K.; Kharangate, C.R.; Asheghi, M.; Goodson, K.E.; Lee, H. A machine learning approach for predicting heat transfer characteristics in micro-pin fin heat sinks. *Int. J. Heat Mass Transf.* **2022**, *194*, 123087. [CrossRef]
14. Yu, C.; Zhu, X.; Li, Z.; Ma, Y.; Yang, M.; Zhang, H. Optimization of elliptical pin-fin microchannel heat sink based on artificial neural network. *Int. J. Heat Mass Transf.* **2023**, *205*, 123928. [CrossRef]
15. Sikirica, A.; Grbčić, L.; Kranjčević, L. Machine learning based surrogate models for microchannel heat sink optimization. *Appl. Therm. Eng.* **2023**, *222*, 119917. [CrossRef]
16. Zohora, F.T.; Akter, F.; Haque, M.A.; Chowdhury, N.M.; Haque, M.R. A novel pin finned structure-embedded microchannel heat sink: CFD-data driven MLP, MLR, and XGBR machine learning models for thermal and fluid flow prediction. *Energy* **2024**, *307*, 132646. [CrossRef]
17. Efatinasab, E.; Irannezhad, N.; Rampazzo, M.; Diani, A. Machine and deep learning driven models for the design of heat exchangers with micro-finned tubes. *Energy AI* **2024**, *16*, 100370. [CrossRef]
18. Aksöz, Z.Y.; Günay, M.E.; Aziz, M.; Tunç, K.M.M. Machine Learning Analysis of Thermal Performance Indicator of Heat Exchangers with Delta Wing Vortex Generators. *Energies* **2024**, *17*, 1380. [CrossRef]
19. Lee, H.; Lee, G.; Kim, K.; Kong, D.; Lee, H. Multimodal machine learning for predicting heat transfer characteristics in micro-pin fin heat sinks. *Case Stud. Therm. Eng.* **2024**, *57*, 104331. [CrossRef]
20. Kuberan, V.; Gedupudi, S. Empirical modeling and hybrid machine learning framework for nucleate pool boiling on microchannel structured surfaces. *Int. J. Heat Mass Transf.* **2025**, *249*, 127163. [CrossRef]
21. Bakır, R.; Khail, A.A.; Bakır, H. Enhancing the prediction of flow characteristics in an inventive plate heat exchanger using deep learning techniques. *Phys. Scr.* **2025**, *100*, 3. [CrossRef]
22. Su, Y.; Zhao, Y.; Wu, J.; Zhang, L. Research on Heat Transfer Coefficient Prediction of Printed Circuit Plate Heat Exchanger Based on Deep Learning. *Appl. Sci.* **2025**, *15*, 4635. [CrossRef]
23. Godasiaei, S.H.; Kamali, H.A. Evaluating Machine Learning as an Alternative to CFD for Heat Transfer Modeling. *Microgravity Sci. Technol.* **2025**, *37*, 6. [CrossRef]
24. Gomathi, B.; Ramanipriya, M.; Anitha, S. Machine learning approach to predict the thermal performance and friction factor of cylindrical heat exchangers with perforated conical ring turbulators. *J. Therm. Anal. Calorim.* **2025**. [CrossRef]
25. Kim, M.H.; Bullard, C.W. Air-side thermal hydraulic performance of multi-louvered fin aluminum heat exchangers. *Int. J. Refrig.* **2002**, *25*, 390–400. [CrossRef]
26. Incropera, F.P.; Dewitt, D.P.; Bergman, T.L. *Fundamentals of Heat and Mass Transfer*, 6th ed.; John Wiley & Sons: Hoboken, NJ, USA, 2007. [CrossRef]
27. Yin, J.M.; Bullard, C.W.; Hrnjak, P.S. R-744 Gas Cooler Model Development and Validation. *Int. J. Refrig.* **2001**, *24*, 692–701. [CrossRef]
28. Ullah, N.; Ishaque, S.; Kim, M.H.; Choi, S. Modeling and Optimization of a Micro-Channel Gas Cooler for a Transcritical CO_2 Mobile Air-Conditioning System. *Machines* **2022**, *10*, 1177. [CrossRef]
29. Chen, T.; Guestrin, C. XGBoost: A scalable tree boosting system. In Proceedings of the ACM SIGKDD International Conference on Knowledge Discovery and Data Mining; Association for Computing Machiner: New York, NY, USA, 2016; pp. 785–794. [CrossRef]
30. Breiman, L. Random Forests. *Mach. Learn.* **2001**, *45*, 5–32. [CrossRef]
31. Boser, B.E.; Guyon, I.M.; Vapnik, V.N. A Training Algorithm for Optimal Margin Classifiers. In Proceedings of the Fifth Annual Workshop on Computational Learning Theory, Pittsburgh, PA, USA, 27–29 July 1992; pp. 144–152.

energies

MDPI

Article

Thermal and Emission Performance Evaluation of Hydrogen-Enriched Natural Gas-Fired Domestic Condensing Boilers

Radosław Jankowski [1,*], Rafał Ślefarski [1], Ireneusz Bauma [1] and Giennadii Varlamov [2]

[1] Institute of Thermal Energy, Poznan University of Technology, 60-965 Poznan, Poland; rafal.slefarski@put.poznan.pl (R.Ś.); ireneusz.bauma@doctorate.put.poznan.pl (I.B.)
[2] Institute of Sustainable Building Materials and Engineering Systems, Riga Technical University, Ķīpsalas 6A-539, LV-1048 Riga, Latvia; varlamovgb@gmail.com
* Correspondence: radoslaw.jankowski@put.poznan.pl; Tel.: +48-616652214

Abstract

The combustion of gaseous fuels in condensing boilers contributes to the greenhouse gas and toxic compound emissions in exhaust gases. Hydrogen, as a clean energy carrier, could play a key role in decarbonizing the residential heating sector. However, its significantly different combustion behavior compared to hydrocarbon fuels requires thorough investigation prior to implementation in heating systems. This study presents experimental and theoretical analyses of the co-combustion of natural gas with hydrogen in low-power-output condensing boilers (second and third generation), with hydrogen content of up to 50% by volume. The results show that mixtures of hydrogen and natural gas contribute to increasing heat transfer in boilers through convection and flue gas radiation. They also highlight the benefits of using the heat from the condensation of vapors in the flue gases. Other studies have observed an increase in efficiency of up to 1.6 percentage points compared to natural gas at 50% hydrogen content. Up to a 6% increase in the amount of energy recovered by water vapor condensation was also recorded, while exhaust gas losses did not change significantly. Notably, the addition of hydrogen resulted in a substantial decrease in the emission of nitrogen oxides (NOx) and carbon monoxide (CO). At 50% hydrogen content, NO_x emissions decreased several-fold to 2.7 mg/m^3, while CO emissions were reduced by a factor of six, reaching 9.9 mg/m^3. All measured NO_x values remained well below the current regulatory limit for condensing gas boilers, which is 33.5 mg/m^3. These results highlight the potential of hydrogen blending as a transitional solution on the path toward cleaner residential heating systems.

Keywords: condensing boiler; hydrogen; nitric oxides; flame emissivity

1. Introduction

Natural gas is the most frequently used fuel for residential heating in the European Union (EU), accounting for about 30.9% of all energy sources. In several countries, this share is close to or exceeds 50% (The Netherlands—66.2%, Italy—49.8%, Hungary—49.2%, Luxembourg—46.2%). The EU is responsible for approximately 34% of energy-related emissions, with a significant share originating from the direct combustion of fossil fuels, including natural gas, in heating appliances. It is estimated that the annual use of gas fuel for residential purposes in the EU results in approximately 220 million tons of CO_2 emissions. Several initiatives are being implemented to reduce CO_2 emissions, including the replacement of solid fuel boilers with heat pumps and electric boilers, the increased use of biomass (wood chips, sawdust, pellets, and briquettes) [1], and the introduction of renewable gaseous fuels (biomethane, biogas, and hydrogen) [2–5].

Hydrogen is increasingly being considered as a viable alternative to natural gas in residential heating systems due to its potential to reduce carbon dioxide emissions. This is supported by key EU documents outlining the policies, strategies, and roadmaps for transitioning to a circular economy. It should be noted that the EU Directive 2024/1788 of 13 June 2024 permits the blending of hydrogen with natural gas; however, it does not specify a reference concentration for H_2 mixed with natural gas. Therefore, several European countries have now introduced their own rules regarding the maximum permissible concentration of hydrogen [6,7]. For example, in Germany, up to 10% hydrogen by volume is allowed in the gas network, provided there are no natural gas compressor stations (CNGs); in France, the limit is 6%; in Austria, 4%; and in Switzerland, 2% [8].

Hydrogen as a fuel differs significantly in its properties from hydrocarbon fuels, which affects the operation of energy devices, including condensing boilers, in several aspects, such as the combustion process, the emission of nitric oxides and carbon monoxide, thermal efficiency, and the safety of device operation. The thermodynamic parameters that differ significantly between H_2 and natural gas (NG) include laminar burning velocity (S_L), adiabatic flame temperature (T_A), flammability limits (FLs), and low heating value (LHV). Chen et al. [9] demonstrated that for combustion process parameters typical of low-power-output boilers (T_{air} = 293 K, P = 1 bar, ϕ = 0.8), the ratio of $S_{L\_H_2}$ to S_{L_NG} is 6.7. The higher velocity of the laminar flame makes hydrogen flame combustion more susceptible to the phenomenon of flashback in premix burners, which can raise serious safety concerns. Additionally, the higher hydrogen adiabatic flame temperature ($T_{A\_H_2}/T_{A\_NG}$ = 1.1) can lead not only to increased nitrogen oxide concentrations in emissions but also to enhanced radiative heat transfer within the combustion chamber. In addition, hydrogen fuel has almost three times less calorific value per cubic meter compared to natural gas, which can limit the power output of heating devices or necessitate their modification [10]. However, the advantages of hydrogen include its wide range of flammability, which under normal atmospheric conditions in the air ranges from 4 to 75% vol. compared to NG (4.3–15% vol.), as well as its low ignition energy of 0.02 mJ, which is much higher for natural gas and reaches 0.28 mJ [11,12]. These properties of hydrogen ensure its stable combustion in much leaner mixtures; however, this feature is not used in small residential heating boilers [13]. Therefore, these distinctive thermodynamic parameters of hydrogen combustion necessitate further research to explore the possibility of its co-combustion with natural gas in heating devices. Cuoci et al. [14] conducted experimental and numerical studies on the operation and emissions of a 30 kW condensing boiler fueled with natural gas mixtures enriched with up to 35% hydrogen by volume. They observed stable operation of the device; however, as the hydrogen content (H_2) increased, NO_x emissions rose, while CO emissions decreased.

However, other studies have indicated a decrease in NO_x emissions at higher concentrations of hydrogen mixed with NG. In experimental studies, Coskun achieved a 37% and 40% reduction in NO_x and CO emissions, respectively, when burning fuel using a 24 kW domestic boiler with a porous burner operating on an NG/H_2 mixture of 20% vol. and 80% vol. [15]. In [16], the authors examined conventional storage water heaters operated on hydrogen-enriched natural gas with up to 30% vol. H_2. They achieved a slight reduction in nitrogen oxide and carbon monoxide emissions. However, the limit for stable operation of the device was only 10% hydrogen by volume in the fuel.

Studies on the co-firing of a mixture of H_2 (up to 45% vol.) and NG in a staged combustion system using a 15 kW domestic boiler showed a significant reduction in NO_x—by more than 10%—with a simultaneous increase in CO and C_xH_y emissions, as well as a slight decrease in thermal efficiency [17]. The possibility of using a mixture of H_2 with low calorific natural gas in selected domestic appliances was presented by Wojtowicz and Jaworski [18]. The combustion process of a mixture containing 13% hydrogen and 87% natural gas by volume in a gas stove, water heater, and gas boilers was analyzed. Fuel replacement resulted in a decrease in boiler efficiency by 0.5 to 1.8, depending on the temperature of the heat carrier, while a 10% increase in efficiency was observed for the water heater. Another observation about the change in the overall efficiency of a medium-sized condensing boiler (2.8 MW) was made by Yang. In his study [19], an increase in the hydrogen content of the fuel to 100% vol. led to an increase in the boiler efficiency compared to natural gas (NG), with an equivalence factor of $\phi = 0.91$. The authors attribute this effect to a decrease in flue gas temperature, resulting in reduced heat loss from the boiler's exhaust gas.

A review of the literature revealed a lack of a comprehensive and comparable experimental database on the co-combustion of hydrogen with natural gas in low-power condensing boilers (second and third generation). This prevents drawing clear and objective conclusions regarding the direct relationship between the increase in installation efficiency and the reduction in harmful emission concentrations as a function of hydrogen content in the NG/H_2 mixture. Moreover, there is a lack of knowledge regarding the influence of hydrogen on heat transfer phenomena within boiler combustion chambers. Therefore, the authors decided to conduct a thermodynamic and environmental assessment of the co-combustion process of hydrogen and natural gas using various hydrogen concentrations (up to 50% vol.) in two types of condensing boilers. The experimental studies were complemented by a theoretical analysis addressing the impact of fuel composition changes on heat transfer mechanisms in condensing boiler systems.

2. Materials and Methods

This study describes the sequence of tests and the methodology for assessing the effect of hydrogen on the performance of one type of condensing gas boiler from the second and third generations, in which a mixture of hydrogen and natural gas (NG) in different proportions was used as fuel. The combustion process in a second-generation boiler occurs in accordance with the manufacturer's specifications from the production stage. The fuel flow is selected according to the heat demand, while the air intake is regulated by adjusting the fan speed according to a programmed curve. In comparison to the second-generation boiler, the third-generation boiler is equipped with an automatic combustion control system that includes an additional ionization electrode and a dedicated controller. The ionization rod signal regulates the air amount by selecting the appropriate fan speed, ensuring that the electrode measurement signal readings are within the specified range. The fuel flow is adjusted to the actual thermal load by a regulation valve. This allows us to ensure that the boiler operation is adjusted to the optimal range of equivalence coefficients, thereby maintaining flame stability. The technical specifications of the tested boilers are presented in Table 1.

Table 1. Technical parameters of the tested condensing boilers.

Device	Nominal Power	Minimal Power	Efficiency [1,2]	NO_x limit	Flame Type
	kW	kW	%	mg/kWh	–
CB_2nd_GEN	25.7	5.4	106.91	37.9	Diffusion
CB_3rd_GEN	21.9	2.8	109.51	33.5	Diffusion

[1]—at water temperature 50/30 °C; [2]—according to EN 15502-1:2021-09 [20].

The experimental research was conducted on a test rig shown in Figure 1. The test setup consists of a fuel supply system, the tested boilers, a thermal energy extraction system, and measuring equipment (thermocouples, mass balance, and flow meters). The natural gas, which was supplied from the gas network, had an average composition of CH_4 = 94.2% vol., C_2H_6 = 4.2% vol., C_3H_8 = 0.4% vol., C_4H_{10} = 0.1% vol., and N_2 = 1.1% vol. This was then mixed with hydrogen in a static mixer. The flow was controlled using two mass flowmeters. The list of measuring instruments is presented in Table 2.

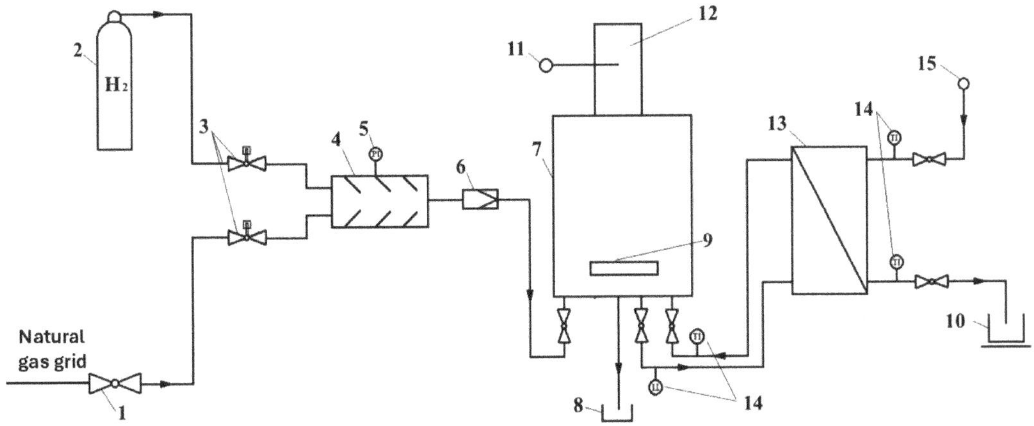

Figure 1. Experimental test rig: 1: natural gas valve; 2: hydrogen vessel; 3: mass flow controllers; 4: static fuel mixer; 5: pressure meter; 6: gas flow meter; 7: boiler; 8: condensate tank; 9: control panel; 10: mass balance; 11: flue gas thermocouple; 12: flue gas measurement port; 13: heat exchanger; 14: temperature sensors; and 15: cooling water connection.

Table 2. List of measurement devices.

Sensor/Device	Measurement	Measurements Range	Accuracy
Gas analyzer NGA2000, Rosemont Inc., Shakopee, MN, USA	Flue gas	O_2: 0–21% CO: 0–100 ppm NO: 0–100 ppm CO_2: 0–25%	±1% FS
Mass flow controller Brooks SLA5853, Brooks Instrument BV, Veenendaal, The Netherlands	NG flow rate	0–300 Nl/min	±0.2% FS
Mass flow controller Bronkhorst EL-FLOW, Bronkhorst High-Tech B.V., Ruurlo, The Netherlands	H_2 flow rate	0–200 Nl/min	±0.5% FS
Manometer MRU DM9200, MRU GmbH, Neckarsulm-Obereisesheim, Germany	Fuel pressure	350 mbar	±1% FS
Temperature sensor RTD PT100, Guenther GmbH, Schwaig, Germany	Temperature	−20 to 100 °C	±1% MV
Mass balance C315.30 Radwag, Radom, Poland	Water	0–30 kg	±0.01 kg

Experimental tests were performed to ensure stable operating conditions, where the monitored parameters (heating water) do not vary by more than ±1 °C over a 10-min time interval for two heat loads: nominal (P_{nom}) and minimal (P_{min}). The measured quantities (temperatures, fuel flow rates, concentrations of nitric oxides, carbon monoxide, oxygen, and carbon dioxide) were recorded at a frequency of 1 Hz and subsequently averaged over time. The hydrogen content in the analyzed mixtures was 10, 20, 30, 40, and 50% by volume. The key parameters of the tested fuels are presented in Table 3, along with their calculated values. For the calculations, pure methane was assumed as the main component of natural gas. Table 4 presents the experimental values measured during the tests.

Table 3. Parameters of the tested fuel mixtures.

Fuel Name	Fuel Composition		LHV	SAR	T_A [1]	S_L [1]	LFL	UFL
	CH_4 % vol.	H_2 % vol.	MJ/m^3	m^3_Air/m^3_Fuel	K	cm/s	%	%
NG	100	0	35.8	9.6	1978	28.4	5.3	15.0
NG_H2_10	90	10	33.3	8.9	1983	30.1	5.1	16.3
NG_H2_20	80	20	30.8	8.2	1992	32.3	5.0	17.9
NG_H2_30	70	30	28.3	7.5	1998	34.8	4.8	19.7
NG_H2_40	60	40	25.8	6.7	2004	38.4	4.7	22.1
NG_H2_50	50	50	23.3	6.0	2011	43.3	4.6	25.0

[1] T_A and S_L values were determined for $\phi = 0.77$ and $T_{in} = 298$ K and P = 1 bar.

Table 4. Selected test parameters.

Device	Power	Temperature				Gas Pressure	Test Duration
		Inlet Water	Outlet Water	NG + H_2	Ambient		
	kW	°C	°C	°C	°C	mbar	Sec.
CB_2nd_Gen	nominal	36	56	15	24	15–25	600
	low	23	30				
CB_3rd_Gen	nominal	35	55				
	low	24	37				

For both condensing boilers, it was possible to test at the rated power using the analyzed fuel mixtures while maintaining similar water temperatures at the boiler inlet and outlet. At the rated power, the minimum outlet water temperature for the CB_2nd_GEN boiler was 30 °C, while the CB_3rd_GEN boiler could operate at an outlet temperature of 37 °C. As a result, the temperature difference between the inlet and outlet water in the third-generation boiler was twice as high as in the second-generation boiler.

Based on measurements of thermodynamic parameters for the studied fuels, calculations were performed to determine the thermal efficiency of the boiler, the heat loss of flue gases at the boiler outlet, and the heat of the condensation of water vapor from flue gases. The effect of hydrogen content in fuel on the emission of NO_x and CO was also determined for the nominal operating parameters of the boiler.

The thermal efficiency of a gas boiler is defined as the ratio of its useful thermal power (Q_{out}) to the heat of the burned fuel (Q_{in}), as shown in Equation (1).

$$\eta_b = \frac{Q_{out}}{Q_{in}} \cdot 100[\%] \quad (1)$$

The heat of combustion of the fuel mixture was determined from Equation (2), while the useful heat transferred to heated water was calculated from Equation (3).

$$Q_{in} = V_f \cdot LHV \quad [\mathrm{W}] \quad (2)$$

$$Q_{out} = m_w \cdot c_w \cdot \Delta T \quad [\mathrm{W}] \quad (3)$$

where V_f denotes the volume flow rate of the fuel [m^3/s]; LHV denotes the lower heating value of the fuel mixture [J/m^3]; m_w denotes the mass flow rate of water; c_w denotes the average specific heat for water [J/kg·K]; and ΔT denotes the water temperature increase [K].

The flue gas heat loss to the environment was determined using the following Equation (4):

$$Q_{fg} = \frac{m_{fg} \sum_{i=1}^{n} g_i h_i \left(T_{fg}\right)}{Q_{in}} \cdot 100\% \quad [\%] \quad (4)$$

where m_{fg} denotes the mass flow rate of flue gases [kg/s]; g_i denotes the mass fraction of flue gas components [–]; h_i denotes the enthalpy of flue gas components at the flue gas temperature [J/kg]; and T_{fg} denotes the flue gas temperature [K].

The emissions measured during the tests were normalized to a reference state corresponding to zero oxygen content in the exhaust gases and recalculated to mg/m^3 of flue gas according to Equations (5) and (6) [21,22].

$$CO_{O2=0\%} = \frac{21 - [O_2]_{ref}}{21 - [O_2]_{mes}} \cdot 1.25[CO]_{mes}\ [mg/m^3_{fg}] \tag{5}$$

$$NO_{xO2=0\%} = \frac{21 - [O_2]_{ref}}{21 - [O_2]_{mes}} \cdot 2.05[NO_x]_{mes}\ [mg/m^3_{fg}] \tag{6}$$

where $[O_2]_{ref}$ denotes the reference oxygen concentration [%]; $[O_2]_{mes}$ denotes the measured oxygen concentration [%]; $[NO_x]_{mes}$ denotes the measured NO_x emission concentration [ppmv]; and $[CO]_{mes}$ denotes the measured CO emission concentration [ppmv].

The heat flux transmitted in the combustion chamber, which heats water, includes the radiative heat flux from the flame and flue gases, the convective heat flux, and the condensation payload. The chemical composition of the fuel affects several thermodynamic parameters that describe the process of heat transfer to the working fluid (water) in the boiler, including flame temperature, gas and air mass flow rates, radiative coefficients, the degree of diffusion, and thermal conductivity. The calculation method for determining the heat energy transferred to the coolant in the condensing boiler is described by Equations (7)–(12). This enabled the theoretical analysis of the effect of changes in fuel composition on the heat exchange process indicators in the condensing boiler.

The convective heat flux was determined using the periodic ratio over the range 2300 < Re < 10,000 [23]

$$Q_c = 0.00263F\frac{k \cdot Pr^{0.35}}{d} \cdot Re^{0.8} \cdot (T_{fg} - T_w)\ [W] \tag{7}$$

where F denotes the heat exchange area [m^2]; k denotes the thermal conductivity coefficient [W/m·K]; Re denotes the Reynolds number [–]; Pr denotes the Prandtl number [–]; d denotes the characteristic length [m]; and T_w denotes the boiler wall temperature [K].

The radiant heat flux transmitted by the flame was calculated according to Equation (8) [24]. The value of the flame emission coefficient (ε_{fl}) for the analyzed fuels was determined using the model described in [25,26] and is given in Equation (9).

$$Q_{R,fl} = 5.67F_{fl}\frac{1}{\frac{1}{\varepsilon_{fl}} + \frac{F_{fl}}{F}\left(\frac{1}{\varepsilon_w} - 1\right)}\left[\left(\frac{T_{fl}}{100}\right)^4 - \left(\frac{T_w}{100}\right)^4\right]\ [W] \tag{8}$$

$$\varepsilon_{fl} = \sum_{i=1}^{n} a_i[1 - \exp(-k_i XPL] \tag{9}$$

where F_{fl} denotes the flame area [m^2]; ε_{fl} denotes the flame emissivity coefficient [–]; ε_w denotes the wall emissivity coefficient [–]; a_i denotes the weighting factor [–]; k_i denotes the absorption coefficient [bar^{-1} m^{-1}]; L denotes the path length [m]; p denotes the total pressure [bar]; X denotes the sum of the molar fraction of absorbing species [–]; and T_{fl} denotes the adiabatic flame temperature [K].

The amount of heat exchange that takes place between the gas layer with a temperature of (T_{fg}) and the surrounding wall of the furnace chamber with a temperature of T_w, taking into account the emissivity of the wall, can be described by Equation (10) [27],

$$Q_{R,fg} = 5.67\mathrm{F}(\varepsilon_w + 1)\left[\varepsilon_{fg(T_{fg})}\left(\frac{T_{fg}}{100}\right)^4 - \varepsilon_{fg(T_w)}\left(\frac{T_w}{100}\right)^4\right]\ [\mathrm{W}] \quad (10)$$

where F denotes the heat exchange area [m^2]; ε_{fg} denotes the flue gas emissivity coefficient [–]; ε_w denotes the wall emissivity coefficient [–]; T_{fg} denotes the flue gas temperature [K]; and T_w denotes the wall temperature [K].

For condensing boilers, latent heat from the condensation of water vapor contained in the flue gases must also be included in the balance of energy supplied to the heat carrier. The amount of energy from the condensation process is determined based on the ratio (11) proposed by Osakabe in [28],

$$Q_{cond} = F \cdot h_c \cdot L_w \left(c_{fg} - c_w\right)\ [M] \quad (11)$$

where F denotes the heat exchange area [m^2]; h_c denotes the mass transfer coefficient [m/s]; L_w denotes the latent heat [J/kg]; c_{fg} denotes the steam mass concentration per unit volume of flue gas [–]; and c_w denotes the mass concentration of saturated steam at the wall temperature [–].

The mass transfer coefficient for flue gases is determined based on Sherwood ratios, where the characteristic length (H) is assumed to be equal to the height of the combustion chamber of the mixture [29],

$$h_c = 0.664\frac{D}{H}\, Re^{1/2} Sc^{1/3}\ [m/s] \quad (12)$$

where D denotes the mass diffusivity [m^2/s]; H denotes the characteristic length [m]; Re denotes the Reynolds number [–]; and Sc denotes the Schmidt number [–].

When assessing the effect of changes in the chemical composition of the fuel on the heat transfer phenomena in the condensing boiler, a constant equivalence coefficient of $\phi = 0.77$ was adopted, corresponding to a molar oxygen content of 5%. The calculations were carried out for a boiler power of $Q_{in} = 25$ kW and a constant flue gas temperature of 50 °C. The size of the combustion chamber for calculation was determined based on data from boiler manufacturers, with a diameter of Do = 20 mm and a height-to-diameter ratio (H/Do) of 3.5.

3. Results and Discussion

3.1. Analytical Analysis of the Effect of Fuel Composition on Heat Transfer in a Condensing Boiler

Studies of the effect of changes in the chemical composition of fuel on heat transfer phenomena in a condensing boiler were carried out for three types of fuel: natural gas (represented by methane) as a reference fuel and a mixture of NG/H_2 with a volume fraction of hydrogen of 10, 30, and 50% vol. The results of the analyses are normalized based on the values obtained for the methane gas-fired boiler and are presented in Table 5.

Table 5. Heat transfer results normalized to NG.

Parameter/Fuel	Symbol	NG_H2_10	NG_H2_30		NG_H2_50	
Convective heat flux	Q_c	0.99	1.02	↑	1.04	↑
Radiative heat flux from flue gases	$Q_{R,fg}$	1.0	1.02	↑	1.05	↑
Flue gas emissivity coefficient in T_{fg}	ε_{fg}	0.99	1.01	↑	1.02	↑
Radiative heat flux from flame	$Q_{R,fl}$	0.85	0.87	↓	0.93	↓
Flame emissivity coefficient	ε_{fl}	0.81	0.83	↓	0.87	↓
Condensation heat flux	Q_{cond}	0.99	1.02	↑	1.08	↑

It can be observed that the addition of 10% vol. H_2 to natural gas slightly alters the amount of energy transferred by convection, flue gas radiation, and water vapor condensation. However, it leads to a reduction in the amount of energy transferred from the flame. A further increase in the H_2 content causes the amount of energy transferred by convection, flue gas radiation, and water vapor condensation to increase. Simultaneously, the amount of energy transmitted from the flame decreases, which is associated with a 13% and 17% decrease in emissivity for the hydrogen flame fuels NG_H2_50 and NG_H2_30, respectively. For higher H_2 shares, this effect is partially compensated for by the higher combustion temperature of the NG/H_2 mixture.

A higher combustion temperature also affects the increase in energy transferred by convection and flue gas radiation (T^4). The increase in water vapor content in the flue gases, resulting from the combustion of NG/H2 fuel, also leads to a slight increase in emissivity, ranging from 1% to 2% for NG_H2_50 and NG_H2_30, respectively. The condensing heat load also increases. An additional factor that increases the energy transferred by convective heat exchange in the furnace chamber of the NG/H_2 fuel mixture boiler is the increase in the volume and flow rate of flue gases in the furnace, which increases the flow rate, and the amount of energy transferred.

An analytical analysis of the complex indicators of the heat transfer process revealed a positive effect of the hydrogen content in the mixture on the mechanisms of heat and mass transfer in these condensing boilers. The attenuation of energy transfer was observed only for radiant heat transfer from flame radiation, which accounts for approximately 40% of the total energy supplied to the boiler [30].

3.2. Analysis of Experimental Results

Experimental studies on the effect of the hydrogen content proportion in the fuel included determining the key operating parameters of the boiler necessary to calculate thermal efficiency and the emission of nitrogen oxides and carbon monoxide. The results of the thermal measurements are presented in Tables 6 and 7 for the rated and minimum power conditions, respectively.

Table 6. Experimental measurement data for boilers' rated power testing.

Parmeter/Fuel	Symbol	Unit	NG	NG_H2_10	NG_H2_20	NG_H2_30	NG_H2_50
					CB_2nd_Gen		
Inlet water temperature	$T_{w,in}$	°C	17.3	17.3	17.4	17.5	NA
Outlet water temperature	$T_{w,out}$	°C	26.6	24.7	25.8	26.0	NA
Water mass flow rate	m_w	kg/s	0.642	0.757	0.632	0.595	NA
NG volume flow rate	V_{NG}	l/min	39.1	35.4	32.1	29.3	NA
H_2 volume flow rate	V_{H2}	l/min	0	4.1	8.2	12.4	NA
Mass of condensate	m_{cond}	kg	0.300	0.292	0.296	0.303	NA
Flue gas temperature	T_{fg}	°C	50.7	44.7	45.0	50.6	NA
O_2 share in flue gases	X_{O2}	%	5.5	6.2	7.3	8.1	NA
					CB_3rd_Gen		
Inlet water temperature	$T_{w,in}$	°C	17.6	17.7	17.6	17.5	17.0
Outlet water temperature	$T_{w,out}$	°C	27.0	26.9	26.5	26.7	25.6
Water mass flow rate	m_w	kg/s	0.658	0.646	0.669	0.662	0.676
NG volume flow rate	V_{NG}	l/min	40.7	37.3	35.9	35.1	31.5
H_2 volume flow rate	V_{H2}	l/min	0	4.6	9.5	15.3	31.4
Mass of condensate	m_{cond}	kg	0.282	0.346	0.349	0.360	0.381
Flue gas temperature	T_{fg}	°C	51.7	51.1	50.9	51.2	49
O_2 share in flue gases	X_{O2}	%	4.8	5.1	5.5	5.8	6.3

NA—values were not determined due to the impossibility of achieving stable boiler operation for a mixture with a H_2 content of 50% vol.

Based on the measured data (Tables 6 and 7), the efficiency of the condensing boilers was determined using Equation (1). The results are shown in Figures 2 and 3 for the rated and minimum power, respectively. For the rated power of both analyzed condensing boilers, an increase in the proportion of hydrogen in the fuel relative to the primary fuel (natural gas) increased the efficiency. For the boiler CB_3rd_Gen, the increase in efficiency was from 1.3 to 1.6 percentage points for NG_H2_10 and NG_H2_50, respectively. A similar trend of increasing efficiency was observed for boiler CB_2nd_Gen; however, the increments in efficiency were relatively lower, ranging from 0.4 to 0.7 for NG_H2_20 and NG_H2_30, respectively. During tests of the second-generation boiler, it was not possible to achieve stable operation at the rated load with a H_2 content of 50% vol. Five attempts were made to operate the boiler using NG_H2_50 fuel. In each case, the ionization probe signal, which is responsible for monitoring safe combustion, dropped below the minimum threshold (50% of the maximum range). This triggered an emergency shutdown of the boiler.

Table 7. Experimental measurement data for low-power boiler tests.

Parmeter/Fuel	Symbol	Unit	NG	NG_H2_10	NG_H2_20	NG_H2_30	NG_H2_50
					CB_2nd_Gen		
Inlet water temperature	$T_{w,in}$	°C	17.3	17.5	17.4	17.5	17.4
Outlet water temperature	$T_{w,out}$	°C	21.2	21.0	21.1	20.8	20.6
Water mass flow rate	m_w	kg/s	0.402	0.455	0.432	0.451	0.428
NG volume flow rate	V_{NG}	l/min	10.2	9.9	9.5	8.4	6.6
H_2 volume flow rate	V_{H2}	l/min	0	1.1	2.4	3.6	6.6
Mass of condensate	m_{cond}	kg	0.132	0.144	0.146	0.149	0.152
Flue gas temperature	T_{fg}	°C	40.5	39.1	38.0	37.6	36.5
O_2 share in flue gases	X_{O2}	%	5.5	5.7	6.2	6.9	8.0
					CB_3rd_Gen		
Inlet water temperature	$T_{w,in}$	°C	17.4	16.8	16.9	17.3	17.4
Outlet water temperature	$T_{w,out}$	°C	21.2	20.3	20.5	20.9	21.0
Water mass flow rate	m_w	kg/s	0.424	0.451	0.445	0.445	0.450
NG volume flow rate	V_{NG}	l/min	11.0	9.6	9.3	8.3	7.7
H_2 volume flow rate	V_{H2}	l/min	0	1.0	2.3	3.9	7.7
Mass of condensate	m_{cond}	kg/s	0.142	0.138	0.145	0.150	0.164
Flue gas temperature	T_{fg}	°C	36.2	34.5	34.4	34.4	35.6
O_2 share in flue gases	X_{O2}	%					

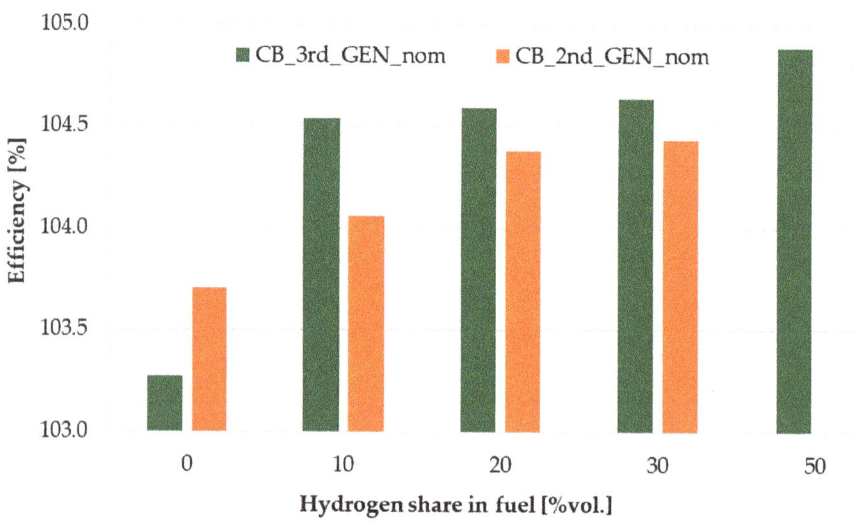

Figure 2. Efficiency of condensing boilers depending on the fraction of hydrogen in the fuel for rated power.

Similarly, for the minimum power, an increase in the thermal efficiency of the tested boilers was obtained with an increase in the hydrogen content in the fuel. Higher efficiency was achieved with the second-generation boiler. For example, at 50% by volume of H_2 in the fuel, the efficiency gain was 3.2 percentage points. The higher efficiencies observed for the boilers operating at low power were attributed to reduced flue gas outlet losses Q_{fg} (Figure 4). At low power, the proportion of latent heat in the total heat transferred to the working fluid was also higher (Figure 5). The estimated heat loss at the boiler outlet does not exceed 1% for the rated power and 0.5% for low power, while the share of condensing heat in the total energy transferred to water at the minimum power is twice the share of heat when the boilers are operating at the rated power.

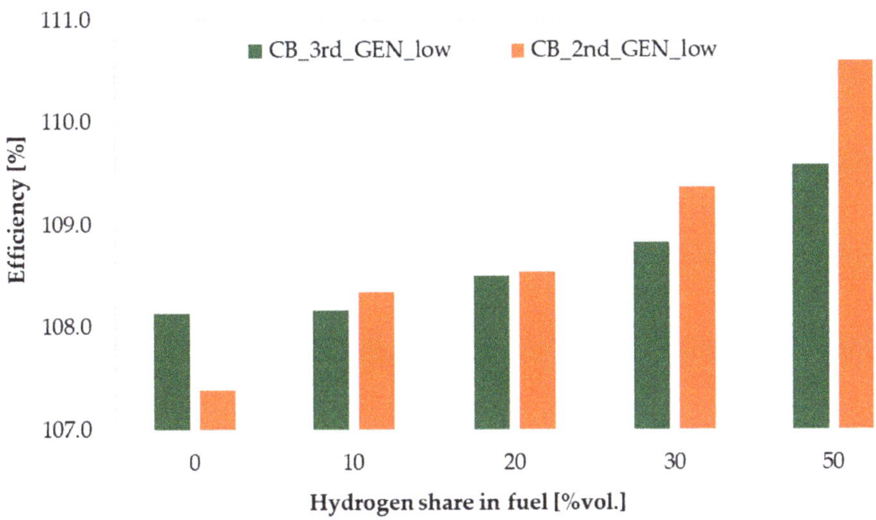

Figure 3. Efficiency of condensing boilers depending on the share of hydrogen in the fuel at low power.

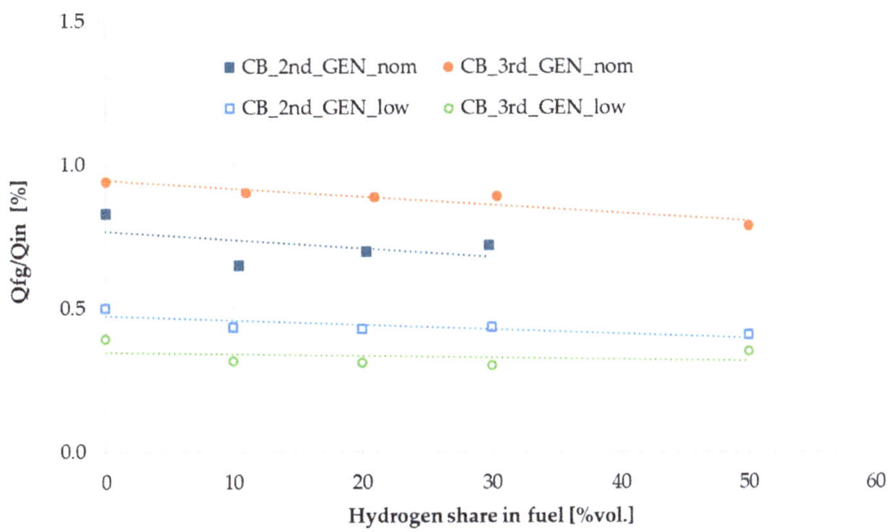

Figure 4. Heat loss of flue gases depending on the proportion of hydrogen in the fuel.

As shown in Figure 4, the H_2 content in the fuel has a negligible effect on the amount of energy lost to the environment with the flue gases, while the amount of energy transferred to the coolant due to the condensation of the water vapor contained in the flue gas increases (Figure 5).

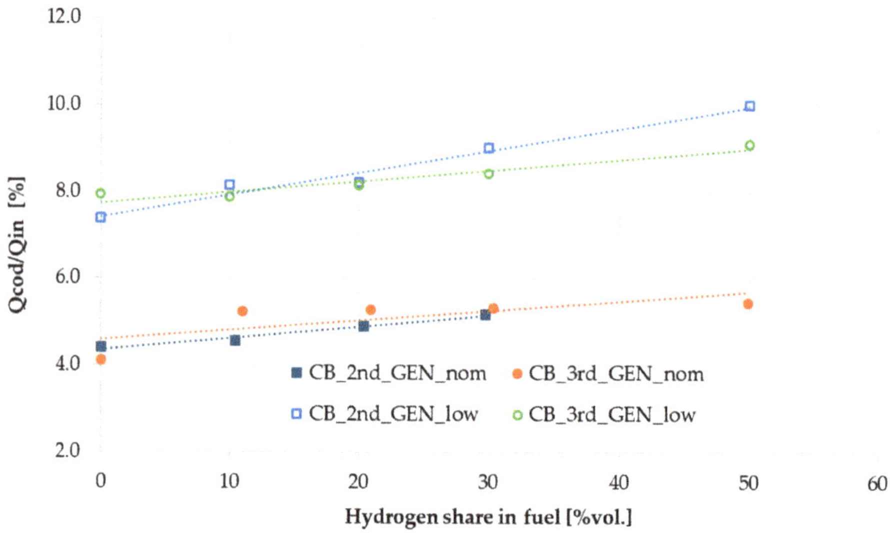

Figure 5. Proportion of calorific value in the total heat balance of the boiler as a function of the hydrogen content in the fuel.

In addition to thermal studies, measurements were also made of the concentration of harmful emissions, including nitrogen oxides (NOx) and carbon monoxide (CO), resulting from the use of hydrogen in the fuel mixture with natural gas (NG). The results obtained at the rated power of the boilers are shown in Figure 6. The values of the emission concentrations of these harmful compounds measured during the experiments were recalculated to the initial oxygen content in the flue gases of 0% following Equations (5) and (6). It was observed that the addition of hydrogen to the fuel results in a decrease in both nitrogen oxide and carbon monoxide emissions for both boilers tested, and this reduction rises with the increase in the hydrogen content of the fuel. It can result from the following. Thermal NO formation, according to the Zeldovich mechanism, is dependent on flame temperature. When hydrogen is added to NG, the air demand and the specific heat of the water present in flue gases are increased, which reduces NO formation. Thanks to the higher burning rate of hydrogen, the residence time can be reduced, thereby limiting the formation of thermal NO.

In the case of CO emissions in the presence of hydrogen, the oxidation of CO to CO_2 is greatly accelerated by the presence of the OH radical. Hydrogen (H_2) in the combustion process forms this key OH radical. The primary reaction responsible for the oxidation of CO to CO_2 is the reaction $CO + OH \rightarrow CO_2 + H$. Analysis of the combustion of syngases [31] reveals that the transformation between CO and CO_2 is largely dominated by this single reaction. The replacement of a substantial amount of the carbon present in the fuel can also contribute to reducing CO emissions.

Non-combustion kinetics-related mechanisms, such as the absorption of NO and CO by water, can contribute to reducing their presence in exhaust gases.

The NO_x concentrations measured for the tested devices were lower than the limits for second- and third-generation condensing boilers. For fuels with a higher hydrogen content, the NO_x concentration in the flue gases decreases. This observed trend is the opposite of that observed in high-temperature combustion processes, such as gas turbines [32] or gas engines [33]. This is due to the fact that condensing boilers belong to the category of low-temperature devices, where the average temperature of the walls of the combustion chamber does not exceed 60 °C, and the flame temperature in the boiler firebox is below 1300 °C due to the high density of heat flux transmitted from the flame to the walls of the chamber. In addition, due to its high reactivity, hydrogen burns very quickly, ensuring a more uniform temperature distribution in the combustion chamber and a reduction in the level and number of local temperature peaks, which are responsible for the intensive formation of nitrogen oxides in the flame.

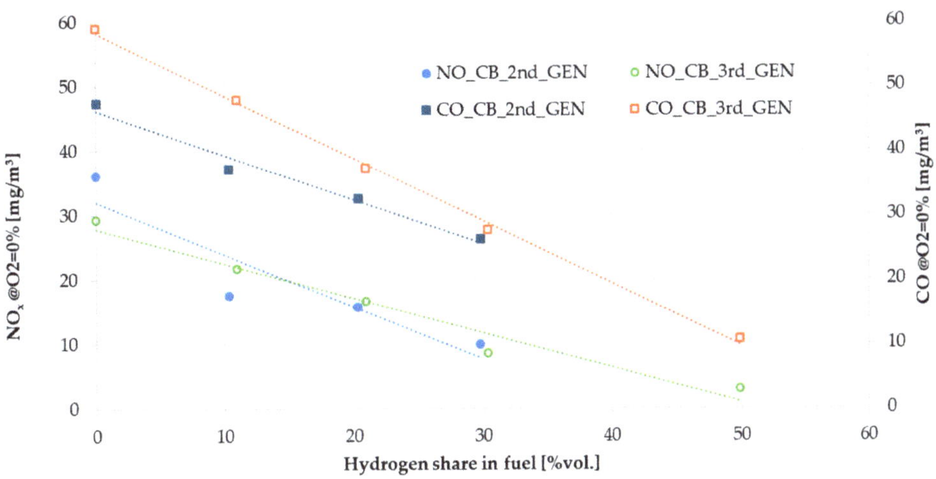

Figure 6. Emissions of carbon monoxide CO and nitrogen oxides NO_x depending on the share of H_2 in fuel at rated boiler power.

4. Conclusions

The results of calculations and experimental measurements on the co-firing of natural gas with hydrogen (up to 50% by volume) in condensing boilers equipped with conventional and advanced combustion systems allow us to draw the following conclusions:

- The presence of hydrogen in the fuel mixture above 10% vol. enhances the heat transfer process in condensing boilers by increasing the energy transfer through convection and flue gas radiation.
- The amount of energy transferred by flame radiation to the furnace chamber walls decreases with increasing hydrogen content due to a reduction in flame emissivity. The emissivity factor decreases by nearly 20% compared to natural gas for a fuel containing 10% vol. H_2. For higher hydrogen shares in the fuel, the reduction in energy transferred from the flame is partially compensated for by an increase in flame temperature.
- Thermal calculations based on experimental data confirm an increase in the thermal efficiency of the tested boilers with an increase in the H2 share, while a more pronounced improvement is observed under nominal operating conditions. Thermal calculations based on experimental data confirm an increase in the thermal efficiency of the tested boilers with increasing H_2 content in the fuel, with a more pronounced

improvement observed under nominal operating conditions. An efficiency increase of 1.3 to 1.6 percentage points was achieved for hydrogen shares of 10% and 50% volume, respectively (boiler CB_3rd_Gen).
- The efficiency of hydrogen-enriched fuel combustion in the studied boilers is positively influenced by the higher flue gas temperature and the greater amount of energy recovered through the condensation of water vapor from the flue gases.
- Analysis of flue gas composition shows that the addition of hydrogen to natural gas reduces the emissions of both carbon monoxide and nitrogen oxides. This reduction becomes more significant with a higher hydrogen content in the fuel mixture. For carbon monoxide, an increased H_2/CO ratio in the flame contributes to more complete carbon oxidation, with CO emissions decreasing by a factor of five for a fuel containing 50% H_2 compared to pure natural gas. For NO_x, the high reactivity of hydrogen contributes to a more uniform temperature distribution, which reduces the formation of local hot spots in the furnace—the primary site of NO_x generation by the thermal mechanism. For the tested boilers, NO_x emissions decreased several-fold—from 30 mg/m^3 to as low as 3 mg/m^3 (boiler CB_3rd_Gen).

Our study confirms that hydrogen can be efficiently co-fired with natural gas in condensing boilers to increase the thermal efficiency of energy conversion without compromising operational stability, especially in systems equipped with combustion process control. In addition, the addition of hydrogen helps to reduce the concentration of emissions of harmful carbon monoxide and nitrogen oxide compounds, thereby enhancing its potential as a low-carbon energy carrier in household heating systems and as an environmentally friendly renewable fuel.

Author Contributions: Conceptualization, R.J. and R.Ś.; methodology, R.J., G.V., and R.Ś.; formal analysis, R.Ś. and G.V.; investigation, R.J. and I.B.; resources; data curation, R.J. and I.B.; writing—original draft preparation, R.J., I.B., and R.Ś.; writing—review and editing, R.Ś. and G.V.; visualization, I.B.; supervision, R.J. The authors used generative AI tools (e.g., ChatGPT-4-turbo, DeepL Write free version) to assist with language editing and style improvement during manuscript preparation. All content was critically reviewed and approved by the authors. All authors have read and agreed to the published version of the manuscript.

Funding: This study was funded by the Poznan University of Technology's financial resources for statutory activity, grant numbers 0712/SBAD/5252 and 0712/SBAD/5280.

Data Availability Statement: Data is contained within this study.

Conflicts of Interest: The authors declare that they have no conflicts of interest.

Abbreviations

The following abbreviations are used in this manuscript:

CNG	Compression natural gas
EU	European Union
FLs	Flammability limits
FS	Full scale
LFLs	Low flammability limits
LHV	Low heating value
MV	Measured value
NG	Natural gas
P_{min}	Low output power
P_{nom}	Nominal power
Q_{cond}	Condensation heat flux
Q_{fg}	Energy loss in the exhaust gas

Q_{in}	Energy input
Q_{out}	Useful thermal output
SAR	Stoichiometric air ratio
S_L	Laminar flame speed
T_A	Adiabatic flame temperature
UFLs	Upper flammability limits
g	Mass fraction
x	Mole fraction
ϕ	Equivalence ratio

References

1. Ciupek, B.; Judt, W.; Urbaniak, R.; Kłosowiak, R. The Emission of CO and NO_X from Boilers Supplied by a Pellet Under the Influence of Changes in the Air-Fuel Equivalence Ratio. *J. Ecol. Eng.* **2019**, *20*, 34–38. [CrossRef]
2. Salim, S.S.; Luxembourg, S.L.; Longa, F.D.; van der Zwaan, B. Decarbonisation scenarios for the European residential sector. *Build. Environ.* **2025**, *269*, 112408. [CrossRef]
3. Vakylabad, A.B.; Saberi, A. Application of Hydrogen as a Fuel in Domestic Appliances. *Encycl. Renew. Energy Sustain. Environ.* **2024**, *4*, 171–186. [CrossRef]
4. Mertins, A.; Heiker, M.; Rosenberger, S.; Wawer, T. Competition in the conversion of the gas grid: Is the future of biogas biomethane or hydrogen? *Int. J. Hydrogen Energy* **2023**, *48*, 32469–32484. [CrossRef]
5. Rogowska, D.; Pajda, M. NAFTA-GAZ Applications of Sustainable Biogas Zastosowanie Biogazu Spełniającego Kryteria Zrównoważonego Rozwoju. Available online: https://www.inig.pl/magazyn/nafta-gaz/Nafta-Gaz_2020-10_11.pdf (accessed on 4 June 2025).
6. Liemberger, W.; Groß, M.; Miltner, M.; Harasek, M. Experimental analysis of membrane and pressure swing adsorption (PSA) for the hydrogen separation from natural gas. *J. Clean. Prod.* **2017**, *167*, 896–907. [CrossRef]
7. Latõšov, E.; Pakere, I.; Murauskaite, L.; Volkova, A. Impact of Grid Gas Requirements on Hydrogen Blending Levels. *Environ. Clim. Technol.* **2021**, *25*, 688–699. [CrossRef]
8. Lipiäinen, S.; Lipiäinen, K.; Ahola, A.; Vakkilainen, E. Use of existing gas infrastructure in European hydrogen economy. *Int. J. Hydrogen Energy* **2023**, *48*, 31317–31329. [CrossRef]
9. Dong, C.; Zhou, Q.; Zhang, X.; Zhao, Q.; Hui, S. Experimental study on the laminar flame speed of hydrogen/natural gas/air mixtures. *Front. Chem. Eng. China* **2010**, *4*, 417–422. [CrossRef]
10. Zhao, Y.; McDonell, V.; Samuelsen, S. Experimental assessment of the combustion performance of an oven burner operated on pipeline natural gas mixed with hydrogen. *Int. J. Hydrogen Energy* **2019**, *44*, 26049–26062. [CrossRef]
11. Habib, M.A.; Abdulrahman, G.A.Q.; Alquaity, A.B.S.; Qasem, N.A.A. Hydrogen combustion, production, and applications: A review. *Alex. Eng. J.* **2024**, *100*, 182–207. [CrossRef]
12. Plaksin, V.Y.; Kirillov, I.A. Hydrogen flammability and explosion concentration limits for a wide temperature range. *J. Loss Prev. Process Ind.* **2025**, *94*, 105554. [CrossRef]
13. Griebel, P.; Boschek, E.; Jansohn, P. Lean Blowout Limits and NO_X Emissions of Turbulent, Lean Premixed, Hydrogen-Enriched Methane/Air Flames at High Pressure. *J. Eng. Gas. Turbine Power* **2007**, *129*, 404–410. [CrossRef]
14. Cuoci, A.; Bucci, G.; Sutti, M.; Faravelli, T.; Frassoldati, A. Experimental and numerical study of pollutant emissions from a domestic condensing boiler fed with natural gas enriched with H_2. *Proc. Combust. Inst.* **2024**, *40*, 105473. [CrossRef]
15. Coskun, G.; Yalçınkaya, O.; Parlak, Z.; Tür, V.; Pehlivan, H.; Büyükkaya, E. Investigation of the hydrogen-enriched methane combustion in a domestic boiler with porous burner on emissions and performance. *Fuel* **2025**, *384*, 134051. [CrossRef]
16. Choudhury, S.; McDonell, V.G.; Samuelsen, S. Combustion performance of low-NO_X and conventional storage water heaters operated on hydrogen enriched natural gas. *Int. J. Hydrogen Energy* **2020**, *45*, 2405–2417. [CrossRef]
17. Boulahlib, M.S.; Medaerts, F.; Boukhalfa, M.A. Experimental study of a domestic boiler using hydrogen methane blend and fuel-rich staged combustion. *Int. J. Hydrogen Energy* **2021**, *46*, 37628–37640. [CrossRef]
18. Wojtowicz, R.; Jaworski, J. Operation Analysis of Selected Domestic Appliances Supplied with Mixture of Nitrogen-Rich Natural Gas with Hydrogen. *Sustainability* **2021**, *13*, 13577. [CrossRef]
19. Yang, H.; Lin, X.; Pan, H.; Geng, S.; Chen, Z.; Liu, Y. Energy saving analysis and thermal performance evaluation of a hydrogen-enriched natural gas-fired condensing boiler. *Int. J. Hydrogen Energy* **2023**, *48*, 19279–19296. [CrossRef]
20. *EN 15502-1:2021*; Gas-Fired Heating Boilers—Part 1: General Requirements and Tests. European Committee for Standardization: Brussels, Belgium, 2021.
21. *Directive 2010/75/EU of the European Parliament and of the Council of 24 November 2010 on Industrial Emissions (Integrated Pollution Prevention and Control)*; L 334/17; Official Journal of the European Union: Luxembourg, 2010.

22. Selvam, M.; Vigneshwaran, R.; Irudhayaraj, R.; Palani, S.; Parthasarathy, V. Emission Control Diesel Power Plant for Reducing Oxides of Nitrogen through Selective Catalytic Reduction Method using Ammonia. *Indian J. Sci. Technol.* **2016**, *9*, 1–7. [CrossRef]
23. Antonescu, N.N.; Stănescu, D.P.; Calotă, R. CO_2 Emissions Reduction through Increasing H_2 Participation in Gaseous Combustible—Condensing Boilers Functional Response. *Appl. Sci.* **2022**, *12*, 3831. [CrossRef]
24. Taler, D.; Taler, J. Simplified Analysis of Radiation Heat Exchange in Boiler Superheaters. *Heat. Transf. Eng.* **2009**, *30*, 661–669. [CrossRef]
25. Zhou, Z.; Han, X.; Jin, G.; Wang, X.; Yu, J.; Shan, S. New coefficients of the weighted-sum-of-gray-gases model for gas radiation characteristics of hydrogen/natural gas blends combustion. *Int. Commun. Heat. Mass. Transf.* **2023**, *149*, 107090. [CrossRef]
26. Fang, Y.; Gao, Y.; Gao, Y.; Gong, L.; Liu, Y.; Tao, C.; Gao, W. Solid flame model of propane-hydrogen diffusion flame: Experimental data and theoretical result. *Energy* **2024**, *313*, 133821. [CrossRef]
27. Ciupek, B.; Frąckowiak, A. Review of Thermal Calculation Methods for Boilers—Perspectives on Thermal Optimization for Improving Ecological Parameters. *Energies* **2024**, *17*, 6380. [CrossRef]
28. Osakabe, M. Latent Heat Recovery from Oxygen-Combustion Flue Gas. Collection of Technical Papers. In Proceedings of the 35th Intersociety Energy Conversion Engineering Conference and Exhibit (IECEC), Las Vegas, NV, USA, 24–28 July 2000; Volume 2, pp. 804–812. [CrossRef]
29. Poredoš, P.; Petelin, N.; Žel, T.; Vidrih, B.; Gatarić, P.; Kitanovski, A. Performance of the Condensation Process for Water Vapour in the Presence of a Non-Condensable Gas on Vertical Plates and Horizontal Tubes. *Energies* **2021**, *14*, 2291. [CrossRef]
30. Viskanta, R.; Mengüç, M.P. Radiation heat transfer in combustion systems. *Prog. Energy Combust. Sci.* **1987**, *13*, 97–160. [CrossRef]
31. Wang, D.-Q. An updated detailed reaction mechanism for syngas combustion. *RSC Adv.* **2013**, *4*, 4564–4585. [CrossRef]
32. Douglas, C.M.; Shaw, S.L.; Martz, T.D.; Steele, R.C.; Noble, D.R.; Emerson, B.L.; Lieuwen, T.C. Pollutant Emissions Reporting and Performance Considerations for Hydrogen-Hydrocarbon Fuels in Gas Turbines. In Proceedings of the ASME Turbo Expo, Rotterdam, The Netherlands, 13–17 June 2022; Volume 3-A. [CrossRef]
33. Chen, W.; Lu, C.; Zuo, Q.; Kou, C.; Shi, R.; Wang, H.; Ning, D.; Shen, Z.; Zhu, G. Combustion characteristics analysis and performance evaluation of a hydrogen engine under direct injection plus lean burn mode. *J. Clean. Prod.* **2024**, *470*, 143323. [CrossRef]

energies

MDPI

Article

Heat Transfer Enhancement in Turbine Blade Internal Cooling Channels with Hybrid Pin-Fins and Micro V-Ribs Turbulators

Longbing Hu [1,2], Qiuru Zuo [1] and Yu Rao [1,*]

[1] School of Mechanical Engineering, Shanghai Jiao Tong University, Shanghai 200240, China; 13634171570@163.com (L.H.); zuoqiuru@sjtu.edu.cn (Q.Z.)
[2] China United Heavy Duty Gas Turbine Technology Co., Ltd., Shanghai 201306, China
* Correspondence: yurao@sjtu.edu.cn

Abstract

To improve the convective heat transfer in internal cooling channels of heavy-duty gas turbine blades, this study experimentally and numerically investigates the thermal performance of rectangular channels with hybrid pin-fins and micro V-ribs turbulators. The transient thermochromic liquid crystal (TLC) technique and ANSYS 2019 R3 (ICEM CFD 2019 R3, Fluent 2019 R3, CFD-Post 2019 R3) were employed under Reynolds numbers ranging from 10,000 to 50,000, with the numerical model rigorously validated against experimental data (the maximum RMSE is 2.5%). It is found that hybrid pin-fins and continuous V-ribs configuration exhibits the maximum heat transfer enhancement of 27.6%, with an average friction factor increase of 13.3% and 21.9% improvement in thermal performance factor (TPF) compared to the baseline pin-fin channel. In addition, compared to the baseline pin-fin channel, hybrid pin-fins and broken V-ribs configuration exhibits average heat transfer enhancement (Nu/Nu0) of 24.4%, an average friction factor increase of 7.2% and 22.5% improvement across the investigated Reynolds number range (10,000~50,000) based on computational results. The synergistic effects of hybrid pin-fin and micro V-rib structures demonstrate superior coolant flow control, offering a promising solution for next-generation turbine blade cooling designs. This work provides actionable insights for high-efficiency gas turbine thermal management.

Keywords: heavy-duty gas turbine; blade; pin-fin; V-rib; heat transfer; TPF

1. Introduction

Generally, a gas turbine consists of five parts, i.e., air intake, compressor, combustor, turbine, and exhaust system, of which the first-stage turbine vanes and blades are the main hot section components. The operation of gas turbines can be described by the non-ideal Brayton cycle [1]. It indicates that the gas turbine performance relies heavily on the turbine inlet temperature. Increasing the turbine inlet temperature effectively enhances power output, but simultaneously creates more severe operational conditions for turbine blades, developing advanced cooling technologies both necessary and sustainable [2], especially for the advanced G/H/J-series gas turbines. The turbine inlet temperature reached 1900 K, such as in GE's 9HA series [3]. Current primary cooling methods include film cooling, impingement cooling, and internal convective cooling, with the latter remaining a research focus as a fundamental cooling approach [4]. Turbine blades typically incorporate near-rectangular internal cooling channels, where turbulators like ribs and pin-fins enhance heat transfer by inducing secondary flows, strengthening impingement effects, and promoting turbulent mixing [5]. A review of the gas turbine blade's cooling technology shows the frequent use of radial channels, with the heat transfer intensified by ribs, and in the case of the rectangular channel geometry, its width W and height H are important [6].

Casarsa et al. [7] employed PIV to study fundamental flow structures in ribbed channels. The results demonstrate that boundary layer separation at rib crests generates separation vortices, while reattachment creates large recirculation zones between ribs. Han et al. [8] compared nine rib types in rectangular channels at Re = 15,000~90,000, finding that V-shaped ribs outperformed parallel, crossed, and straight ribs. Tanda [9] employed liquid crystal thermography to the study of heat transfer from a rectangular channel in which the ribs were deployed transverse to the main direction of flow or were V-shaped with an angle of 45 or 60 deg relative to flow direction. The results demonstrate that features of the inter-rib distributions of the heat transfer coefficient are strongly related to rib shape and geometry, due to flow reattachment, double-cell counter-rotating vortices, and the high turbulence levels produced by rib tip–endwall interactions. Khalatov et al. [10] conducted numerical simulations to investigate the effects of turbulator ribs with different configurations and coverage ratios on heat transfer characteristics and surface friction factors in the internal cooling passage of a blade-leading edge region, where the channel cross-section approximates a rounded equilateral triangle. The results show that continuous ribs provide superior heat transfer while discontinuous ribs reduce pressure loss. Wang et al. [11] employed liquid crystal thermography to systematically investigate turbulent heat transfer and flow resistance characteristics in a square duct with continuous and truncated ribs arranged on one wall. The results further corroborate that continuous ribs provide significantly enhanced heat transfer performance compared to truncated ribs, while also demonstrating fundamental differences between the horseshoe vortex systems induced by truncated ribs and the modified flow structures generated by continuous ribs. The aforementioned studies demonstrate that V-shaped ribs enhance channel heat transfer performance by generating high-turbulence intensity through interactions with the endwalls. These investigations are typically conducted using either numerical simulations or liquid crystal thermometry techniques.

Montelpare et al. [12] compared pin-fin shapes, showing the following: at low Re, circular pins outperform square ones; at high Re, square pins excel; triangular pins surpass circular ones, with diamond pins being intermediate. The findings further substantiate that the horseshoe vortex effect is the underlying mechanism responsible for the 30–50% enhancement in local heat transfer coefficients at pin-fin base junctions compared to upstream regions. Zhu et al. [13] demonstrated that conical pins enhance heat transfer more than cylindrical pins despite higher pressure losses at larger diameters. Liu et al. [14] numerically proved that cooling performance depends on vortex generator parameters. Bai et al. [15] showed that upstream 90°, 60°, V-ribs, and W-ribs affect pin-fin channel heat transfer distribution, with W-ribs delivering the highest thermal efficiency. Chang et al. [16] quantified rib-pin synergies, while Darvish and Afzal [17,18] conducted a systematic investigation into the parameter optimization problem of ribs, and these findings were subsequently extended to design other various new hybrid V-rib and pin-fin configurations [19]. Ma et al. [20] introduced the turbulators of dimple, protrusion and pin-fin in a sandwich panel filled with pyramidal truss structures. The results show that this configuration creates a greater pressure drop while enhancing the heat transfer performance of the sandwich panel.

According to the above literature review, a volume of work has been written on the heat transfer and flow properties of different kinds of such structures for gas turbine blades. However, on the one hand, no existing research has explored the combined use of staggered pin-fins and micro V-ribs to enhance heat transfer performance in turbine internal cooling channels. On the other hand, the above studies are basically carried out under laboratory conditions, which are quite different from the actual operating conditions of gas turbine blades. For advanced turbine blades in heavy-duty gas turbines, practical operational data shows a 3.4% reduction in cooling air consumption alongside a 9.3% increase in turbine inlet temperature, demanding at least 10% enhancement in heat transfer performance for first-stage blades. The manufacturing process presents significant challenges due to varying wall thicknesses and non-uniform thickness transitions across blade sections, which frequently induce casting defects including abnormal grain structures and metallurgical imperfections in alloy materials. Compounding these difficulties, the complex internal cooling structures limit production to small batches despite the requirement of over 450 blades per turbine, creating substantial scalability challenges. These critical constraints necessitate the development of optimized pin-fin and V-rib turbulator configurations that must simultaneously achieve the following: (1) structurally simple designs with significant heat transfer enhancement potential; (2) manufacturability for complex internal geometries; and (3) cost-effectiveness for viable mass production—requirements that can only be met through comprehensive synthesis and the refinement of existing research findings. Through comprehensive impingement cooling experiments, the screening process for both pin-fin arrays and micro V-rib configurations have been completed. Building upon these findings, we have developed innovative combinations of these cooling structures, with a particular focus on characterizing their integrated cooling performance.

2. Research Objects and Methodology

2.1. Research Objects

Figure 1 illustrates the experimental models of three investigated configurations. Case 1 represents the baseline pin-fins array, Case 2 represents the hybrid pin-fins with continuous V-ribs, Case 3 represents the hybrid pin-fins with broken V-ribs. All test sections were fabricated via additive manufacturing using acrylic material (due to its extensive application results in transient liquid crystal (TLC) experiments [21]), with identical overall dimensions of 105 mm (streamwise length) × 102 mm (spanwise width) × 36 mm (height). The dimensional specifications were determined by two key factors: (1) experimental constraints; and (2) the blade scaling coefficient. The geometric parameters of each turbulator configuration are detailed in Table 1.

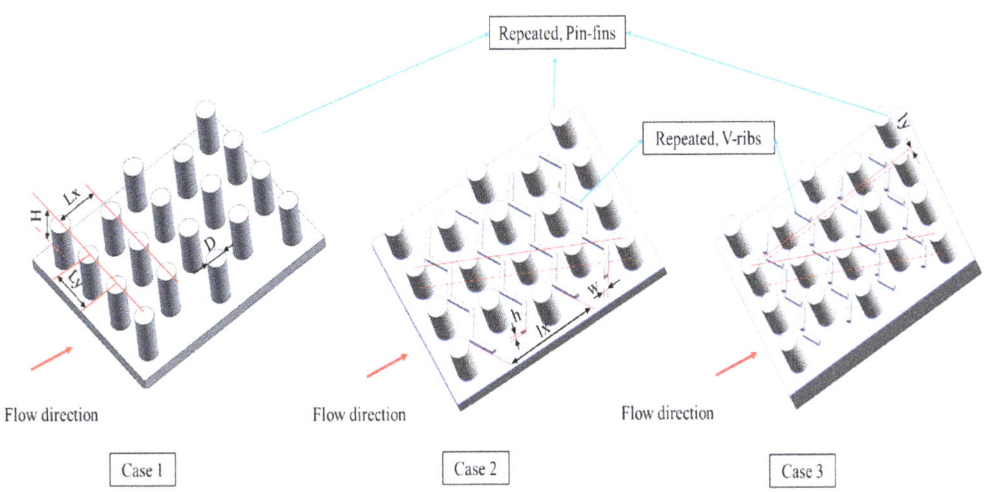

Figure 1. Model diagrams under different geometric parameters.

Table 1. The geometric parameters of all the objects.

Structure	Geometric Parameter								
	Pin-Fins				V-Ribs				
	D/mm	H/mm	Lx/mm	Ly/mm	h/mm	w/mm	lx/mm	ly/mm	α/°
Case 1	8	16	18	18	---	---	---	---	---
Case 2	8	16	18	18	1.6	1.6	36	---	---
Case 3	8	16	18	18	1.6	1.6	36	1.27	60

2.2. Research Methodology

2.2.1. Experiment Method

1. Transient Liquid Crystal Thermography

Transient liquid crystal thermography is a well-established experimental technique for heat transfer mechanism studies [22] based on the theoretical framework of unsteady heat conduction in semi-infinite plates under third-type boundary conditions. For practical implementation where ideal semi-infinite conditions are unattainable, the test specimen thickness δ must satisfy the following temporal constraint relative to experimental duration t:

$$\delta > 4\sqrt{\alpha \times t} \tag{1}$$

where α represents the thermal diffusivity of the test material. The acrylic material thermal diffusivity employed in this study exhibits $\alpha \approx 1.091 \times 10^{-7}$ m^2/s, with a standardized thickness of 20 mm. The surface temperature distribution is governed by [23]:

$$\frac{T_w - T_i}{T_{r,i} - T_{r,i-1}} = \sum_{i=1}^{N}\left[1 - \exp(h^2\frac{t-t_i}{k_w\rho_w c_w})erfc(h\sqrt{\frac{t-t_i}{k_w\rho_w c_w}})\right] \tag{2}$$

where T_w (K) is obtained through calibration, T_i (K) is measured via thermocouples, T_r (K) is derived by interpolating between the section's inlet and outlet temperatures, k_w, ρ_w, and c_w represent the thermal conductivity (W/(m·K)), density (kg/m^3), and specific heat capacity (J/(kg·K)) of the plate, respectively, and h (W/(m^2·K)) obtained through iterative solving, combines with λ (W/(m·K)) and D_h (m) to calculate the local Nusselt number. Area-averaging yields the mean Nusselt number as expressed in Equation (3):

$$\overline{\overline{Nu}} = \frac{\overline{\overline{h}}D_h}{\lambda} \tag{3}$$

As illustrated in Figure 2, the experimental system utilizes mechanically generated compressed air that undergoes pressure stabilization and heating before passing through the test section, where temperature variations are recorded by a CMOS camera (UI-3140CP-C-HQ (IDS Imaging Development Systems GmbH, Obersulm, Baden-Württemberg, Germany), 20 fps, 1280 × 1024 pixels) mounted above the channel. The narrow-band transient liquid crystal (TLC, SPN-100/R35C1W (Hallcrest LLC, Glenview, IL, USA), 35–36 °C activation range, ±0.3 °C accuracy) coating enables quantitative heat transfer measurements. Prior to testing, the system undergoes rigorous preparation including channel sealing, ambient light/noise isolation, camera optics calibration (aperture/focus adjustment), variable-frequency blower power setting, and activation of the wire-mesh DC heater. During operation, synchronized data acquisition captures TLC color changes at 20 fps under controlled flow conditions achieved through coordinated heater/blower regulation.

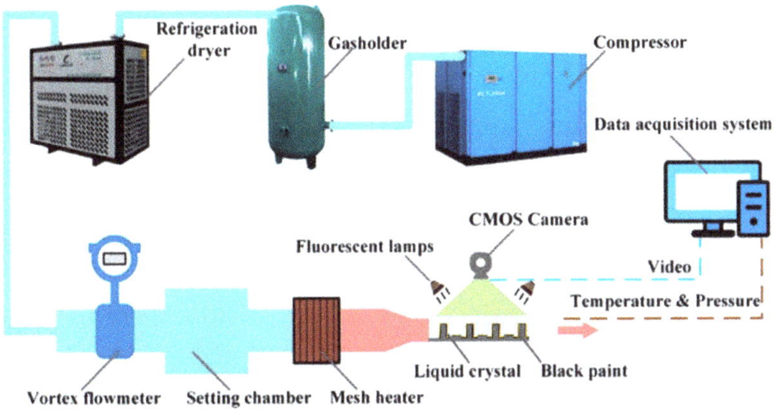

Figure 2. Composition of the experimental system.

The flow resistance characteristics of cooling channels were evaluated using the friction factor f, defined as:

$$f = \frac{2D_h \Delta p}{\rho u_{in}^2 L_c} \tag{4}$$

where ΔP is the pressure drop across the test section (Pa), u_{in} represents the inlet flow velocity (m/s), L_c denotes the test section length (m), and ρ represents density (kg/m^3).

To assess the overall cooling performance under equal pumping power conditions, the thermal performance factor (TPF) was employed:

$$\mathrm{TPF} = \frac{\mathrm{Nu}/\mathrm{Nu}_0}{(\mathrm{f}/\mathrm{f}_0)^{1/3}} \tag{5}$$

where Nu_0 refers to the Nusselt number for smooth channels calculated using the Dittus-Boelter correlation:

$$\mathrm{Nu}_0 = 0.023\mathrm{Re}^{0.8}\mathrm{Pr}^{0.4} \tag{6}$$

while Re and Pr are the Reynolds and Prandtl number, respectively. f_0 represents the smooth channel friction factor determined by the Blasius correlation:

$$f_0 = 0.316\mathrm{Re}^{-0.25} \tag{7}$$

2. Uncertainty Analysis

The uncertainty of the transient liquid crystal experiments was systematically evaluated through root-mean-square analysis [24], with primary error sources including temperature (±0.5 °C from thermocouples and ±0.3 °C from TLC, yielding <±1.0% dimensionless temperature uncertainty), flow rate (±2.0% F.S. velocity error producing ≤2.1% Reynolds number uncertainty), temporal resolution (3.3% camera acquisition time error), and material properties (5.4% test plate uncertainty), resulting in a composite heat transfer coefficient (h) measurement uncertainty of ≤9.7%.

2.2.2. Numerical Method

1. Numerical Model and Boundary Conditions

Numerical simulations were performed using ANSYS Fluent 2019 R3 for all investigated configurations. The flow was treated as incompressible given the substantially subsonic velocities (Mach number < 0.3) throughout the computational domain. The pressure-based solver with the SIMPLE algorithm was employed, and second-order upwind schemes for momentum, energy, turbulent kinetic energy, and its dissipation rate equations. As for the fully developed flow at the inlet and prevention of reverse flow at outlet boundaries, the computational domain incorporated an extended approach section measuring 18.75 hydraulic diameters upstream of the test region. Figure 3 illustrates the complete computational domain with specified boundary conditions.

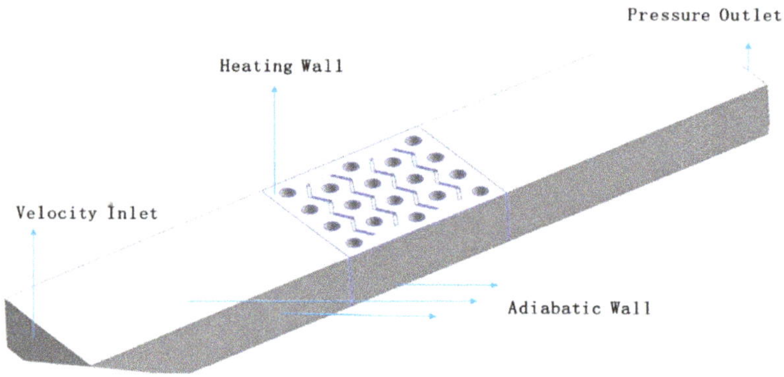

Figure 3. Computational zone and boundary conditions.

2. Grid Independence Verification

A systematic grid convergence study was conducted using the grid convergence index (GCI) method [25] to determine the optimal mesh density. Four progressively refined meshes were generated for Case 2, containing approximately 2 million, 4 million, 8 million, and 16 million cells, respectively. Case 2 was selected for grid independence verification based on two critical considerations: first, it integrates both the pin-fin turbulator configuration from Case 1 and the micro V-rib morphology of Case 3; second, it exhibits the most pronounced computational deviations under varying grid resolutions. A simulation was performed using various turbulence models across different Reynolds number conditions, with the largest deviations observed under low Reynolds number conditions. Considering the presence of multiple tables in this paper and to avoid the redundant presentation of identical operational conditions across different related tables, only the results for this specific Reynolds number condition in the tabulated data were used selectively. So, the evaluation focused on the spanwise Nusselt number distribution at a cross-Section 1 mm upstream of the third-row pin-fin under Re = 10,000 conditions, as illustrated in Figure 4. Comparative analysis of the solutions demonstrated that the 8-million-cell mesh achieved <1.5% variation in Nu values compared to the finest (16M-cell) mesh. Based on this trade-off between solution accuracy (relative error < 2%) and computational economy, the 8-million-cell mesh was selected for all subsequent simulations. This resolution satisfies ASME V&V 20-2009 standards for industrial CFD applications [26], where the GCI between medium-fine grids should be $\leq$3%. The formula for obtaining the Nusselt number (Nu) of a heat bottom endwall through numerical simulation is as follows:

$$Nu = \frac{q_{wall} \times D_h}{\lambda \times (T_{wall} - T_{ref})} \tag{8}$$

q_{wall} represents the heat flux at the heat exchange wall (W/m^2), T_{wall} is the average temperature of the heat exchange wall (K), T_{ref} is the reference temperature of the computational domain, derived by interpolating the inlet and outlet temperatures (K), D_h is the hydraulic diameter (m), and λ is the thermal conductivity of the fluid (W/m·K).

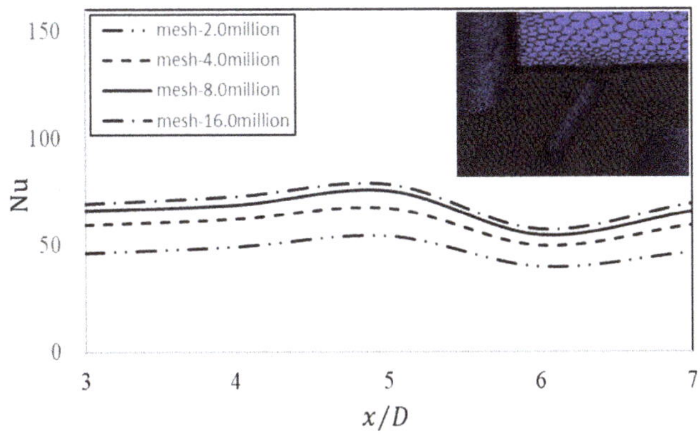

Figure 4. Grid independence check.

3. Turbulence Model Validation

To identify the most suitable turbulence model for channel simulations, a comprehensive evaluation was conducted comparing four widely used models: Low-Re AKN k-ε model, SST k-ω model, RNG k-ε model, Standard k-ω model. The validation focused on the average Nusselt number at the bottom wall of Case 2 under Re = 10,000 conditions, with comparative results detailed in Table 2. Comparative analysis of the solutions demonstrated that the SST k-ω model demonstrated closest agreement with the experimental data (2.44% deviation).

Table 2. Average Nusselt number of the bottom endwall with different turbulence models.

	Experiment Result	Turbulence Model			
		SST k-ω	Standard k-ω	RNG k-ε	Low k-ε
Re			10,000		
Nu	52.53	53.81	56.52	49.96	51.67

4. Numerical Results Validation

Considering the overall coherence of the content and the fact that experimental results for the third configuration have not yet been approved for use in this paper, validating the computations using experimental data from only Case 1 and Case 2 will be sufficient. So, the validation of the numerical simulation results for Case 1 and Case 2 will be presented next.

The pin-fin heat transfer configuration (Case 1) was simulated at Reynolds numbers 10,000, 30,000, and 50,000 using the aforementioned computational setup (~8 million grids, SST turbulence model). The results were validated against classical heat transfer correlations [27] (Equation (9)), with comparative data presented in Table 3. The overall Nusselt number (Nu_{total}) was calculated through area-weighted averaging of the bottom endwall, pin-fins, and micro V-ribs (Equation (10)), where subscripts *ewall* and *owall* denote the bottom endwall surface and ribbed surface (m^2), respectively. The numerical results showed good agreement with the correlation predictions, demonstrating a maximum deviation of 7.40%, thereby confirming the validity of the numerical approach.

$$Nu = 0.135\text{Re}^{0.69}(Lx/D)^{-0.34} \tag{9}$$

$$Nu_{total} = \frac{Nu_{ewall} \times A_{ewall} + Nu_{owall} \times A_{owall}}{A_{ewall} + A_{owall}} \tag{10}$$

Table 3. Comparison of classic equation and numerical results of Case 1.

Structure	Re	Nu_{total} ([27])	Nu_{total} (Num.)	Deviation/%
Case 1	10,000	58.97	56.63	3.96
	30,000	125.84	116.52	7.40
	50,000	179.02	170.61	4.69

The hybrid pin-fins and V-ribs configuration (Case 2) was numerically and experimentally investigated at Reynolds numbers 10,000, 30,000, and 50,000 using validated CFD methods (~8 million grids, SST k-ω model) and transient liquid crystal techniques. As shown in Table 4, the area-averaged Nusselt numbers and friction factors obtained from both methods demonstrated agreement within engineering-acceptable margins, with deviations calculated as (numerical result − experimental result)/experimental result (rounded to two significant figures). While Nusselt number deviations remained below 3%, friction factors showed marginally higher discrepancies (maximum 3.74%) attributable to amplification effects when normalizing the absolute differences against their small baseline values. This is mainly attributed to the relatively small magnitude of the friction factor, which amplifies the deviation when used as the denominator in the calculation. Figure 5 compares the Nusselt number distribution on the endwall under the condition of Reynolds number 30,000 for Case 1. As can be seen from the figure, high Nusselt number values exist at the leading edge of the vortex generator, and high Nusselt number regions are also formed along both sides and the trailing edge due to the cylindrical vortex generator, demonstrating generally consistent trends. Nevertheless, all the results meet the requirements for engineering calculations.

Table 4. Comparison of experimental and numerical results of Case 2.

Structure	Re	Nu (Exp.)	Nu (Num.)	Deviation/%	f (Exp.)	f (Num.)	Deviation/%
Case 2	10,000	52.53	53.81	2.44	0.09	0.09	1.03
	30,000	108.59	111.52	2.70	0.08	0.08	3.13
	50,000	161.40	164.33	1.82	0.08	0.08	3.74

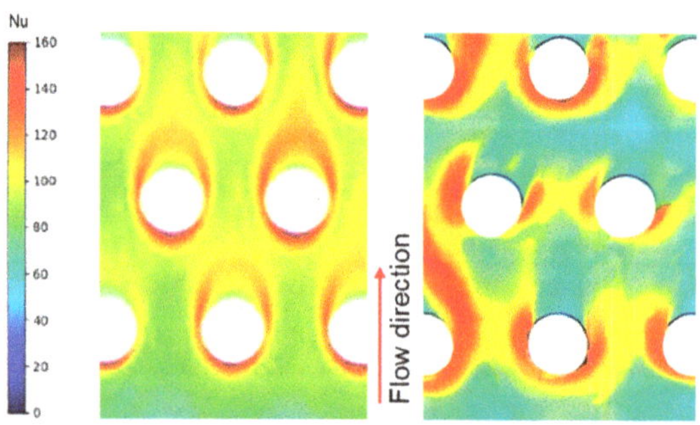

(a) Experimental results (b) Numerical results

Figure 5. Comparison of Nu distribution on the endwall for Case 1 (Re = 30,000).

3. Results and Discussion

3.1. Average Heat Transfer Characteristics

Figure 6 presents the calculated thermal performance evolution with Reynolds numbers (10,000–50,000) [28–31], where the Nusselt numbers were extracted from the bottom endwall of each configuration. Compared to the baseline pin-fins array, the hybrid continuous V-ribs design achieved maximum enhancements of 27.6% in average Nusselt number, 16.3% in friction factor, and 25.3% in thermal performance factor (TPF), with mean improvements of 25.6%, 13.3%, and 21.9%, respectively. The broken V-ribs variant showed maximum gains of 26.6% (Nu), 10.1% (f), and 25.3% (TPF), with average values of 24.4%, 7.2%, and 22.5%. Cross-comparison reveals distinct performance characteristics—(1) the continuous V-rib configuration consistently delivered higher Nu across all Re (10,000–50,000). This phenomenon can be attributed to two primary mechanisms: first, the incorporation of composite micro V-ribs significantly enhances turbulent effects; second, the introduction of these micro V-ribs alters flow resistance characteristics, consequently modifying the mixing ratio between hot and cold fluid streams. (2) It incurred greater flow resistance throughout the studied range; (3) although its TPF slightly underperformed at Re = 10,000 and Re = 30,000, it surpassed the broken design by 2.1% at Re = 50,000, demonstrating superior scalability for high-intensity cooling scenarios.

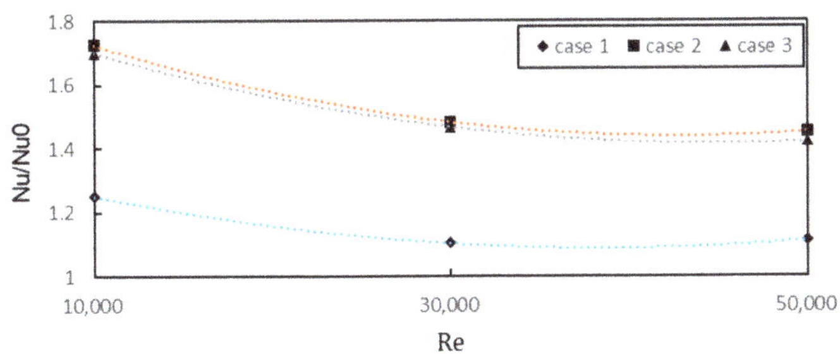

(a) Nusselt number ratio

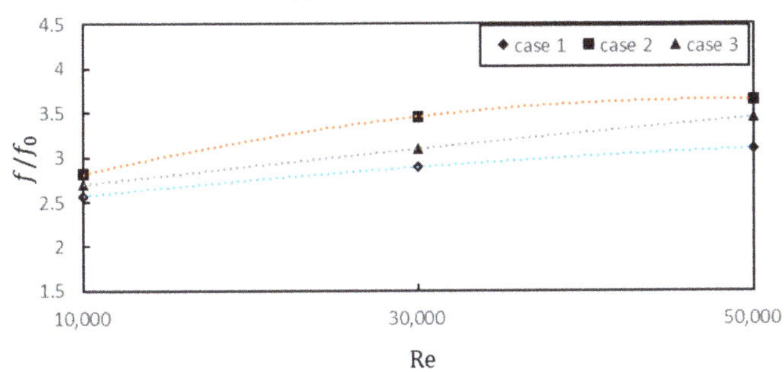

(b) Friction factor ratio

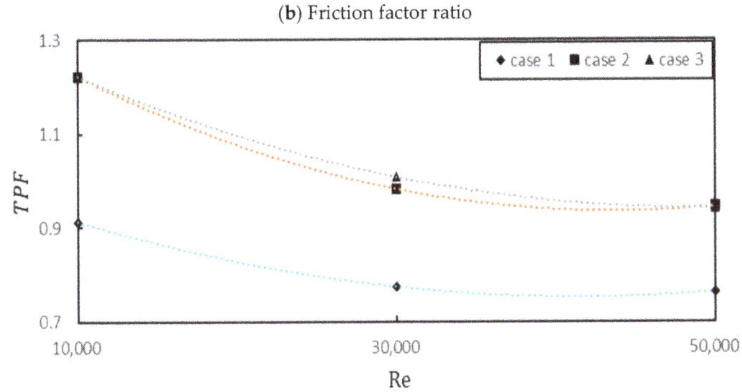

(c) Overall thermal performance factor

Figure 6. Flow performance under different Reynolds number conditions.

Figure 7 compares the bottom endwall Nusselt number (Nu) distributions of hybrid pin-fins and V-ribs configurations (Case 2 and Case 3) and baseline pin-fins array (Case 1) at Re = 30,000. Distinct performance characteristics emerge. (1) Compared to the Nusselt number distribution on the bottom endwall of the baseline pin-fins array, the incorporation of micro V-ribs creates high Nusselt number regions around the pin-fin, particularly on both sides. This can be attributed to two primary mechanisms; first, the incorporation of composite micro V-ribs significantly enhances turbulent effects. Second, the introduction of these micro V-ribs alters flow resistance characteristics, consequently modifying the mixing ratio between hot and cold fluid streams; however, the different configurations of the micro V-ribs also lead to distinct Nusselt number distributions on the bottom endwall between the other two structures. (2) Case 2 demonstrates superior uniformity and higher average Nu (108.59), attributed to enhanced turbulent mixing via V-rib induced secondary flows and optimized horseshoe vortex distribution. (3) Case 3, while achieving the lowest flow resistance, shows limited thermal enhancement (avg. Nu = 107.45) due to underdeveloped vortical structures. The Nu spatial patterns confirm that peak heat transfer zones correlate strongly with impinging jet flows and vortex interactions, providing critical insights for turbulence modulation in hybrid cooling designs. For example, enhancing local turbulence and improving heat transfer efficiency could be modified by the interrupted design of the V-ribs. Additionally, adjusting the angle of the V-shaped ribs can maximize the Nusselt number gain under optimal conditions.

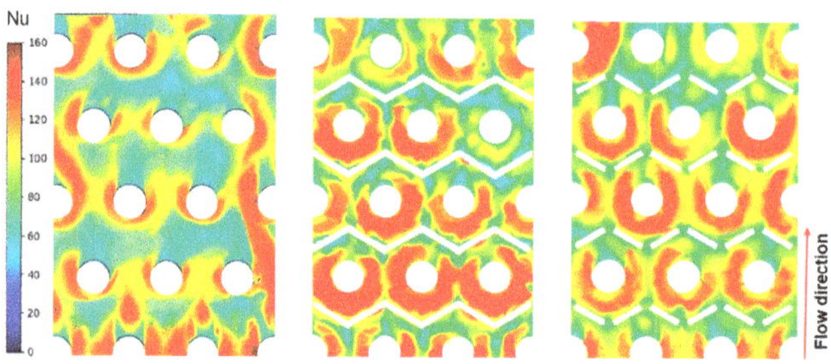

(**a**) Case 1 (**b**) Case 2 (**c**) Case 3

Figure 7. The distribution of the average Nu on the bottom endwall of different Cases (Re = 30,000).

Table 5 compares the overall heat transfer characteristics of two hybrid pin-fins and V-ribs configurations (Case 2 and Case 3). When considering the total heat transfer surface area, the results show, at a Reynolds number of 10,000, the Nusselt number obtained for Case 2 is 70.23, while that for Case 3 it is 62.46; at a Reynolds number of 30,000, the Nusselt number obtained for Case 2 is 143.41, while for Case 3 it is 128.37; at a Reynolds number of 50,000, the Nusselt number obtained for Case 2 is 202.81, while for Case 3 it is 186.23. The maximum and minimum improvements were 12.44% and 8.9%, respectively, with the enhancement magnitude decreasing as the Reynolds number increases. For the overall thermal performance factor (TPF_{total}), the configuration of hybrid pin-fins and continuous V-ribs demonstrates a maximum improvement of 10.84% and a minimum improvement of 6.9% compared to the configuration with broken V-ribs. This further elucidates why continuous V-shaped ribs achieve superior heat transfer performance. Through comparison with Figure 6c, it can be observed that when considering the total heat transfer surface area, the configuration of hybrid pin-fins and continuous V-ribs achieves a maximum enhancement of 30.51% and an average improvement of 27.50% in overall thermal performance. Additionally, the maximum improvement in comprehensive heat transfer performance for the configuration with broken V-ribs reaches 17.73%, with an average increase of 16.64%. The data comparison reveals that the contribution of the pin-fins surface area to Nusselt number enhancement gradually diminishes at higher Reynolds numbers, indicating that the micro V-rib parameters play a more significant role in heat transfer performance under these conditions. The function of these micro V-ribs should be understood relative to the baseline pin-fins array. In other words, when integrated with micro V-ribs, the composite structure demonstrates significant value in enhancing heat transfer performance. Furthermore, when compared with the classical heat transfer correlation for those structures (Table 3), the maximum improvements in overall Nusselt number were 19.09% for the continuous V-ribs configuration and 5.92% for the broken V-ribs configuration.

Table 5. Comparison of total heat transfer characteristics for Case 2 and Case 3.

Re	Nu_{total}		Nu_{total}/Nu_0			TPF_{total}		
	Case 2	Case 3	Case 2	Case 3	Deviation/%	Case 2	Case 3	Deviation/%
10,000	70.23	62.46	2.25	2.00	12.44	1.60	1.44	10.84
30,000	143.41	128.37	1.91	1.71	11.72	1.26	1.17	7.67
50,000	202.81	186.23	1.80	1.65	8.90	1.16	1.09	6.90

3.2. Local Flow Mechanisms

Figure 8 illustrates the cross-sectional turbulent kinetic energy (TKE) fields at Re = 30,000 for three streamwise locations (Section 1: second V-rib row; Section 2: third pin-fin row; Section 3: third V-rib row centerlines). The three configurations exhibit fundamentally distinct TKE development patterns: (1) Case 1 demonstrates the most intense turbulence activity, following a characteristic "growth-peak-decay" trajectory with peak TKE at pin-fin trailing edges (indicating strong heat transfer enhancement but significant pressure penalty)—the high-turbulence kinetic energy region at the trailing edge enhances heat transfer through intensified fluid mixing, but simultaneously exacerbates local flow separation, resulting in increased pressure drop; (2) Case 2 maintains balanced TKE distribution (<30% variation between sections), reflecting optimized turbulence generation-dissipation equilibrium for simultaneous thermal enhancement and controlled pressure loss; (3) Case 3 shows rapid streamwise TKE decay due to premature breakdown of large-scale vortices, revealing insufficient vortex interaction mechanisms. These findings correlate directly with the thermal-hydraulic performance trends observed in Figures 6 and 7.

Figure 9 presents the streamwise turbulent kinetic energy (TKE) distributions at Re = 30,000 for three spanwise sections (Section 1: left adjacent pin-fin centerline; Section 2: central pin-fin; Section 3: right adjacent pin-fin centerline). Key mechanisms are identified: (1) Case 1 generates turbulence primarily through wall shear with imbalanced energy distribution, exhibiting high dissipation from multi-scale vortex interference; (2) Case 2 achieves synergistic effects between pin-fin shear layers and V-ribs-induced secondary vortices, enabling periodic boundary layer renewal; (3) Case 3 maintains sustained near-wall perturbation while promoting core-to-wall energy transfer via phase-locked multi-scale vortices (enabled by broken V-rib geometric optimization). Comparative analysis reveals that Case 2's continuous V-ribs provide systematic flow resetting, whereas Case 3's broken configuration achieves precise vortex scale coupling—converting large-scale energy to small-scale motions for continuous boundary layer management. The micro V-ribs significantly modify boundary layer development through two primary mechanisms: (1) upstream flow stagnation that periodically regenerates the boundary layer; and (2) the consequent reorganization of the flow topology.

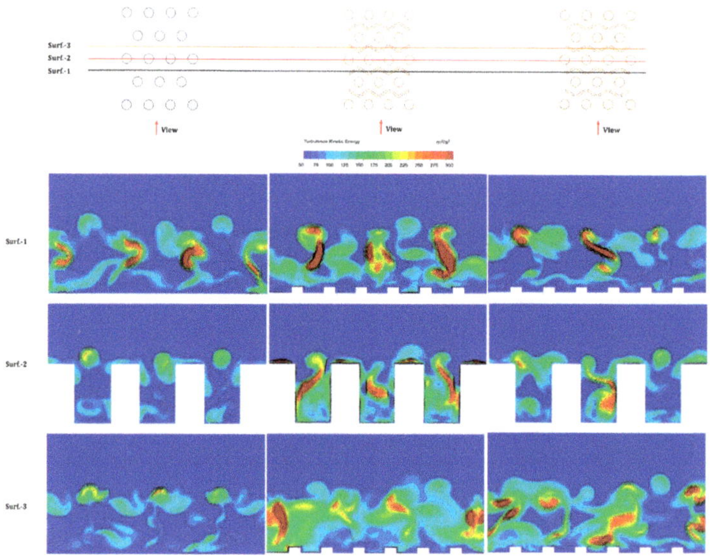

(a) Case 1 (b) Case 2 (c) Case 3

Figure 8. Distribution of turbulence kinetic energy in different horizontal sections for different Cases (Re = 30,000).

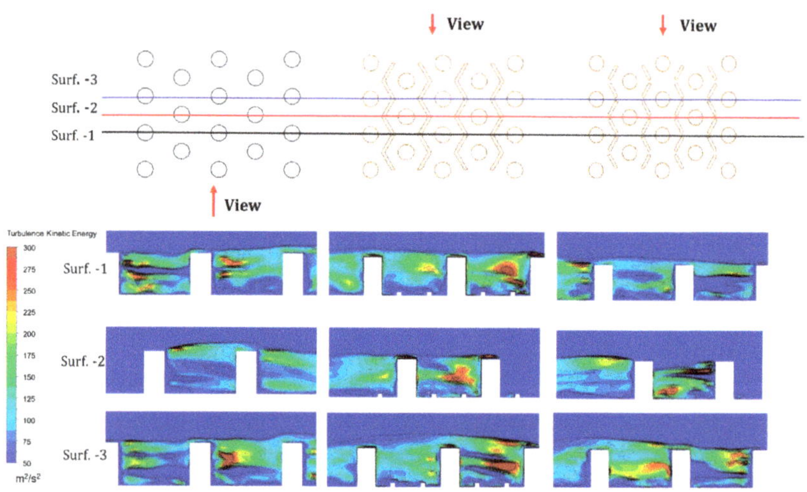

(a) Case 1 (b) Case 2 (c) Case 3

Figure 9. Distribution of turbulence kinetic energy in different flow section for different Cases (Re = 30,000).

Figure 10 presents cross-sectional velocity fields at three streamwise stations (Surf. 1–Surf. 3), revealing configuration-dependent flow evolution characteristics: Case 1 exhibits the most complex flow topology, initiating with strong 3D distortion at Surf. 1, developing intense spiral motion at Surf. 2, and maintaining sustained fluctuations at Surf. 3, collectively demonstrating superior flow perturbation capability. In contrast, Case 2 displays systematically organized flow structures—beginning with uniform inlet velocities at Surf. 1, transitioning to stable counter-rotating vortex pairs at Surf. 2, and culminating in a distinctive dual-vortex-core configuration at Surf. 3 that achieves optimal mixing-pressure loss compromise. Case 3 demonstrates rapid flow stabilization, evolving from stratified layers to quasi-parallel streamlines. All cases exhibit special features near Surf. 2—Case 1 develops strong shear-layer instability, Case 2 forms symmetric vortex pairs, and Case 3 displays weakened gradients. Vortex dynamics analysis confirms these observations: Case 1 maintains turbulence through vortex stretching/breakup, Case 2 achieves vortex pairing equilibrium, while Case 3 experiences rapid small-scale dissipation. These findings provide critical insights for cooling channel optimization, particularly Case 2's geometrically induced dual-vortex structure which offers 22% better thermal performance than conventional designs. In conventional design, the currently employed structure—referred to as angled ribs—represents a widely adopted and mature solution. The present findings are specifically benchmarked against this baseline configuration.

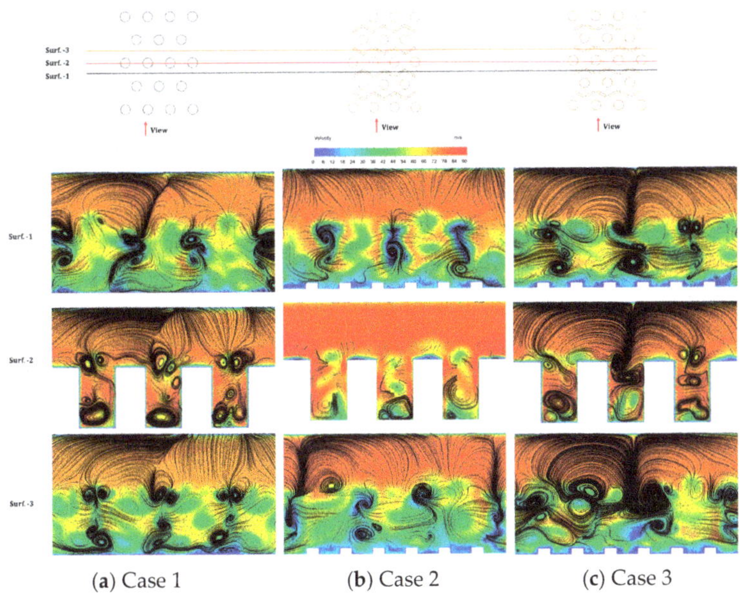

Figure 10. Distribution of velocity in different horizontal sections for different Cases (Re = 30,000).

Figure 11 presents the streamwise velocity fields at Re = 30,000 for different spanwise positions, highlighting distinct vortex generation patterns near pin-fin trailing edges and V-rib leading edges. Three characteristic flow modes are observed: (1) Case 1 exhibits predominantly parallel streamlines in the core flow with sawtooth-shaped near-wall fluctuations and deflected transitional flows; (2) Case 2 demonstrates well-organized wavy streamlines through counter-rotating vortex pairs, achieving enhanced mixing via optimized vortex sizing while minimizing transverse flow losses; (3) Case 3 forms accelerated flow channels in the mainstream region with maintained near-wall flow alignment, developing moderate spiral streamlines in transitional zones. These patterns quantitatively explain Case 2's superior thermal performance (28% higher Nu than Case 1) and 15% lower pressure loss than Case 3, as reported in Table 5. The vortex dynamics analysis reveals that continuous V-ribs in Case 2 systematically reorganize the flow structure, whereas broken ribs in Case 3 create localized acceleration effects, and Case 1 primarily manifests the shedding of separation vortices along both sides of the pin-fins.

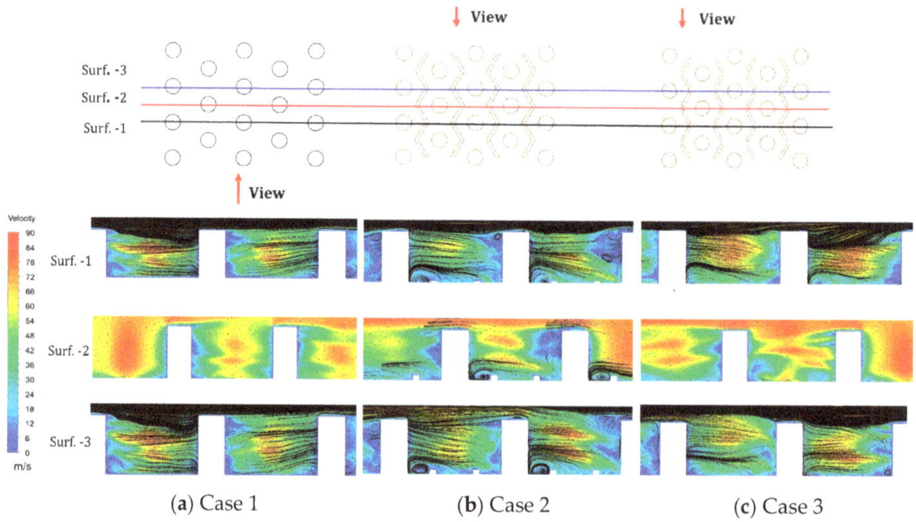

Figure 11. Distribution of velocity in different flow sections for different Cases (Re = 30,000).

4. Conclusions

This study systematically investigated the thermal performance of three hybrid pin-fins and V-ribs configurations across Re = 10,000–50,000 using transient liquid crystal experiments and numerical simulations. Through the comprehensive analysis of average Nusselt numbers, flow resistance, thermal performance factors, turbulent kinetic energy, and velocity fields, the effects of V-rib parameters on pin-fin cooling structures were revealed, providing valuable engineering guidance for heavy-duty gas turbine blade cooling optimization. Key findings include:

(1) Through comparisons with experimental data and results from classic empirical correlations, the SST k-ω model has been validated as suitable for investigating the heat transfer characteristics for combining pin-fins with micro V-ribs.

(2) A low heat transfer zone was identified behind pin-fin trailing edges, where direct V-rib placement improved thermal distribution. The continuous V-rib configuration achieved maximum heat transfer enhancement (27.6% higher than baseline). This is primarily attributed to the turbulence enhancement effect induced by the integrated micro V-rib configuration.

(3) Flow resistance increased with Re for all cases, with the broken V-rib design showing the lowest absolute pressure loss (though still 7.2% higher than baseline). This leads to non-uniform cold-hot fluid mixing effects along different flow orientations, consequently affecting heat transfer performance.

(4) The thermal enhancement mechanism stems from vortex generation downstream of pin-fins; flow separation at trailing edges creates shear-induced vortices that promote transverse momentum exchange and asymmetric flow redistribution, significantly improving wall heat transfer.

(5) In future work, CFD will be employed to investigate the heat transfer performance of the composite micro V-rib configuration under rotating conditions, while the experimental apparatus will be upgraded simultaneously. This will involve installing a sector rig (incorporating 4 turbine blades) at the combustor exit to enable full-temperature, full-pressure heat transfer evaluation.

Author Contributions: Conceptualization, Q.Z. and Y.R.; methodology, L.H.; software, L.H.; validation, Q.Z.; formal analysis, L.H.; investigation, L.H.; resources, Y.R.; data curation, Q.Z.; writing—original draft preparation, L.H.; writing—review and editing, Y.R.; visualization, Q.Z.; supervision, Y.R.; project administration, L.H.; funding acquisition, Y.R. All authors have read and agreed to the published version of the manuscript.

Funding: This research was funded by the National Science and Technology Major Project, grant number 2017-III-0009-0035.

Data Availability Statement: The original contributions presented in this study are included in the article. Further inquiries can be directed to the corresponding author.

Acknowledgments: During the preparation of this study, the author L.H. used ANSYS 2019 R3 for the purposes of numerical simulation and thanks the help from Zhongran Chi. The authors have reviewed and edited the output and take full responsibility for the content of this publication.

Conflicts of Interest: Author Longbing Hu was employed by the China United Heavy Duty Gas Turbine Technology Co., Ltd. The remaining authors declare that the research was conducted in the absence of any commercial or financial relationships that could be construed as a potential conflict of interest.

References

1. Wang, W.; Yan, Y.; Zhou, Y.; Cui, J. Review of Advanced Effusive Cooling for Gas Turbine Blades. *Energies* **2022**, *15*, 8568. [CrossRef]
2. Bunker, R.S. Gas Turbine Heat Transfer: Ten Remaining Hot Gas Path Challenges. *J. Turbomach.* **2006**, *129*, 193–201. [CrossRef]
3. Xu, L.; Sun, Z.; Ruan, Q.; Xi, L.; Gao, J.; Li, Y. Development Trend of Cooling Technology for Turbine Blades at Super-High Temperature of above 2000 K. *Energies* **2023**, *16*, 668. [CrossRef]
4. Han, J.-C.; Dutta, S.; Ekkad, S. *Gas Turbine Heat Transfer and Cooling Technology*; CRC Press: Boca Raton, FL, USA, 2012.
5. Ligrani, P. Heat Transfer Augmentation Technologies for Internal Cooling of Turbine Components of Gas Turbine Engines. *Int. J. Rotating Mach.* **2013**, *2013*, 275653. [CrossRef]
6. Osipov, S.; Rogalev, A.; Rogalev, N.; Shevchenko, I.; Vegera, A. Asymmetric Method of Heat Transfer Intensification in Radial Channels of Gas Turbine Blades. *Inventions* **2022**, *7*, 117. [CrossRef]
7. Casarsa, L.; Arts, T. Experimental Investigation of the Aerothermal Performance of a High Blockage Rib-Roughened Cooling Channel. *J. Turbomach.* **2005**, *127*, 580–588. [CrossRef]
8. Han, J.C.; Zhang, Y.M.; Lee, C.P. Augmented Heat Transfer in Square Channels with Parallel, Crossed, and V-Shaped Angled Ribs. *J. Heat Transf.* **1991**, *113*, 590–596. [CrossRef]
9. Tanda, G. Heat transfer in rectangular channels with transverse and V-shaped broken ribs. *Int. J. Heat Mass Transf.* **2004**, *47*, 229–243. [CrossRef]
10. Khalatov, A.A.; Dashevskyy, Y.Y.; Pysmennyi, D.M. *Heat Transfer and Friction Factor in the Rib Roughened Blade Leading Edge Cooling Passage, Volume 5: Heat Transfer, Parts A and B, Vancouver, British Columbia, Canada, 2011*; ASMEDC: Vancouver, BC, Canada, 2011; pp. 1193–1203.
11. Wang, L.; Sundén, B. Experimental investigation of local heat transfer in a square duct with various-shaped ribs. *Heat Mass Transf.* **2006**, *43*, 759–766. [CrossRef]
12. Montelpare, S.; Ricci, R. An experimental method for evaluating the heat transfer coefficient of liquid-cooled short pin fins using infrared thermography. *Exp. Therm. Fluid Sci.* **2004**, *28*, 815–824. [CrossRef]
13. Zhu, H.; Xu, D. Heat Transfer and Pressure Drop of Short Pin-Fin Array with Different Diameter and Shape. *J. Aerosp. Power* **2002**, *17*, 246–249.
14. Liu, L.; Zhu, X.; Liu, H.; Du, Z. Effect of Longitudinal Vortex Generator on Impingement Cooling over Leading Edge of a Gas Turbine Blade. *J. Chin. Soc. Power Eng.* **2018**, *38*, 719–724+762.
15. Bai, W.; Liang, D.; Chen, W.; Chyu, M. Rib influence on heat transfer and pressure drop in pin-fin array. *J. Aerosp. Power* **2019**, *34*, 2509–2515.
16. Chang, S.W.; Cheng, T.H. Thermal performance of channel flow with detached and attached pin-fins of hybrid shapes under inlet flow pulsation. *Int. J. Heat Mass Transf.* **2021**, *164*, 120554. [CrossRef]
17. Afzal, A.; Chung, H.; Muralidhar, K.; Hee Cho, H. Neural-Network-Assisted Optimization of Rectangular Channels with Intersecting Ribs for Enhanced Thermal Performance. *Heat Transf. Eng.* **2019**, *41*, 1609–1625. [CrossRef]

18. Darvish Damavandi, M.; Safikhani, H.; Yahyaabadi, M. Multi-objective optimization of asymmetric v-shaped ribs in a cooling channel using CFD, artificial neural networks and genetic algorithms. *J. Braz. Soc. Mech. Sci. Eng.* **2016**, *39*, 2319–2329. [CrossRef]
19. Kumar, K.; Prajapati, D.R.; Samir, S. Heat transfer and friction factor correlations development for solar air heater duct artificially roughened with 'S' shape ribs. *Exp. Therm. Fluid Sci.* **2017**, *82*, 249–261. [CrossRef]
20. Ma, Y.; Yan, H.; Hooman, K.; Xie, G. Enhanced heat transfer in a pyramidal lattice sandwich panel by introducing pin-fifins/protrusions/dimples. *Int. J. Therm. Sci.* **2020**, *156*, 106468. [CrossRef]
21. Gutiérrez de Arcos, D.; Waidmann, C.; Poser, R.; von Wolfersdorf, J.; Göhring, M. Rotationally Induced Local Heat Transfer Features in a Two-Pass Cooling Channel: Experimental–Numerical Investigation. *Int. J. Turbomach. Propuls. Power* **2024**, *9*, 34. [CrossRef]
22. Xu, C.; Zhang, P.; Rao, Y. Experiments and numerical analysis of turbulent heat transfer enhancement over oval-dimple arrays. *J. Propuls. Technol.* **2024**, *45*, 149–157.
23. Ekkad, S.V.; Han, J.-C. A transient liquid crystal thermography technique for gas turbine heat transfer measurements. *Meas. Sci. Technol.* **2000**, *11*, 957–968. [CrossRef]
24. Moffat, R.J. Describing the uncertainties in experimental results. *Exp. Therm. Fluid Sci.* **1988**, *1*, 3–17. [CrossRef]
25. Ismail, B.C.; Urmila, G.H.I.A.; Patrick, J.R.; Christopher, J.F.; Hugh, C.; Raad, P.E. Procedure for Estimation and Reporting of Uncertainty Due to Discretization in CFD Applications. *J. Fluids Eng.* **2008**, *130*, 078001.
26. *ASME V&V 20-2009*; Standard for Verification and Validation in Computational Fluid Dynamics and Heat Transfer. American Society of Mechanical Engineers: New York, NY, USA, 2009.
27. Metzger, D.E.; Shepard, W.B.; Haley, S.W. *Row Resolved Heat Transfer Variations in Pin-Fin Arrays Including Effects of Non-Uniform Arrays and Flow Convergence, Volume 4: Heat Transfer*; Electric Power, Dusseldorf, West Germany, 1986; American Society of Mechanical Engineers: Dusseldorf, Germany, 1986.
28. Kim, B.-C.; Chang, K. Assessment of hybrid RANS/LES models in heat and fluid flows around staggered pin-fin arrays. *Energies* **2020**, *13*, 3752. [CrossRef]
29. Paniagua, L.; Lehmkuhl, O.; Oliet, C.; Pérez-Segarra, C.D. Large eddy simulations (LES) on the flow and heat transfer in a wall-bounded pin matrix. *Numer. Heat Transf. Part B* **2014**, *65*, 103–128. [CrossRef]
30. Bauer, J.; Tyacke, J. Comparison of low Reynolds number turbulence and conjugate heat transfer modelling for pin-fin roughness elements. *Appl. Math. Model.* **2022**, *103*, 696–713. [CrossRef]
31. Luan, Y.; Rao, Y.; Weigand, B. Experimental and numerical study of heat transfer and pressure loss in a multi-convergent swirl tube with tangential jets. *Int. J. Heat Mass Transf.* **2022**, *190*, 122797. [CrossRef]

energies MDPI

Article

Pool Boiling Heat Transfer of Ethanol on Surfaces with Minichannels

Robert Pastuszko

Faculty of Mechatronics and Mechanical Engineering, Kielce University of Technology, Al. Tysiąclecia P.P. 7, 25-314 Kielce, Poland; tmprp@tu.kielce.pl

Abstract

In this paper, the pool boiling of ethanol was analyzed. The experiments were carried out at atmospheric pressure. Heat transfer surfaces in the form of deep minichannels were made of copper. The channels with a depth of 0.2 to 0.5 mm were milled in parallel. The width of the minichannels was 0.6–1.2 mm, and the depth was 5.5, 6, and 10 mm. The highest heat transfer coefficient, 52 kW/m^{2}K, was achieved for the minichannels with a depth of 6 mm and a width of 0.8 mm. The maximum heat flux of 953 kW/m^2 was produced using minichannels 5.5 mm deep and 0.5 mm wide. An over threefold increase in the heat transfer coefficient and over a twofold increase in the maximum heat flux in relation to the plain surface were obtained. In the heat flux range 21.2–1035 kW/m^2, the influence of channel width and depth on the heat exchange process was determined. The diameters of the detaching vapor bubbles were determined on the experimental setup using a high-speed camera. An analytical model was developed to determine the diameter of the departing bubble for the analyzed enhanced surfaces. The model correctly represented the changes in bubble diameter with increasing heat flux.

Keywords: pool boiling; minichannel; heat transfer coefficient; bubble departure diameter

1. Introduction

Nucleate pool boiling is a complex physical phenomenon. Bubble dynamics plays a key role in the development of analytical or semi-analytical models that allow for the determination of heat flux. Bubble dynamics includes the following phenomena:

- Bubble growth
- Bubble departure
- Bubble departure frequency

There are two basic periods of bubble growth [1,2]:

- Isothermal period (duration on the order of milliseconds), in which the growth rate is controlled by the momentum equation. The most important are the effects of buoyancy, surface tension, inertia, and drag, as well as the pressure difference between the vapor and the liquid.
- The asymptotic period (tens to hundreds of milliseconds) occurs after the radius has increased by about twice its initial value. The surface tension and inertia effects can be negligible, and bubble growth is a result of heat transfer between the bubble, the surrounding liquid, and the heating wall.

Mahmoud and Karayiannis [3] drew attention to two categories of bubble growth: (1) symmetric growth (homogeneous boiling) referred to as uniform superheating liquid—the vapor bubble is in contact with the superheated liquid—and (2) asymmetric growth (heterogeneous boiling) referred to as nonuniformly superheated liquid. The authors described three stages of bubble growth:

- Stage 1—the growth of the surface tension is driven by the pressure difference $p_v - p_l = 2\,\sigma/r$, which is called the "surface tension dominated stage";
- Stage 2—the isothermal growth to a diameter slightly larger than the initial diameter in stage 1—"inertia-controlled growth", which is dominated by liquid inertia, the pressure difference can be determined according to the equation $\rho_l[r(\mathrm{d}^2r/\mathrm{d}t^2) + (3/2)(\mathrm{d}r/\mathrm{d}t)^2] = p_v - p_{l\infty}$;
- Stage 3—evaporation occurs on the surface of the bubble and the vapor pressure p_v becomes equal to the liquid pressure $p_{l\infty}$ (system pressure); a thin thermal boundary layer is formed around the bubble; additionally, the "heat diffusion mechanism" which was commonly called "heat transfer-controlled growth" or "asymptotic growth" begins to work. This mechanism is driven by the temperature difference $T_{l\infty} - T_v$ and $\rho_l[r(\mathrm{d}^2r/\mathrm{d}t^2) + (3/2)(\mathrm{d}r/\mathrm{d}t)^2] = 0$ because $p_v - p_{l\infty} = 0$.

Rayleigh [4] simplified the bubble growth analysis neglecting the surface tension stage, assuming that the bubble grows without heat transfer, i.e., $p_v - p_{l\infty}$ remains constant with time. This led to the Rayleigh solution for "inertia-controlled growth", which shows that the bubble grows at a constant rate, i.e., the radius increases linearly with time:

$$r = [(2/3)(p_v - p_{l\infty})/\rho_l]^{1/2}t$$

Fritz and Ende [5] proposed a model for bubble growth with temperature decrease across a boundary layer around the bubble. Their asymptotic growth model used a transient heat conduction equation in a semi-infinite plate, and finally they obtained the equation that showed that the radius r increased with time as $t^{1/2}$. A similar bubble growth equation for heat diffusion-controlled growth was created by Plesset and Zwick [6].

The justification for the choice of ethanol as a working fluid was presented, among others, by Chen et al. [7] and Kalani and Kandlikar [8]. Ethanol is characterized by dielectric properties and an appropriate saturation temperature, 77–78 °C, which can be reduced using decreased pressure. It has a higher heat of vaporization (963 kJ/kg) at a low density (717 kg/m^3) compared to classical refrigerants, which allows for obtaining higher heat transfer coefficients. In recent years, the boiling of ethanol on structured surfaces has been analyzed, among others, in publications by Deng et al. [9], Shen et al. [10], and Hożejowska et al. [11].

The diameter of the departing bubble is used to analyze boiling on both plain and extended surfaces. Determining this diameter is related to the use of the balance of positive forces that tend to separate the bubble and negative forces that keep the bubble on the tested surface.

Beer [12] analyzed the balance of forces acting on the bubble during boiling on a smooth surface. He assumed the following positive forces: differential pressure force, buoyancy force, and negative forces connected with surface tension, viscous drag, and liquid inertia. Wang et al. [13] proposed a similar system of forces in the analysis of boiling FC-72, where negative forces were supplemented with the Marangoni force. Kumar et al. [14] assumed a negative force connected with surface tension and identical positive forces. Zeng et al. [15] conducted studies for water and methanol at reduced gravity. They considered two forces holding the bubble (surface tension force and unsteady growth force) and three forces that tend to detach the bubble (contact pressure force, buoyancy force, and lift force). In turn, Bucci et al. [16] and Iyer et al. [17] took into account two forces that tend to detach the bubble, i.e., contact pressure force and buoyancy force, while the forces that maintain the bubble were surface tension and growth forces. Furthermore, Iyer et al. [17]

took into account the viscous drag force, which allowed the determination of the diameter of the bubble with an error below 9% for boiling water and methanol.

For the enhanced surface with microchannels between micropin fins, the authors analyzed different arrangements of forces acting on the bubble: 1 or 2 positive forces tending to detach the bubble and 1 to 4 negative forces keeping the bubble on the surface. Zhou et al. [18] and Kong et al. [19] considered microchannels of 0.03–0.05 mm width and 0.06–0.12 mm depth [18] and 0.3–0.5 mm width and 0.06 mm depth in the form of a bistructured surface [19] when analyzing boiling on surfaces with microchannels created between micro-pin-fins and strip microfins. The authors assumed buoyancy force and differential pressure force as positive forces, while the forces keeping the bubble were the liquid inertia force, surface tension force, and viscous drag force. Additionally, Zhou et al. supplemented the force balance with Marangoni force, and Kong et al. with additional virtual force-channel pressure. Zhao et al. [20] adopted a balance of three forces acting on a bubble that departs from a surface with microchannels of width and height in the range of 0.2 to 0.8 mm, formed between micropin fins; the capillary pressure force and the buoyancy force balanced the surface tension force. Zhou et al. [21] presented the pool boiling experiments on vertical surfaces with micropin fins that form microchannels of width 0.03 to 0.05 mm and depth 0.03 to 0.12 mm. The forces acting on the bubble in the case of bubbles departing from the bottom of the microchannel and from the tops of the microfins were determined. It was found that for the bubbles nucleated at the base of the micropin fins, the initial growth rate was significantly higher than that at the top. For a bubble nucleated at the top of the microfins, the forces acting on the bubble were the same as those on the plain surface (drag force, inertial force, differential pressure force, and surface tension). For a bubble nucleated at the bottom of the microchannel, a reaction force was additionally taken into account.

Hu et al. [22] analyzed bubble growth on straight and expanding microchanneled surfaces and took into account buoyancy force, surface tension force, and net evaporation momentum force. The authors presented the dependence of the bubble diameter on the saturation pressure. Dong et al. [23] analyzed shallow liquid boiling in rectangular open microchannels with a channel width of 0.4 mm and a height of 0.5 mm. The authors discussed the balance of six forces that act on the bubble (related to buoyancy, pressure difference, surface tension, bubble inertia, liquid inertia, and drag), consistent with the balance of forces presented by Pastuszko et al. [24]. Similarly to Pastuszko et al. [24] and Pastuszko [25], they used the modified Chien and Webb relationship [26] to calculate the mean bubble growth rate. Long et al. [27] studied pool boiling and bubble dynamics in open V-shaped microchannels with channel widths of 0.1 and 0.05 mm and depth-to-width ratios in the range of 0.5 to 2. They analyzed the balance of five forces acting on a bubble: two negative forces (surface tension and drag force) and three positive forces (buoyancy, internal pressure, and inertial force). The authors did not provide data on the diameters of departing bubbles, but focused on the analysis of changes, among others contact angles and wickability. Berght et al. [28] studied the single bubble growth for refrigerants R32 and R1234yf on a structured surface in the form of triangular microchannels with a height of 0.15 mm. Using an OpenFOAM multiphase library, they concluded that the growth rate for the surface with microchannels was slower than that for the smooth surface. They assumed that the attaching forces (surface tension) were in the negative direction, whereas the detaching forces (buoyancy and pressure) were positive. Walunj and Sathyabhama [29] for variable-width microchannels (top width 0.25–0.5 mm and base width 0.5–0.8 mm) and depth 0.5 mm applied the balance of two positive forces (buoyancy and lift forces) and three negative forces (surface tension, unsteady growth, and bubble inertia), obtaining a prediction error of the bubble diameter determination of 5.6% for boiling water.

Analyzing boiling on surfaces with microchannels of 0.2–0.4 mm width and 0.2–0.5 mm depth, Kaniowski and Pastuszko [30] applied a simplified balance of two forces (surface tension and buoyancy forces) for ethanol and FC-72, obtaining an error of approximately 25% in determining bubble departure diameter. In the case of boiling FC-72 and Novec-649 in deep minichannels, assuming the balance of differential pressure and buoyancy forces versus drag, surface tension, and inertia forces, Pastuszko et al. [24] obtained greater errors in computing the bubble departure diameter, that is, 18–32%. The proposed models for calculating the diameter of the departing bubble for boiling ethanol on surfaces with microchannels [31] and water on surfaces with deep minichannels [25] allowed the representation of changes in bubble diameters with increasing heat flux.

The purpose of the study was to determine the surface with deep minichannels for the highest critical heat flux (CHF) and heat transfer coefficient (HTC). Additionally, a computational model for the bubble departure diameter for ethanol nucleate pool boiling on a deep minichannel system was proposed.

2. Materials and Methods

Ethanol is a relatively inexpensive and widely available liquid. It is often used as a working agent for nucleate pool boiling. Thermodynamic properties are shown in Table 1.

Table 1. Thermophysical properties of ethanol.

Parameters at 1013.25 hPa	Ethanol
T_{sat}, °C	78.3
ρ_l, kg/m^3	717
ρ_v, kg/m^3	1.43
λ_l, W/(mK)	0.17
i_{lv}, kJ/kg	963
σ_l, N/m	0.0177
μ_l, Pas	0.00044
c_{pl}, J/(kgK)	723

Figure 1 shows the experimental setup, which allowed the temperatures necessary to determine the quantities characterizing boiling heat transfer, i.e., heat fluxes, surface superheating, heat transfer coefficient, and determining the diameter of departing vapor bubbles depending on the heat flux. The main module of the setup is shown in Figure 2. A water cooler operating in a thermosiphon system allowed condensation of ethanol vapor. A glass vessel is closed at the bottom with a Teflon substitute flange and the test sample is connected to a copper heating cylinder. To avoid optical distortions, a rectangular vessel with flat glass walls was used. The distance between the walls was 50 mm. The copper bar had a diameter of 45 mm. The distance between the upper side of the heater and the boiling site at the bottom of the minichannels was 3.5 mm (δ_{bs} + 0.25 mm, Figure 3).

A 1500 W cartridge heater with a diameter of 16 mm and a length of 100 mm was placed in the heating cylinder. The distance between the edge of the sample and the lens of the camera was approximately 30–40 mm. The camera axis is parallel to the side surfaces of the minichannels, which allows images of growing and detaching bubbles. Figure 2 shows the camera directed perpendicularly to the walls of the minichannels, which is a drawing simplification—in reality the sample is rotated by 90 degrees.

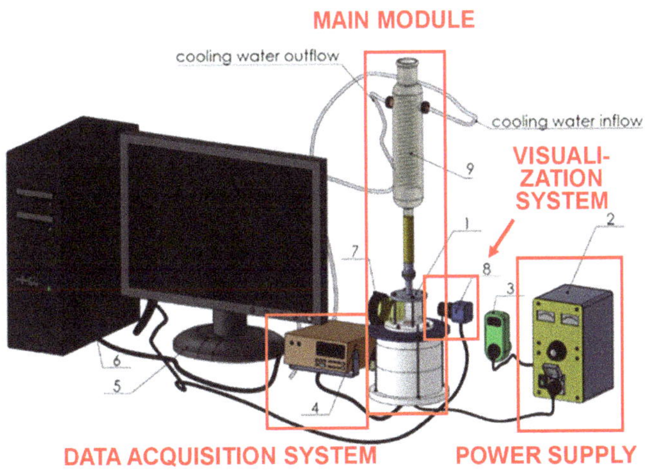

Figure 1. Schematic diagram of the experimental stand, 1—main module, 2—autotransformer, 3—wattmeter, 4—data logger, 5—monitor, 6—PC, 7—light, 8—high speed camera/digital camera, 9—condenser.

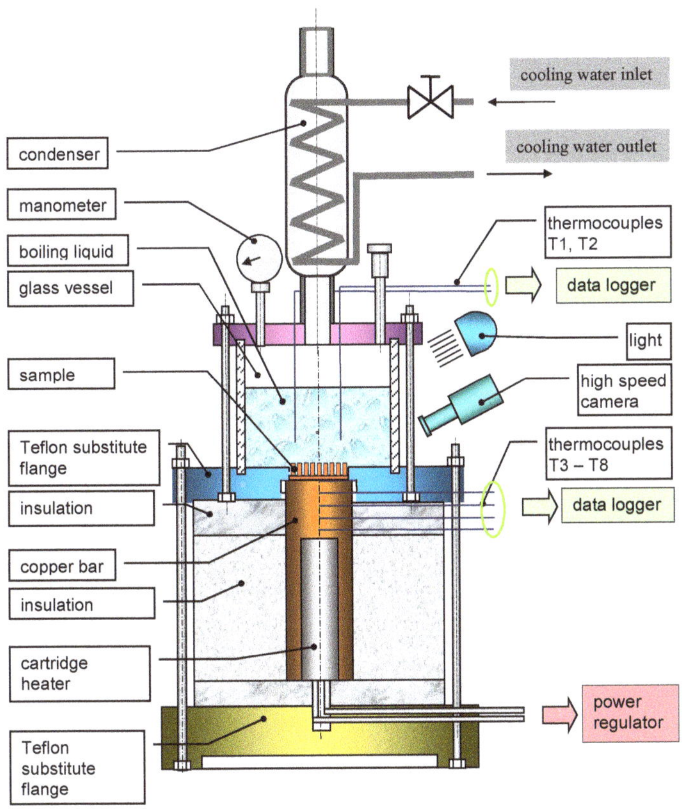

Figure 2. The main module of the measurement system.

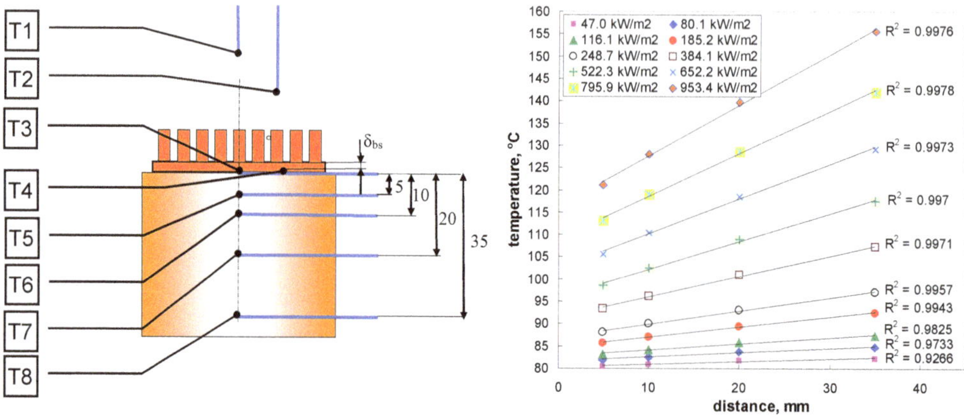

(a) (b)

Figure 3. (**a**) Thermocouple arrangement, (**b**) Temperature distribution for the sample DMC-0.5-5.5.

The camera axis was tilted at an angle of 20–30° to the horizontal, so the diameters of the bubble were determined in a plane perpendicular to the camera axis. The diameter of the departure bubble was determined as the arithmetic mean of the maximum and minimum bubble diameter measurements. Taking into account the constant minichannel pitch (2 ± 0.1 mm) and relating it to the measurements of the pitch and diameter in the images, the actual average diameter of the departure bubble was determined. Assuming that the bubble diameter was approximately twice the minichannel pitch, the uncertainty in the maximum and minimum diameters was assumed to be 0.2 mm. The combined uncertainty in the diameter of the departure bubble was 0.14 mm.

The autotransformer was used to regulate the heat flux supplied to the copper bar. The time required for the temperature to stabilize the heating cylinder and the sample was approximately 15 min with increasing heat flux and 20 min with decreasing heat flux. The FLUKE Hydra Series II measurement data acquisition system was used to read and record the temperature of eight thermocouples. This time is required to reach steady state after a step change in power supplied to the copper bar.

To measure the temperature in the heating cylinder and the boiling liquid, K-type thermocouples (NiCr-NiAl) with a diameter of 0.5 mm were used. The arrangement of the thermocouples is shown in Figure 3a. The sample with minichannels was connected to the copper bar with a layer of tin. Before actual measurements, the thermocouples were calibrated using the Altek 422 calibrator. The calibration procedure was carried out by the calibrator with all thermocouples used in the range of 70–170 °C. For subsequent analysis, the calibrated thermocouples were connected to a data logger. The temperature differences observed did not exceed 0.1 K. Given the sensitivity of the logger (0.1 K) and the accuracy of the thermocouples for direct measurement of the temperature difference (assumed to be ±0.2 K), the uncertainty of the heat flux and the heat transfer coefficient were calculated taking this value as the uncertainty of the independent variable.

The measurements were repeated if the temperature difference under the sample (reading from thermocouples T3 and T4, Figure 3) was greater than 0.2 K. It was assumed that the difference in the heat flux and HTC values obtained during the increase and decrease in the heat flux should not exceed the calculated combined uncertainties in the measurement of the heat flux and heat transfer coefficients.

An example graph of temperature changes read for thermocouples placed in the cylinder axis is shown in Figure 3b. The linear distribution with a coefficient of determination R^2 close to 1 confirms one-dimensional heat flow.

The thermal conductivity of the copper samples was 380 W/(mK). Dimensions and photos of the samples are shown in Figure 4. The minichannels were made with a disc milling cutter with a width of 0.5, 0.6, 0.8, 1.0, and 1.2 mm and a constant pitch of 2 mm. The geometric parameters of the minichannels and the values characterizing the extended surface, i.e., the aspect ratio of the fin (w/h) and the surface extension coefficient φ are given in Table 2. The active surface of the sample was 27 × 27 mm^2.

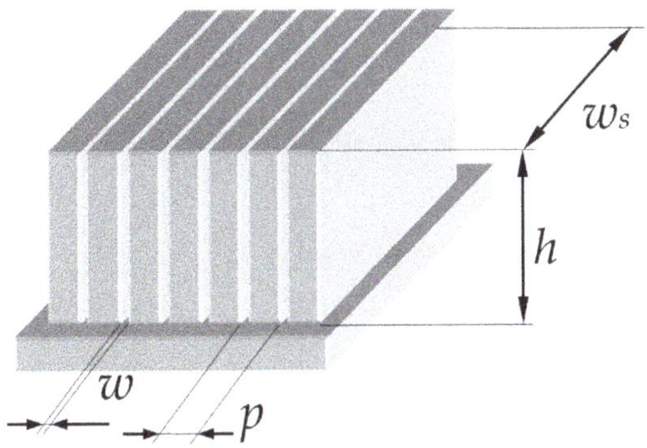

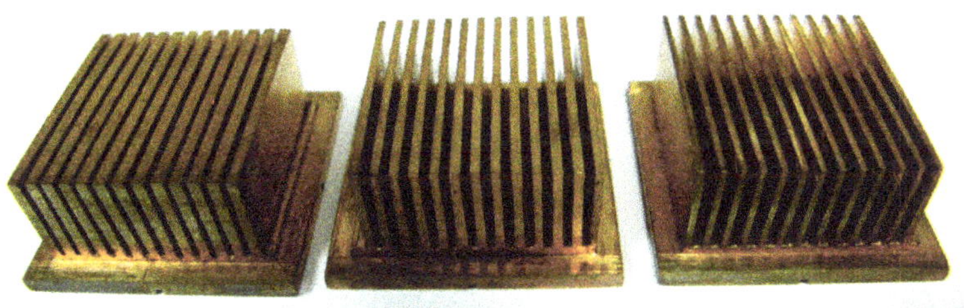

Figure 4. Dimensions and photos of the tested surfaces.

Table 2. Surface codes and specifications.

Sample code	W, mm	h, mm	p, mm	φ	w/h	Bo	α_{max}, kW/m^2K
DMC-0.5-5.5	0.5	5.5	2.0	6.5	0.09	0.10	45.7
DMC-0.8-6.0	0.8	6.0	2.0	7	0.13	0.27	52
DMC-0.6-10	0.6	10	2.0	11	0.06	0.15	42.4
DMC-1.0-10	1.0	10	2.0	11	0.10	0.42	47.8
DMC-1.2-10	1.2	10	2.0	11	0.12	0.60	42.4

Creating channels in copper using milling is associated with the possibility of inaccuracies, especially in the case of deep minichannels. After the surface was fabricated, the channel depths were checked with a caliper and their widths were checked with a feeler gauge. A tolerance of 0.03 to 0.05 mm was assumed.

Roughness measurements were performed using a Leica (Wetzlar, Germany) DCM8 confocal microscope. The arithmetic mean deviation of the roughness profile, Ra, was 0.46–0.47 μm for the minifin tops, while the values for the minichannel bottoms ranged from 0.50 to 0.69 μm. Increasing roughness increases the density of nucleation centers, which contributes to an increase in HTC at lower heat fluxes and an increase in CHF. These changes are significant at roughnesses greater than 2–3 μm. For the analyzed DMC surfaces, it can be assumed that the mechanism of bubble nucleation and initial bubble growth in the corner at the bottom of the minichannel dominates, resulting in the formation of bubbles with diameters of 2–6 mm. The few small bubbles with diameters of 0.2–0.3 mm visible in the visualization photos are formed as a result of nucleation in microcavities on the surface of the bottom of the minichannels, without contact with the minifin walls.

To develop the pool boiling mechanism for DMC surfaces, it is important to visualize the dynamics of bubble growth. The images were recorded using a digital monochrome camera PHOT MV-D1024-160-CL (Photonfocus, Lachen, Switzerland), which recorded images at a speed of 428 frames per second at a resolution of 500 × 250 pixels. Visualization was also performed using the RX-10 camera (Sony Corp., Tokyo, Japan).

The copper bar was surrounded by a thick insulating layer, which ensured one-dimensional heat conduction. Relationship (1) takes into account the increase in heat flux caused by the reduction in the sample base cross-section compared to the copper bar cross-section:

$$q = \lambda_{Cu}\frac{T_{T8} - T_{T5}}{\delta_{T8-T5}} \cdot \frac{\pi d_{cyl}^2}{4{w_s}^2} \tag{1}$$

The wall superheat was referred to the surface of the bottoms of the minichannels; therefore, it was necessary to extrapolate the temperature read from the thermocouples T3 and T4 to the distance δ_{bs} (Figure 3).

$$\Delta T = \frac{T_{T3} + T_{T4}}{2} - q\frac{\delta_{bs}}{\lambda_{Cu}} - \frac{T_{T1} + T_{T2}}{2} \tag{2}$$

The heat transfer coefficient was defined according to Newton's law:

$$\alpha = \frac{q}{\Delta T} \tag{3}$$

where

- T_{T1} to T_{T4}—thermocouple temperatures,
- δ_{bs}—the thickness between the base of the sample and the bottom of the minichannel,
- λ_{Cu}—a copper heat conductivity coefficient,
- δ_{T8-T5}—the distance between thermocouples T8 and T5,
- d_{cyl}—the external diameter of the copper cylinder to which the sample is soldered.

The diameters of the bubbles d_b were measured in two directions x and y. They were determined for at least 30 consecutive departing bubbles with an average value of 8–10 nucleation sites. Diameters were determined with constant heat flux q. The departing bubble was treated as two rotating semi-ellipsoids with a vertical and a horizontal rotation axis. The bubble diameter can be determined according to the relationship [32]:

$$d_b = \left(x^2 y\right)^{0.33} \tag{4}$$

The dimensionless number relating to the flow resistance in the minichannel space is the Bond number, which can be defined as

$$\text{Bo} = \left(\frac{w}{L}\right)^2 \tag{5}$$

where L is the capillary length:

$$L = \sqrt{\frac{\sigma}{g(\rho_l - \rho_v)}} \tag{6}$$

The increase in the heat transfer surface is one of the factors that increases the heat flux. The surface enhancement factor (or extension coefficient) can be defined as the ratio of the total extended surface area to the base (smooth) surface area [33]:

$$\varphi = \frac{A_{ext}}{A_{bs}} = \frac{2h}{p} + 1 \tag{7}$$

Experimental studies were performed in the range from ONB (onset of nucleate boiling) to CHF (critical heat flux). The tested samples contained surfaces with deep minichannels with dimensions presented in Table 1. The boiling curves were determined for increasing and decreasing heat flux. Before starting the measurement series, a power of approximately 300 W was supplied to the heater for 20–30 min, which gave a heat flux of approximately 400 kW/m^2 in order to degas the tested surfaces and the vessel.

The analysis of measurement uncertainty was performed in a way similar to the work of Pastuszko [25] using the total differential error.

The combined standard uncertainties in the measurement of the heat flux and heat transfer coefficients were defined as the total differential error dependent on the following:

- The uncertainty in determining the thermal conductivity coefficient $u(\lambda)$ = 1 W/mK,
- The uncertainty in determining the temperature difference on the heating cylinder $u(\Delta T_{T5\text{–}T8})$ = 0.2 K;
- the uncertainty in determining the temperature difference $u(\Delta T_{sat})$ = 0.2 K, where $\Delta T_{sat} = (T_{T3} + T_{T4})/2 - (T_{T1} + T_{T2})/2$;
- The uncertainty in determining the distance between the temperature sensors $u(\delta_{T5\text{–}T8})$ = 0.25 mm;
- The uncertainty in determining the diameter of the heating cylinder $u(d_{cyl})$ = 0.25 mm;
- The uncertainty in determining the side of the sample $u(a)$ = 0.25 mm.

The following equation shows the relationship:

$$u(q) = \sqrt{\left(\frac{\partial q}{\partial \lambda}u(\lambda)\right)^2 + \left(\frac{\partial q}{\partial \Delta T_{\mathrm{T5-T8}}}u(\Delta T_{\mathrm{T5-T8}})\right)^2 + \left(\frac{\partial q}{\partial \delta_{\mathrm{T5-T8}}}u(\delta_{\mathrm{T5-T8}})\right)^2 + \left(\frac{\partial q}{\partial d_{cyl}}u(d_{cyl})\right)^2 + \left(\frac{\partial q}{\partial a}u(a)\right)^2} \tag{8}$$

The uncertainty of the heat transfer coefficient was determined as follows:

$$u(\alpha) = \sqrt{\left(\frac{\partial \alpha}{\partial q}u(q)\right)^2 + \left(\frac{\partial \alpha}{\partial \Delta T}u(\Delta T)\right)^2} \tag{9}$$

where the uncertainty in the superheat measurement was calculated according to the equation:

$$u(\Delta T) = \sqrt{\left(\frac{\partial \Delta(\Delta T)}{\partial \lambda}u(\lambda)\right)^2 + \left(\frac{\partial \Delta(\Delta T)}{\partial \Delta T_{sat}}u(\Delta T_{sat})\right)^2 + \left(\frac{\partial \Delta(\Delta T)}{\partial \delta_{bs}}u(\delta_{bs})\right)^2 + \left(\frac{\partial \Delta(\Delta T)}{\partial q}u(q)\right)^2} \tag{10}$$

Changes in measurement uncertainties with increasing heat flux and HTC are shown in Figures 5 and 6, respectively. The relative combined standard uncertainties in the measurement of the heat flux and heat transfer coefficients are inversely proportional to the heat flux and HTC. For increasing heat flux in the range of 17–950 kW/m^2, the relative uncertainty of the determination of the heat flux varied between 17% and 2% with increasing heat flux (Figure 5), while the relative uncertainty of the heat transfer coefficient changed from 35 to 5% with increasing heat transfer coefficient (Figure 6). The uncertainties of HTC determination are high at the lowest heat flux and heat transfer coefficients because of the small superheats at these values.

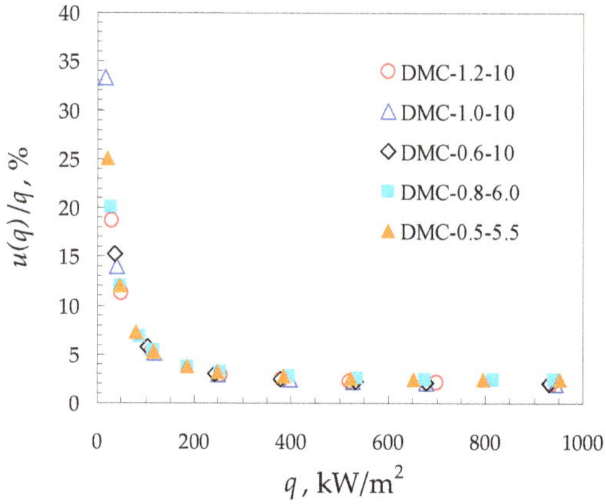

Figure 5. Relative uncertainties at various heat fluxes.

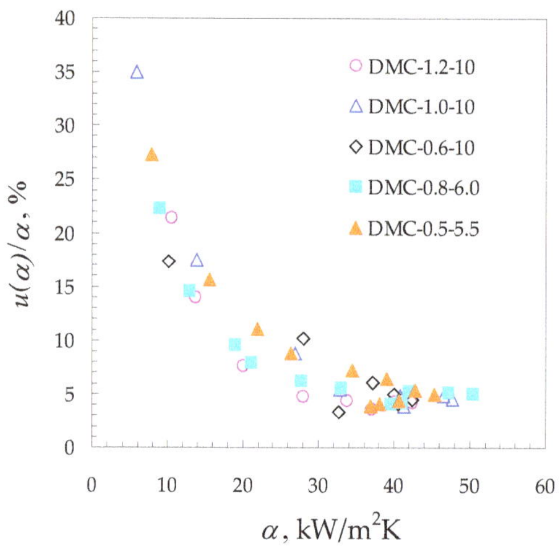

Figure 6. Relative uncertainties in different HTCs.

3. Results—Boiling Curves

The onset of nucleate boiling occurs at the moment of reaching the saturation temperature corresponding to the atmospheric pressure and observing the separation of steam bubbles. The high-speed camera was used as an indicator of ONB. The surface of the DMC wall superheated at ONB was 2.8–3.6 K. The heat flux of 20.3 kW/m^2 for the surface of DMC-0.5-5.5 corresponds to a superheat of 2.8 K. These are significantly lower values than those obtained during ethanol boiling, e.g., on the perforated micromesh surface (superheat of 10–12 K at ONB [7]).

Figures 7 and 8 show the influence of minichannel geometry on the heat transfer process. For surfaces with minichannels of depths 5.5 to 6 mm and 10 mm, an approximately twofold increase in the critical heat flux was observed. Changes in the depth and width of the minichannels have a small effect on the values of the obtained CHF. The increase in heat transfer intensity on extended surfaces occurs with an increase in the heat exchange surface, as well as with an increase in the frequency of bubble detachment and the density of nucleation centers. The maximum heat transfer coefficients obtained are in the range of 42 to 52 kW/m^{2}K, with higher values (46 to 52 kW/m^{2}K) obtained for surfaces with shallower minichannels (5.5 to 6 mm). This can be explained by a smaller temperature drop in the case of lower fins, which results in obtaining greater superheat at the fin tips, i.e., at the minichannel outlets.

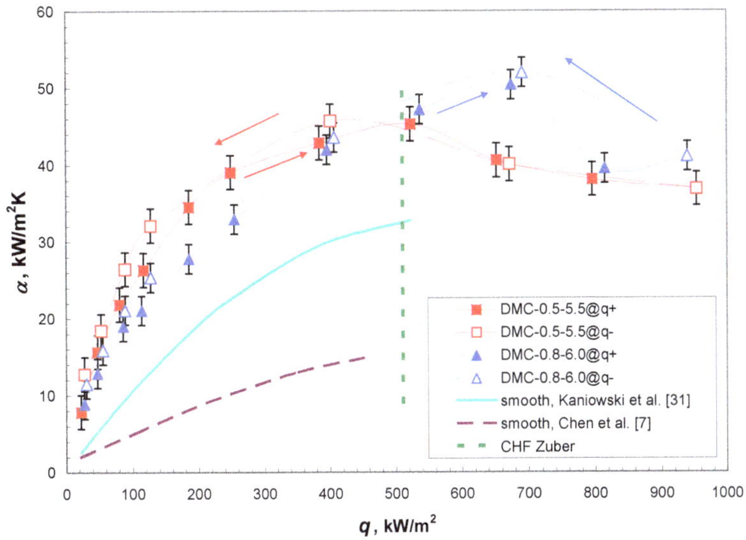

Figure 7. Pool boiling curves for ethanol at different minichannel widths, and depth of the minichannel 5.5–6 mm; arrows show the direction of increasing and decreasing heat flux, the colors are related to the color of the sample marking in the legend.

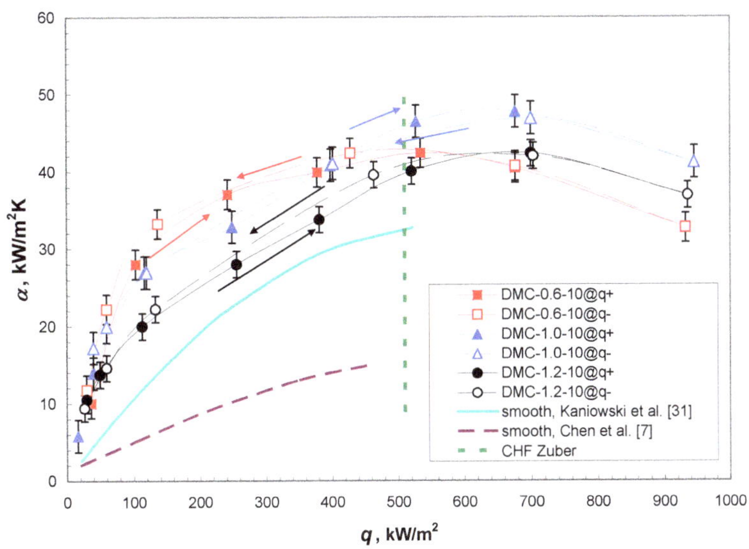

Figure 8. Pool boiling curves for ethanol at different minichannel widths, and depth of minichannel 10 mm; arrows show the direction of increasing and decreasing heat flux, the colors are related to the color of the sample marking in the legend.

The small space between the minifins that form the walls of the minichannel causes an increase in capillary pressure, allowing the liquid to be sucked into the lower part of the channel, which helps to replenish the liquid and prevents the minichannel spaces from drying out. For heat fluxes below 500 kW/m^2, both in the case of minichannels with a depth of 5.5–6 mm and 10 mm, it is more beneficial to use the smallest width of minichannels, i.e., 0.6 mm. The high capillary pressures occurring at this small width will contribute to the intensive inflow of liquid into the minichannel space, allowing for the obtained heat transfer coefficients of about 40 kW/m^{2}K at a heat flux of 300 kW/m^2. For surfaces with minichannels of this width, after exceeding the heat flux of 500 kW/m^2, a gradual decrease in HTC of 20–25% can be observed. A more advantageous solution, guaranteeing an increase in the heat transfer coefficient at higher heat fluxes, is the use of minichannels with a width increased to 0.8–1 mm. In the case of DMC with a depth of 6 mm, an HTC of up to 52 kW/m^{2}K can be obtained at a heat flux of about 700 kW/m^2. Slightly lower HTC values (approximately 47 kW/m^{2}K) at the same heat flux were obtained for minichannels with a depth of 10 mm. Using a channel with a width of 0.6 mm at a depth of 10 mm results in a significant decrease in the heat transfer coefficient after exceeding 500 kW/m^2. Despite the large superheat of the fins forming the channel walls, the significant friction flow resistance that is formed blocks the release of vapor [34], which leads to drying out of the minichannel space. A significant increase in superheat, especially at the bottom of the minichannel, i.e., at the base of the minifins, with a small increase in the heat flux will cause a gradual decrease in the heat transfer coefficient.

According to Jaikumar and Kandlikar [35], increasing the channel width results in better liquid flow to the channel, which limits drying out; however, excessive increases in width, despite the improvement in the intensity of the vapor flow from the bottom of the minichannel, also result in a decrease in the thickness of the minifins. The reduced thickness of the fins that limit the minichannel causes an intensive temperature drop at their height, because the superheat at the channel outlet may not be sufficient to maintain nucleate boiling. According to Winter and Weibel [36], with the decrease in the width of the interfin space, i.e., at the same time as the width of the minichannel, a stable vapor layer will not be formed on the surface of the minifin base until larger heat fluxes appear. In turn, Huang et al. [37] analyzed the fin array with fins of constant thickness of 1 mm predicted critical heat flux for varying heights (3–10 mm) and spacings (0.3–2 mm). Maximum CHF values were obtained for fins of about 4 mm height with the smallest interfin space widths (0.3–0.6 mm). However, it should be noted that, with a constant fin thickness, reducing the spacing between the fins or increasing the fin height increases the total available heat transfer surface. In the case of the analyzed DMC surfaces with a constant minichannel pitch, i.e., simultaneous fins, reducing the minichannel width results in an increase in the aspect ratio of the fin, $(p\text{-}w)/h$, while the surface extension coefficient φ remains constant. With a similar minichannel width and increasing depth, the liquid flow resistance in the minichannel spaces increases, which can be observed as a slight decrease in CHF.

When studying heat transfer during boiling on extended surfaces, fins are used to form minichannels with widths ranging from 0.5 to 8.5 mm and depths between 0.5 and 15 mm. According to Winter and Wiebel [36], at channel widths smaller than the capillary length, there is confinement of vapor between the fins. The capillary length for ethanol is 1.55 mm; therefore, the author assumed $w < L$. Additionally, a smaller width increases capillary pressure and the intensity of liquid inflow into the minichannel. According to Chan et al. [34], greater channel depths limit the coalescence of large bubbles, which prevents the entire developed surface from being covered by a "vapor blanket". The author of this paper wanted to determine whether, in the case of 10 mm deep minichannels, this leads to increased HTC and CHF.

The analysis of surfaces with minichannels with depths of 5–10 mm is related to the reference of the channel dimensions to the capillary length L, which for ethanol has a value of approximately 1.55 mm. If both dimensions related to the space between the fins, that is, the height of the fin (minichannel depth) and the width of the interfin space (channel width) exceed the dimension L, then the fins forming a given minichannel system can be treated as isolated [36]. For DMC surfaces $h > L$ and $w < L$, the height of the boiling regimes along the minifin and superheat of the channel bottom are strongly affected by the confinement of the vapor. The difference in the obtained HTC values with the increase and decrease in the heat flux is within the range of the calculated measurement uncertainties. The exception is the DMC-0.8-6.0 surface, for which after reaching maximum heat flux and decreasing q from 940 to 690 kW/m^2, hysteresis related to the increase in HTC by approximately 8 kW/m^{2}K was obtained. Hysteresis disappeared with a further decrease in the heat flux below 690 kW/m^2. Hysteresis is generally considered an unfavorable phenomenon, which prevents thermal stabilization of systems that emit high heat fluxes. The effect of hysteresis is significant in the case of boiling on surfaces with a porous structure. In the case of surfaces with deep minichannels, residual hysteresis related to the increase in HTC was observed only for the DMC-0.8-6 sample in the first stage of heat flux reduction after reaching CHF. Because this phenomenon did not occur for the other tested surfaces and the differences in HTC during heat flux increases and decreases were within the measurement uncertainty range, it can be assumed that in the case of boiling on surfaces with deep minichannels, it is of negligible significance.

The line of the critical heat flux shown in Figures 7 and 8 is calculated according to the Zuber formula [38]:

$$q_{\mathrm{CHF}} = 0.131 {\rho_v}^{0.5} i_{lv} [\sigma g(\rho_l - \rho_v)]^{0.25} \tag{11}$$

A distinctive highest value of CHF was obtained with DMC surfaces—approximately a doubling of CHF was achieved. A large channel flow cross-section contributes to easy flooding with liquid and vapor removed even at high superheats and heat fluxes.

The differences in the maximum heat flux obtained for individual surfaces are small, with a slight advantage of minichannels with a depth of 5.5–6 mm. A smaller channel width (0.5 mm) gives a greater fin thickness at a constant pitch, which in combination with a smaller height increases the fin efficiency. Additionally, the higher capillary pressure in the narrower channel ensures an intensive inflow of liquid into the minichannel space. As a result, a surface with such a combination of depth and width has the ability to remove the largest heat fluxes.

The author compared the performance of DMP surfaces and other enhancement structures for ethanol boiling using data with the maximum HTC and CHF presented by Chen et al. [7]. The comparison presents data for 14 micro/nanostructured surfaces. Three of the surfaces presented allow for obtaining higher HTCs (perforated micromesh surface, microchannel, and nanofiber-covered surface), one has a similar maximum HTC value, while ten have lower values. With respect to CHF, DMC surfaces provide values approximately 10–15% lower than the three best and at least 45% higher than the remaining ten.

Different trends are observed for the DMC surfaces tested during boiling of working fluids with low saturation temperatures, i.e., FC-72 and Novec-649. The best performance is observed using deeper minichannels (10 mm) with thicknesses of 0.6 and 1.0 mm [24]. Reducing the depth to 5.5–6 mm is unfavorable for these fluids. It can be assumed that similar phenomena will occur in the case of ethanol boiling at reduced pressure, but this requires a series of measurements on a modified experimental setup.

4. Results—Bubble Departure Diameter

4.1. Bubble Growth Rate

Figure 9 shows boiling images for four heat fluxes for surface DMC-0.5-5.5. Figures 10–12 show bubble growth for three samples with minichannel depths of 10 mm for selected heat fluxes.

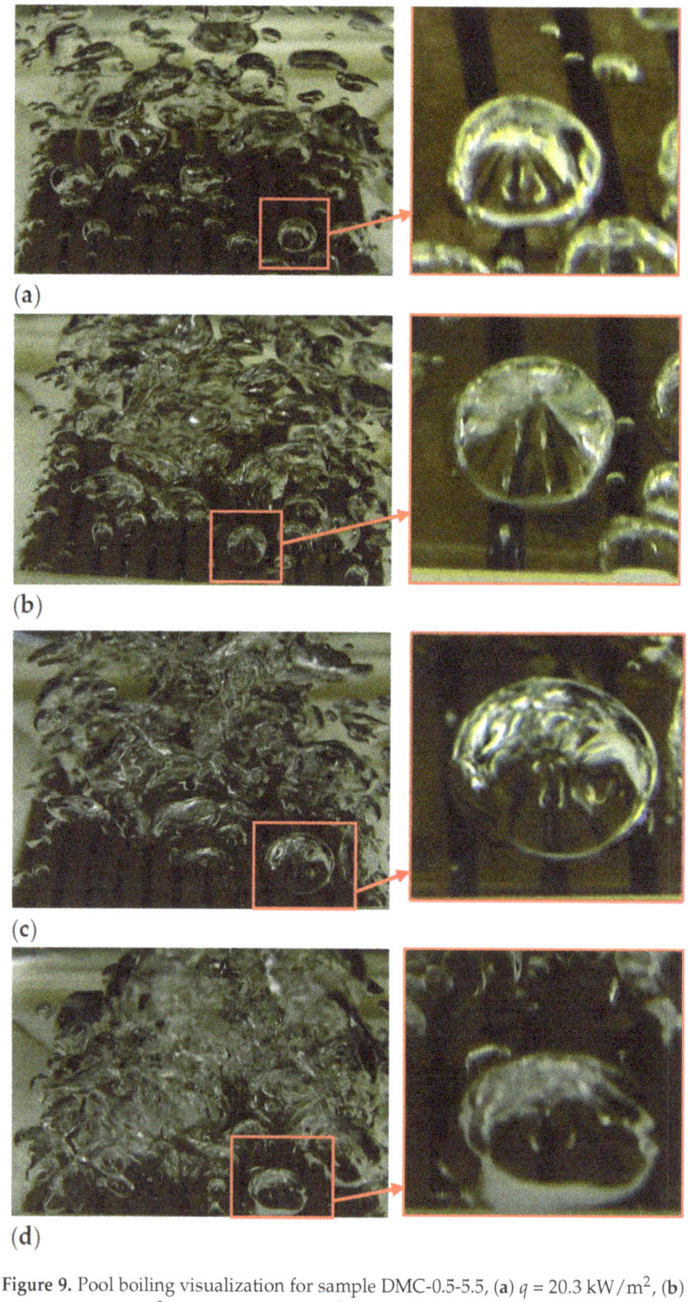

(a) (b) (c) (d)

Figure 9. Pool boiling visualization for sample DMC-0.5-5.5, (**a**) q = 20.3 kW/m^2, (**b**) q = 73.5 kW/m^2, (**c**) q = 106.4 kW/m^2, (**d**) q = 169.7 kW/m^2.

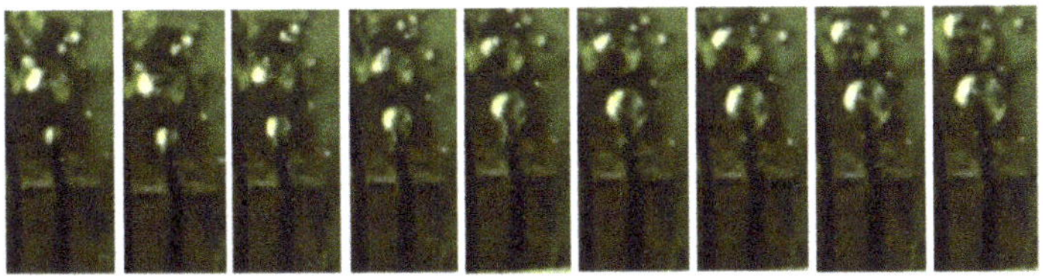

Figure 10. Bubble growth, sample DMC-0.6-10, q = 58.3 kW/m^2.

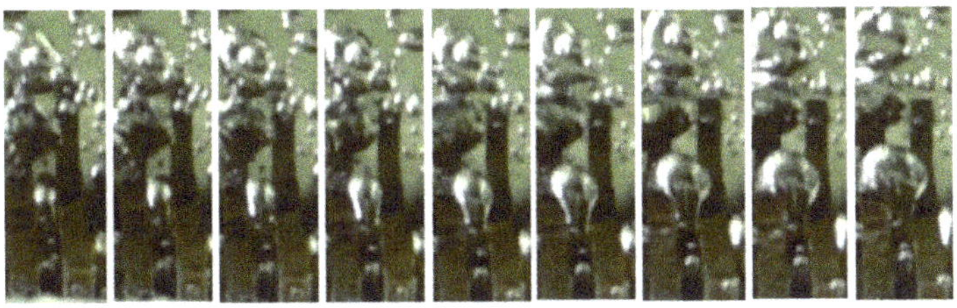

Figure 11. Bubble growth, sample DMC-1.0-10, q = 45.6 kW/m^2.

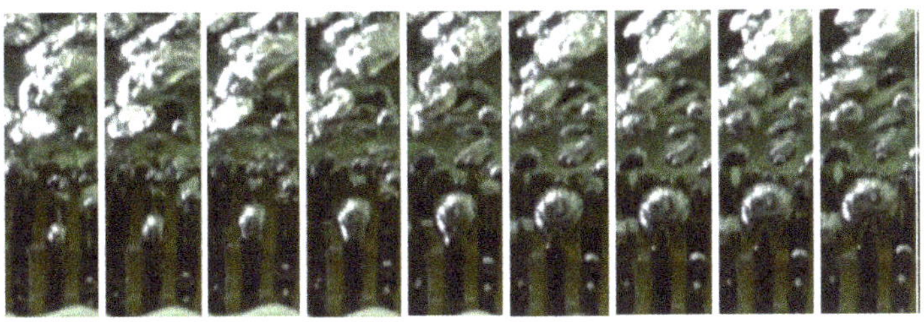

Figure 12. Bubble growth, sample DMC-1.2-10, q = 50.7 kW/m^2.

Determining the diameter of a detaching bubble based on the balance of forces acting on it requires knowledge of the bubble growth rate dr/dt and the acceleration $\mathrm{d}^2r/\mathrm{d}t^2$. On plain surfaces, the asymptotic bubble growth rate is proportional to the square root of the growth time $t^{1/2}$. This relationship was presented by Plesset and Zwick [6] and Han and Griffith [2]. Ghazvini et al. [39] concluded that traditional growth models were established based on a plain surface, while pool boiling on the fins was not considered. For the surface with microchannels of width 0.25–0.8 mm and depth 0.5 mm, Walunj and Sathyabhama [29] assumed a linear dependence of the bubble growth rate on time for the inertia-driven mechanism. They assumed a simple relationship $r(t) = at$, where a was a function of the fluid property and the wall temperature. In the case of flat surfaces, the intensity of bubble growth decreases towards the end of the growth period. For surfaces with minichannels, a constant linear increase in the radius may be caused by the intensive inflow of vapor from the channel space between the fins to the growing bubble. This article analyzes changes in the radius of the growing bubble for the surfaces listed in Table 2, in the superheat range of up to 3.9–5.6 K. The limitation of the maximum superheat results from the difficulty of observing individual bubbles at heat flux exceeding 100–200 kW/m^2. Example frames of the bubble growth recording for minichannels with a depth of 10 mm are shown in Figures 10–12. Figures 13–17 show the experimentally obtained changes in the size of the radius of the growing bubble for four superheats. For the data presented, linear interpolation was used: the obtained coefficient of determination obtained for linear regression ranged from approximately 0.85 to 1. The graphs show the values of the coefficients of determination and the equation of the trend line. The slope of the line (gradient) is also the average value of the growth rate, which was used in the calculation model to determine the drag force and the pressure difference force. The growth rate took values from about 0.02–0.03 m/s at the smallest superheats (1.4–3.1 K) to about 0.12 m/s at the largest analyzed superheats (3.9–5.6 K). The best fit (coefficients of determination) was obtained for larger superheats.

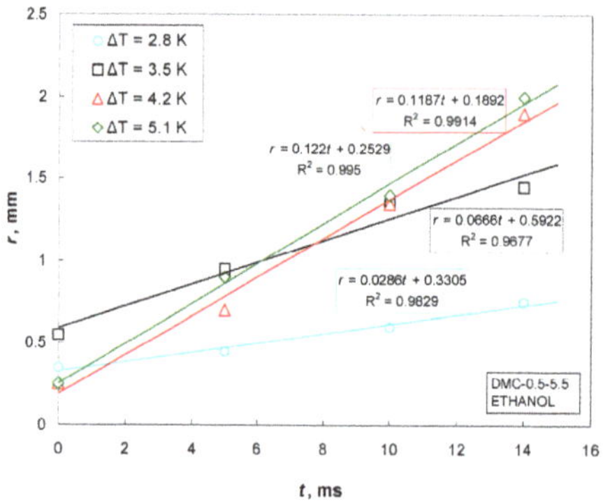

Figure 13. Variation of the bubble equivalent radius during bubble growth and linear approximation for surface DMC-0.5-5.5.

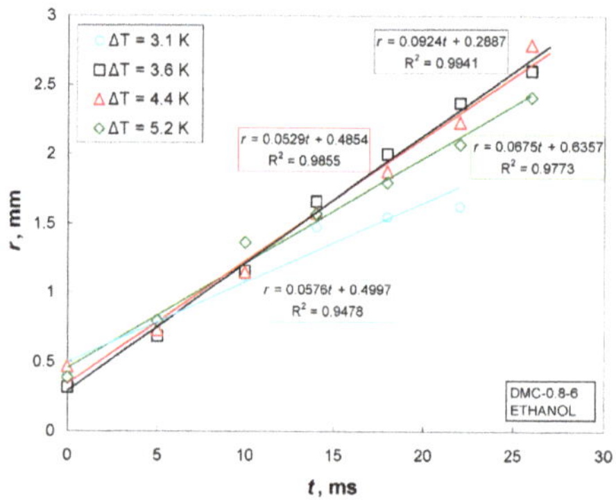

Figure 14. Variation of the bubble equivalent radius during bubble growth and linear approximation for surface DMC-0.8-6.

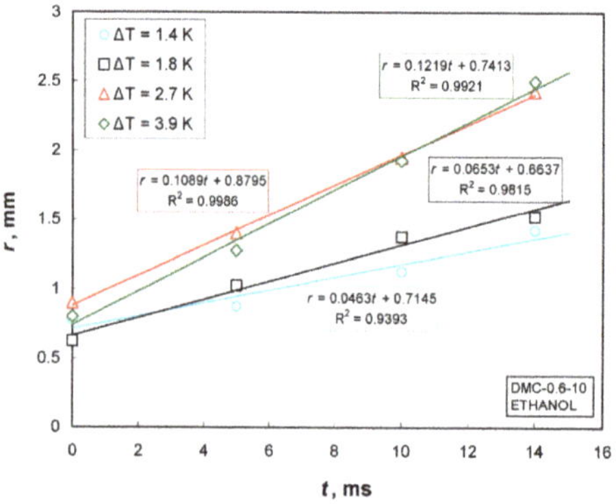

Figure 15. Variation of the bubble equivalent radius during bubble growth and linear approximation for surface DMC-0.6-10.

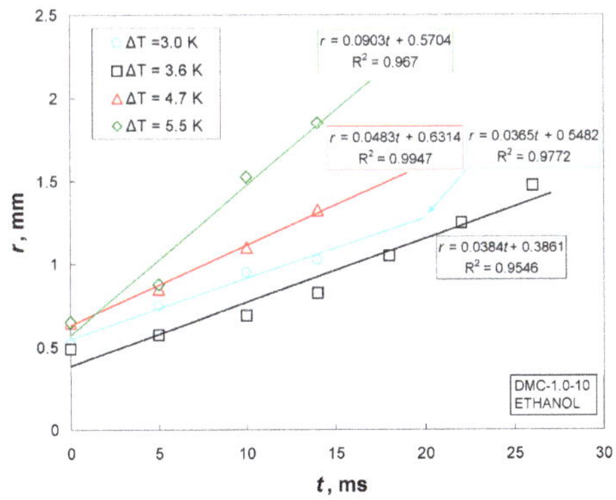

Figure 16. Variation of the bubble equivalent radius during bubble growth and linear approximation for surface DMC-1.0-10.

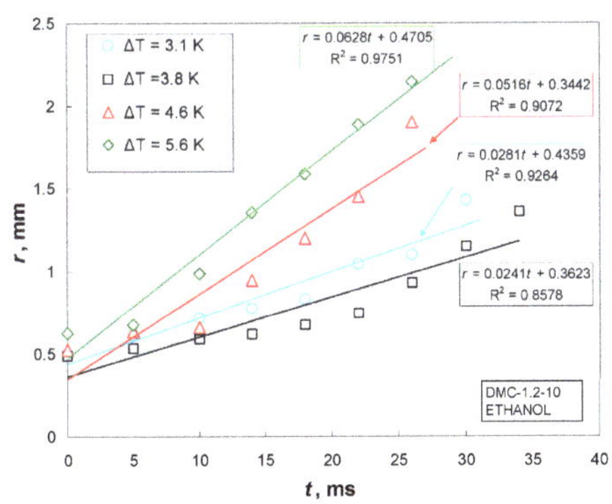

Figure 17. Variation of the bubble equivalent radius during bubble growth and linear approximation for surface DMC-1.2-10.

The three phases of bubble growth described in the introduction refer to boiling on a plain surface. In the case of pool boiling in vertical minichannels, analyzed in this article, the measurements showed bubble growth linearly with time, i.e., the dominance of stage 2 ("inertia controlled growth"). For boiling on a flat surface, this is the initial stage of bubble growth. This growth can be described by the Reyleigh equation [3,4] in the following form:

$$r = \frac{2}{3}\left(\frac{\rho_v h_{fg} \Delta T}{\rho_l T_{sat}}\right)^{1/2} t \tag{12}$$

For example, the growth rate calculated from the above equation for superheating of 4.2 K and 5.1 K is 0.12 m/s and 0.133 m/s. Using measurement interpolation, 0.119 m/s and 0.122 m/s were obtained, respectively (DMC-0.5-5.5, Figure 13). Greater discrepancies appear for smaller superheats. At higher superheats, due to the merging of bubbles (coalescence) and their irregular shapes, it is impossible to determine the changes in diameter in relation to a single, isolated bubble.

4.2. Forces Balance

In this paper, the balance of four forces was adopted to compute the diameter of the departing bubble on the surface with minichannels, two of which tend to detach (the buoyancy force and pressure difference force), and two forces hold the bubble (drag force and surface tension force), Figure 18.

$$F_{bu} + F_p = F_{st} + F_d \tag{13}$$

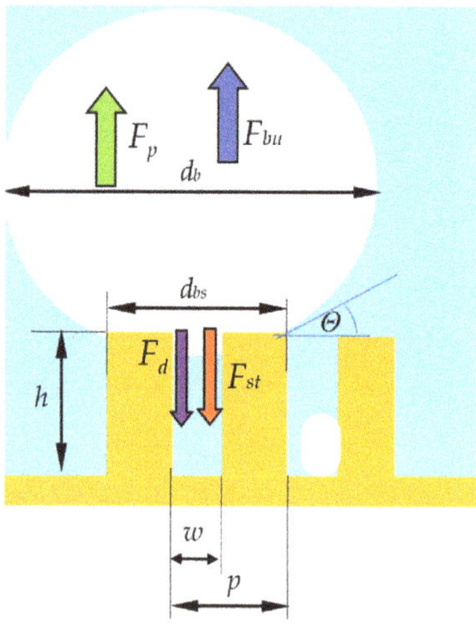

Figure 18. The balance of forces.

4.2.1. Buoyancy Force

The departing bubble has the shape of an elongated vertically truncated spheroid, but, assuming a spherical shape for simplicity, the buoyancy force is determined according to the following formula:

$$F_{b_u} = \frac{\pi d_b^3}{6} g(\rho_l - \rho_v) \tag{14}$$

4.2.2. Pressure Difference Force

The pressure difference force [12,13] depends on the capillary pressure and the vapor pressure:

$$F_p = \left(\frac{C_d \rho_l}{8} \left(\frac{dr}{dt} \right)^2 + \frac{4\sigma}{d_b} \right) A_c \tag{15}$$

The bubble growth rate dr/dt was assumed based on experimental data (Figures 13–17). The drag coefficient, C_d, was calculated according to Beer [12]:

$$C_d = \frac{5360}{\mathrm{Re}^{0.79}} \tag{16}$$

This relationship was also used by Wang et al. [13] and Wu et al. [40]. The Reynolds number was determined using the following formula:

$$\mathrm{Re} = \frac{\frac{dr}{dt} d_b}{\nu} \tag{17}$$

The contact surface area between the minifin's top and the bubble is the area of two segments of a circle with a radius corresponding to half the diameter of the bubble base d_{bs}. Due to the small width of the interfin space (channel) compared to the width of the fin, it was assumed that the length of the segment chord corresponds to its diameter. Finally, the contact surface area is the surface of a circle with diameter d_{bs}, reduced by the area of a rectangle with sides corresponding to the diameter d_{bs} and the width of the minichannel w:

$$A_c = \frac{\pi d_{bs}^2}{4} - 2d_{bs}w \tag{18}$$

The diameter of the bubble base corresponds to the sum of the microchannel width and the thickness of two microfins, giving $d_{bs} = 2p\text{-}w$ (Figure 18).

4.2.3. Surface Tension Force

The surface tension force can be calculated according to the following formula:

$$F_{st} = \sigma L_c \sin\Theta \tag{19}$$

The contact line L_c consists of two horizontal arcs with radii corresponding to half the diameter of the bubble base (d_{bs}), placed at the tops of adjacent microfins, closed by two chords with a length approximately corresponding to the diameter of d_{bs} (Figure 18):

$$L_c = \pi d_{bs} - 2w + 2d_{bs} \tag{20}$$

The diameter of the bubble base d_{bs} was determined according to the explanation in Formula (12). Furthermore, it was assumed that the contact angle $\Theta = 13°$. A static contact angle value of 13° was entered based on measurements using the Biolin Scientific's Attension Theta Tensiometer. Since the surface tension force depends on the value of the contact angle, the bubble departure diameter calculation results are sensitive to changes in θ. For DMC-0.5-5.5 surfaces in the superheat range of 3.5 to 5.1 K, which corresponds to a heat flux range of 74 to 170 kW/m^2, reducing the contact angle value to 8° results in a reduction of the determined d_b value from 2.4 to 1.1%. Increasing the contact angle value to 18° results in an increase in the calculated d_b value of 2.2 to 1%.

4.2.4. Drag Force

The drag force is related to the resistance of the liquid to the expansion of the vapor bubble. The drag coefficient C_d and the bubble growth rate, dr/dt, were calculated similarly to the pressure difference force:

$$F_d = \frac{C_d \rho_l}{2}\left(\frac{dr}{dt}\right)^2 \frac{\pi d_b^2}{4} \tag{21}$$

4.3. Bubble Departure Diameters

Figure 19 shows a comparison of the bubble diameters measured experimentally and computed based on the theoretical model presented, for individual surfaces. The graphs also show models developed previously by the author and coworkers [24] and a simple computational model by Cooke and Kandlikar [41]. For the balance of dynamic forces, the authors [24] assumed that the calculation of the diameter of the bubble is based on a balance of six forces (buoyancy, surface tension, pressure difference, drag, liquid inertia, and bubble inertia). In the case of the static force balance analysis, only the surface tension force and the buoyancy force were taken into account. The original relationship given by Cooke and Kandlikar is the following:

$$d_b = \frac{w}{\cos\frac{180° + \Theta_v}{2}} \tag{22}$$

which gives d_b values less than zero. It has been corrected in the following form:

$$d_b = \frac{w}{\cos\frac{90^\circ + \Theta_v}{2}} \quad (23)$$

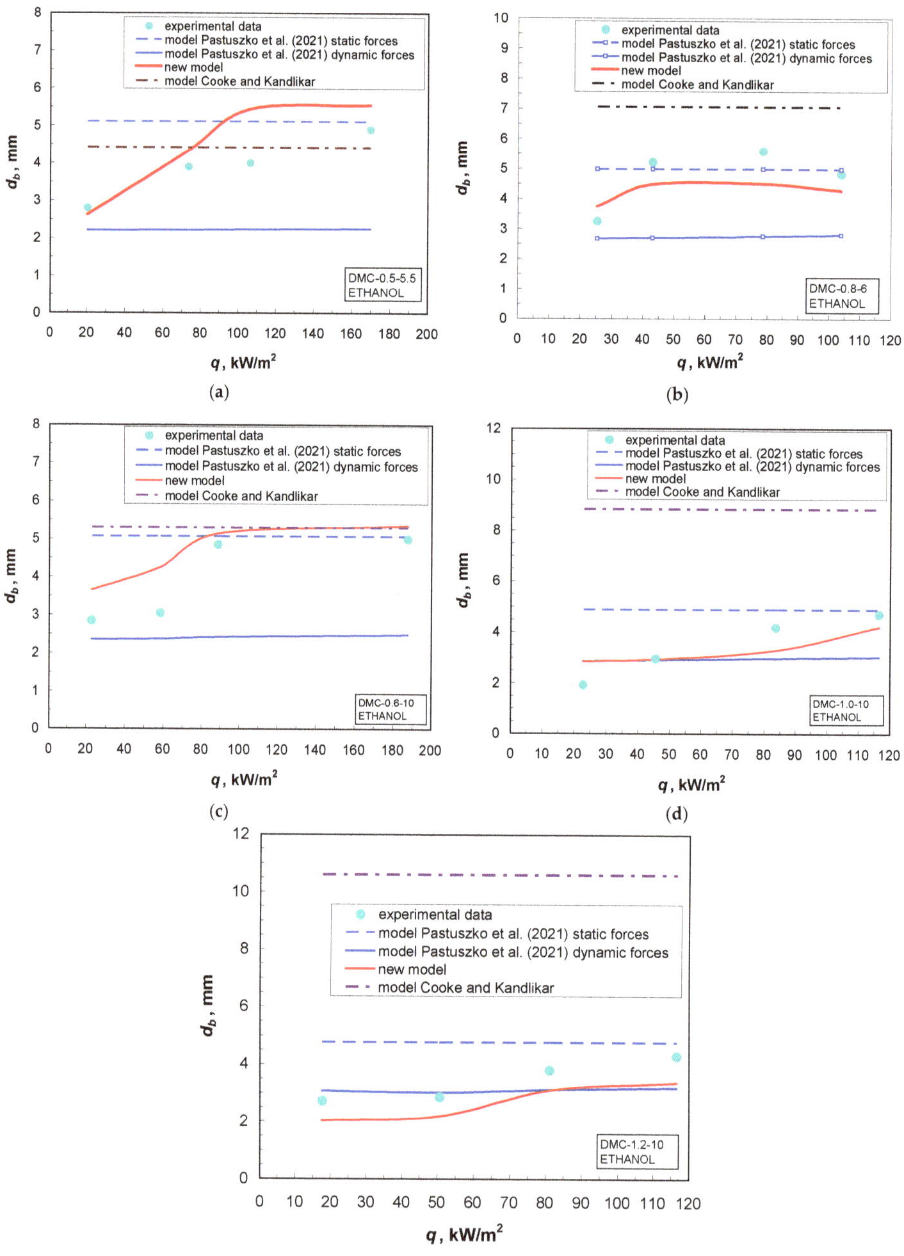

Figure 19. Comparison of the measured and predicted bubble departure diameters for deep minichannels with the previous models of the author and coworkers [24] and the Cooke and Kandlikar model [41]; (**a**) DMC-0.5-5.5, (**b**) DMC-0.8-6, (**c**) DMC-0.6-10, (**d**) DMC-1.0-10, (**e**) DMC-1.2-10.

The corrected relationship presented was used to calculate the bubble departure diameter for the contact angle Θ_v referring to the vertical sides of the minichannel. Calculations were performed for the contact angle values of $\Theta_v = 90^\circ - \Theta$.

A small bubble diameter can be observed, 2–3.5 mm at the lowest heat flux (22–30 kW/m^2). An increase in the heat flux to approximately 70–190 kW/m^2 results in stabilization of the bubble diameter in the range of 4.2–5.6 mm. The proposed calculation model correctly reflects the trend related to the increase in the bubble departure diameter for the heat flux range considered. The best agreement of the calculations with the experimental data was obtained for a greater depth of the minichannels, i.e., 10 mm. The relative error in determining the diameter does not exceed 17% for $q > 40$ kW/m^2. The model of Pastuszko et al. [24] is consistent with the experimental data in the range of the highest heat flux and for minichannels with widths of 0.5–1 mm, it is close to the current model. The Cooke and Kandlikar model [41] presents the experimental data well and can be used for fast calculations only for the smallest minichannel widths, that is, 0.6 mm for heat fluxes greater than 70–80 kW/m^2. For larger minichannel widths, a significant (3–4 times) overprediction is obtained. However, the model of Pastuszko et al. related to dynamic forces gives good accuracy in the range of the lowest heat flux (20–30 kW/m^2). For the DMC-1.0-10 surface, almost perfect agreement of the new model with the dynamic forces model was obtained in the range of low and medium heat flux, 20 to 80 kW/m^2. A similar trend occurs for the largest minichannel width (sample DMC-1.2-10), but in the range of medium and largest heat fluxes, i.e., from about 70 to 120 kW/m^2.

For similar DMC surfaces spreading heat during water boiling, the proposed model using the balance of five forces [25] enabled the determination of the diameter of departing bubbles with errors of up to 25%. Also, the models developed by the author and coworkers for these structures [24] gave bubble departure diameter prediction errors of up to 32% (boiling FC-72) and 24% (boiling Novec-649).

HTC does not appear in Formulas 13-21 used to determine the diameter of the departure bubble. When comparing the calculated and experimental values, which are related to the heat flux, the uncertainty of the heat flux determination is important. For the analyzed range q = 20–180 kW/m^2 (Figure 19), Δq = 5.6–7 kW/m^2.

The possible sources of discrepancy between the predicted bubble diameters and the experimental data are as follows:

- Changes in the bubble departure diameters at different locations (outlets) of the minichannel
- Non-spherical shape of bubbles
- Failure to meet the assumption of a linear dependence of the radius of the growing bubble on time.

5. Conclusions

This paper presents the results of experimental and theoretical studies of ethanol nucleate pool boiling on surfaces with deep minichannels (DMC). Experiments were performed from the onset of boiling (ONB) to the boiling crisis (CHF) at atmospheric pressure. For the tested surfaces, an increase in heat transfer was observed in comparison to that for a plain smooth surface, with the heat transfer coefficient (HTC) and the critical heat flux (CHF) depending on the depth and width of the minichannel. The maximum HTCs obtained were more than three times higher than for the plain surface for the Chen et al. data [7], reaching a value of 52 kW/m^{2}K for the DMC-0.8-6.0 sample. The highest HTC was obtained for the sample with a low surface extension $\varphi = 7$, that is, for minichannels with a width of 0.8 mm and a depth of 6 mm. The critical (maximum) heat fluxes for all tested surfaces were similar and about twice as high as those for the smooth plain surface.

On the basis of the measurements carried out, the following general recommendations can be given to obtain the highest heat transfer coefficients during ethanol pool boiling of ethanol:

- At high heat fluxes (above 500 kW/m^{2}K), the analyzed minichannels with a depth of 5.5 to 10 mm should be 0.8 to 1 mm wide, that is, approximately 1/2 to 2/3 of the capillary length for ethanol;
- At lower heat fluxes (below 500 kW/m^{2}K), it is more beneficial to use narrower minichannels (0.5–0.6 mm), that is, about a third of the capillary length;
- Due to similar values of the heat transfer coefficients in the case of lower and higher HTC values, it is more optimal to use minichannels with a depth of 5.5–6 mm in terms of lower material consumption;
- There are two main possible applications for the analyzed DMC surfaces in terms of heat removal from electronic components or electronic subassemblies:
- Direct cooling, also known as two-phase immersion cooling—cooling of electronic systems connected to the DMC surface, immersed in a dielectric fluid;
- Indirect cooling—the use of a heat pipe or thermosyphon with a DMC surface as an evaporator to remove large heat fluxes from electronic systems.

For the analyzed DMC surfaces, one can assume inertia-controlled growth of the bubble: the author presented a method of bubble departure calculation assuming a constant bubble growth rate. The developed model allowed determining the diameter of the departing bubble on surfaces with deep minichannels of width 0.6–1.2 mm with an average relative error of 23.5% in the heat flux range of 22–190 kW/m^2 and below 17% in the range of 40–190 kW/m^2. The model showed satisfactory agreement with the experimental data and a correct trend of increasing bubble diameter with increasing heat flux. The increase in the growth rate influenced the increase in the diameter of the departing bubble.

Funding: This research received no external funding.

Institutional Review Board Statement: Not applicable.

Informed Consent Statement: Not applicable.

Data Availability Statement: The data presented in this study are available on request from the corresponding author.

Conflicts of Interest: The author declares no conflicts of interest.

Nomenclature

A	area, m^2
Bo	Bond number
C_d	drag coefficient
c_p	specific heat, J/(kgK)
CHF	critical heat flux, W m^{-2}
DMC	deep minichannel
d	diameter, m
F	force, N
g	gravitational acceleration, m s^{-2}
HTC	heat transfer coefficient, W m^{-2}K^{-1}
h	minichannel depth, m
i_{lv}	Enthalpy of vaporization, kJ/kg
L	capillary length, m
L_c	lenght of the contact line
q	heat flux, Wm^{-2}

p	pitch, m
R^2	coefficient of determination
r	radius, m
Re	Reynolds number
T	temperature, K
t	time, s
u	uncertainty
w	width, m
x, y	distance, m
Greek letters	
α	heat transfer coefficient, W $m^{-2}K^{-1}$
Δ	error, uncertainty
ΔT	superheat referred to the minifin base, K
δ	thickness, m
Θ	contact angle, rad
φ	surface extension coefficient
λ	thermal conductivity, W m^{-1} K^{-1}
ν	kinematic viscosity, m^2/s
ρ	density, kg/m^3
σ	surface tension, N/m
Subscripts	
b	departing bubble
bs	base
bu	buoyancy
Cu	copper
c	contact line
cyl	cylinder
d	drag
ext	extended
l	liquid
max	maximum
p	pressure difference
s	sample
Sn	tin
sat	saturated
st	surface tension
T1,. . ., T8	thermocouple number
v	vapor, vertical

References

1. Cieśliński, J. *Modeling of Pool Boiling;* Wydawnictwo Politechniki Gdańskiej: Gdańsk, Poland, 2005. (In Polish)
2. Han, C.-Y.; Griffith, P. The mechanism of heat transfer in nucleate pool boiling—Part I: Bubble initiaton, growth and departure. *Int. J. Heat Mass Transf.* **1965**, *8*, 887–904.
3. Mahmoud, M.M.; Karayiannis, T.G. Bubble growth models in saturated pool boiling of water on a smooth metallic surface: Assessment and a new recommendation. *Int. J. Heat Mass Transf.* **2023**, *208*, 124065. [CrossRef]
4. Rayleigh, J.W.S. *Boiling Heat Transfer*, 2nd ed.; Tong, L.S., Tang, Y.S., Eds.; CRL Press: New South Wales, Australia, 2010.
5. Fritz, W.; Ende, W. Über den verdampfungsvorgang nach kinematographischen aufnahmen an dampfblasen. *Phys. Zeitschr.* **1936**, *37*, 391–401.
6. Plesset, M.S.; Zwick, S.A. The growth of vapor bubbles in superheated liquids. *J. Appl. Phys.* **1954**, *25*, 403–500. [CrossRef]
7. Chen, Y.; Li, P.; Zou, Q.; Liu, X.; Yang, R. Enhancing pool boiling with separated liquid-vapor pathways on perforated micromesh surface. *Int. J. Heat Mass Transf.* **2025**, *244*, 126949. [CrossRef]
8. Kalani, A.; Kandlikar, S.G. Enhanced Pool Boiling with Ethanol at Subatmospheric Pressures for Electronics Cooling. *J. Heat Transf.* **2013**, *135*, 111002. [CrossRef]

9. Deng, D.; Feng, J.; Huang, Q.; Tang, Y.; Lian, Y. Pool Boiling Heat Transfer of Porous Structures with Reentrant Cavities. *Int. J. Heat Mass Transf.* **2016**, *99*, 556–568. [CrossRef]
10. Shen, B.; Hamazaki, T.; Ma, W.; Iwata, N.; Hidaka, S.; Takahara, A.; Takahashi, K.; Takata, Y. Enhanced Pool Boiling of Ethanol on Wettability-Patterned Surfaces. *Appl. Therm. Eng.* **2019**, *149*, 325–331. [CrossRef]
11. Hożejowska, S.; Kaniowski, R.; Pastuszko, R. Application of the Trefftz method for pool boiling heat transfer on open microchannel surfaces. *Heat Transf. Eng.* **2021**, *43*, 362–370. [CrossRef]
12. Beer, H. Das dynamische Blasenwachstum beim Sieden von Flüssigkeiten an Heizflächen. *Forsch. Ing-Wes.* **1971**, *37*, 85–90. [CrossRef]
13. Wang, X.; Wu, Z.; Wei, J.; Sundén, B. Correlations for Prediction of the Bubble Departure Radius on Smooth Flat Surface during Nucleate Pool Boiling. *Int. J. Heat Mass Transf.* **2019**, *132*, 699–714. [CrossRef]
14. Kumar, N.; Ghosh, P.; Shukla, P. Development of an Approximate Model for the Prediction of Bubble Departure Diameter in Pool Boiling of Water. *Int. Commun. Heat Mass Transf.* **2021**, *127*, 105531. [CrossRef]
15. Zeng, L.Z.; Klausner, J.F.; Mei, R. A Unified Model for the Prediction of Bubble Detachment Diameters in Boiling Systems—I. Pool Boiling. *Int. J. Heat Mass Transf.* **1993**, *36*, 2261–2270. [CrossRef]
16. Bucci, M.; Buongiorno, J.; Bucci, M. The Not-so-Subtle Flaws of the Force Balance Approach to Predict the Departure of Bubbles in Boiling Heat Transfer. *Phys. Fluids* **2021**, *33*, 017110. [CrossRef]
17. Iyer, S.; Kumar, A.; Coventry, J.; Lipiński, W. Modelling of Bubble Growth and Detachment in Nucleate Pool Boiling. *Int. J. Therm. Sci.* **2023**, *185*, 108041. [CrossRef]
18. Zhou, J.; Zhang, Y.; Wei, J. A Modified Bubble Dynamics Model for Predicting Bubble Departure Diameter on Micro-Pin-Finned Surfaces under Microgravity. *Appl. Therm. Eng.* **2018**, *132*, 450–462. [CrossRef]
19. Kong, X.; Zhang, Y.; Wei, J. Experimental Study of Pool Boiling Heat Transfer on Novel Bistructured Surfaces Based on Micro-Pin-Finned Structure. *Exp. Therm. Fluid Sci.* **2018**, *91*, 9–19. [CrossRef]
20. Zhao, Z.; Ma, X.; Li, S.; Yang, S.; Huang, L. Visualization-Based Nucleate Pool Boiling Heat Transfer Enhancement on Different Sizes of Square Micropillar Array Surfaces. *Exp. Therm. Fluid Sci.* **2020**, *119*, 110212. [CrossRef]
21. Zhou, J.; Xu, P.; Qi, B.; Zhang, Y.; Wei, J. Effects of micro-pin-fins on the bubble growth and movement of nucleate pool boiling on vertical surfaces. *Int. J. Therm. Sci.* **2022**, *171*, 107186. [CrossRef]
22. Hu, Y.; Fu, D.; Hong, S.; Gao, Z.; Dang, C.; Wang, S. Experimental investigation on pool boiling performance of expanding-microchanneled surface at sub-atmospheric pressure environment. *Int. Commun. Heat Mass Transf.* **2025**, *161*, 108408. [CrossRef]
23. Dong, Y.; Ibrahim, A.; Su, R.; Jiao, B.; Hu, X.; Hao, Y. Study on bubble behaviors and heat transfer at shallow liquid boiling over open rectangular microchannels. *Appl. Therm. Eng.* **2024**, *254*, 123900. [CrossRef]
24. Pastuszko, R.; Kaniowski, R.; Dadas, N.; Bedla-Pawlusek, M. Pool boiling enhancement and a method of bubble diameter determination on surfaces with deep minichannels. *Int. J. Heat Mass Transf.* **2021**, *179*, 121713. [CrossRef]
25. Pastuszko, R. Determining boiling heat transfer and bubble diameter for water in deep minichannels. *Int. J. Heat Mass Transf.* **2024**, *233*, 126009. [CrossRef]
26. Chien, L.-H.; Webb, R.L. A Nucleate Boiling Model for Structured Enhanced Surfaces. *Int. J. Heat Mass Transf.* **1998**, *41*, 2183–2195. [CrossRef]
27. Long, J.; Liu, Z.; Lin, H.; Li, Y.; Cao, Z.; Zhang, Z.; Xie, X. Pool boiling heat transfer and bubble dynamics over V-shaped microchannels and micropyramids: Does high aspect ratio always benefit boiling? *Appl. Therm. Eng.* **2022**, *201*, 117796. [CrossRef]
28. van den Bergh, W.J.; Whiting, M.; Theodorakis, P.E.; Everts, M. Nucleate pool boiling bubble dynamics for R32 and R1234yf on machined micro-structured surfaces. *Int. J. Therm. Sci.* **2024**, *206*, 109340. [CrossRef]
29. Walunj, A.; Sathyabhama, A. Comparative Study of Pool Boiling Heat Transfer from Various Microchannel Geometries. *Appl. Therm. Eng.* **2018**, *128*, 672–683. [CrossRef]
30. Kaniowski, R.; Pastuszko, R. Pool boiling of ethanol and FC-72 on open microchannel surfaces. *EPJ Web Conf.* **2018**, *180*, 02042. [CrossRef]
31. Kaniowski, R.; Pastuszko, R.; Dragašius, E.; Baskutis, S. Pool Boiling of Ethanol on Copper Surfaces with Rectangular Microchannels. *Energies* **2023**, *16*, 7883. [CrossRef]
32. Kim, J.; Oh, B.D.; Kim, M.H. Experimental Study of Pool Temperature Effects on Nucleate Pool Boiling. *Int. J. Multiph. Flow* **2006**, *32*, 208–231. [CrossRef]
33. Kaniowski, R.; Pastuszko, R. Boiling of FC-72 on Surfaces with Open Copper Microchannel. *Energies* **2021**, *14*, 7283. [CrossRef]
34. Chan, M.A.; Yap, C.R.; Ng, K.C. Pool boiling heat transfer of water on finned surfaces at near vacuum pressures. *J. Heat Transf.* **2010**, *132*, 031501. [CrossRef]
35. Jaikumar, A.; Kandlikar, S.G. Enhanced Pool Boiling Heat Transfer Mechanisms for Selectively Sintered Open Microchannels. *Int. J. Heat Mass Transf.* **2015**, *88*, 652–661. [CrossRef]
36. Winter, M.; Weibel, J.A. The capillary length scale determines the influence of bubble-fin interactions and prediction of pool boiling from heat sinks. *Int. J. Heat Mass Transf.* **2023**, *202*, 123727. [CrossRef]

37. Huang, Y.; Sarma, B.; Weibel, J.A. A predictive model for fin array boiling heat transfer performance under two-phase immersion cooling. *Int. J. Heat Mass Transf.* **2025**, *239*, 126513. [CrossRef]
38. Zuber, N. Nucleate Boiling. The Region of Isolated Bubbles and the Similarity with Natural Convection. *Int. J. Heat Mass Transf.* **1963**, *6*, 53–78. [CrossRef]
39. Ghazvini, M.; Hafez, M.; Mandin, P.; Kim, M. Experimental study of bubble growth on novel fin structures during pool boiling. *Int. J. Multiph. Flow* **2023**, *168*, 104568. [CrossRef]
40. Wu, Z.; Cao, Z.; Sundén, B. Saturated pool boiling heat transfer of acetone and HFE-7200 on modified surfaces by electrophoretic and electrochemical deposition. *Appl. Energy* **2019**, *249*, 286–299. [CrossRef]
41. Cooke, D.; Kandlikar, S.G. Effect of Open Microchannel Geometry on Pool Boiling Enhancement. *Int. J. Heat Mass Transf.* **2012**, *55*, 1004–1013. [CrossRef]

energies

MDPI

Article

A Reduced Order Model of the Thermal Profile of the Rolls for the Real-Time Control System

Dmytro Svyetlichnyy

AGH University of Krakow, Faculty of Metals Engineering and Industrial Computer Science, al. Mickiewicza 30, 30-059 Krakow, Poland; svetlich@metal.agh.edu.pl

Abstract

Effective real-time control systems require fast and accurate models. The thermal profile models of the rolls presented in this paper are proposed for a real-time control system for the design of the rolling schedule. The thermal profile of the roll defines the shape of the roll surface, its convexity, and, finally, the shape of the final product of the flat rolling, its convexity, and flatness. This paper presents accurate semi-analytical and finite element (FE) models, which serve to obtain an accurate solution of the joint thermal and mechanical problem, that is, heat transfer and thermal expansion. The results of the FE simulation are used for training the developed thermal model based on the neural network (NN) and for the creation of a dynamic reduced order model (ROM) of the roll surface profile. The pre-trained NN model gives accurate results and is faster than the FE model, but the model is not very useful for fast calculations in a real-time control system, mainly because the temperature distribution inside the rolls is not explicitly used in further calculations. In contrast, the ROM is fast and accurate and provides surface-shaped results that can be immediately used by other models of the real-time control system. The results of the simulation of the real process are also shown. Calculations of the roll campaign (more than 9 h) by the FEM model last several hours, while by the ROM less than 20 s.

Keywords: reduced order model; flat rolling; thermal model; roll profile

1. Introduction

Modeling of the process becomes more accurate and takes into account more factors and less important phenomena. The complexity and dimension of the models are constantly arising. Many advanced mathematical models are difficult or impossible to use in real-time processes. To reduce computational complexity, for example, in control systems simulations, model order is reduced. Such a model replaces the original complex model and is commonly called a reduced-order model (ROM). Model order reduction consists in an approximation or a reduction in the state spatial dimension or the degree of freedom of the original model. The main requirements for ROM are computational efficiency, a small approximation error, and the conservation of the properties and characteristics of the original model [1].

Model order reduction techniques can be classified into the following classes:

- Data-driven modeling [2,3], neural network [4,5], machine learning [6], and deep learning [7].
- Proper orthogonal decomposition used for computational fluid dynamics and structural analysis [8,9].

- Proper generalized decomposition is used to solve boundary value problems [10,11].
- Reduced basis methods applied for the Navier–Stokes equation [12], finite volume approximations [13], stochastic problems [14], nonlinear steady-state thermal analysis [15], etc.
- Balancing methods [16].
- Simplified physics [17,18].
- Matrix interpolation [19–21].
- Transfer function interpolation [22] and the other.

The rolling process is one of the processes that requires fast and accurate models for efficient online (or real-time) control. These models can be justified as called ROM; however, they are almost never named in such a way.

The development of many advanced steel grades with improved mechanical properties is based on the concept of thermomechanical treatment or thermomechanical control. Recrystallization, precipitation, and phase transformation phenomena form the basis for the production of fine, homogeneous microstructures with improved properties. Computer-assisted control and real-time modeling require ROM development [23].

Hu, et al., in the review [24], stressed that the rolling process is multiscale, multivariable, nonlinear, and unbalanced with strong coupling and a non-steady state. It is difficult to handle high-speed rolling conditions and specification changes in complex products. The main reason is that force parameter predictions are based on traditional mathematical models, and the procedure parameter settings depend on static optimization methods. To obtain accurate control of large-scale and high-speed rolling, the analysis of rolling process rules based on industrial large-scale data should be taken into account to establish dynamic process models, and also a multi-objective real-time calculation method for rolling schedules should be introduced.

A fast, rigid plastic finite element method (FEM) was developed by Zhang et al. [25] for online application in strip rolling. They then used a refined neural network to generate an initial guess for the Newton–Raphson iteration, then the Hessian matrix is divided into subdomains for parallel computing, Brent's method is adopted, the energy functional is partitioned for parallel computing, and, finally, the energy method is proposed for predicting the rolling force. They showed that fast rigid-plastic FEM can meet both computational time and accuracy requirements [25].

Larkiola et al. [26] noted that applications of neural networks in steel rolling were published in 1991, and, since then, the number of publications has steadily increased. Most applications used a backpropagation algorithm for training. Using this model, it is possible to investigate whether new products of a certain width, strength, and thickness can be produced and determine optimal mill settings. Another application is to predict the mechanical properties of the steel strip and the temporal roll force using neural network models and data processing. The rolling force can be predicted with good accuracy and can be used to determine the mill pre-settings.

Kwak et al. [27] developed a real-time model for hot strip rolling to accurately predict roll force and rolling power. The model is based on the multiple studies of finite element (FE) process simulations and the selection of nondimensional parameters characterizing the thermomechanical behavior of the strip.

Lee and Lee [28] and Son et al. [29] applied a long-term learning method using a neural network to improve the accuracy of rolling force prediction in a hot rolling mill. Implementation of this model allows us to considerably reduce the thickness error at the head-end part of the strip. The predicted rolling force agrees very closely with the practical rolling force, and the thickness error of the strip is considerably reduced.

Maurya et al. [30] proposed an artificial neural network model to predict the thermal deformation of machine-tool spindles and a genetic algorithm (GA)-based model for the optimization of the input parameters. Hsieh et al. [31] proposed a cooling control method to reduce the impact of heat on the spindle by using a thermal suppression technique accompanied by the adaptive neuro-fuzzy inference system to predict the static thermal behavior of a spindle.

Alaei et al. [32] developed an artificial NN model to predict the thermal expansion of the work roll crown. Profile and shape control are used to maintain the dimensional quality of the rolled strip. They used a full three-dimensional model based on the finite difference method under a transient condition. The computation time for this model was more than 15 s. Due to the long calculation time of accurate analysis models, the online application of these models was impossible. Therefore, the results of the model were used for the training of the NN. The NN model is accurate enough, and its computation time is less than 0.1 s, making it possible for an online application.

John et al. [33] proposed a hybrid model with the combination of a predictive artificial NN and a genetic algorithm to minimize flatness defects in strips. The genetic algorithm is used to optimize several parameters that affect the flatness of the strip using NN as the internal loop for calculations. The predictive model has been tested, and the flatness values are minimized for a set of selected strips.

Yang et al. [34] applied a genetic algorithm to optimize the cold rolling schedule. The analysis and comparison of the optimized schedule with the existing schedule were presented. The performance of the optimal rolling schedule is satisfactory.

An analysis of the publication shows that the ROM has become an important tool to improve real-time control of the rolling processes. Despite the rapid development, evolution, and renewal of ROM in recent years, the rolling process remains somewhat away from such general development. ROM is a very effective tool that can and should be used for the rolling process, which can improve the quality of the final product. An analysis of NN applied for modeling of rolling process shows that the feedforward neural network (FNN) with the backpropagation algorithm is mainly used. FNN considers states and processes information in a single forward direction. However, a recurrent neural network (RNN) is more suitable for modeling the process. RNN introduces feedback loops, allowing them to retain a memory of past inputs and process sequential data more effectively. RNN deals with tasks that involve sequences of data, such as time-series prediction. RNN is probably used only in [32], although the type of NN is not declared directly there. Also, the application ROM with the transfer function, which seems very natural for dynamic processes, is very difficult to find in the scientific literature related to the rolling process.

The author participates in the development of the real-time control system that offers real-time design of rolling schedule and aids in controlling that process. The real-time system of rolling schedule design is developed for reverse and continuous mills and contains several modules, including models of roll bending, roll wear, and thermal profile of the roll. These models serve to control the convexity and flatness of the final product. The system of rolling schedule design also contains a flow stress model, a rolling force and torque, a microstructure evolution model, and others.

The objective of this paper is the presentation of the models of the thermal profile of the roll and the way in which the transformation of the full-order FEM model into an efficient reduced-order model is performed.

2. Research Structure

Figure 1 presents a flowchart of research connected with the development, study, identification, testing, verification, and simulation of thermal and thermomechanical models presented in this paper. There are three kinds of models: Finite Element Models (FEM), MetaModel based on Neural Network (MMNN), and Reduced-Order Models (ROM) based on Transfer Functions (TF—TF ROM). Blocks colored in yellow present thermal models, those colored in green present thermomechanical models, and models of thermal profile, roll, and sheet convexity. Thermal models, analytical and semianalytical solutions, FEM, MMNN, and TF ROM are considered in detail in Section 3. The thermal model allows us to obtain the temperature distribution, but does not solve the titled problem of thermal profile. However, thermal models allowed us to compare two proposed approaches, MMNN and TF ROM, and to choose the kind of model more suitable for the thermal profile.

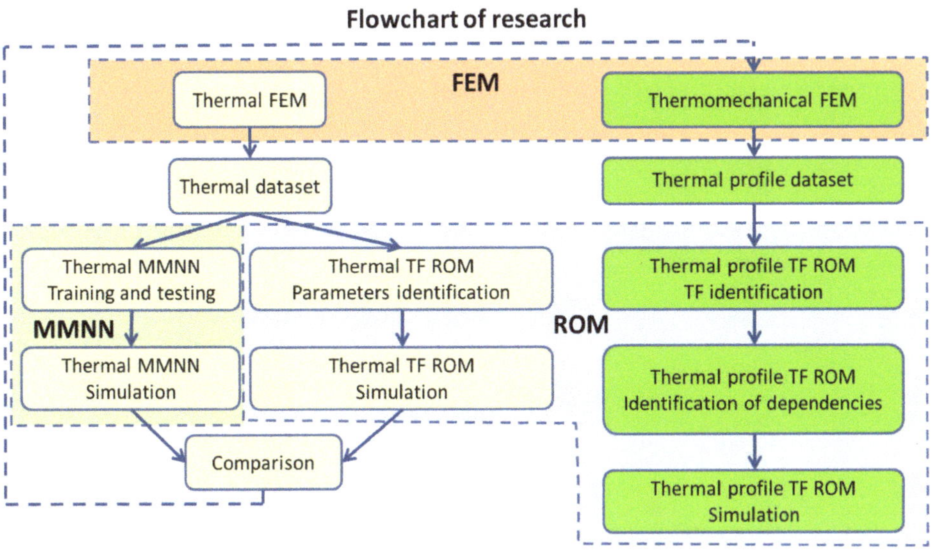

Figure 1. Flowchart of research.

The approach accepted for thermal MMNN is similar to the spatial discrete method used for partial differential equations (for example, finite difference method with an explicit calculation scheme). As can be seen in Section 3.3, every node takes information about the current and previous value of itself and neighboring nodes. TF ROM applies ordinary differential equations of the first, second, or higher order for every node without consideration of neighboring nodes, independently of them.

Section 4 is devoted to the analysis of these two approaches. Firstly, several FEM simulations were performed, and a dataset was created. Then, the dataset was used for training and testing of MMNN and identification of parameters of transfer functions. Finally, MMNN and TF ROM were compared, and TF ROM was chosen for further study thermal profile model. The arguments used are as follows. A network with nodes used MMNN for the considered problem requires at least 20 different NNs, and the choice of them is untrivial. The time of training the whole network with hundreds of nodes is very time-consuming. Thus, the approach was considered inappropriate, a dead-end, and of academic interest only. On the other hand, identification of the transfer function for the node is fast, simple, and independent of the other nodes of the modeled space. That is one of the causes of the choice of TF ROM, instead of MMNN ROM.

Section 5 presents the thermal profile model: FEM and TF ROM. For this problem, a recurrent neural network can likely be studied along with TF ROM. Identification, verification, and simulations of TF ROM and dependences on process conditions, material properties, and roll parameters are presented in Section 6.

3. Thermal Models

Thermal models can be classified as empiric, analytical, semi-analytical, numerical, and ROMs (or metamodels). Empirical models are not considered here due to their low usability.

3.1. Analytical and Semianalytical Solutions

Analytical models or solutions are based on a physical model but are limited to simple geometry, stationary states, and constant conditions. For more complex tasks, they use Green functions. Problems of one-dimensional linear symmetric and axisymmetric problems are described by the following equations:

$$\frac{\lambda}{\rho c_p}\frac{\partial^2 \vartheta}{\partial x^2} = \frac{\partial \vartheta}{\partial t} \tag{1}$$

$$\frac{\lambda}{\rho c_p}\left(\frac{\partial^2 \vartheta}{\partial r^2} + \frac{1}{r}\frac{\partial \vartheta}{\partial r}\right) = \frac{\partial \vartheta}{\partial t} \tag{2}$$

with initial and boundary conditions, for example, for an axisymmetric problem:

$$\vartheta(r) = 0 \tag{3}$$

$$\frac{\partial \vartheta(0,t)}{\partial r} = 0 \forall t \geq 0 \tag{4}$$

$$\frac{\partial \vartheta(R,t)}{\partial r} = -\frac{\alpha}{\lambda}\vartheta(R,t)\ \forall t > 0; \tag{5}$$

where ϑ—excess ambient temperature, x—linear coordinate, r—coordinate along the roll radius, t—time, λ—heat conduction coefficient, ρ—material density, c_p—specific heat capacity, α—heat transfer coefficient, and R—roll radius.

A solution of Equation (1) at time t has the following form:

$$\vartheta(x, t+\Delta t) = \sum_{n=1}^{\infty}\left[\frac{\beta_n \cos(\beta_n x)}{\beta_n + \sin\beta_n \cos\beta_n} exp\left(-\beta_n^2 \frac{4\lambda\Delta t}{\rho c_p h^2}\right)\int_0^1 \vartheta(x,t)\cos\beta_n x dx\right] \tag{6}$$

A coefficient β_n in (6) should be determined from the characteristic equation of a given relationship:

$$cot\beta = \frac{2\beta\lambda}{\alpha h} \tag{7}$$

where h—length of the analyzed domain.

Calculation time and accuracy with a semi-analytical solution depend on several parameters in (6). They are n, i.e., the number of first terms of a series that approximates the temperature, n_n—the number of nodes that affect the precision of calculating the integral in the equation, and Δt—the time step. The rational choice of these parameters makes the semi-analytical solution more efficient than most numerical solutions.

The analytical solution of the axisymmetric problem (2)–(5) can be presented as follows:

$$\vartheta\left(\frac{r}{R}, t\right) = \sum_{n=1}^{\infty} A_n J_0\left(\frac{\mu_n r}{R}\right) exp\left(-\mu_n^2 \mathrm{Fo}\right) \tag{8}$$

where $\mathrm{Fo} = \frac{\lambda t}{\rho c_p R^2}$—Fourier number, μ_n—roots of the characteristic equation:

$$\frac{J_0(\mu)}{J_1(\mu)} = \frac{\mu}{Bi} \quad (9)$$

where J_0 and J_1—Bessel functions of first-type zero- and second-order, $\mathrm{Bi} = \frac{\alpha R}{\lambda}$—Biot number, A_n—factors calculated from the following:

$$A_n = \frac{2Bi}{\left(\mu_n^2 + Bi^2\right) J_0(\mu_n)} \quad (10)$$

Both solutions, in general, can be presented as a sum of exponents, and these properties will be used in the thermal and thermal profile models presented in the latter section:

$$\vartheta(t) = \theta_0 \left[1 - \sum_{n=1}^{\infty} k_n exp\left(-\frac{t}{T_n}\right)\right] \quad (11)$$

where k_n—gain factor, T_n—time constant, and J_0—input temperature.

Analytical and semi-analytical solutions are efficient for simple one-dimensional problems, but the thermal problem for the rolls of rolling mills cannot be reduced to one-dimensional problems.

3.2. Finite Element Model

Heat conduction and then thermal expansion of the rolls can be presented as a two-dimensional axisymmetric problem. Due to symmetry, a quarter of the roll was modeled. A typical solution can be obtained with the use of the finite element method (FEM). Figure 2 presents the coarse mesh of the FEM model with several control points marked with the letters *A*–*J* (the color of the points means nothing).

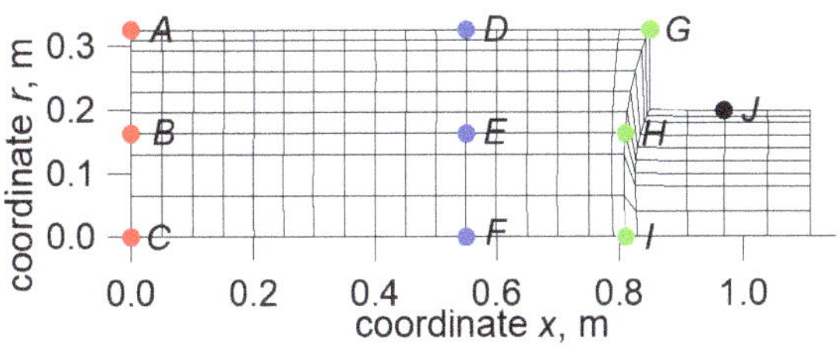

Figure 2. Mesh of the roll of the FE model.

The nonstationary thermal problem leads to a set of equations:

$$\mathbf{Ht} + \mathbf{C}\frac{\partial \boldsymbol{T}}{\partial t} + \mathbf{p} = 0 \quad (12)$$

where **T**—vector of nodal temperatures. The matrices **H** and **C** and the vector **p** are defined as follows:

$$\mathbf{H} = \int_V \left[\lambda_x \frac{\partial \mathbf{N}^T}{\partial x}\frac{\partial \mathbf{N}}{\partial x} + \lambda_r \frac{\partial \mathbf{N}^T}{\partial r}\frac{\partial \mathbf{N}}{\partial r}\right] dV + \int_S \alpha \mathbf{N}^T \mathbf{N} dS \quad (13)$$

$$\mathbf{C} = \int_V \mathbf{N}^T \rho c_p \mathbf{N} dV \quad (14)$$

$$\mathbf{p} = -\int_V Q\mathbf{N}^T dV - \int_S (\alpha T_0 - q)\mathbf{N}\, dS; \quad (15)$$

where **N**—matrix of shape functions. A further solution is based on the assumption of linear changes in nodal temperatures between t_0 and t_1 and the Galerkin integration scheme:

$$\left(2\mathbf{H}+\frac{3}{\Delta \mathrm{t}}\mathbf{C}\right)T_1+\left(2\mathbf{H}-\frac{3}{\Delta \mathrm{t}}\mathbf{C}\right)T_0+3\mathbf{p}=0 \tag{16}$$

Equation (15) is a set of linear equations, which allows the calculation of the vector of the nodal temperatures $\mathbf{T}_1$ after time Δt for the known temperatures $\mathbf{T}_0$. The solution described above is used in the present work for the calculations of the temperature field in the rolls.

3.3. Metamodel with Neural Network

The author proposed to build such a structure of a thermal metamodel, in which a node of the FEM-like mesh is replaced by an artificial neural network (NN). This model can be treated in different ways, for example, as a finite difference method with an explicit calculation scheme and replacement of finite difference equations with a neural network, or as cellular automata with transition rules using a neural network, or as a modified Lattice Boltzmann method with a neural network. It was decided to name this model a metamodel with neural network (MMNN). Figure 3 presents schematically the mesh with node y, for which a neural network was built.

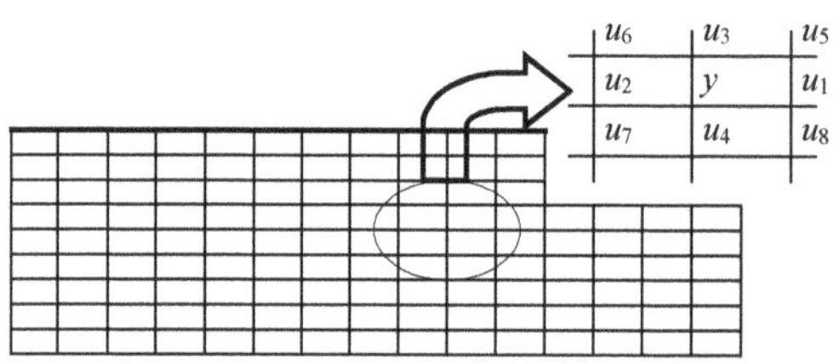

Figure 3. Mesh of the metamodel of the roll with node y and neighboring nodes used in NN.

The basic structure of NN is shown in Figure 4. NN contains memory that can remember and take into account two previous states. This MMNN can be treated as ROM only partially and only in comparison with FEM. Explicit calculations in the proposed structure of MMNN can be easily parallelized, which additionally allows for a huge reduction in calculation time.

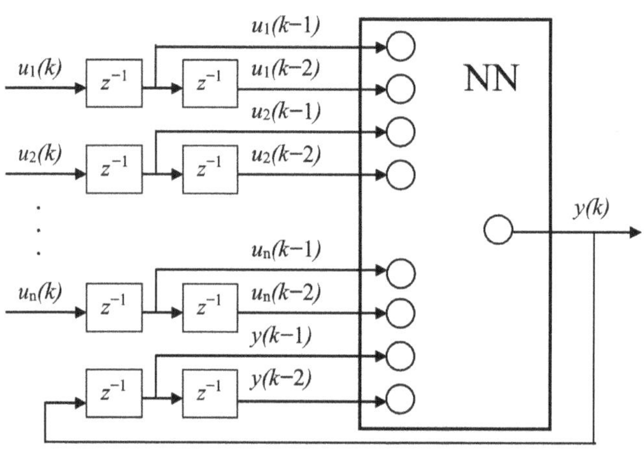

Figure 4. Basic structure of MMNN for a node.

NNs with various configurations were tested, and the optimum configuration was determined. The NN can consist of four layers: input, output, and two hidden layers. Several variants of structures were studied. The number of previous states was determined first. The comparison of networks that account for one and two previous states did not show a visible difference. Further analysis has shown that the maximum number of inputs is 9. For the internal nodes, the inputs are the temperatures of all neighboring nodes and the node itself. Symmetry allows for a reduction in the number of inputs to 6. The relevant heat transfer coefficient, as well as the temperature of the hot plate and the cooling medium (water or air), are the additional inputs for the surface nodes. The number of neurons in the hidden layer was also adjusted as a result of training and testing.

3.4. Thermal ROM Based on the Transfer Functions

The general analytical solution (11) can be transformed into the form of a transfer function $G(s)$ by applying an integral Laplace transform (or Laplace–Carson transform). Then, the solution can be presented as follows:

$$G(s) = \sum_{n=1}^{\infty} \frac{k_n}{T_n s + 1} \approx \sum_{n=1}^{N} \frac{k_n}{T_n s + 1} \tag{17}$$

Since the solution should not theoretically depend on the selected method, it can be said that analytical and numerical methods should give the same results. Thus, it can be stated that the results that cannot be obtained by analytical methods, but which can be obtained by numerical methods (e.g., FEM), can be presented in the same form, i.e., in the form of a transfer function.

The accuracy of solutions (11) and (17) depends on the order of the solution N (the number of components of the sum or terms of the series). The order of solution N, the gain factors k_n, and the time constants T_n can be found from the numerical solution.

4. Results of Thermal Model Simulations

This section contains results of FEM simulations, MMNN training, and verification.

4.1. Results of Thermal FEM Simulation

The results of the FEM simulation are presented in two forms: a temperature distribution at a fixed time and temperature changes at representative points. Figure 5 presents the temperature distribution in the roll after rolling strips of various widths. The rolling process was simulated until the temperature distribution reached a steady state. The results of the simulations of the widths of the rolling strip are presented in Figure 5: 600, 1000, and 1600 mm. The distributions for all three cases are similar in relation to the edge of the strip; some differences occur in the center of the roll for the narrow strip and at the edge of the roll for the wide strip. It can be said that the temperature field around the edge of the strip is independent of the width of the strip. For a strip width greater than 800 mm, the temperature distribution in the center of the roll length remains the same. When the width exceeds 1200 mm, changes appear in the neck of the roll. Parameters such as the heat transfer coefficient α, conductivity λ, and roll diameter D do not affect the shape of the steady state of the temperature distribution.

Changes in representative points A–J (Figure 1) were monitored during the simulation of the process with a step change in the boundary condition on the surface. A step change in surface temperature was 100 °C. The calculated temperature changes for two widths of the strip are shown in Figure 6. The coordinates r and x of the representative points are shown. The differences in the transient processes for various points are clearly seen in Figure 6. The delay in response increases with increasing distance from the surface and outside the edge of the strip. Analysis of the results for various widths shows the similarity of the temperature changes related to the edge of the strip. It can be concluded that not only static characteristics but also dynamic ones, when related to the edge of the strip, show insensitivity to the strip width.

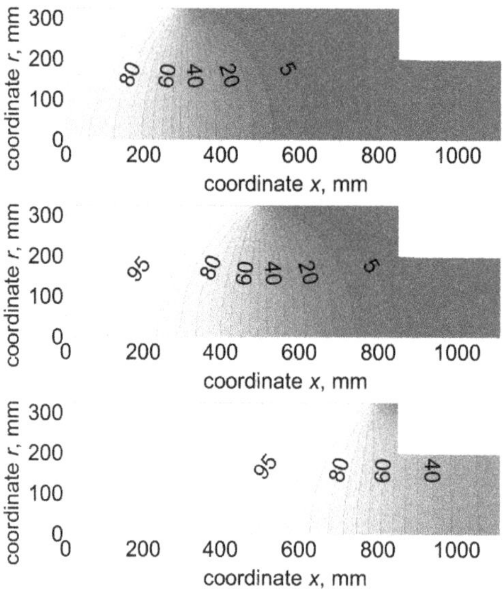

Figure 5. Temperature distribution in the roll after rolling strips with various widths.

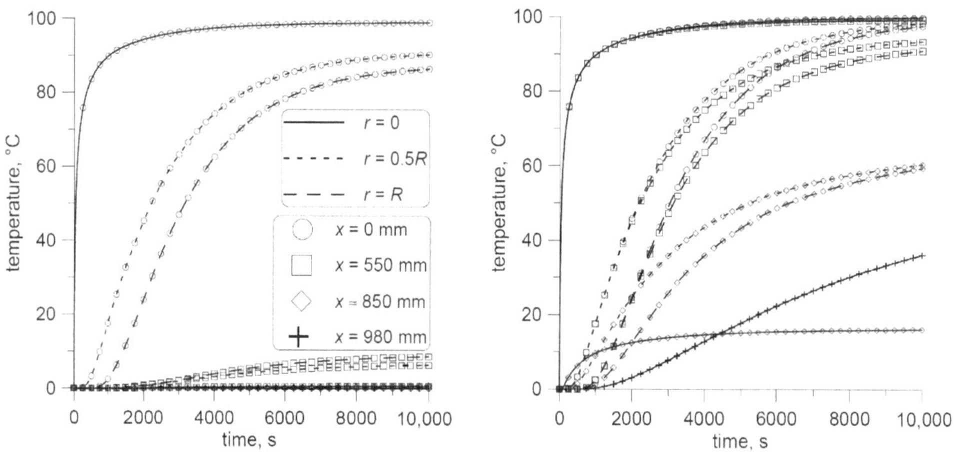

Figure 6. Changes in temperature at representative points for various strip widths: (**a**) 600 mm, (**b**) 1600 mm.

Unlike the static characteristic, the dynamic is sensitive to the heat transfer coefficient α, the conductivity λ, and the roll radius R. An increase in α, λ, or a decrease in R accelerates the temperature changes (these results are not presented in this paper). The influence of various parameters on the dynamic characteristic can be investigated by an analytical solution (8) assuming time constants:

$$T = \frac{t}{\mu_1^2 Fo} = \frac{R^2}{a\mu_1^2} = \frac{R^2 \rho c_p}{\lambda \mu_1^2} \tag{18}$$

where t—time, Fo—Fourier number, μ_1—the first root of the characteristic Equation (9).

Parameters that control the Fourier number (a, λ, R, and l) directly influence the time constants T, while the influence of the parameter α, which controls the Biot number, is much weaker. An increase in Biot number involves a slight increase in roots μ and a decrease in the largest (main) time constant T. Since parameters such as conductivity λ and roll radius R control both Fourier and Biot numbers, their influence on the time constants T is slightly lower than that calculated from the Fourier number only.

4.2. Results of Training and Verification of MMNN

To obtain data for learning, testing, and verifying the network, several FEM calculations were carried out, containing several heating and cooling cycles. In these processes, the temperatures, the width of the strip, the heat transfer coefficient, the conductivity, the roll radius R, and other parameters were varied. Some cycles were selected for teaching, others for testing the network; finally, one of the processes was left for verification. The results of the NN testing and verification for one node are shown in Figure 7.

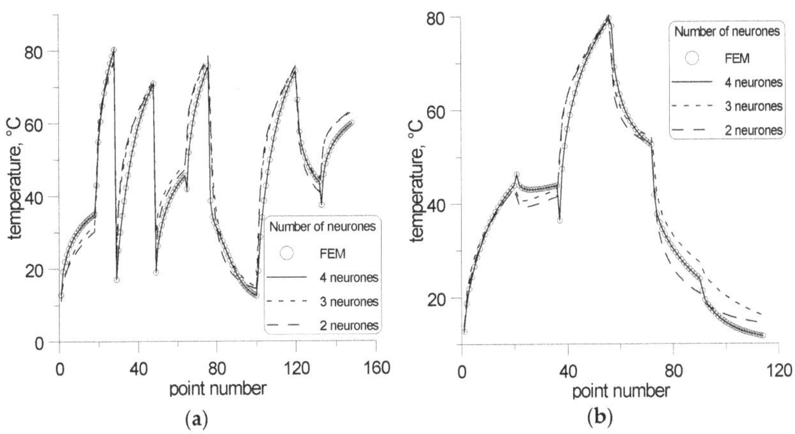

Figure 7. Results of the testing (**a**) and verification (**b**) of the networks.

In Figure 7, it is seen that two neurons in the hidden layer do not give good results. Three hidden neurons give good training results, but testing still remains unsatisfactory. Four hidden neurons give good results for both datasets. However, signs of overtraining were observed for this network. An increase in the number of hidden neurons to 5 leads to larger differences in the accuracy obtained for training, testing, and verification.

The typical results of the training, testing, and verification of NN are shown in Table 1. Simple networks with two or three hidden neurons show similar accuracy in training, testing, and verifying datasets. The difference between these sets appears for the four hidden neurons. At the beginning of training (case 1), the difference in accuracy between the training and testing sets is clearly seen. When the network is properly trained (case 2), the accuracy of both sets increases and is closer to each other. Further training (case 3) leads to an increase in the accuracy of the training set and a decrease in the testing set. This phenomenon is characterized by overtraining of the network. Finally, the structure of the

MMNN for the node contains NN with one hidden layer and four neurons in the hidden layer (Figure 8).

Table 1. The results of training and testing various configurations of recurrent networks.

Dataset	Factor	2 Neurons	3 Neurons	4 Neurons (Case 1)	4 Neurons (Case 2)	4 Neurons (Case 3)
training	RMS error *	0.0229	0.0109	0.0073	0.0051	0.0031
	Good pct **	38.10	57.50	73.80	86.90	95.00
testing	RMS error	0.0215	0.0103	0.0181	0.0077	0.0450
	Good pct	28.40	66.20	35.80	80.40	9.50
verification	RMS error	0.0234	0.0081	0.0102	0.0048	0.0245
	Good pct	37.70	73.70	70.20	90.40	36.00

(* RMS error—root mean square error; ** Good pct—percentage of data points with root mean square error less than 0.01, [%]).

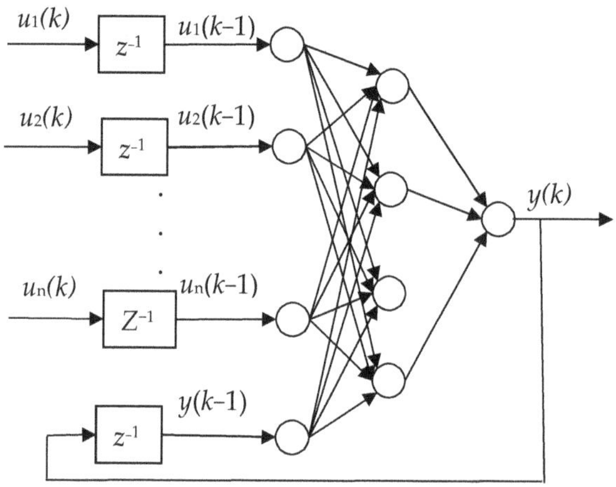

Figure 8. Structure of the MMNN for node with NN with one hidden layer.

MMNN resented in this section was implemented on a GPU that allowed one to obtain a temperature distribution in a much shorter time than the online (real-time) control system requires. Each real-time step (20 s) is calculated in approximately 0.1 s. However, this model was not used in the roll calculations of the thermal profile due to the need to introduce a temperature distribution into the thermal expansion model. A different model described below was used for the thermal model of the thermal profile. So, the model described in this subsection has mainly an academic character and, for its implementation, requires too many FEM calculations and teaching of NNs.

4.3. *Identification and Verification of Thermal ROM*

As shown in Section 3.4, the temperature at an arbitrary point in the roll can be presented in the form (17). The temperature transient function or the response to the unit step function obtained from the FEM simulations is used to identify the ROM parameters (transfer functions), i.e., order N, gain factors k_n, and time constants T_n. MATLAB (version R2022b) Control Identification Tools were used here. Data for learning, testing, and verifying the network previously obtained with FEM simulations were also used for the identification of ROM parameters.

Figure 9 presents the result of the ROM compared to the results of the FEM simulations. Temperature changes are shown for representative points A, B, C, D, and E (see Figure 2). For representative point C (Figure 9), the results are plotted for three transfer functions of the first, second, and third orders, and for the other point, the transfer function of the second order only. The transfer function for point C with root mean square error is as follows:

$$G_{C1} = \frac{1.3254}{6412.6s+1};\ \chi = 7.435\ ^\circ\text{C} \tag{19}$$

$$G_{C2} = \frac{4.034}{1801.7s+1} - \frac{3.059}{1245.6s+1};\ \chi = 1.068\ ^\circ\text{C} \tag{20}$$

$$G_{C3} = \frac{2.188}{2063.3s+1} - \frac{1.851}{691.7s+1} + \frac{0.639}{363.4s+1};\ \chi = 0.208\ ^\circ\text{C}; \tag{21}$$

$$G_{C4} = \frac{2.016}{2149.2s+1} - \frac{2.235}{559.2s+1} + \frac{1.684}{309.5s+1} - \frac{0.485}{198.1s+1};\ \chi = 0.0353\ ^\circ\text{C}. \tag{22}$$

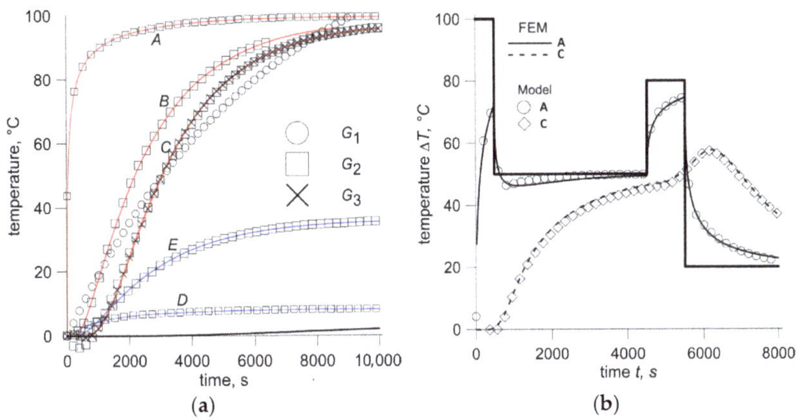

Figure 9. Comparison of the results of the thermal FEM model and the ROM: (**a**) identification, (**b**) verification.

The accuracy of the second-order transfer function of can be considered sufficient for most points (see the results for points A, B, D, and E in Figure 9), although for some points, the third-order transfer function of should be taken. The transfer functions for the other representative points are as follows:

$$G_{A2} = \frac{0.55}{68.8s+1} + \frac{0.45}{1015.8s+1}; \tag{23}$$

$$G_{B2} = \frac{1.45}{1699.3s+1} - \frac{0.45}{458.2s+1}; \tag{24}$$

$$G_{D2} = \frac{0.0465}{1750s+1} + \frac{0.0049}{207s+1} \tag{25}$$

$$G_{E2} = \frac{0.561}{4635s+1} - \frac{0.235}{1898s+1}. \tag{26}$$

The verification of the model consisted of modeling the process in which the thermal boundary condition was changed several times by step and comparing the modeling results of the two models. Temperature changes on the roll surface and the modeling results for representative points A and C are shown in Figure 9b), and show good agreement between the results of the two models.

The time of calculation for one real-time step (20 s) by the ROM presented in this section is below 0.01 s. However, this model (as well as MMNN) was not used in the calculations of the thermal profile of the roll due to the need to introduce a temperature distribution into the thermal expansion model.

5. Models of the Thermal Profile of the Roll

In this section, two models of the roll thermal profile are presented. The first model is the thermal expansion FEM model based on the data obtained from the thermal FEM model, although, in fact, the thermal and thermal expansion FEM models were then joined into one FEM model. The second model is the ROM based on the transfer functions.

5.1. Thermal Expansion FEM Model

The roll profile is calculated by a solution of linear stiffness equations for deformations caused by thermal expansion. The linear stiffness equation is the following:

$$\mathbf{Kd} = \mathbf{f} \tag{27}$$

where **K**—stiffness matrix, **d**—vector of nodal displacements, **f**—vector of forces.

The stiffness matrix **K** and the vector of forces **f** can be calculated as follows:

$$\mathbf{K} = \int_V \boldsymbol{B}^T \boldsymbol{C}\boldsymbol{B} dV \tag{28}$$

$$\mathbf{f} = \int_V \boldsymbol{B}^T \frac{E\alpha\vartheta}{1-2v} 1 dV \tag{29}$$

where **B**—matrix of derivatives of shape functions, **C**—constitutive matrix (Hook's matrix), and **f**—vector of forces. E—Young modulus, ν—Poisson coefficient, and α—thermal expansion coefficient, $\mathbf{1} = \{1,1,10\}^T$.

Then, the thermomechanical FE model contains two modules: the thermal FEM model (12)–(16), which calculates changes in temperature distribution during the process, and thermal expansion FEM (27)–(29), which calculates deformations based on temperature distribution. As a result, changes in displacement (deformation) of an arbitrary point are presented as transient functions, that is, time dependencies of displacement on the step changes in input variables (boundary conditions).

5.2. Thermal Profile ROM with Transfer Functions

The temperature distribution in the roll and the thermal expansion coefficient α are the main factors determining the thermal profile of the roll. Young's modulus E and the Poisson coefficient ν, which significantly influence the value of thermal stresses, do not influence the roll profile. The influence of the thermal expansion coefficient α is linear. The smaller the distance to the point from the surface, the stronger and more localized the influence of its temperature on the roll diameter.

When the temperature distribution is known, the influence of the temperature of each node on the roll diameter and the surface profile can be determined (for example, by a thermal expansion FEM model). Thus, the roll profile can be calculated using an additivity rule. This can simplify the calculations of the roll thermal profile. However, the large number of nodes and the dependence of nodal temperatures on surface temperature and several process and material parameters significantly limit the task of determining nodal temperatures for different conditions.

Therefore, another approach was suggested. The profile of the roll surface can be presented as a combined influence of the temperature at single nodes. The nodal temperatures can be calculated using the transfer functions (17), which are the sum of simple transfer functions. Therefore, the profile of the roll surface can be presented with the use of transfer functions of appropriate order (or the number of simple transfer functions). Then, data for identification of transfer functions can be obtained from the FEM simulations, taking into account that the model of the profile of the roll surface does not require temperature distribution, and two FEM models are joined, and only the results of the following profile are needed for the ROM.

Therefore, the ROM of the thermal profile with transfer functions can be presented by (17) or as follows:

$$G_x = \frac{\Delta r_x}{\vartheta_r(x)} \approx \sum_{n=1}^{N} \frac{k_n(x, R, b, \alpha, a \ldots)}{T_n(x, R, b, \alpha, a \ldots)s + 1} \tag{30}$$

The outputs Δr_x of (30) are the changes in the coordinate r (along the roll radius) of the points on the roll surface, which are defined by the coordinate x (along the roll axis). The input of (30) is the temperature distribution on the roll surface as a function of the coordinate x. The temperature of the surface of the rotated roll is calculated taking into account the heating with hot metal and the cooling with water and air. Gain factors and time constants are dependent on several parameters (coordinate x, roll radius R, width of rolling strip b, thermal diffusivity a, heat transfer coefficient α, etc.) and are independent of temperature. The determination of the order of the transfer function and the identification of the parameters of the dependences of the gain factors and time constants is the essence of the ROM identification.

6. Identification and Verification of Thermal Profile ROM

6.1. Identification of Dynamic Characteristic of the ROM

Identification of the thermal profile ROM was performed on the database created with FEM simulations for different conditions. This ROM was applied to different rolls for reverse and continuous mills with different roll sizes. In this paper, the roll with a diameter D = 650 mm and length l = 1700 mm is analyzed. The parameters of the model are varied in the following bounds:

- Roll diameter D = 615–685;
- Strip width b = 600–1600 mm;
- Thermal conductivity λ = 14–40 W/mK;
- Heat transfer coefficient a = 500–4000 W/m^{2}K.

An example of FEM and ROM simulations is presented in Figure 10. It shows changes in the roll profile Δr for selected points on the roll surface. Coordinate x represents the distance between the point and the middle of the roll length. It is seen in this figure that changes in the roll profile depend on the location of the point.

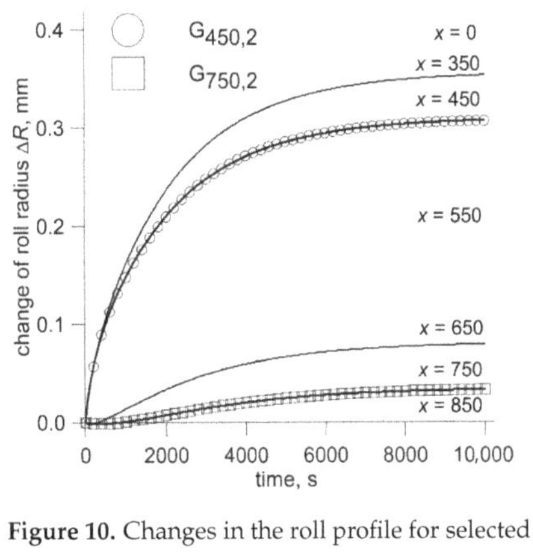

Figure 10. Changes in the roll profile for selected points on the roll surface.

The second-order transfer function was established to be satisfactory for an accurate prediction of changes in the thermal profile of the roll. The same results can be obtained by some modification of (17) or (30) as shown below:

$$G_x = \frac{\Delta r_x}{\vartheta_r(x)} \approx \frac{k_1}{T_1 s+1} + \frac{k_2}{T_2 s+1} = \frac{k}{T_1 s+1} \cdot \frac{Ts+1}{T_2 s+1} \tag{31}$$

Four parameters are necessary to determine the transfer functions in both cases. These include the same time constants T_1 and T_2 in both cases and the coefficient k and the time constant T in the second case, instead of two coefficients k_1 and k_2 in the first case. The coefficient $k(x)$ can be treated as a static characteristics that directly show the shape of the roll surface. The roll profile always tends to the profile determined by the coefficient k. The time constants T_1, T_2, and T are the parameters of the dynamic characteristics that show how long the transient process is.

Some results of the identification of parameter functions $k(x,R,b,\alpha,a\ldots)$, $T_1(x,R,b,\alpha,a\ldots)$, $T_2(x,R,b,\alpha,a\ldots)$, and $T(x,R,b,\alpha,a\ldots)$ are presented in Figures 11–13. The coordinate $x = 0$ refers to the edge of the strip that almost eliminates the effect of a different strip width.

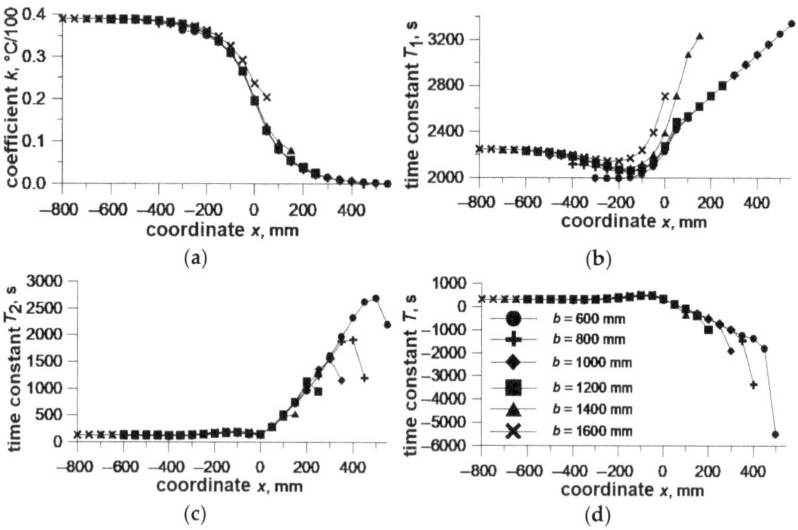

Figure 11. Parameter functions for different strip widths: k (**a**), T_1 (**b**), T_2 (**c**), and T (**d**).

An analysis of the changes in the parameters shows that the coefficient k is the least sensitive to most parameters. Some time constants are strongly dependent on some parameters, and others are almost independent.

6.2. Roll Convexity

The roll diameter, conductivity, and heat transfer coefficients are the parameters that do not change during one roll campaign or only change slightly. The width of the strip is the main variable in the process. In the coordinate system connected to the edge of the strip, the coefficient k is almost constant. Thus, it can be assumed that this coefficient does not change in the middle of the roll and at its edge. The largest changes in this coefficient are observed in the previous and next locations of the edge of the strip. An increase in width involves an increase in high-temperature contact and an additional roll expansion. On the contrary, a decrease in width results in a decrease in high-temperature contact and a decrease in roll expansion. In this case, the roll profile tends to that determined by the coefficient k, but the time constants evaluated from previous relationships cannot be applied. This is related to the fact that the relationships that describe time constants can be divided into two parts. The first part deals with the contact zone and influences the dynamic characteristics in this zone. The second part deals with the area beyond the contact zone and accounts for the mutual influence of one zone on another.

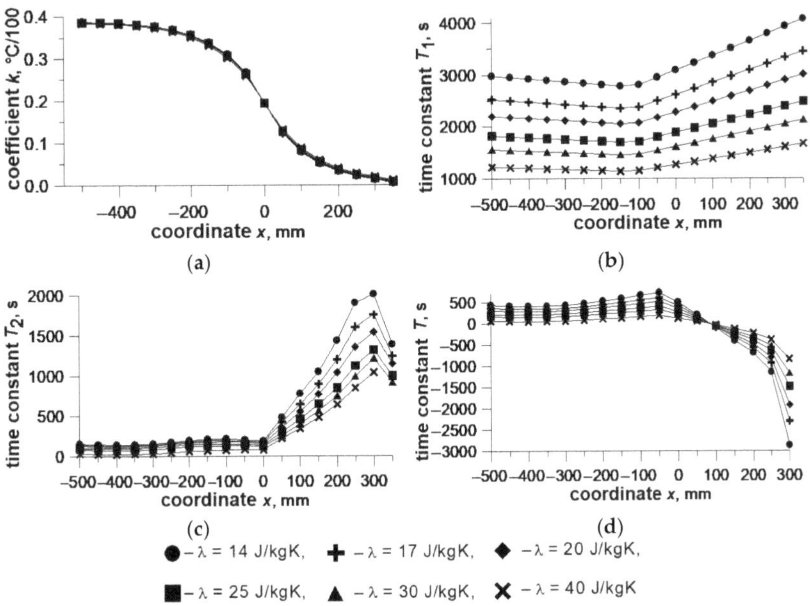

Figure 12. Parameter functions for different thermal conductivities: k (**a**), T_1 (**b**), T_2 (**c**), and T (**d**).

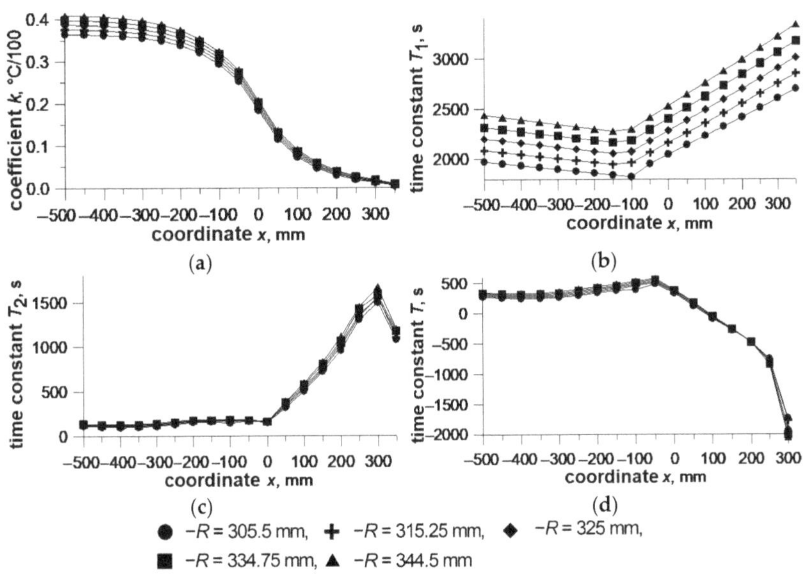

Figure 13. Parameter functions for different roll radii: k (**a**), T_1 (**b**), T_2 (**c**), and T (**d**).

Roll convexity is a variable that is used in the real-time control system at a higher level to calculate the convexity of the rolling strip and in the subsystem controlling the flatness of the strip. Roll convexity is determined by roll diameters at two points: in the middle of the roll and at the edge of the strip. Then, only these two values have to be calculated. The thermal expansion in the middle of the roll and the time constants for this point are almost insensitive to changes in width. The roll expansion at the edge is almost constant. However, a change in the width of the strip leads to a rapid change in the coefficient k for the edge of the strip, while the time constants do not change. This means that the dynamic model of roll convexity has a variable characteristic, which is a dependence of k on the coordinate x. This characteristic is needed for the calculation of the roll profile at the edge of the strip caused by the change in width. Thus, dynamic models should contain two terms with constant input and an artificially changing output signal. The transient process due to the change in the width comprises two segments of the exponential function (time constants T_2 and T are small compared to T_1) with a constant asymptote and small steps in the direction dependent on the direction of the change in the strip width.

The results of the calculations for the whole roll campaign, which was designed for ROM testing, are shown in Figure 14. These results were obtained from the FEM model and ROM with the artificial NN for the parameter functions and with a discretization of the strip width and the average values of temperature and strip thickness. The changes in the roll profile are shown for selected points on the roll surface. Figure 14a shows that FEM and ROM give similar results for the roll profile. When the width of the strip changes, there is a rapid change in the roll profile. The change in strip thickness can also be seen in Figure 14a for a time near 1000 and 2700 s when the width of the strip does not change. The reduction leads to a change in the time of contact, and consequently to a change in the average temperature and the heat transfer coefficient. Also, the roll convexities calculated by the two models are close to each other.

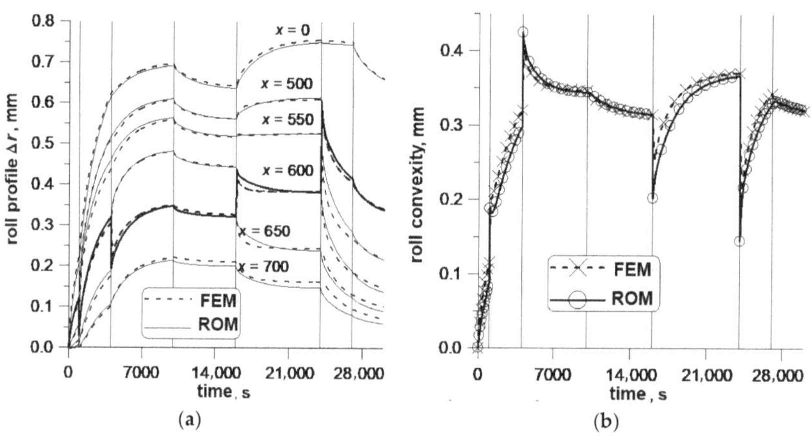

Figure 14. Changes calculated by FEM model and ROM during the campaign: (**a**)—roll profile, (**b**)—roll convexity.

Other results are presented in Figure 14. Here, data from the real roll campaign (over 9 h, 683 strips) were applied for calculations by the FEM model and two variants of ROM, with discretization of the strip width and without such a discretization. The horizontal size of the finite element was 100 mm, and the same discretization level was applied for the first ROM. The strip width was rounded, and it introduces a round-off error. Then, the FEM model and the first variant of ROM have the same round-off error, while the second variant of ROM is free of this error. The discretization (rounding) of the width of the strip produces unjustified jumps in the roll profile, marked by the letter 'a' in Figure 15. This is the case, small changes in the strip width caused a change in the rounded width in the model by the length of the finite element (100 mm). Comparison of the FEM model and discrete ROM shows good agreement in changes in roll convexity, but the results have additional round-off error, whereas the continuous ROM shows somewhat different results, but they are more accurate because they are free of this round-off error.

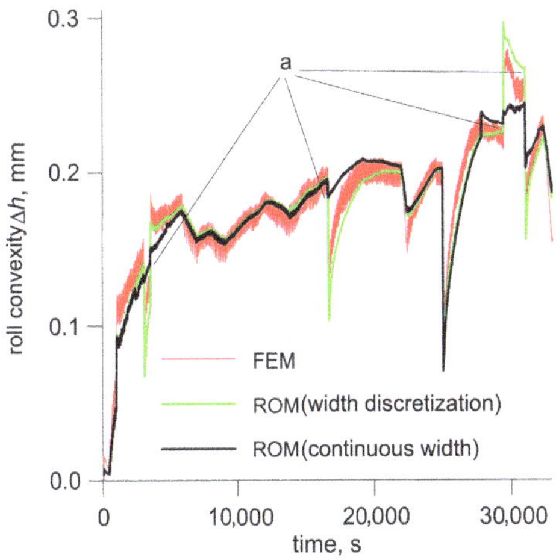

Figure 15. Changes in roll convexity calculated by the FEM model and ROM for the real campaign.

Calculations of the whole campaign by the FEM model last several hours, while those by ROM last several seconds. A real-time step used in the real-time system for updating roll convexity is equal to 20 s; this real-time step is simulated by ROM less than 0.01 s. Calculations of the entire campaign by the ROM last less than 20 s. The ratio of the real process time to the ROM simulation time is approximately 1650.

7. Conclusions

The paper presents developed ROMs based on the transfer functions for calculating temperature distribution, thermal profile of the roll (shape of the roll surface), and roll convexity. Novelty of the proposed ROM is the application of transfer functions for a fast calculation of the shape of the roll surface, the convexity of the roll surface, and the rolling sheet (strip). The ROM of the convexity of the rolling sheet can be applied to the real-time control of the convexity and flatness of the final rolling product. Elements of the ROM were implemented into the control system of two rolling mills. Analysis of the results of the calculations confirms the high efficiency of the proposed ROMs and their feasibility for application in real-time control systems. ROM predicts the thermal profile of the roll with reasonably good accuracy in a very short time. This model, combined with the other models (which calculate roll bending and roll wear), allows predictions of the plate, sheet, and strip profile and flatness during rolling. The results of the calculations presented in the paper confirm the good predictive capabilities of the model. Very short computing times permit an application of this model in real-time control systems. It is planned to connect the FE model with the identification of ROM parameters in one computing block, which will allow the input of the basic parameters of the roll, its material, and possible rolling conditions, and the receipt of the complete ready dependencies of the ROM parameters at the output, which can be feasible for direct application of the ROM.

Funding: This work was supported by the Ministry of Science and Higher Education, Poland, Grant AGH University of Krakow, no. 16.16.110.663.

Institutional Review Board Statement: Not applicable.

Data Availability Statement: The original contributions presented in this study are included in the article material. Further inquiries can be directed to the author.

Acknowledgments: During the preparation of this manuscript, the author used AI Writefull, version v2023.6.0-vsto, for the purposes of the text edition. The author has reviewed and edited the output and takes full responsibility for the content of this publication.

Conflicts of Interest: The author declares that there are no conflicts of interest. The funders had no role in the design of the study; in the collection, analysis, or interpretation of the data; in the writing of the manuscript; or in the decision to publish the results.

References

1. Keiper, W.; Milde, A.; Volkwein, S. *Reduced-Order Modeling (ROM) for Simulation and Optimization: Powerful Algorithms as Key Enablers for Scientific Computing*; Springer: Cham, Switzerland, 2018; ISBN 9783319753188.
2. Li, J.; Wang, X.; Zhao, J.; Yang, Q.; Qie, H. Predicting Mechanical Properties Lower Upper Bound for Cold-Rolling Strip by Machine Learning-Based Artificial Intelligence. *ISA Trans.* **2024**, *147*, 328–336. [CrossRef]
3. Maurya, S.N.; Dezfoli, A.R.A.; Lin, L.S. Data-Driven Approach for Optimizing the Czochralski Process and Predictive Modeling: A Finite Element and Machine Learning Analysis. *Int. J. Adv. Manuf. Technol.* **2025**, *138*, 3077–3087. [CrossRef]
4. Fukami, K.; Hasegawa, K.; Nakamura, T.; Morimoto, M.; Fukagata, K. Model Order Reduction with Neural Networks: Application to Laminar and Turbulent Flows. *SN Comput. Sci.* **2021**, *2*, 467. [CrossRef]
5. Fukagata, K. Reduced Order Modeling of Fluid Flows Using Convolutional Neural Networks. *J. Fluid Sci. Technol.* **2023**, *18*, JFST0002. [CrossRef]
6. Lu, Y.; Li, H.; Saha, S.; Mojumder, S.; Al Amin, A.; Suarez, D.; Liu, Y.; Qian, D.; Liu, W.K. Reduced Order Machine Learning Finite Element Methods: Concept, Implementation, and Future Applications. *CMES—Comput. Model. Eng. Sci.* **2021**, *129*, 1351–1371. [CrossRef]
7. Vu-Quoc, L.; Humer, A. Deep Learning Applied to Computational Mechanics: A Comprehensive Review, State of the Art, and the Classics. *Comput. Model. Eng. Sci.* **2023**, *137*, 1069–1343. [CrossRef]
8. Berkooz, G.; Holmes, P.; Lumley, J.L. The Proper Orthogonal Decomposition in the Analysis of Turbulent Flows. *Annu. Rev. Fluid Mech.* **1993**, *25*, 539–575. [CrossRef]
9. Lu, K.; Jin, Y.; Chen, Y.; Yang, Y.; Hou, L.; Zhang, Z.; Li, Z.; Fu, C. Review for Order Reduction Based on Proper Orthogonal Decomposition and Outlooks of Applications in Mechanical Systems. *Mech. Syst. Signal Process.* **2019**, *123*, 264–297. [CrossRef]
10. Néron, D.; Ladevèze, P. Proper Generalized Decomposition for Multiscale and Multiphysics Problems. *Arch. Comput. Methods Eng.* **2010**, *17*, 351–372. [CrossRef]
11. Chinesta, F.; Ladeveze, P.; Cueto, E. A Short Review on Model Order Reduction Based on Proper Generalized Decomposition. *Arch. Comput. Methods Eng.* **2011**, *18*, 395–404. [CrossRef]
12. Deparis, S. Reduced Basis Error Bound Computation of Parameter-Dependent Navier-Stokes Equations by the Natural Norm Approach. *SIAM J. Numer. Anal.* **2009**, *46*, 2039–2067. [CrossRef]
13. Haasdonk, B.; Ohlberger, M. Reduced Basis Method for Finite Volume Approximations of Parametrized Linear Evolution Equations. *M2AN (Math. Mode.l Numer. Anal.)* **2008**, *42*, 277–302. [CrossRef]
14. Boyaval, S.; Le Bris, C.; Lelièvre, T.; Maday, Y.; Nguyen, N.C.; Patera, A.T. Reduced Basis Techniques for Stochastic Problems. *Arch. Comput. Methods Eng.* **2010**, *17*, 435–454. [CrossRef]
15. Noor, A.K.; Balch, C.D.; Shibut, M.A. Reduction Methods for Non-Linear Steady-State Thermal Analysis. *Int. J. Numer. Methods Eng.* **1984**, *20*, 1323–1348. [CrossRef]
16. Benner, P.; Gugercin, S.; Willcox, K. A Survey of Projection-Based Model Reduction Methods for Parametric Dynamical Systems. *SIAM Rev.* **2015**, *57*, 483–531. [CrossRef]
17. Blazer, S., Jr.; Marchetti, B.; Zhou, X.-D.; Monti, A.; Wendel, C.; Santarelli, M. Electrochemical Models: Methods and Applications for Safer Lithium-Ion Battery Operation. *J. Electrochem. Soc.* **2022**, *169*, 100501. [CrossRef]
18. Amsallem, D.; Zahr, M.J.; Farhat, C. Nonlinear Model Order Reduction Based on Local Reduced-Order Bases. *Int. J. Numer. Methods Eng.* **2012**, *92*, 891–916. [CrossRef]
19. Hendryx Lyons, E.P. The Discrete Empirical Interpolation Method in Class Identification and Data Summarization. *Wiley Interdiscip. Rev. Comput. Stat.* **2024**, *16*, e1653. [CrossRef] [PubMed]

20. Antil, H.; Gupta, M.; Price, R. A Note on Dimensionality Reduction in Deep Neural Networks Using Empirical Interpolation Method. *arXiv* **2023**. [CrossRef]
21. Ahmadi-Asl, S.; Caiafa, C.F.; Cichocki, A.; Phan, A.H.; Tanaka, T.; Oseledets, I.; Wang, J. Cross Tensor Approximation Methods for Compression and Dimensionality Reduction. *IEEE Access* **2021**, *9*, 150809–150838. [CrossRef]
22. Feng, L. Review of Model Order Reduction Methods for Numerical Simulation of Nonlinear Circuits. *Appl. Math. Comput.* **2005**, *167*, 576–591. [CrossRef]
23. Buchmayr, B. Thermomechanical Treatment of Steels—A Real Disruptive Technology Since Decades. *Steel Res. Int.* **2017**, *88*, 1700182. [CrossRef]
24. Hu, Z.; Wei, Z.; Sun, H.; Yang, J.; Wei, L. Optimization of Metal Rolling Control Using Soft Computing Approaches: A Review. *Arch. Comput. Methods Eng.* **2021**, *28*, 405–421. [CrossRef]
25. Zhang, S.H.; Zhang, G.L.; Liu, J.S.; Li, C.S.; Mei, R.B. A Fast Rigid-Plastic Finite Element Method for Online Application in Strip Rolling. *Finite Elem. Anal. Des.* **2010**, *46*, 1146–1154. [CrossRef]
26. Larkiola, J.; Myllykoski, P.; Korhonen, A.S.; Cser, L. The Role of Neural Networks in the Optimisation of Rolling Processes. *J. Mater. Process. Technol.* **1998**, *80–81*, 16–23. [CrossRef]
27. Kwak, W.J.; Lee, J.H.; Hwang, S.M.; Kim, Y.H. A Precision On-Line Model for the Prediction of Roll Force and Roll Power in Hot-Strip Rolling. *Metall. Mater. Trans. A Phys. Metall. Mater. Sci.* **2002**, *33*, 3255–3272. [CrossRef]
28. Lee, D.; Lee, Y. Application of Neural-Network for Improving Accuracy of Roll-Force Model in Hot-Rolling Mill. *Control Eng. Pract.* **2002**, *10*, 473–478. [CrossRef]
29. Son, J.S.; Lee, D.M.; Kim, I.S.; Choi, S.G. A Study on On-Line Learning Neural Network for Prediction for Rolling Force in Hot-Rolling Mill. *J. Mater. Process. Technol.* **2005**, *164–165*, 1612–1617. [CrossRef]
30. Maurya, S.N.; Luo, W.J.; Panigrahi, B.; Negi, P.; Wang, P.T. Input Attribute Optimization for Thermal Deformation of Machine-Tool Spindles Using Artificial Intelligence. *J. Intell. Manuf.* **2024**, *36*, 2387–2408. [CrossRef]
31. Hsieh, M.C.; Maurya, S.N.; Luo, W.J.; Li, K.Y.; Hao, L.; Bhuyar, P. Coolant Volume Prediction for Spindle Cooler with Adaptive Neuro-Fuzzy Inference System Control Method. *Sens. Mater.* **2022**, *34*, 2447–2466. [CrossRef]
32. Alaei, H.; Salimi, M.; Nourani, A. Online Prediction of Work Roll Thermal Expansion in a Hot Rolling Process by a Neural Network. *Int. J. Adv. Manuf. Technol.* **2016**, *85*, 1769–1777. [CrossRef]
33. John, S.; Sikdar, S.; Swamy, P.K.; Das, S.; Maity, B. Hybrid Neural GA Model to Predict and Minimise Flatness Value of Hot Rolled Strips. *J. Mater. Process. Technol.* **2008**, *195*, 314–320. [CrossRef]
34. Yang, J.; Che, H.; Dou, F.; Zhou, T. Genetic Algorithm-Based Optimization Used in Rolling Schedule. *J. Iron Steel Res. Int.* **2008**, *15*, 18–22. [CrossRef]

energies

MDPI

Article

Environmental and Economic Optimisation of Single-Family Buildings Thermomodernisation

Anna Sowiżdżał, Michał Kaczmarczyk *, Leszek Pająk, Barbara Tomaszewska, Wojciech Luboń and Grzegorz Pełka

Faculty of Geology, Geophysics and Environmental Protection, AGH University of Krakow, Mickiewicza 30, 30-059 Kraków, Poland; ansow@agh.edu.pl (A.S.); pajakl@agh.edu.pl (L.P.); bts@agh.edu.pl (B.T.); lubon@agh.edu.pl (W.L.); pelka@agh.edu.pl (G.P.)
* Correspondence: mkz@agh.edu.pl

Abstract

This study offers a detailed environmental, energy, and economic evaluation of thermal modernisation options for an existing single-family home in southern Poland. A total of 24 variants, combining different heat sources (solid fuel, biomass, natural gas, and heat pumps) with various levels of building insulation, were analysed using energy performance certification methods. Results show that, from an energy perspective, the most advantageous scenarios are those utilising brine-to-water or air-to-water heat pumps supported by photovoltaic systems, reaching final energy demands as low as 43.5 kWh/m^{2}year and primary energy demands of 41.1 kWh/m^{2}year. Biomass boilers coupled with solar collectors delivered the highest renewable energy share (up to 99.2%); however, they resulted in less notable reductions in primary energy. Environmentally, all heat pump options removed local particulate emissions, with CO_2 reductions of up to 87.5% compared to the baseline; biomass systems attained 100% CO_2 reduction owing to renewable fuels. Economically, biomass boilers had the lowest unit energy production costs, while PV-assisted heat pumps faced the highest overall costs despite their superior environmental benefits. The findings highlight the trade-offs between ecological advantages, energy efficiency, and investment costs, offering a decision-making framework for the modernisation of sustainable residential heating systems.

Keywords: energy auditing; energy efficiency; renewable energy sources; environmental protection

1. Introduction

To achieve climate neutrality, the need to transform our entire economy to reduce greenhouse gas emissions, in particular in the heat and power generation sector, has been raised [1] This requires the development of integrated energy, water, and environmental systems towards climate neutrality for sustainable development [2], especially in the context of climate mitigation ambitions, which should lead to carbon neutrality [3]. Developing energy generation based on renewable energy sources (RES) is also indispensable. Moreover, apart from increasing the share of renewable energy in electricity and heat production, another important task is to develop regulations favouring the development of local, sustainable energy areas within energy clusters or cooperatives [4]. Broader energy efficiency initiatives remain essential, including promoting the development of energy-efficient buildings and enhancing energy efficiency, with a primary focus on reducing energy consumption through energy renovation.

An energy assessment of buildings makes it possible to determine their energy intensity, which is the starting point for planning an energy transition. Forecasting future energy demand in the context of heating buildings is therefore important. In the broader context, the analysis of energy consumption in buildings provides valuable information on potential economic shocks and environmental impacts [5,6]. From a technological point of view, research in this area has been conducted by, among others, Tettey et al. (2016) [7], Guarino et al. (2016) [8], Jiang et al. (2021) [9], Gibbons and Javed (2022) [10]. The development of technologies for building energy management is a critical aspect in this context, especially for HVAC systems [11–13], and future optimisation will be related to the application of artificial intelligence algorithms [14,15] and building energy management [16].

Replacing heat sources in buildings in areas that take measures to improve energy efficiency is often a fundamental step towards success. However, these investments become much more effective if accompanied by measures to ensure appropriate building thermal insulation standards [17]. To operate efficiently (from both environmental and economic points of view), the heating systems must be installed in buildings with a favourable balance of heat losses and gains. Ensuring adequate thermal insulation of buildings reduces the energy demand for heating or cooling them to the minimum possible values [18]. Depending on the needs, ceilings and walls should be insulated and windows replaced. Many buildings constructed in the 1980s, 1990s, or earlier pose considerable energy renovation problems. Many buildings constructed according to the so-called old standards and technical requirements require significant financial outlays to improve their thermal insulation. It is, therefore, necessary to support energy renovation measures in private buildings to enable heating systems to work efficiently. Initiatives taken by local authorities and the refurbishment of public buildings used by all residents help raise the general public's environmental awareness. Authorities play an important role in disseminating information about energy renovation measures and, above all, in actively and effectively raising funds to subsidise such measures [19]. In addition to active solutions such as efficient heating systems and renewable energy technologies, passive design strategies play a crucial role in reducing building energy demand. Measures including optimised orientation, appropriate glazing, improved airtightness, thermal mass utilisation, and effective natural ventilation can significantly lower the heating and cooling loads. When integrated with active systems, these approaches contribute to achieving low-or nearly zero-energy standards while improving indoor comfort and reducing operational costs [20].

As indicated by Błazy et al. (2021) [21], the demand for primary energy in a building is influenced by its proper thermal modernisation, especially the thermal insulation of external partitions. Similar conclusions were drawn by Lis and Ujma (2016) [22]. In the case of the research by Błazy et al. (2021) [21], the authors focused on the environmental assessment of the effects of thermal modernisation, specifically air quality. The research was carried out for two voivodships, Śląskie and Małopolskie. The authors proposed four scenarios to show the relationship between the emission reduction value and the level of co-financing for thermomodernisation. Finally, they concluded that the higher the level of co-financing, the greater the willingness of stakeholders to undertake thermal modernisation measures; thus, the more significant the effects of improving air quality. This is an obvious conclusion, and it should be considered universal. This article does not consider any level of co-financing resulting from the desire to show actual investment costs. It should be stated directly that in the case of the analysed facility, similar to other facilities of this type that are not insulated, the costs of thermal modernisation are very high, and only a small part of society can afford such an expense.

It is worthwhile to refer to the Energy Performance Certificate (EPC) determination methodology used in this article to calculate a building's useful energy requirements.

Indeed, it is a method that also allows the setting of energy efficiency targets for buildings [23–25] and certainly provides valuable information on energy efficiency and building performance. This is all the more reason to strive to make the results presented in energy performance certificates as accurate as possible and reflect the real impact of the building on the energy system, the environment, and the economic sector, as Kaczmarczyk [6,16] called for in his articles. Conticelli et al. (2024) [26] and Manso-Burgos et al. (2023) [27] presented a method using EPCs to support urban planning. In both cases, the importance of EPCs as analytical tools for diagnosing energy efficiency problems at the city level was highlighted. Also, from the point of view of environmental quality, this is crucial [28].

Dzikuć (2017) [29] conducted research in Zielona-Góra (Lubuskie Voivodeship) to determine what primarily affects air quality. The author emphasises that even though Zielona Góra is located in an area with few industrial plants, the air quality is unsatisfactory. He sees the reasons primarily in local pollutant emissions coming mainly from households heated with solid fuels, followed by transport. Similar studies were then conducted for the entire Lubuskie Voivodeship, drawing similar conclusions (Dzikuć et al., 2021) [30]. This is confirmed by the fact that the processes of energy combustion of fuels, especially coal, are the primary source of anthropogenic emissions of pollutants. Over 75% of NOx and SO_2 emissions, approximately 70% of CO emissions, over 75% of dust emissions, and over 90% of CO_2 emissions originate from the combustion of conventional fuels [31]. The situation in which solid fuels are still the dominant fuel is mainly explained by the lack of an appropriate number of financial instruments aimed at households that would allow for investments in the thermal modernisation of buildings, including the use of renewable energy sources. It is important to note that assessing the environmental impact of buildings throughout their life cycle is crucial in the context of sustainability. This was pointed out by Piccardo and Gustavsson (2021) [32], Alvarez Florez et al. (2023) [33], and Ramon et al. (2023) [34]. The latter highlights the importance of climate change in long-term energy consumption analyses. Their study showed, among other things, that the demand for cooling buildings will increase in the future, which will affect the energy balance and the need to modify energy-management strategies. These conclusions are somewhat identical to those obtained in this article, regarding building heating.

It is natural that not only single-family buildings should be an area of interest in thermal modernisation. For example, research on thermal modernisation of multi-family buildings was conducted in Lithuania by Staniunas et al. (2013) [35], and in Poland, e.g., by Basińska et al. (2015) [36]. The authors presented a comparative analysis of the profitability ratios of investments in thermomodernisation to meet WT2021, i.e., one of the variants also analysed in this article. The authors compared the cost method with the most commonly used economic assessment tools, i.e., SPBT and NPV. They indicated that the method of global costs for the assessment of thermal modernisation is better than SPBT or NPV because, in their opinion, it allows the building assessment process to be carried out from the future assumed time perspective. Considering economic factors, the authors concluded that there is a cost-effectiveness limit, indicating the optimal variant despite the possibility of using greater insulation thickness or better quality materials [36]. Szulgowska-Zgrzywa et al. (2022) [37] drew attention to thermal modernisation in multi-family buildings erected before World War II. The authors considered the effects of thermal modernisation to be energy consumption, pollutant emissions, energy costs, and comfort of use. At the same time, they drew attention to a significant issue, which is the wealth of society. Their conclusions show that the impact of human factors on the energy intensity of buildings is greater than that estimated based on theoretical assumptions at the building design stage. The modernisation activities analysed by the authors indicated that the average reduction in energy costs after modernisation in the original state was 41%, and the decrease in operating expenses was only 2%.

Solutions to improve air quality are sought not only in the context of replacing heat sources. Many studies have been conducted on the implementation of district heating solutions based on renewable energy sources. Such examples include research by Hajto and Kaczmarczyk (2022) [38], who analysed the possibility of improving air quality using geothermal heating systems. Thermal modernisation measures alone are not sufficient to achieve climate neutrality. An interesting proposal that goes beyond the scope of thermal modernisation and falls within the scope of energy management was proposed by Liu et al. (2021) [39]. They developed a short-term model for forecasting building energy consumption 24 h in advance using a neural network and a Multi-Input Multi-Output strategy. First, it is desirable to increase the energy autonomy of the building based on the use of renewable energy sources (e.g., increasing self-consumption from PV installations). Andrews and Jain (2022) [40] also draw attention to the problem of discontinuity of energy generation in zero-emission sources, pointing out that the flexibility of energy demand is necessary to achieve success in a sustainable and reliable energy transformation. The authors claim that the current comparative methods focusing on annual energy consumption fail. They considered the impact of energy consumption time on emissions under rapidly changing power grid operating conditions. The authors based their conclusions on an analysis of the energy consumption of 306 primary and secondary schools in Southern California, USA. From the point of view of the progressive electrification of our lives, including the electrification of heating, it is difficult to disagree with such a statement. Shimoda et al. (2020) [41] argue that to develop a decarbonised society, two opposing requirements must be met: reducing the demand for energy and creating flexibility in the demand for it. This responds to fluctuations in electricity production from renewable sources. Renewable energy sources are significant factors [5].

Climate neutrality is tantamount to phasing out emissions of all greenhouse gases [1]. In the fuel and energy sectors, climate neutrality means zero life cycle greenhouse gas emissions (net life cycle assessment). One of the most important issues in this context is low stack emissions. It is defined as a phenomenon involving the emission of combustion products of solid, liquid, and gaseous fuels into the atmosphere from emission sources located at 40 m or less. These encompass different types of emissions, including traffic emissions, emissions resulting from heat production for central and water heating purposes, and industrial emissions [42]. The combustion products most frequently taken into account in quantitative assessments are carbon dioxide, carbon monoxide, sulphur dioxide, nitrogen oxides, polycyclic aromatic hydrocarbons, e.g., benzo(a)pyrene, and dioxins, as well as heavy metals, PM10, PM2.5, and frequently unidentified pathogens floating on dust particles. Pollution is further aggravated by the still unresolved problem of burning waste in domestic stoves. In Poland, the main sources of low-stack emissions are heat production and water heating (82.3%), 9.6% of the pollution originates from transport, 5.4% from industrial emissions, and other sources of low-stack emissions account for 2.7% [42,43]. In particular, the southern part of Poland is considered one of the most polluted areas in the European Union. This is due to climate conditions, as the heating season in Poland lasts from September to the end of April [44]. Addressing this problem requires various measures, such as replacing non-ecological boilers in homes, improving insulation, enhancing public transport, and limiting older vehicles. Some answers to this issue were a case of air pollution in Kraków and changes observed according to the implementation of a solid fuel ban. Kaczmarczyk and Sowiżdżał (2024) [28] analysed the data, which showed impressive effects on air quality improvements and potential in thermo-modernisation and ecological energy source utilisation in urban areas.

Local initiatives aimed at building energy renovations and installing renewable energy sources are becoming increasingly popular. However, these measures are perceived as capital-intensive. As a result, their implementation requires a thorough assessment of the energy demand of the building and specific individual targets, which can be achieved through energy audits. In this context, interesting research has been presented by Kaczmarczyk (2024) [6]. In assessing building energy performance, both the efficiency of its operation and its environmental impact play a decisive role in determining the overall energy intensity of the residential sector and shaping strategies for energy transition. Reliable planning of such measures requires an accurate determination of a building's energy demand. In this study, a static calculation model was applied to conduct a multi-scenario evaluation of the analysed single-family building, considering various heating system configurations. This approach, based on the methodology for preparing energy performance certificates, was extended to include an assessment of the efficiency of individual energy systems and their associated pollutant emissions. For each of the twenty-four examined scenarios, values of final and primary energy demand, fuel consumption, and emissions were calculated. The findings revealed a lack of direct correlation between the primary energy indicator commonly used in building energy assessments and both the actual energy intensity and environmental burden of the building. Regarding the model building, which represents an individual customer, the issue of "efficient individual heating and cooling" has been considered. According to European Union regulations, this term refers to a separate heating and cooling supply option that, compared to efficient district heating and cooling, measurably reduces the input of non-renewable primary energy required to supply one unit of delivered useful energy within a relevant system boundary or requires the same input of non-renewable primary energy but at a lower environmental cost, taking into account the energy required for extraction, conversion, transport, and distribution. In many cases, the achievement of this goal must be preceded by a so-called "substantial refurbishment", which means a refurbishment whose cost exceeds 50% of the capital cost for a new comparable unit.

Solid fuels, especially coal, are commonly used as energy carriers in Poland, accounting for most of the national energy mix. According to data from the Central Statistical Office [45], in 2021, 42.5% of all households were heated by solid fuel boilers. Burning solid fuels results in the emission of harmful substances into the atmosphere. The amount of these emissions depends primarily on the fuel combustion technology and quality. The increasingly noticeable effects of low-stack emissions, especially in the municipal and household sectors, make replacing outdated conventional stoves a crucial factor in improving the quality of life of residents of Polish municipalities.

Additionally, the thermal energy required for heating buildings accounts for as much as 65.1% of the total energy consumption by households in Poland, broken down by energy carriers and their types of use. This figure highlights the significant share of heating in household energy consumption [45]. Therefore, in newly constructed houses, considerable emphasis is placed on limiting heat loss through penetration and ventilation, which translates into lower heating costs. In buildings that do not meet high energy standards, it is necessary to carry out energy renovations, including external wall, ceiling, and roof insulation, replacing old windows, and upgrading the heating installation. This may involve replacing elements that distribute heat throughout the building (pipes, radiators) and replacing the existing heating source with a new, higher-efficiency, or more environmentally friendly system.

The purpose of this paper is to indicate environmentally friendly and energy-efficient alternatives for heating and hot water preparation in a model single-family building. The proposed methodology can be implemented in other buildings and locations, which adds value to this article. The added value of this article lies in its multivariate analysis of the use of different green energy sources, which contributes to the understanding of the effects of modernisation work. This is particularly important from the point of view of the investor and those responsible for energy planning in the municipality. The presented modernisation variants, the analysis of their ecological impact, and the economic effects possible from an investment point of view provide an auxiliary tool in the decision-making process of reducing the energy demand of buildings, justifying the investment decisions made.

2. Research Methodology

To this end, the thermal performance of the building was determined using an energy audit and thermal imaging. The feasibility of implementing solutions to reduce energy consumption, such as installing thermal insulation, mechanical ventilation with heat recovery, or heating system refurbishment, was analysed, as well as the feasibility of replacing a heat source with an environmentally friendly solution. Environmentally friendly solutions for electricity generation were selected, including the equipment and components required for refurbishment, and an economic analysis of the installation was conducted.

The study was carried out using Audytor OZC 7.0 Pro software developed by SANKOM. It is a tool that enables the generation of building energy performance certificates following the standards and regulations in force in Poland. The guidelines and calculation methodology implemented are based on the following documents:

- ISO 6946 "Building components and building elements–Thermal resistance and thermal transmittance–Calculation methods"–the standard for calculating thermal transmittance coefficients of multilayer walls [46].
- ISO 13370 "Thermal performance of buildings–Heat transfer via the ground–Calculation methods"–the standard for calculating thermal transmittance of building elements in contact with the ground [47].
- ISO 10077-1 "Thermal performance of windows, doors and shutters–Calculation of thermal transmittance" [48].
- ISO 12831 "Heating systems in buildings. Method for calculation of the design heat load"–the standard for calculating the heat load of a building [49].
- ISO 13788 "Hygrothermal performance of building components and building elements. Internal surface temperature to avoid critical surface humidity and interstitial condensation. Calculation methods"–the standard for analysing the humidity of building elements [50].
- Journal of Laws [Dz. U.] of 2015 item 376: Regulation of the Minister of Infrastructure and Development of 27 February 2015 on the methodology for determining the energy performance of a building or part of a building and certificates [51].
- Journal of Laws [Dz. U.] of 2023 item 697: Regulation of the Minister of Development and Technology of 13 April 2023 changing Regulation of the Minister of Infrastructure and Development of 27 February 2015 on the methodology for determining the energy performance of a building or part of a building and energy performance certificates [52].

The methodology used to calculate primary energy in this study involved assessing the annual demand for non-renewable primary energy for the technical systems of the building and dividing it by the area of the heated or cooled space. The yearly energy demand was divided into specific components, including the demand for heating, domestic hot water, cooling, and built-in lighting. Each element was calculated based on the annual demand for final energy for the respective systems, which was then adjusted using specific coefficients to account for the non-renewable energy input required for energy production and delivery. The auxiliary energy required to operate the technical systems was also considered.

Final energy was determined by calculating the total annual final energy demand for the systems and dividing it by the heated or cooled area. The total energy demand for buildings with simple technical systems included all technical systems, and the final energy was adjusted accordingly. Lastly, usable energy was calculated by assessing the actual energy required to maintain the desired indoor conditions and normalised by the building's heated or cooled area. This step-by-step approach allowed for a comprehensive assessment of the energy performance of the building, accounting for both the energy used and the efficiency of energy conversion processes. The methodology used is utilitarian and generally available in the aforementioned standards and regulations; therefore, it is replicable in other cases.

The analysed building is located in southern Poland in climate zone 3 (according to ISO 12831 [49]). The design external temperature during the heating season is −20 °C, and the average annual external temperature is 7.6 °C. The meteorological station closest to the building analysed is located in Nowy Sącz. The model is a four-story single-family house (Figure 1). The total area is 265.4 m^2, the area of rooms with controlled air temperature is 191.98 m^{2,} and the usable area is 188.26 m^2. The total volume of the building is 529.8 m^{3,} and the volume of rooms with controlled air temperature is 453.3 m^3. The building has a south-facing gabled roof with a pitch of approximately 30°. The internal temperatures in the building were determined based on the guidelines contained in the Journal of Laws [Journal of Laws U.] of 2015 item 376 [51], which determines the heat demand of rooms depending on their function and purpose, and ultimately determines the heat demand of the entire building, concerning the design outside temperature. Based on these guidelines, the amount of energy required to heat domestic water was calculated. These issues are independent of the individual preferences of building users, which is consistent with the regulations and calculation methods used in this article.

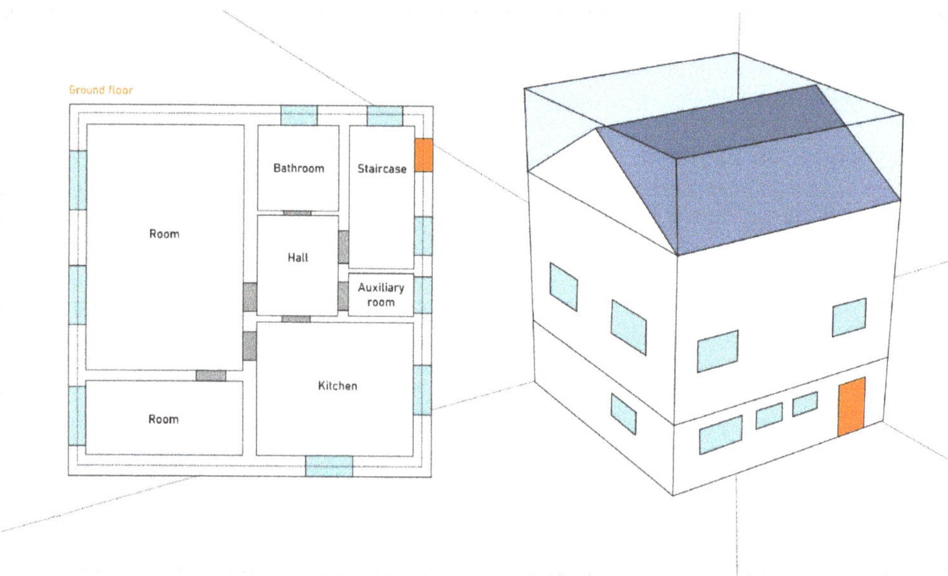

Figure 1. 3D view of the model building analysed and plan of one of the floors.

The building was constructed in the 1970s, and as it stands, it is under-insulated, with a useful energy demand of 207.7 kWh/m^{2}year. The design heat loss by penetration is 15,245.6 W, the design heat loss by ventilation is 2619.8 W, and the design heat load of the building is 17,865.4 W. Thermal needs, both concerning central heating and domestic hot water preparation, are met using a solid-fuel boiler, with the fuel consisting of 50% biomass and 50% of hard coal. However, these percentages are related to central heating. In the case of domestic hot water preparation, the needs of building users are met using biomass. With the energy needs met in this manner, the final energy demand for this building is 389.3 kWh/m^{2}year, and the primary energy demand is 214 kWh/m^{2}year. It should be emphasised that final energy takes into account the demand for useful energy and the efficiency of the building's energy systems. At the same time, primary energy also takes into account the so-called non-renewable primary energy input factor. In the analysed case, this is partially biomass, for which the input factor is 0.2; hence, the value of primary energy is lower than the final energy. The share of renewable energy sources is 62.8% due to the use of biomass. The exact methodology for calculating the data presented above is described in Section 2.2. An extract from the energy performance certificate relating to the useful, final, and primary energy values is shown in Table 1.

Table 1. Extract from the energy performance certificate.

Energy Performance Indicator	Rated Building	Requirements for a New Building Pursuant to Technical and Construction Regulations
Annual useful energy demand	EU = 207.7 kWh/m^{2}year	
Annual final energy demand	EK = 389.3 kWh/m^{2}year	
Annual primary energy demand	EP = 214.8 kWh/m^{2}year	EP = 70.0 kWh/m^{2}year
Unit CO_2 emissions	E_{CO2} = 0.051 t CO_2/m^{2}year	
Share of renewable energy sources in annual final energy demand	U_{RES} = 62.8%	

2.1. Energy Analysis

For the model building analysis, 24 options for energy source switching and energy renovation works were assessed, and energy performance certificates were generated for each option. The basis for determining the number of variants was the desire to compare all available ecological forms of heat production for central heating and hot water needs. To enable the performance of these works, an on-site inspection was carried out before their commencement, which consisted of reading design documentation, verifying whether the building permit design corresponds to the actual state of affairs, and discussing with building owners to obtain any missing information. Options P0–P7 relate to the current state of affairs regarding the building's useful energy demand, with P0 being the baseline option. P1–P7 are options in which the building structure is not altered, but the heat source is replaced to analyse how such a measure would change the final and primary energy values. Analogously, analysis was conducted concerning options T0–T7 and M0–M7, but for the options marked with the "T" symbol, energy renovation of the building was carried out to meet the technical conditions in force at the time of the study, i.e., WT2017 (Journal of Laws [Dz. U.] of 2017 item 2285) [53]. In the case of the options marked with the "M" symbol, the building was optimised to meet the technical conditions that will apply from 2021 onwards (WT2021) (Journal of Laws [Dz. U.] of 2017 item 2285) [53]. It is essential to understand the differences between the technical conditions mentioned. They set requirements for newly constructed buildings and buildings undergoing thermal modernisation using public financial resources (subsidies) regarding the maximum value of primary energy. For single-family buildings, this value, according to WT2017, was 95 kWh/m^2 year, and according to WT2021, it is 70 kWh/m^{2}year. Additionally, the maximum allowable heat-transfer coefficients for building partitions have changed. A summary of all options is presented in Table 2.

Table 2. Summary of energy source switching and energy renovation options analysed.

Variants			Type of Installation
P0	T0	M0	Solid fuel boiler (50% coal, 50% biomass)
P1	T1	M1	Biomass boiler
P2	T2	M2	Biomass boiler + solar collectors
P3	T3	M3	Gas boiler
P4	T4	M4	Gas boiler + solar collectors
P5	T5	M5	Heat pump brine/water (COP = 3.3)
P6	T6	M6	Heat pump brine/water (COP = 3.3) + PV
P7	T7	M7	Heat pump air/water (COP 2.6) + PV

Option designations are as follows: P0—baseline option. P1–P7—options in which the building structure is not altered in any way, but the heat source is replaced to analyse how such a measure would change the final and primary energy values. T0–T7—heat sources as for the "P" options, but the building is subject to energy renovation to meet the technical conditions in force at the time of the study, i.e., WT2017. M0–M7—optimisation to meet the technical conditions that will apply from 2021 onwards (WT2021).

It should be noted that for options involving a 50% biomass and 50% hard coal mix, it is assumed that 100% of domestic hot water is generated using biomass. These values were adopted based on discussions with the facility owners during the site inspection. Additionally, it has been assumed that solar collector installations accounted for 40% of domestic hot water preparation, which is a typical value for Polish weather conditions. Of note is also the fact that the building is equipped with high-temperature radiator heating (80/60 °C); therefore, in the energy renovation options adopted, it was assumed that the operating parameters of heat pump-based systems would be as follows: a flow temperature of 55 °C and a return temperature of 45 °C. This is because no conversion of the central heating system from radiator to underfloor heating is assumed, and, of course, also because the heat demand of the building and its rooms will be reduced, allowing the existing system to be used with a lower flow temperature.

In the simulations, the coefficient of performance (COP) of the heat pumps was assumed to be a constant value based on typical operating conditions. Specifically, a COP of 3.3 was used for brine-to-water heat pumps, and 2.6 for air-to-water heat pumps. These values correspond to the operational characteristics of the heat pumps under the conditions described in this study. The fixed COP assumption reflects standard operation with flow temperatures suitable for high-temperature radiators (80/60 °C reduced to 55/45 °C after renovation). Although COP typically varies seasonally with outdoor temperatures, this study uses static values to maintain consistency and allow comparison across all scenarios. These values ensure compatibility with the building's heating system and facilitate direct comparisons between variants, simplifying modelling and aligning with expected performance for the specific climate zone and building features. Future research could include dynamic COP variations affected by seasonal temperature changes to provide more detailed and accurate insights.

In all cases, the share of RES should be understood as the percentage of RES in the total energy utilisation of the building for heating purposes. To meet the technical conditions stipulated in WT2017, it was necessary to carry out an energy renovation of walls and floors that did not meet the required U_{max} thermal transmittance coefficient value. To this end, the ground floor was insulated with 10 cm-thick expanded polystyrene foam, the external walls were insulated with 15 cm-thick expanded polystyrene foam, the ceiling under the unheated attic was insulated with 22 cm-thick mineral wool, the roof was insulated with 30 cm-thick mineral wool, and the external doors and windows were replaced. A summary of energy renovation works, including thermal transmittance coefficients before and after energy renovation, is shown in Table 3.

Table 3. Summary of energy renovation works for options T0–T7 (WT2017).

No.	Type of Thermomodernisation	U_o (Before Thermomodernisation) [W/(m^2 K)]	U_o (After Thermomodernisation) [W/(m^2 K)]	U_{max} [W/(m^2 K)]
1	Thermal insulation of the floor on the ground with 10 cm of polystyrene	0.554	0.236	0.30
2	Thermal insulation of external walls with 15 cm polystyrene	0.932	0.227	0.23
3	Thermal insulation of the ceiling under the unheated attic with 22 cm mineral wool	0.729	0.179	0.18
4	Roof thermal insulation with 30 cm mineral wool	4.946	0.176	0.18
5	Replacement of external doors	2.500	1.500	1.50
6	Windows replacement	1.500	1.100	1.10

Similarly, to achieve the WT2021 standard, energy renovation work involving the same measures was carried out. However, it was necessary to increase the thickness of the thermal insulation and use windows and doors with correspondingly lower thermal transmittance coefficients. Table 4 summarises the work carried out.

Table 4. Summary of energy renovation works for options M0–M7 (WT2021).

No.	Type of Thermomodernisation	U_o (Before Thermomodernisation) [W/(m^2 K)]	U_o (After Thermomodernisation) [W/(m^2 K)]	U_{max} [W/(m^2 K)]
1	Thermal insulation of the floor on the ground with 10 cm polystyrene	0.554	0.236	0.30
2	Thermal insulation of external walls with 18 cm polystyrene	0.932	0.197	0.20
3	Thermal insulation of the ceiling under the unheated attic with 30 cm mineral wool	0.729	0.140	0.15
4	Roof thermal insulation with 35 cm mineral wool	4.946	0.150	0.15
5	Replacement of external doors	2.500	1.100	1.10
6	Windows replacement	1.500	0.900	0.90

2.2. *Economic Analysis*

Several factors were taken into account to determine the economic effects. Reference was made to the costs of thermomodernisation works (investment costs) and operating costs. In the case of expenses incurred for the thermal modernisation of the building, the costs based on the average values of materials and work are listed in Tables 5 and 6. As can be seen, the difference in the costs of modernisation work between the technical conditions of 2017 and 2021 is 7405.13 Euro. This results from using different insulating materials to meet the required heat transfer coefficients for individual partitions.

Table 5. Costs of energy renovation works for options T0–T7 (WT2017).

No.	Type of Thermomodernisation Single Action	Area [m^2]	Cost [EUR/m^2]	Total Costs [EUR]
1	Thermal insulation of the floor on the ground with 10 cm of polystyrene	67.93	43.00	2920.99
2	Thermal insulation of external walls with 15 cm polystyrene	96.85	57.00	5520.45
3	Thermal insulation of the ceiling under the unheated attic with 22 cm mineral wool	77.95	57.00	4443.15
4	Roof thermal insulation with 30 cm mineral wool	278.12	47.50	13,210.70
5	Replacement of external doors	1.90	276.00	524.40
6	Windows replacement	34.95	193.50	6762.83
7	TOTAL	–	–	33,382.85

Table 6. Costs of energy renovation works for options M0–M7 (WT2021).

No.	Type of Thermomodernisation Single Action	Area [m^2]	Cost [EUR/m^2]	Total Costs [EUR]
1	Thermal insulation of the floor on the ground with 10 cm of polystyrene	67.93	43.00	9290.99
2	Thermal insulation of external walls with 18 cm polystyrene	96.85	58.50	5665.73
3	Thermal insulation of the ceiling under the unheated attic with 30 cm mineral wool	77.95	59.50	4638.03
4	Roof thermal insulation with 35 cm mineral wool	278.12	50.00	13,906.00
5	Replacement of external doors	1.90	276.00	524.40
6	Windows replacement	34.95	193.50	6762.83
7	TOTAL	–		40,787.98

An economic analysis was carried out based on the energy demand determined for some of the options. In defining the fuels analysed, the following assumptions were made (concerning their Q_w calorific values and net purchase prices of energy carriers), and on this basis, the consumption of the energy carrier in question was subsequently determined in measurement units given below in Table 7.

Table 7. Assumptions of selected fuel parameters taken into account in the economic analysis.

No.	Type of Fuel	Calorific Value Q_w	Net Price [EUR]
1	firewood, birch, moisture content 0%	15.6 MJ/kg [m^3/(m^{2}year)]	96.67 per m^3
2	hard coal	26 MJ/kg [Mg/(m^{2}year)]	333.33 per Mg
3	wood chips with moisture content 20–60%, density 150–400 kg/m^3 (275 kg/m^3 assumed) [kg/(m^{2}year)]	6–16 MJ/kg (11 MJ/kg assumed)	48.33 per Mg
4	electricity	[kWh/(m^{2}year)]	0.23 per kWh
5	solar energy	[kWh/(m^{2}year)]	–
6	natural gas	48 TJ/Gg (~34.23 MJ/m^3) [m^3/(m^{2}year)]	0.86 per m^3

To determine the fixed costs of using the energy source, an estimate of the required capital expenditure is necessary. Based on experience and market research, the net capital expenditure rates for the technologies analysed were adopted as follows: biomass-fired boilers–EUR 217.39 per kW, solid-fuel boilers–EUR 173.91 per kW, solar collectors–EUR 1021.74 per kW, natural gas-fired boilers–EUR 147.83 per kW, brine-to-water heat pumps (including the installation of the lower heat source)–EUR 1086.96 per kW, photovoltaic cells–EUR 1086.96 per kW, and air-source heat pumps (including the installation of the lower heat source)–EUR 804.35 per kW. The depreciation period for the above installations, which is necessary to estimate fixed costs, was assumed to be 15 years. The capital expenditure figures stated here do not consider the costs associated with upgrading the boiler room, but only represent the cost of the heating source. It was assumed that the costs of upgrading the boiler room would be similar for all types of heating sources. It should be noted that the present cost analysis does not account for differences in the service life of individual components. This discrepancy can have a significant impact on the results of a life cycle cost assessment, particularly when comparing investment options with markedly different replacement intervals. Since the scope of this study did not include a payback period analysis or complete life cycle economic modelling, the calculations presented are based solely on uniform depreciation periods for all technologies. Future research should incorporate technology-specific lifespans to provide a more precise economic comparison over the entire operational horizon of the analysed systems.

2.3. *Environmental Analysis*

The environmental analysis aimed to determine the pollutant emissions of the model building from the combustion of solid fuels in the baseline option and to compare these emissions with those of the other energy renovation options. The analysis and calculations were carried out using data from the building's energy audit, annual useful energy demand, and emission factors for fuels calculated by the National Centre for Emissions Management–KOBiZE [54]. The indicators were based on values applicable during the project's implementation period. Although it is recognised that the carbon intensity of Poland's electricity mix has decreased in recent years due to the rising share of renewable energy sources, dynamic modelling of this trend was beyond the scope of the current analysis. Future research could include time-dependent emission factors to account for the expected decarbonisation pathways of the national grid. The reduction in the emissions of individual substances compared to the baseline was also determined. The following pollutants were taken into account: total particulate matter (also broken down into PM10 and PM2.5), carbon dioxide (CO_2), carbon monoxide (CO), nitrogen oxides (NO_x), sulphur dioxide (SO_2), and benzo(a)pyrene (BaP).

The amount of existing emissions and the degree of the expected environmental effect depend on several factors. The most important factors among these are the types of energy carriers used for central heating and hot water preparation, the amount of fuel consumed, and its physical and chemical parameters.

To calculate the pollutant emissions for heat production from fuel combustion, pollutant emission factors from fuel combustion for sources with a nominal heat capacity of up to 5 MW [54] were applied. For pollutant emissions from electricity generation, factors for electricity [55] were applied, as shown in Table 8. The emission factor value depends on the fuel type and technological solutions used in the heating source. For the P0 baseline option, emission factors for traditional coal-fired and wood-fired boilers were used. For options P1, P2, M1, M2, T1, and T2, emission factors for a manually loaded wood-fired boiler that met the Ecodesign Framework Directive 2009/125/EC requirements were used. For options P3, P4, M3, M4, T3, and T4, emission factors for natural gas were used, and for options involving heat pumps (P5–P7, M5–M7, and T5–T7), emission factors for electricity for the end customer (mixed electricity production) were used according to KOBiZE (2020) [55]. The energy provided by solar thermal and photovoltaic installations has emission factors of zero for all pollutants analysed. For energy renovation options involving a photovoltaic (PV)-powered heat pump, it was assumed that 70% of the annual electricity is supplied by the PV installation and 30% comes from the electricity grid. This is due to the limitations in the possibility of installing PV systems on roofs with greater electrical power. Before performing the calculations, the authors conducted a site visit and audit. Based on this, the technical condition of the building, including the roof, its orientation, pitch, and shading, was assessed. Therefore, a value of 70% was adopted. No local low-stack emissions are present for energy renovation options involving heat pumps (P5–P7, T5–T7, and M5–M7). Therefore, when these options are selected, the problem of low-stack emissions at the site is completely eliminated.

Table 8. Emission factors W for the energy carriers and combustion technologies used in the baseline and energy renovation options [54,55].

No.	Pollutant	Emission Factor *W*				
		Coal–Traditional Boiler with Manual Loading (g/GJ)	Wood–Traditional Boiler with Manual Loading (g/GJ)	Wood–Boiler with Manual Loading–Eco-Design (g/GJ)	Fuel Gas (g/GJ)	Electricity (kg/MWh)
1	TSP	350	350	40	0.5	0.029
2	PM10	312	333	38	0.5	No data
3	PM2,5	242	315	36	0.5	No data
4	CO_2	96,370	0	0	57650	719
5	CO	2500	3000	440	30	0.233
6	NO_x	160	80	120	50	0.576
7	SO_2	410	15	11	0.4	0.511
8	BaP	0.35	0.13	0.015	0.0000008	No data

To calculate individual emissions based on the emission factors per unit of fuel consumed, the following formula was used:

$$E = \frac{Q \times W}{1000} [\text{g/GJ; Kg/MWh}]$$

where:

Q—seasonal energy consumption [GJ/year, MWh/year]
E—seasonal substance emissions [kg/year]
W—emission factor [g/GJ, kg/MWh]

3. Results

Calculation results for the different options are presented in Tables 9–11 and Figures 2–4. The analysis of final energy consumption, which is the most important figure from the building owner's point of view, indicates that the most efficient solutions are those based on the use of heat pumps. This applies to all three cases (P5–P7), for which the final energy value ranges from 92.1 to 114.1 kWh/m^{2}year. The difference in the final energy value between the P5 variant and the P6 and P7 variants results from the change in the lower source for the heat pump from ground exchangers to air. Consequently, this causes a decrease in efficiency and an increase in the final energy value for the variant with an air/water heat pump. In the case of primary energy, the options involving heat pumps combined with photovoltaic installations (P6 and P7) exhibit the most favourable values, ranging from 61 to 75 kWh/m^{2}year. The difference in these values is a derivative of the efficiencies of the brine/water and air/water heat pumps and the electricity consumption by the heat pump compressor. However, it should be noted that these are not the options with the highest share of renewables. The highest share of renewables is achieved for the options based on a biomass-fired boiler plus solar collectors, with RES shares of 99–99.2%. For hybrid systems with heat pumps and PV, this value is 94.9–95.5%, which is slightly lower.

For options T0–T7, useful energy demand was 93.9 kWh/m^{2}year, with heating and ventilation accounting for 69.8 kWh/m^{2}year and hot water preparation accounting for 24.1 kWh/m^{2}year. Therefore, both the final and primary energy demands have been more than halved. There is also a slight decrease in the total share of RES, which is 98.1–98.5% for the most favourable options (T1 and T2). The slight reduction in the share of renewable energy sources between the P and T variants is because the demand for heat is reduced. At the same time, there is no change in the electrical energy necessary for the operation of auxiliary devices, such as central heating circulation pumps, and the domestic hot water circulation pump.

Table 9. Analysis results for heat source switching (building left as is) (options P0–P7).

Variant	Final Energy [kWh/m^{2}year]			Primary Energy [kWh/m^{2}year]			RES Share [%]
	Total	Heating and Ventilation	Domestic Hot Water	Total	Heating and Ventilation	Domestic Hot Water	
P0	389.3	321.8	67.6	214.8	197.4	17.4	62.8
P1	422.3	354.7	67.6	94.1	76.8	17.4	99.2
P2	403.8	354.7	49.1	90.7	76.8	13.9	99.0
P3	298.6	249.6	49.0	341.6	285.0	56.5	0.0
P4	286.5	249.6	36.9	320.6	285.0	35.6	2.4
P5	92.1	77.0	15.1	276.3	231.1	45.2	65.7
P6	92.1	77.0	15.1	75.2	61.0	14.1	94.9
P7	114.1	97.0	17.1	90.6	75.0	15.6	95.9

Table 10. Analysis results for heat source switching (options T0–T7).

Variant	Final Energy [kWh/m^{2}year]			Primary Energy [kWh/m^{2}year]			RES Share [%]
	Total	Heating and Ventilation	Domestic Hot Water	Total	Heating and Ventilation	Domestic Hot Water	
T0	181.9	114.3	67.6	93.1	75.7	17.4	68.8
T1	203.2	135.6	67.6	49.0	31.6	17.4	98.5
T2	184.7	135.6	49.1	45.5	31.6	13.9	98.1
T3	138.5	89.5	49.0	158.0	101.5	56.5	0.0
T4	127.4	89.5	38.0	138.9	101.5	37.4	5.8
T5	44.0	28.9	15.2	132.0	86.6	45.5	62.2
T6	44.0	28.9	15.2	40.4	26.0	14.4	90.5
T7	53.2	36.0	17.2	46.8	30.9	15.9	92.2

Table 11. Analysis results for heat source switching (options M0–M7).

Variant	Final Energy [kWh/m^2 year]			Primary Energy [kWh/m^2 year]			RES Share [%]
	Total	Heating and Ventilation	Domestic Hot Water	Total	Heating and Ventilation	Domestic Hot Water	
M0	179.0	111.4	67.6	87.7	70.4	17.4	71.2
M1	190.3	122.8	67.6	46.3	28.9	17.4	98.5
M2	171.8	122.8	49.1	42.8	28.9	13.9	97.9
M3	135.3	86.3	49.0	154.4	97.9	56.5	0.0
M4	124.3	86.3	38.0	135.3	97.9	37.4	5.9
M5	43.5	28.4	15.2	130.6	85.2	45.5	61.3
M6	43.5	28.4	15.2	41.1	26.7	14.4	89.4
M7	52.5	35.2	17.2	47.4	31.5	15.9	91.2

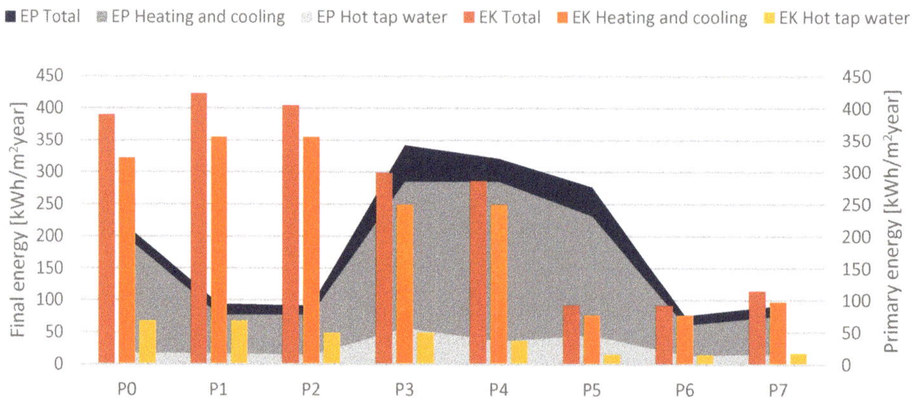

Figure 2. Analysis results for heat source switching (building left as is) (options P0–P7).

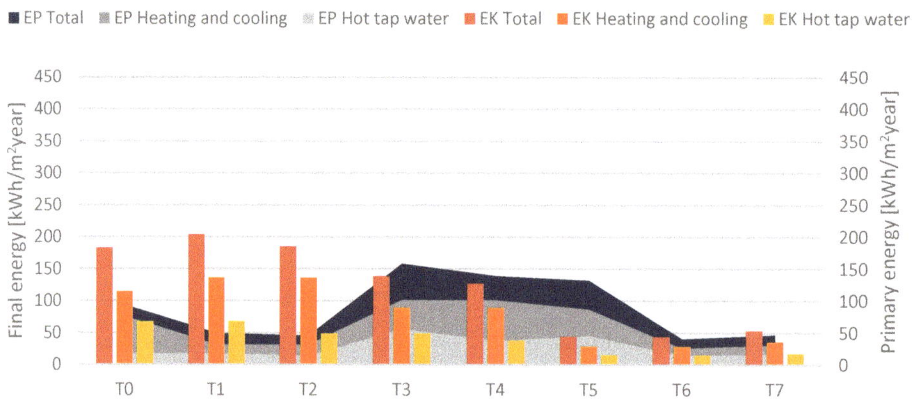

Figure 3. Analysis results for heat source switching (options T0–T7).

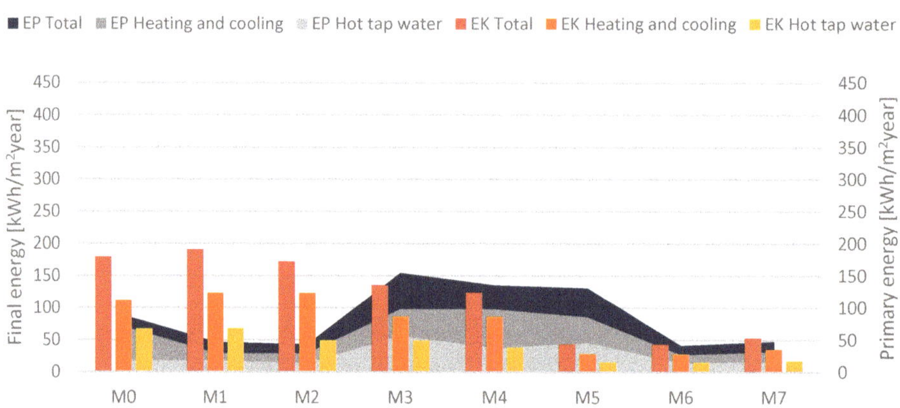

Figure 4. Analysis results for heat source switching (options M0–M7).

For options M0–M7, useful energy demand was 87.2 kWh/m^{2}year, with heating and ventilation accounting for 63.1 kWh/m^{2}year and hot water preparation accounting for 24.1 kWh/m^{2}year, similar to the "P" and "T" options. It should, of course, be noted that these are the most favourable results obtained where, e.g., options P1, T1, and M1 are compared, i.e., those using the same heat production technology for central heating and domestic hot water preparation.

From a technological standpoint, the building materials used for insulation influenced the utility energy results obtained for the individual variants. The thickness of the thermal insulation and heat transfer coefficient directly affect the thermal resistance of the building envelope, and consequently reduce the demand for usable energy. Adapting the building to the technical conditions of WT2021 requires the use of higher-quality materials than those used in the case of WT2017. However, in this case, the energy effects do not show a linear relationship, e.g., with the insulation thickness. Consequently, the obtained energy effects are not necessarily commensurate with the financial outlays incurred for better-quality insulating materials. From the point of view of final energy, the analysis is much simpler, as the difference in the obtained values results directly from the efficiency of the heating devices used.

By analysing all variants in terms of energy, the one characterised by the lowest values of demand for useful energy, final energy, and, consequently, primary energy should be considered sought or desirable. The analysis may differ if economic or ecological factors are taken into account. In the case of the building analysed, it should be stated that, from the energy point of view, the optimal options result in the building meeting the WT2021 technical conditions in conjunction with the use of heat pumps assisted by a photovoltaic installation. The M6 option with the brine-to-water heat pump and the M7 option with the air-to-water heat pump exhibited the lowest final and primary energy values. This results directly from the production of electricity for heat pump operation. The heat pumps themselves, owing to the high COP coefficient, allow for achieving low final energy values. In contrast, the PV installation with a primary energy input index of 0, assuming that it would provide 80% of the electricity required by the heat pump, allowed for a significant reduction in the primary energy value in the variants where it was applied. This assumption was made based on the balance of energy produced and drawn from the grid on an annual basis.

However, it should be noted that regarding the capital expenditure associated with the energy renovation work required, options T6 and T7, which meet the WT2017 technical conditions, may be more viable. They are also based on renewable energy sources, i.e., heat pumps and a photovoltaic installation, and the difference in final and primary energy values compared to options M6 and M7 is small.

3.1. Economic Analysis Results

Figure 5 presents the total net unit energy production costs for the individual options analysed. These costs do not account for any subsidies for purchasing heat sources and energy carriers. From the comparison of results, it can be concluded that the lowest energy production costs are achieved for options M1, M2, P1, P2, T1, and T2. The options involve biomass-fired boilers (M1, P1, and T1) and biomass-fired boilers combined with solar panels (M2, P2, and T2). Using heat pumps fed by grid electricity (options M5 and P3) resulted in somewhat higher or similar (T5) energy production costs to the cost of generating energy from natural gas. Supplementing a heat pump with a photovoltaic installation increases the total cost of energy production. The highest costs are associated with installations involving heat pumps and PV cells (options M6, M7, P6, P7, T6, and T7). It is worth noting that this is one of Poland's most common energy source configurations, especially for new buildings or those undergoing thermal retrofitting.

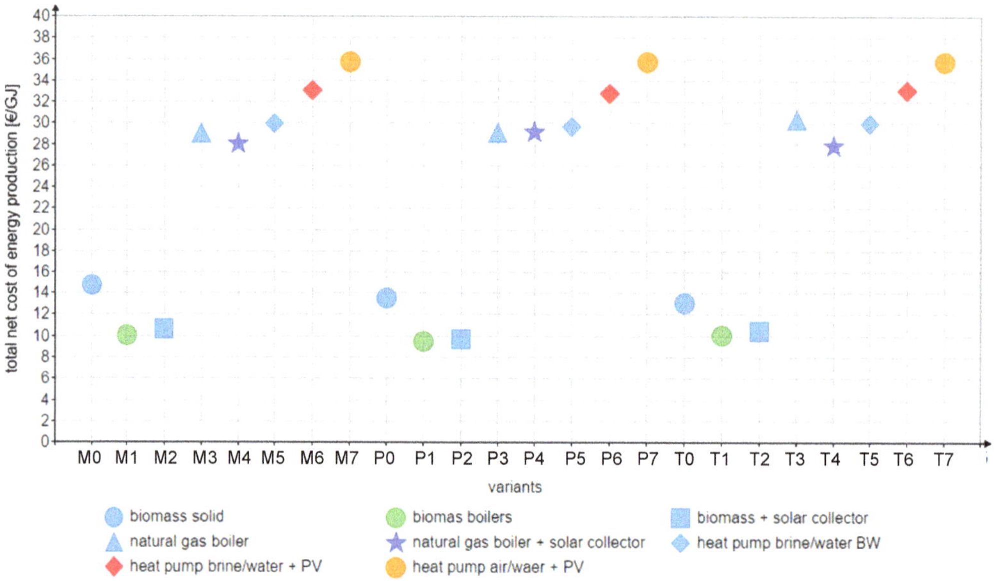

Figure 5. Comparison of total net unit costs of energy generation for individual options [EUR/GJ].

Figure 6 present a summary of these costs. The charts have been prepared assuming an exchange rate of 1 EUR = 4.2 PLN (03.2025). Operating (variable) costs in the options involving the use of PV cells assisting a heat pump and grid-powered heat pumps are lower than variable costs in the options involving the use of natural gas.

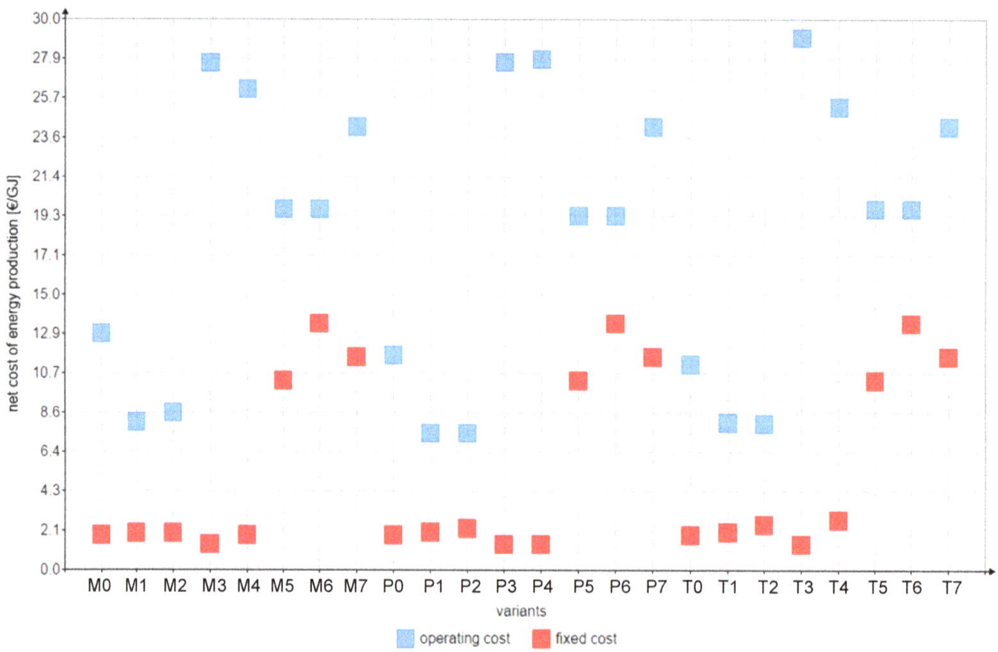

Figure 6. Comparison of net unit fixed and variable costs of energy generation for individual options [EUR/GJ] (values stated do not include subsidies).

Regarding the total unit cost of energy production, biomass- and coal-fired boilers remain the cheapest energy sources (Figure 5). Unfortunately, the assumptions made regarding the purchase costs of primary energy carriers are correct. Heat pumps cannot compete with solid fuel boilers, even when exclusively considering operating costs (Figure 6). The situation looks even worse after fixed costs, which are affected by capital expenditures, are considered.

An economic analysis was presented concerning the unit of energy produced and investment costs per unit of power (kW). In this context, two fundamental differences in investment costs should be indicated when comparing the T6–T7 and M6–M7 variants. The first is the difference in the costs of modernising the building, amounting to approximately EUR 2347.83. The second is the cost of energy installation. In the case of a heat pump, there is a difference of EUR 282.60 per kW between a brine/water heat pump and an air/water heat pump. This is mainly due to the cost of the lower heat source. The heat load of the building after modernisation is approximately 8 kW, which results in a difference of EUR 2260.87. A separate issue is the selection of the power of the PV installation concerning the heat pump energy demand to drive the compressor, which is directly related to the COP coefficient. However, this issue has not been analysed.

3.2. Environmental Analysis Results

Emission volumes for all energy renovation options considered are presented in Table 12, while percentage reductions in emissions for individual energy renovation options compared to the baseline option are presented in Table 13. The analysis has made it possible to draw the following conclusions:

Table 12. Pollutant emissions for individual energy renovation options.

Variant	Type of Installation	Emission (kg/year)							
		TSP	PM 10	PM 2.5	CO_2	CO	NO_x	SO_2	B(a)P
P0	Solid fuel boiler (50% coal, 50% biomass)	83.64	77.62	68.46	8992.48	670.24	26.58	40.44	0.0516
P1	Biomass boiler	7.76	7.37	6.98	0.00	85.36	23.28	2.13	0.0029
P2	Biomass boiler + solar collectors	7.40	7.03	6.66	0.00	81.40	22.20	2.03	0.0028
P3	Gas boiler	0.08	0.08	0.08	8804.64	4.58	7.64	0.06	0.0000
P4	Gas boiler + solar collectors	0.07	0.07	0.07	8395.99	4.37	7.28	0.06	0.0000
P5	Heat pump brine/water	0.35	0.00	0.00	8789.47	2.85	7.04	6.25	0.0000
P6	Heat pump brine/water + PV	0.11	0.00	0.00	2636.84	0.85	2.11	1.87	0.0000
P7	Heat pump air/water + PV	0.13	0.00	0.00	3308.37	1.07	2.65	2.35	0.0000
T0	Solid fuel boiler (50% coal, 50% biomass)	38.37	35.76	31.94	3418.71	311.13	11.61	15.66	0.0221
T1	Biomass boiler	3.51	3.33	3.16	0.00	38.59	10.52	0.96	0.0013
T2	Biomass boiler + solar collectors	3.15	2.99	2.83	0.00	34.63	9.44	0.87	0.0012
T3	Gas boiler	0.03	0.03	0.03	3980.53	2.07	3.45	0.03	0.0000
T4	Gas boiler + solar collectors	0.03	0.03	0.03	3571.88	1.86	3.10	0.02	0.0000
T5	Heat pump brine/water	0.16	0.00	0.00	4028.91	1.31	3.23	2.86	0.0000
T6	Heat pump brine/water + PV	0.05	0.00	0.00	1208.67	0.39	0.97	0.86	0.0000
T7	Heat pump air/water + PV	0.06	0.00	0.00	1495.70	0.48	1.20	1.06	0.0000

Table 12. *Cont.*

Variant	Type of Installation	Emission (kg/year)							
		TSP	PM 10	PM 2.5	CO_2	CO	NO_x	SO_2	B(a)P
M0	Solid fuel boiler (50% coal, 50% biomass)	35.70	33.29	29.79	3090.55	289.98	10.73	14.20	0.0203
M1	Biomass boiler	3.26	3.10	2.93	0.00	35.84	9.77	0.90	0.0012
M2	Biomass boiler + solar collectors	2.90	2.75	2.61	0.00	31.88	8.69	0.80	0.0011
M3	Gas boiler	0.03	0.03	0.03	3696.51	1.92	3.21	0.03	0.0000
M4	Gas boiler + solar collectors	0.03	0.03	0.03	3287.86	1.71	2.85	0.02	0.0000
M5	Heat pump brine/water	0.15	0.00	0.00	3748.63	1.21	3.00	2.66	0.0000
M6	Heat pump brine/water + PV	0.05	0.00	0.00	1124.59	0.36	0.90	0.80	0.0000
M7	Heat pump air/water + PV	0.06	0.00	0.00	1388.98	0.45	1.11	0.99	0.0000

Table 13. Pollutant emissions for individual energy renovation options.

Variant	Type of Installation	Emission Reduction in Relation to the Variant P0 (%)							
		TSP	PM 10	PM 2.5	CO_2	CO	NOx	SO_2	B(a)P
P1	Biomass boiler	90.7	90.5	89.8	100.0	87.3	12.4	94.7	94.4
P2	Biomass boiler + solar collectors	91.2	90.9	90.3	100.0	87.9	16.5	95.0	94.6
P3	Gas boiler	99.9	99.9	99.9	2.1	99.3	71.3	99.8	100.0
P4	Gas boiler + solar collectors	99.9	99.9	99.9	6.6	99.3	72.6	99.9	100.0
P5	Heat pump brine/water	99.6	100.0	100.0	2.3	99.6	73.5	84.6	100.0
P6	Heat pump brine/water + PV	99.9	100.0	100.0	70.7	99.9	92.1	95.4	100.0
P7	Heat pump air/water + PV	99.8	100.0	100.0	63.2	99.8	90.0	94.2	100.0
T0	Solid fuel boiler (50% coal, 50% biomass)	54.1	53.9	53.3	62.0	53.6	56.3	61.3	57.3
T1	Biomass boiler	95.8	95.7	95.4	100.0	94.2	60.4	97.6	97.5
T2	Biomass boiler + solar collectors	96.2	96.1	95.9	100.0	94.8	64.5	97.9	97.7
T3	Gas boiler	100.0	100.0	99.9	55.7	99.7	87.0	99.9	100.0
T4	Gas boiler + solar collectors	100.0	100.0	100.0	60.3	99.7	88.3	99.9	100.0
T5	Heat pump brine/water	99.8	100.0	100.0	55.2	99.8	87.9	92.9	100.0
T6	Heat pump brine/water + PV	99.9	100.0	100.0	86.6	99.9	96.4	97.9	100.0
T7	Heat pump air/water + P	99.9	100.0	100.0	83.4	99.9	95.5	97.4	100.0
M0	Solid fuel boiler (50% coal, 50% biomass)	57.3	57.1	56.5	65.6	56.7	59.6	64.9	60.6
M1	Biomass boiler	96.1	96.0	95.7	100.0	94.7	63.2	97.8	97.6
M2	Biomass boiler + solar collectors	96.5	96.5	96.2	100.0	95.2	67.3	98.0	97.9
M3	Gas boiler	100.0	100.0	100.0	58.9	99.7	87.9	99.9	100.0
M4	Gas boiler + solar collectors	100.0	100.0	100.0	63.4	99.7	89.3	99.9	100.0
M5	Heat pump brine/water	99.8	100.0	100.0	58.3	99.8	88.7	93.4	100.0
M6	Heat pump brine/water + PV	99.9	100.0	100.0	87.5	99.9	96.6	98.0	100.0
M7	Heat pump air/water + PV	99.9	100.0	100.0	84.6	99.9	95.8	97.6	100.0

- Total Suspended Particles (TSP): The energy renovation options utilising gas-fired boilers and heat pumps demonstrate the most significant reductions in TSP emissions. Options P3 and P4 achieve a remarkable 99.9% reduction, while options T3, T4, M3, and M4 approach near-total reductions of nearly 100%, as illustrated in Figure 7.
- Carbon Dioxide (CO_2): The highest reduction of 100% in CO_2 emissions is linked to biomass-fired boiler options (P1–P2, T1–T2, M1–M2). Furthermore, energy renovation options employing heat pumps powered by photovoltaic (PV) installations (P6–P7, T6–T7, M6–M7) result in substantial CO_2 reductions, ranging from 63.2% to 87.5% compared to the P0 baseline option. This analysis assumes a 70% contribution of PV electricity to the heat pump operation.
- Carbon Monoxide (CO): All options involving a switch in heat sources exhibit significant reductions in CO emissions, ranging from 87.3% for biomass-fired boilers to 99.9% for heat pumps powered by photovoltaics.
- Nitrogen Oxides (NO_x): The most effective options for reducing nitrogen oxide emissions are those that employ heat pumps in conjunction with photovoltaics, achieving reductions between 90% and 96.6%. Options utilising gas-fired boilers (P3, P4, T3, T4, M3, and M4) also yield notable reductions, varying from 71.3% to 87.9%.
- Benzo(a)pyrene (BaP): The analysis indicates that all energy renovation options that involve switching heat sources result in a minimum reduction of 94.4% in BaP emissions for biomass-fired boilers, with reductions reaching up to 100% for gas-fired boilers and heat pumps.

Figures 7–11 provide a graphical presentation of emissions of individual pollutants for energy renovation options, with the P0 baseline option highlighted in red.

In conclusion, the analysis of the emission evaluation results for various energy renovation options shows that modern technologies, such as heat pumps and gas boilers, significantly reduce air pollutant emissions, including particulate matter, carbon dioxide, and nitrogen oxides. The most significant emission reductions, approaching nearly 100%, were observed for options utilising heat pumps powered by solar energy and biomass boilers. These results highlight the substantial ecological benefits of implementing efficient heating technologies, which can significantly improve air quality and reduce negative impacts on the natural environment. This is crucial for combating climate change and striving for sustainable development.

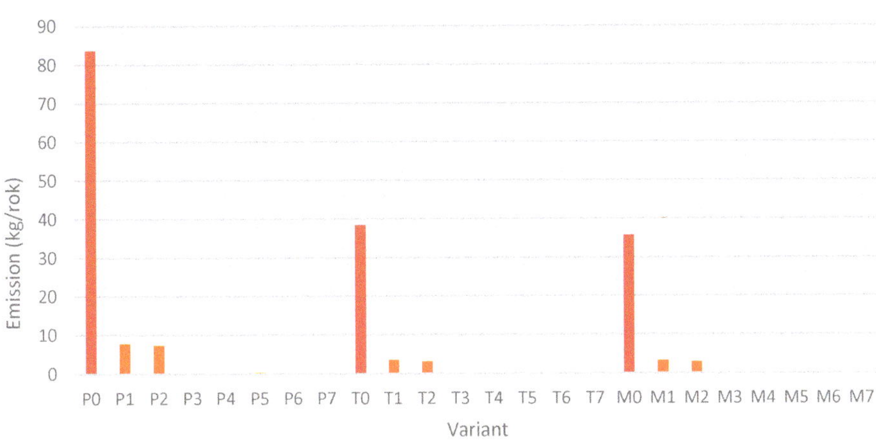

Figure 7. Total particulate matter emissions from individual energy renovation options.

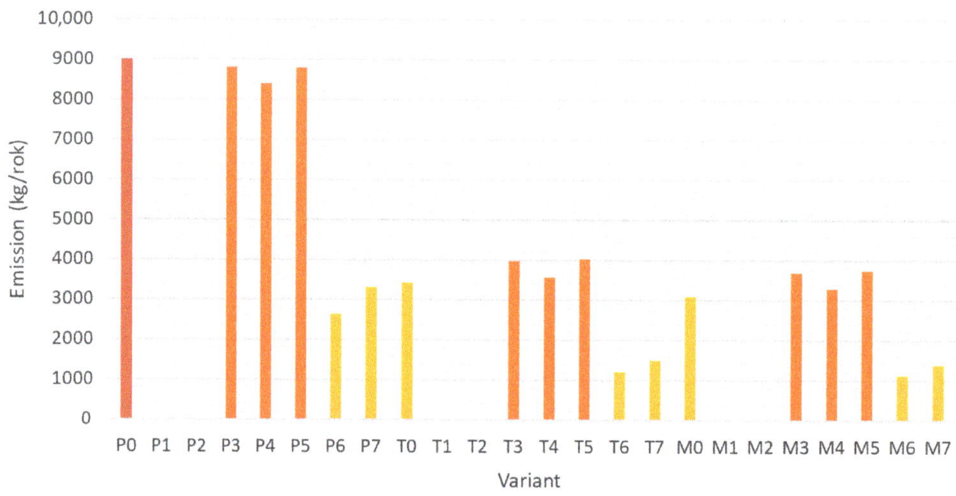

Figure 8. Carbon dioxide emissions from individual energy renovation options.

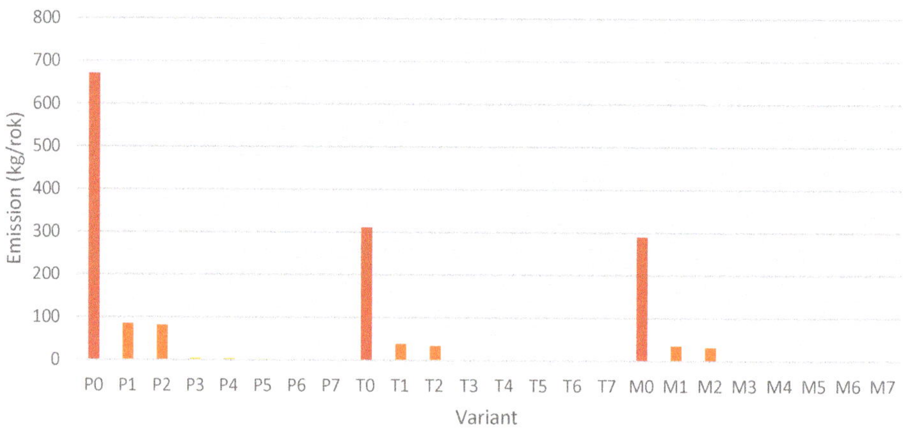

Figure 9. Carbon monoxide emissions from individual energy renovation options.

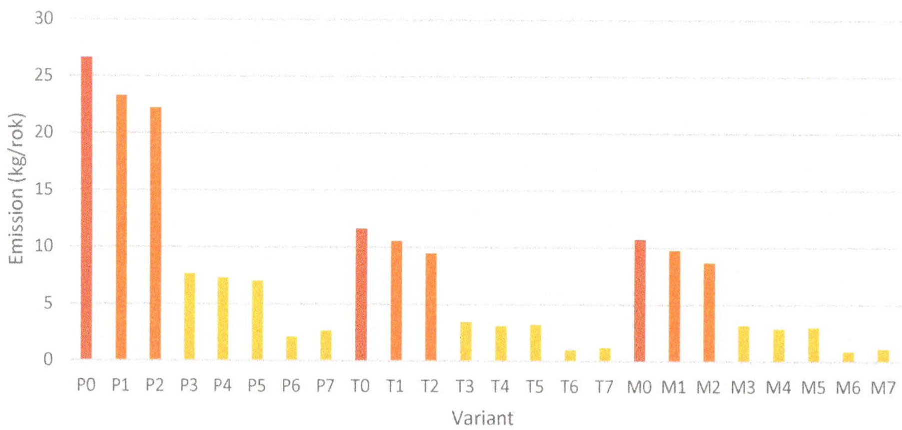

Figure 10. Nitrogen oxide emissions for individual energy renovation options.

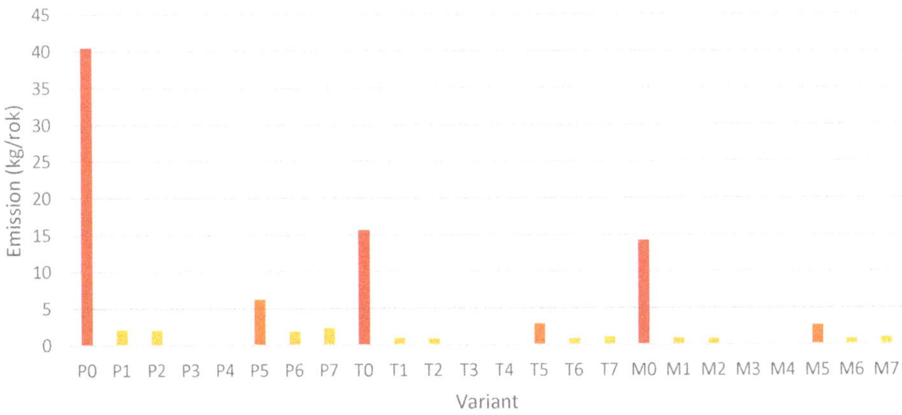

Figure 11. Sulphur dioxide emissions for individual energy renovation options.

4. Conclusions

The most efficient solutions from the analysis involve the use of heat pumps. This applies to all three cases (P5–P7), for which the final energy value ranges from 92.1 to 114.1 kWh/m^{2}year. In the case of primary energy, the options involving heat pumps combined with photovoltaic installations exhibit the most favourable values, ranging from 61 to 75 kWh/m^{2}year.

The options with the highest share of renewables are those based on a biomass-fired boiler plus a solar collector system, with RES shares of 99–99.2%. In the case of options involving energy renovation (T0–T7), both final and primary energy demand have been more than halved. Useful energy demand was 93.9 kWh/m^{2}year, with heating and ventilation accounting for 69.8 kWh/m^{2}year and hot water preparation accounting for 24.1 kWh/m^{2}year. There was also a slight decrease in the total share of RES, which amounted to 98.1–98.5% for the most favourable options. This is due to the percentage change in the proportion of thermal energy to the electrical energy required to drive auxiliary equipment, such as circulation pumps. Options M0–M7 exhibit the most favourable results compared to options P1, T1, and M1, i.e., those using the same heat production technology for central heating and domestic hot water preparation. For options M0–M7, the calculated useful energy demand was 87.2 kWh/m^{2}year, with heating and ventilation accounting for 63.1 kWh/m^{2}year and hot water preparation accounting for 24.1 kWh/m^{2}year, similar to the "P" and "T" options.

From an energy perspective, the optimal options result in the building meeting the WT2021 technical conditions. Options M1, M2, P1, P2, and T1, T2 exhibit the lowest energy generation costs. The options involve biomass-fired boilers (M1, P1, and T1) and biomass-fired boilers combined with solar panels (M2, P2, and T2). All options using heat pumps fed by grid electricity (options M5, P5, and T5) resulted in energy production costs that are slightly higher or similar to the cost of generating energy from natural gas. Supplementing a heat pump with a photovoltaic installation increases the total cost of energy production. Despite the lower capital expenditure associated with using air-source heat pumps, the total unit cost of energy generation for these sources was higher than that of brine-to-water heat pumps. The highest costs are associated with installations involving heat pumps driven by energy from PV cells (options M6, M7, P6, P7, T6, and T7). Based on the assumptions made regarding the purchase costs of primary energy carriers, heat pumps cannot compete with solid fuel boilers, even when exclusively variable costs are considered. Only in the case of natural gas are operating costs similar to those of heat pumps.

The model building selected for analysis currently exhibits a high demand for useful energy (for central heating purposes). The solid fuel boiler currently in use, which serves central heating and hot water preparation purposes, has low energy efficiency (68% when burning coal and 55% when burning wood), which also results in high fuel consumption (almost 3.6 tonnes of coal per year and 8.8 tonnes of wood per year, which gives about 19 spatial meters of wood).

The fuel burnt in the boiler currently results in annual pollutant emissions of around 9 tonnes of CO_2, 670 kg of CO, 40 kg of SO_2, 84 kg of particulate matter, and 52 g of benzo(a)pyrene. Comprehensive energy renovation measures involving heat source switching can significantly reduce both fuel consumption and pollutant emissions. All energy renovation options involving heat pumps (P5–P7, T5–T7, and M5–M7) eliminate pollutant emissions into the atmosphere at the installation site, contributing to the elimination of the low-stack emission problem in the municipality. In the case of the building considered, any energy renovation measure will result in at least a 50% reduction in particulate matter emissions and a 50% reduction in carbon monoxide and benzo(a)pyrene emissions. For most energy renovation options, the reduction in nitrogen oxide emissions is also higher than 50% (only for options P1 and P2, their emissions into the atmosphere are reduced just slightly). Carbon dioxide emissions comparable to the current state will only be present for energy renovation options P3 and P4 (replacing the heat source with a gas-fired boiler without insulating the building) and P5 (using a heat pump supplied with electricity from the power grid without insulating the building). There is at least a 50% reduction in CO_2 emissions for the remaining energy renovation options, and for options with biomass-fired boilers (options P1, P2, T1, T2, M1, and M2), the reduction in CO_2 emissions will be 100%.

Regarding this article, further research should be directed toward a broader spectrum of modelling. An interesting direction in this regard was indicated by Rashad et al. (2022) [56], who presented a similar position as Andrews and Jain (2022) [40], claiming that the static calculations used so far do not provide a detailed answer to questions such as: what is the energy demand for individual purposes in a building, and how does it change during the day, month, and year. The same conclusions, but concerning domestic hot water only, were formulated by Bergel et al. (2016) [57], who claimed that real water consumption is inadequate to that calculated based on applicable guidelines. Andrews and Jain (2022) [40] based their research on the use of TRNSYS software for year-round building energy analysis. A dynamic energy chewing analysis of an academic building in Pisawas was conducted by Franco et al. (2021) [58]. By analysing an HVAC system based on a heat pump, chiller, and mechanical ventilation with heat recovery, they concluded that such a system should be dynamically controlled in response to the presence of building occupants and their needs. At the same time, they pointed to the value of 44% energy savings with this energy management method in the building, of which 33% will be for the ventilation system. Heracleous et al. (2022) [59] analysed educational buildings in Cyprus using dynamic modelling, but in the Integrated Environmental Software Virtual Environment software. The optimal variants of thermal modernisation were identified using the life cycle cost analysis (LCCA) method, confirming that this direction for further research is appropriate. Leiria et al. (2023) [60] and Kaczmarczyk et al. (2025) [61] conduct research based on the readings of smart heat meters for the assessment of forecasted and actual energy consumption values in buildings. Martinez-de-Alegria et al. (2021) [62] searched for ways to optimise energy consumption in existing facilities in Spain. Perhaps, in the context of this article, it is not directly related, but it shows that limiting oneself to thermal modernisation alone is currently insufficient. Dynamic analyses of energy demand and the search for new solutions that increase energy efficiency should be the focus of future research. This requires a lot of interdisciplinarity; however, as indicated by the analyses of

Li et al. (2021) [63], interdisciplinary, interactive research that combines the natural and social environment will attract new research ideas in the context of the energy intensity of buildings.

An important aspect of assessing heating technologies is their compliance with current and upcoming regulatory frameworks, especially the EU Ecodesign Directive (2009/125/EC) and its delegated regulations for space and water heaters (EU) No. 813/2013 and No. 814/2013. The directive establishes minimum seasonal space heating efficiency and maximum allowable pollutant emission levels for boilers and heat pumps sold in the EU. From 2027, more rigorous eco-design standards will come into effect, including higher minimum seasonal efficiency thresholds (SCOP for heat pumps and seasonal efficiency ηs for boilers) and stricter limits on NO_x, particulate matter, and organic gaseous compounds. In this study, the analysed heat pumps, brine-to-water and air-to-water, are technologies that, in their current market configurations, already meet or surpass the anticipated 2027 requirements for seasonal efficiency and local emissions. Likewise, the biomass boilers examined are compliant Eco-design units equipped with high-efficiency combustion and flue gas cleaning systems. However, actual compliance relies on the specific model chosen for installation, and any investment decision should verify conformity with the updated EU product database (EPREL) to ensure compatibility with post-2027 regulatory standards.

Apart from energy issues, aspects that may influence the decision regarding the modernisation of the building are worth mentioning. It is essential that the building provides comfortable conditions for its residents or users. This may include ensuring adequate ventilation, lighting, acoustics, and temperature regulation. Sometimes, the choice may be dictated by aesthetic or architectural considerations. Some solutions may be more visually appealing or better fit into existing infrastructure. While investing in more advanced technologies may be more expensive upfront, they can provide long-term savings or benefits. Analysing investment costs and return on investment can be significant in making decisions. Some solutions may be more durable and require less maintenance over the long term, thereby saving money or reducing the risk of failure. In addition to energy efficiency, other environmental aspects, such as water consumption and impact on local wildlife, can influence the selection of optimal options. Sometimes, your choice may be limited by building regulations, energy standards, or other legal regulations. Not all advanced technologies are always available or profitable in a given region. The availability of building materials and technology may influence this choice. In practice, decisions regarding the construction or renovation of a building often require consideration of many of these factors simultaneously to find the optimal solution that meets various needs and constraints.

Author Contributions: A.S. and M.K.—Conceptualisation, A.S., M.K., L.P. and B.T.—methodology, L.P. and M.K.—software, M.K.—validation, B.T.—formal analysis, M.K., W.L. and G.P.—resources, W.L., G.P. and M.K.—data curation, A.S. and M.K.—writing—original draft preparation, M.K., L.P., B.T., W.L. and G.P.—writing—review and editing, M.K. and L.P.—visualisation, A.S.—supervision, A.S.—project administration, A.S.—funding acquisition. All authors have read and agreed to the published version of the manuscript.

Funding: The project was co-financed by the funds of the National Centre for Research and Development within the framework of the research and development programme Social and economic development of Poland in the conditions of globalising markets GOSPOSTRATEG/contract No Gospostrateg1/385085/21/NCBR/19. This research project was supported by the program "Excellence initiative–research university" for the AGH University of Krakow. This research was funded by a statutory research program at the Faculty of Geology, Geophysics, and Environmental Protection AGH University of Krakow, Poland, statutory work No. 16.16.140.315.

Data Availability Statement: The data that support the findings of this study are available from the corresponding author, [M.K.], upon reasonable request.

Conflicts of Interest: The authors declare no conflicts of interest. The funders had no role in the design of the study; in the collection, analyses, or interpretation of data; in the writing of the manuscript, or in the decision to publish the results.

Nomenclature

B(a)P	benzo(a)pyrene
CO	carbon monoxide
NO_x	nitrogen oxides
CO_2	carbon dioxide
COP	heat pump coefficient of performance
E_{CO2}	carbon dioxide emission
EK	final energy
EP	primary energy
EU	useful energy
EPC	Energy Performance Certificate
GHG	greenhouse gases
LCCA	life cycle cost analysis
NPV	net present value
PM10	particulate matter $\leq$ 10 µg
PM2.5	particulate matter $\leq$ 2.5 µg
PV	photovoltaic
RES	renewable energy source
SO_2	sulphur dioxide
SPBT	simple payback time
U_{RES}	share of renewable energy sources in annual final energy demand
Q	seasonal energy consumption [GJ/year, MWh/year]
Q_w	calorific value
W	emission factor [g/GJ, kg/MWh]
WT2021	technical conditions for new buildings created from 2021
WT2017	technical conditions for buildings that have been created in 2017–2020

References

1. Capros, P.; Zazias, G.; Evangelopoulou, S.; Kannavou, M.; Fotiou, T.; Siskos, P.; De Vita, A.; Sakellaris, K. Energy-system modelling of the EU strategy towards climate-neutrality. *Energy Policy* **2019**, *134*, 110960. [CrossRef]
2. Kilkis, S.; Krajacic, G.; Duic, N.; Rosen, M.A.; Al-Nimr, M.A. Advances in integration of energy, water and environment systems towards climate neutrality for sustainable development. *Energy Convers. Manag.* **2020**, *225*, 113410. [CrossRef]
3. Salvia, M.; Reckien, D.; Pietrapertosa, F.; Eckersley, P.; Spyridaki, N.A.; Krook-Riekkola, A.; Olazabal, M.; De Gregorio Hurtado, S.; Simoes, S.G.; Geneletti, D.; et al. Will climate mitigation ambitions lead to carbon neutrality? An analysis of the local-level plans of 327 cities in the EU. *Renew. Sustain. Energy Rev.* **2021**, *135*, 11025. [CrossRef]
4. Oudes, D.; Stremke, S. Spatial transition analysis: Spatially explicit and evidence-based targets for sustainable energy transition at the local and regional scale. *Landsc. Urban Plan.* **2018**, *169*, 1–11. [CrossRef]
5. Kaczmarczyk, M.; Sowiżdżał, A.; Tomaszewska, B. Energetic and Environmental Aspects of Individual Heat Generation for Sustainable Development at a Local Scale—A Case Study from Poland. *Energies* **2020**, *13*, 454. [CrossRef]
6. Kaczmarczyk, M. Building energy characteristic evaluation in terms of energy efficiency and ecology. *Energy Convers. Manag.* **2024**, *306*, 118284. [CrossRef]
7. Tettey, U.; Dodoo, A.; Gustavsson, L. Primary energy implications of different design strategies for an apartment building. *Energy* **2016**, *104*, 132–148. [CrossRef]
8. Guarino, F.; Cellura, M.; Longo, S.; Gulotta, T.; Mistretta, M.; Tumminia, G.; Ferraro, M.; Antonucci, V. Integration of building simulation and life cycle assessment: A TRNSYS application. *Energy Procedia* **2016**, *101*, 360–367. [CrossRef]

9. Jiang, Z.; Risbeck, M.J.; Ramamurti, V.; Murugesan, S.; Amores, J.; Zhang, C.; Lee, Y.M.; Drees, K.H. Building HVAC control with reinforcement learning for reduction of energy cost and demand charge. *Energy Build.* **2021**, *239*, 110833. [CrossRef]
10. Gibbons, L.; Javed, S. A review of HVAC solution-sets and energy performance of nearly zero-energy multi-story apartment buildings in Nordic climates by statistical analysis of environmental performance certificates and literature review. *Energy* **2022**, *238*, 121709. [CrossRef]
11. Zhou, S.L.; Shah, A.A.; Leung, P.K.; Zhu, X.; Liao, Q. A comprehensive review of the applications of machine learning for HVAC. *DeCarbon* **2023**, *2*, 100023. [CrossRef]
12. Zhang, F.; Saeed, N.; Sadeghian, P. Deep learning in fault detection and diagnosis of building HVAC systems: A systematic review with meta analysis. *Energy AI* **2023**, *12*, 100235. [CrossRef]
13. Liang, X.; Chen, K.; Chen, S.; Zhu, X.; Jin, X.; Du, Z. IoT-based intelligent energy management system for optimal planning of HVAC devices in net-zero emissions PV-battery building considering demand compliance. *Energy Convers. Manag.* **2023**, *292*, 117369. [CrossRef]
14. Wang, C.; Ferrando, M.; Causone, F.; Jin, X.; Zhou, X.; Shi, X. An innovative method to predict the thermal parameters of construction assemblies for urban building energy models. *Build. Environ.* **2022**, *224*, 109541. [CrossRef]
15. Askeland, M.; Georges, L.; Korpas, M. Low-parameter linear model to activate the flexibility of the building thermal mass in energy system optimization. *Smart Energy* **2023**, *9*, 100094. [CrossRef]
16. Kaczmarczyk, M. Energy environmental matrix for buildings energy performance certificate evaluation. *Energy Build.* **2025**, *341*, 115859. [CrossRef]
17. Wi, S.; Kang, Y.; Yang, S.; Kim, Y.U.; Kim, S. Hazard evaluation of indoor environment based on long-term pollutant emission characteristics of building insulation materials: An empirical study. *Environ. Pollut.* **2021**, *285*, 117223. [CrossRef]
18. Anh, L.-D.H.; Pasztory, Z. An overview of factors influencing thermal conductivity of building insulation materials. *J. Build. Eng.* **2021**, *44*, 102604. [CrossRef]
19. Edelenbosch, O.Y.; Rovelli, D.; Levesque, A.; Marangoni, G.; Tavoni, M. Long term, cross-country effects of buildings insulation policies. *Technol. Forecast. Soc. Change* **2021**, *170*, 120887. [CrossRef]
20. Lim, T.; Yim, W.S.; Kim, D.D. Evaluation of Daylight and Cooling Performance of Shading Devices in Residential Buildings in South Korea. *Energies* **2020**, *13*, 4749. [CrossRef]
21. Błazy, R.; Błachut, J.; Ciepiela, A.; Łabuz, R.; Papież, R. Thermal Modernization Cost and the Potential Ecological Effect—Scenario Analysis for Thermal Modernization in Southern Poland. *Energies* **2021**, *14*, 2023. [CrossRef]
22. Lis, A.; Ujma, A. Redukcja emisji pyłów zawieszonych w wyniku poprawy izolacyjności cieplnej przegród i zmiany nośnika energii. Reducing of particulate matter emissions as a result of walls thermal insulation improvement and energy carriers changes. *Constr. Optimazed Energy Potential* **2016**, *1*, 47–54.
23. Kim, Y.; Yu, K.H. Study on the certification policy of zero-energy buildings in Korea. *Sustainability* **2020**, *12*, 5172. [CrossRef]
24. Yousefi, M.; Hajizadeh, A.; Soltani, M.N.; Hredzak, B.; Kianpoor, N. Profit assessment of home energy management system for buildings with A-G energy labels. *Appl. Energy* **2020**, *277*, 115618. [CrossRef]
25. Andelkovic, A.S.; Kljajić, M.; Macura, D.; Munćan, V.; Mujan, I.; Tomić, M.; Stepanov, B. Building energy performance certificate—A relevant indicator of actual energy consumption and savings? *Energies* **2021**, *14*, 3455. [CrossRef]
26. Conticelli, E.; Falcioni, S.; Marzani, G.; Morini, G.L.; Tondelli, S. Assessing energy efficiency at urban scale through the use of energy performance certificates: An application in the Emilia-Romagna region, Italy. *Cities* **2024**, *145*, 104728. [CrossRef]
27. Manso-Burgos, A.; Ribo-Perez, D.; Van As, J.; Montagud-Montalva, C.; Royo-Pastor, R. Diagnosis of the building stock using Energy Performance Certificates for urban energy planning in Mediterranean compact cities. Case of study: The city of Valencia. in Spain. *Energy Convers. Manag. X* **2023**, *20*, 100450. [CrossRef]
28. Kaczmarczyk, M.; Sowiżdżał, A. Environmental friendly energy resources improving air quality in urban area. *Energy Rep.* **2024**, *11*, 3383–3394. [CrossRef]
29. Dzikuć, M. Problems associated with the low emission limitation in Zielona Góra (Poland): Prospects challenges. *J. Clean. Prod.* **2017**, *166*, 81–87. [CrossRef]
30. Dzikuć, M.; Piwowar, A.; Szufa, S.; Adamczyk, J.; Dzikuć, M. Potential and Scenarios of Variants of Thermo-Modernization of Single-Family Houses: An Example of the Lubuskie Voivodeship. *Energies* **2021**, *14*, 191. [CrossRef]
31. Piotrowska-Woroniak, J.; Woroniak, G. Redukcja emisji zanieczyszczeń w wyniku termomodernizacji zabytkowych obiektów sakralnych. Reduction of emission pollution as a result of thermomodernisation historic sacral buildings. *Civ. Environ. Eng.* **2014**, *5*, 73–77.
32. Piccardo, C.; Gustavsson, L. Implications of different modelling choices in primary energy and carbon emission analysis of buildings. *Energy Build.* **2021**, *247*, 111145. [CrossRef]
33. Alvarez Florez, L.; Pean, T.; Salom, J. Hourly based methods to assess carbon footprint flexibility and primary energy use in decarbonized buildings. *Energy Build.* **2023**, *294*, 113213. [CrossRef]

34. Ramon, D.; Allacker, K.; Trigaux, D.; Wouters, H.; Lipzig, N.P.M. Dynamic modelling of operational energy use in a building LCA: A case study of a Belgian office building. *Energy Build.* **2023**, *278*, 112634. [CrossRef]
35. Staniunas, M.; Medineckiene, M.; Zavadskas, E.; Kalibatas, D. To modernize or not: Ecological-economical assessment of multi-dwelling houses modernization. *Archiv. Civ. Mech. Eng.* **2013**, *13*, 88–98. [CrossRef]
36. Basińska, M.; Koczyk, H.; Kosmowski, A. Assessment of thermo modernization using the global cost method. *Energy Procedia* **2015**, *78*, 2040–2045. [CrossRef]
37. Szulgowska-Zgrzywa, M.; Piechurski, K.; Stefanowicz, E. Multi-criteria assessment of the scenarios of changing the heating system in apartments in historical buildings in Wroclaw (Poland)—Case study. *Energy Build.* **2022**, *254*, 111611. [CrossRef]
38. Hajto, M.; Kaczmarczyk, M. The potential to improve air quality by increasing the use of deep geothermal energy. *Geol. Geophys. Environ.* **2022**, *48*, 147–175. [CrossRef]
39. Liu, J.; Zhang, Q.; Dong, Z.; Li, X.; Li, G.; Li, K. Quantitative evaluation of the building energy performance based on short-term energy predictions. *Energy* **2021**, *223*, 120065. [CrossRef]
40. Andrews, A.; Jain, R.K. Beyond Energy Efficiency: A clustering approach to embed demand flexibility into building energy benchmarking. *Appl. Energy* **2022**, *327*, 119989. [CrossRef]
41. Shimoda, Y.; Yamaguchi, Y.; Iwafune, Y.; Hidaka, K.; Meier, K.; Yagita, Y.; Kawamoto, H.; Nishikiori, S. Energy demand science for a decarbonized society in the context of the residential sector. *Renew. Sustain. Energy Rev.* **2020**, *132*, 110051. [CrossRef]
42. Kaczmarczyk, M.; Kaczmarczyk, M.A.; Pełka, G.; Luboń, W.; Będkowska, A.; Piechowicz, Ł.; Ciapała, B.; Blok, M. *Niska Emisja od Przyczyn Występowania do Sposobów Eliminacji [Low-Stack Emissions: Causes and Methods of Elimination]*; Geosystem Burek, Kotyza S.C.: Kraków, Poland, 2015.
43. Kaczmarczyk, M.; Kaczmarczyk, M.A.; Pełka, G.; Luboń, W.; Będkowska, A.; Ciapała, B.; Malik, D.; Podlewska, E.; Zboina, M. *Niska Emisja—Efektywność Energetyczna w Gminach i Samorządach [Low-Stack Emissions: Energy Efficiency in Municipalities and Local Governments]*; Globenergia Sp. z o.o.: Kraków, Poland, 2017.
44. POP. Program Ochrony Powietrza Dla Województwa Małopolskiego, Urząd Marszałkowski Województwa Małopolskiego [Air Protection Programme for the Małopolska Province, Marshal's Office of the Małopolska Province], Kraków. 2017. Available online: https://powietrze.malopolska.pl/program-ochrony-powietrza (accessed on 6 August 2025).
45. GUS. *2024: Zużycie Nośników Energii w Gospodarstwach Domowych w 2021 r.*; Główny Urząd Statystyczny: Warszawa, Poland, 2024.
46. *ISO 6946*; "Building Components and Building Elements—Thermal Resistance and Thermal Transmittance—Calculation Methods"—The Standard for Calculating Thermal Transmittance Coefficients of Multilayer Walls. ISO: Geneva, Switzerland, 2017.
47. *ISO 13370*; Thermal Performance of Buildings—Heat Transfer via the Ground—Calculation Methods. ISO: Geneva, Switzerland, 2017.
48. *ISO 10077-1*; Thermal Performance of Windows, Doors and Shutters—Calculation of Thermal Transmittance. ISO: Geneva, Switzerland, 2017.
49. *EN 12831:2006*; Heating systems in buildings—Method for calculating the design heat load. ISO: Geneva, Switzerland, 2006.
50. *ISO 13788*; Hydrothermal Performance of Building Components and Building Elements. Internal Surface Temperature to Avoid Critical Surface Humidity and Interstitial Condensation. Calculation Methods. ISO: Geneva, Switzerland, 2012.
51. Journal of Laws [Dz. U.] of 2015 Item 376: Rozporządzenie Ministra Infrastruktury i Rozwoju z Dnia 27 Lutego 2015 r. w Sprawie Metodologii Wyznaczania Charakterystyki Energetycznej Budynku lub Części Budynku oraz Świadectw [Regulation of the Minister of Infrastructure and Development of 27 February 2015 on the Methodology for Determining the Energy Performance of a Building or Part of a Building and Certificates]. Available online: https://isap.sejm.gov.pl/isap.nsf/DocDetails.xsp?id=WDU20150000376 (accessed on 6 August 2025).
52. Journal of Laws [Dz. U.] of 2023 Item 697: Regulation of the Minister of Development and Technology of 13 April 2023 Changing Regulation of the Minister of Infrastructure and Development of 27 February 2015 on the Methodology for Determining the Energy Performance of a Building or Part of a Building and Energy Performance Certificates. Available online: https://isap.sejm.gov.pl/isap.nsf/DocDetails.xsp?id=WDU20230000697 (accessed on 6 August 2025).
53. Journal of Laws [Dz. U.] of 2017 Item 2285: Rozporządzenie Ministra Infrastruktury i Budownictwa z Dnia 14 Listopada 2017 r. Zmieniające Rozporządzenie w Sprawie Warunków Technicznych, Jakim Powinny Odpowiadać Budynki i Ich Usytuowanie [Regulation of the Minister of Infrastructure and Construction of 14 November 2017 Amending the Regulation on Technical Conditions to be Met by Buildings and Their Location]. Available online: https://isap.sejm.gov.pl/isap.nsf/DocDetails.xsp?id=WDU20170002285 (accessed on 6 August 2025).
54. KOBiZE, 2021, Wskaźniki Emisji Zanieczyszczeń ze Spalania Paliw dla Źródeł o Nominalnej Mocy Cieplnej do 5 MW, Zastosowane do Automatycznego Wyliczenia Emisji w Raporcie do Krajowej Bazy za 2020 r. [Emission Factors for Pollutants Produced by Fuel Combustion for Sources with Nominal Thermal Power of up to 5 MW, Used for Automatic Emission Calculation in the Report to the National Database for 2020]. Available online: https://krajowabaza.kobize.pl/docs/MATERIAL_wskazniki_male_kotly_2020.pdf (accessed on 6 August 2025).

55. KOBiZE, 2020, Wskaźniki Emisyjności CO_2, SO_2, NOx, CO i Pyłu Całkowitego dla Energii Elektrycznej na Podstawie Informacji Zawartych w Krajowej Bazie o Emisjach Gazów Cieplarnianych i Innych Substancji za 2019 rok [CO_2, SO_2, NOx, CO and Total Particulate Matter Emission Factors for Electricity Based on Information Contained in the National Database on Greenhouse Gas and Other Substance Emissions for 2019]. Available online: https://www.kobize.pl/uploads/materialy/materialy_do_pobrania/wskazniki_emisyjnosci/Wskazniki_emisyjnosci_grudzien_2020.pdf (accessed on 6 August 2025).
56. Rashad, M.; Żabnieńska-Góra, A.; Norman, L.; Jouhara, H. Analysis of energy demand in a residential building using TRNSYS. *Energy* **2022**, *254*, 124357. [CrossRef]
57. Bergel, T.; Kotowski, T.; Woyciechowska, O. Daily water consumption for household purposes and its variability in a rural household. *J. Ecol. Eng.* **2016**, *17*, 47–52. [CrossRef]
58. Franco, A.; Miserocchi, L.; Test, D. A method for optimal operation of HVAC with heat pumps for reducing the energy demand of large-scale non residential buildings. *J. Build. Eng.* **2021**, *43*, 103175. [CrossRef]
59. Heracleous, C.; Michael, A.; Savvides, A.; Hayles, C. A methodology to assess energy-demand savings and cost-effectiveness of adaptation measures in educational buildings in the warm Mediterranean region. *Energy Rep.* **2022**, *8*, 5472–5486. [CrossRef]
60. Leiria, D.; Johra, H.; Marszal-Pomiarnowska, A.; Pomianowski, M.Z. A methodology to estimate space heating and domestic hot water energy demand profile in residential buildings from low-resolution heat meter data. *Energy* **2023**, *263*, 125705. [CrossRef]
61. Kaczmarczyk, M.; Książek, R.; Hałaj, E.; Gdowska, K.; Kapłan, R.; Pełka, G.; Luboń, W. Assessing discrepancies in heat demand: A case study of diverse energy management systems within the energy performance certificate framework in a student's dormitory. *Energy Builds* **2025**, *329*, 115235. [CrossRef]
62. Martínez-de-Alegría, I.; Río, R.M.; Zarrabeitia, E.; Alvarez, I. Heating demand as an energy performance indicator: A case study of buildings built under the passive house standard in Spain. *Energy Policy* **2021**, *159*, 112604. [CrossRef]
63. Li, L.; Sun, W.; Hu, W.; Sun, Y. Impact of natural and social environmental factors on building energy consumption: Based on bibliometrics. *J. Build. Eng.* **2001**, *37*, 102136. [CrossRef]

energies

MDPI

Article

Thermomechanical Analysis of the GTM 400 MOD Turbojet Engine Nozzle During Kerosene and Hydrogen Co-Combustion

Łukasz Brodzik [1,*], Bartosz Ciupek [1,*], Andrzej Frąckowiak [1] and Dominik Schroeder [2]

1 Institute of Thermal Energy, Faculty of Environmental Engineering and Energy, Poznan University of Technology, 5 M. Sklodowska-Curie Square, 60-965 Poznan, Poland; andrzej.frackowiak@put.poznan.pl
2 Faculty of Environmental Engineering and Energy, Poznan University of Technology, 5 M. Sklodowska-Curie Square, 60-965 Poznan, Poland; dominik.schroeder@student.put.poznan.pl
* Correspondence: lukasz.brodzik@put.poznan.pl (Ł.B.); bartosz.ciupek@put.poznan.pl (B.C.)

Abstract

This study investigated the thermomechanical behaviour of the nozzle of a GTM 400MOD miniature turbojet engine during combustion of aviation kerosene and co-combustion of kerosene with hydrogen. Numerical analysis was based on experiments conducted on a dedicated test rig at engine speeds ranging from 31,630 rpm to 65,830 rpm, providing data on the temperature and dynamic pressure at the nozzle outlet. These data served as input to numerical analyses using the ANSYS Fluent, Steady-State Thermal, and Static Structural modules to evaluate exhaust gas flow, temperature distribution, and stress and strain states. The paper performed a basic analysis with additional simplifications, and an extended analysis that took into account, among other things, thermal radiation in the flow. The results of the basic analysis show that, at comparable thrust levels, co-firing and pure kerosene combustion yield similar nozzle temperature distributions, with maximum wall temperatures ranging from 978 K to 1090 K, which remain below the allowable limit of 1193 K (920 °C). Maximum stresses reached approximately 261 MPa, close to but not exceeding the yield strength of 316 stainless steel. Maximum nozzle deformation did not exceed 0.8 mm. Small dynamic pressure fluctuations were observed; For example, at 31,630 rpm, co-firing increased the maximum dynamic pressure from 1.56 × 104 Pa to 1.63 × 104 Pa, while at 47,110 rpm, it decreased from 4.05 × 104 Pa to 3.89 × 104 Pa. The extended analysis yielded similar values for the nozzle temperature and pressure distributions. Stress and strain increased by more than 76% and 78%, respectively, compared to the baseline analysis. The results confirm that hydrogen co-firing does not significantly alter the nozzle thermomechanical loads, suggesting that this emission-free fuel can be used without negatively impacting the nozzle's structural integrity under the tested conditions. The methodology, combining targeted experimental measurements with coupled CFD and FEM simulations, provides a reliable framework for assessing material safety margins in alternative fuel applications in small turbojet engines.

Keywords: miniature turbojet engine; combustion; aviation kerosene; hydrogen; thermomechanical analysis

1. Introduction

Modern aviation engineering faces increasing challenges in optimizing combustion processes and reducing harmful emissions from aircraft engines. One of the most promising research directions is the development and implementation of alternative aviation fuels that can lower the environmental footprint while maintaining or improving propulsion efficiency. Hydrogen is of particular interest due to its high energy content per unit mass and the absence of carbon in its molecular structure, which eliminates direct carbon dioxide emissions during combustion. When co-combusted with conventional fuels such as aviation kerosene, hydrogen can contribute to a reduction in nitrogen oxides (NO_x) emissions, improve combustion stability, and potentially enhance overall engine performance.

Despite these advantages, the use of hydrogen in aviation presents significant technical challenges. These include its influence on combustion temperature, flame characteristics, and the resulting thermal and mechanical loads on engine components. Understanding these effects is crucial for ensuring operational safety, material durability, and optimal engine efficiency. Miniature turbojet engines provide an effective and cost-efficient platform for experimental and numerical studies on hydrogen and kerosene co-combustion, enabling detailed analysis of flow, heat transfer, and structural behaviour under controlled conditions.

Intensive research is being conducted on fuels with reduced greenhouse gas emissions that maintain or improve the energy efficiency of aircraft engines [1–3]. In particular, studies focus on the co-combustion of fossil fuels such as aviation kerosene (e.g., JET A-1) with hydrogen, aiming to reduce CO_2 and NO_x emissions while preserving engine performance and reliability [4,5]. Miniature turbojet engines, such as the GTM 400 MOD, are widely used for analyzing thermomechanical processes during combustion due to their compact size and simplified design. For example, Yan et al. [6] developed a multispectral radiation thermometry method for measuring turbine blade temperatures without assuming emissivity, achieving deviations of less than 50 K compared with conventional thermocouples. Li et al. [7] improved turbojet performance using a supersonic preconditioner with microchannels, increasing the Mach number to 3.35 and thrust by 39.8%. Sogut [8] analysed hybrid propulsion systems for UAVs, reporting an average energy efficiency of 38 % and identifying significant potential for optimization.

Experimental platforms allow precise assessment of how different fuel mixtures affect engine operation, particularly regarding combustion stability and component durability. Beltrán et al. [9] showed that advanced micromixing techniques can reduce NO_x emissions during hydrogen combustion, while highlighting gaps in material selection and burner geometry design that remain barriers to industrial adoption. The exhaust nozzle plays a critical role in exhaust gas expansion and thrust generation [10], and must withstand high thermal and mechanical stresses, especially when operating with fuels that alter flame temperature and flow characteristics [11]. Strategies such as nozzle profiling, high-temperature coatings, and active cooling [12,13] can improve durability.

Numerical methods, including computational fluid dynamics (CFD) and finite element analysis (FEA), have become essential tools for these studies. CFD enables accurate modelling of exhaust flows and their influence on performance and emissions, while FEA predicts thermal stresses and potential structural damage. Recent work has combined CFD with optimization algorithms [14] and rotor-motion modelling [15] to improve prediction accuracy, while studies on air–fuel ratio effects [16] have advanced understanding of combustion efficiency.

Research into green gaseous fuels, including hydrogen, has demonstrated performance benefits. Sekar [17] reported that injecting a hydrogen–biogas mixture into a turbojet engine increased maximum thrust by 4.5 % and reduced fuel consumption by 2.2 %, with potential to mitigate NO_x emissions through optimized injection strategies. Aygun et al. [18] used multi-objective optimization methods to evaluate small turbojet engine (STJE) performance under varying turbine inlet temperature, compressor pressure ratio, and ambient conditions, identifying trade-offs between thrust and specific fuel consumption. Wang et al. [19]

proposed a multi-stage precooling–compression cycle to enhance high-speed turbojet performance, while Cican et al. [20] evaluated alcohol–kerosene blends in micro turbojets, finding reductions in CO_2 emissions but with efficiency trade-offs.

Other relevant studies include Lee et al. [21], who developed an integrated simulation model for micro gas turbines with secondary flow and combustion efficiency effects, achieving performance prediction errors below 5 %. Xu [22] examined particulate number emissions from micro-turbojets, identifying higher non-volatile PM compared with micro-piston engines, and Cican et al. [23] explored exhaust nozzle chevron geometries for noise reduction and improved shear layer mixing.

However, the literature provides limited data on stresses generated in the nozzle during kerosene–hydrogen co-combustion. Most studies address combustion characteristics, emissions, or mixing processes without assessing structural impacts under realistic operating conditions. This study addresses that gap by experimentally measuring outlet nozzle temperature and dynamic pressure, and by performing coupled CFD–FEA simulations to evaluate temperature distribution, stress, and deformation for kerosene combustion and kerosene–hydrogen co-combustion at comparable thrust levels. The results provide new insight into the thermomechanical implications of hydrogen use in turbojet propulsion.

This paper involved both basic and extended numerical analysis. The basic analysis takes into account a smaller number of phenomena occurring during gas flow through the nozzle. Some of the coefficients related to steel properties were also simplified, i.e., not related to temperature. More detailed information is included in the Methods section.

2. Methods

Numerical studies were performed on the exhaust nozzle geometry of the JETPOL (Poznan, Poland) GTM400 MOD turbojet engine, shown in Figure 1. This is a miniature single-flow engine fuelled with JET A-1 kerosene and hydrogen. The analysis was performed for rotational speeds of 31,630 rpm, 47,110 rpm, 64,200 rpm, and 65,830 rpm. For the first two speeds, the simulation assumed the engine was fuelled with kerosene, and then with kerosene and hydrogen. For the last two speeds, the lower value corresponds to kerosene combustion, and the higher value corresponds to hydrogen combustion. A more detailed description of the engine and hydrogen system is included in [24]. The experiment, along with kerosene and hydrogen consumption values for assumed engine speeds, is presented in [5].

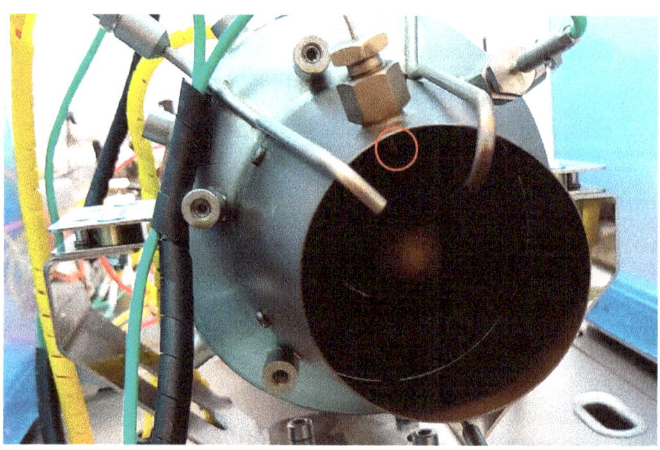

Figure 1. Engine exhaust nozzle with the location of the temperature sensor marked with a red circle. [own source].

In the first stage of the analysis, the flow through the exhaust nozzle was simulated as shown in Figure 2 and Table 1. The ANSYS Fluent (ver. R1, 2025) computational environment was used for the calculations. The goal was to determine the thermal load distribution on the inner wall of the exhaust nozzle.

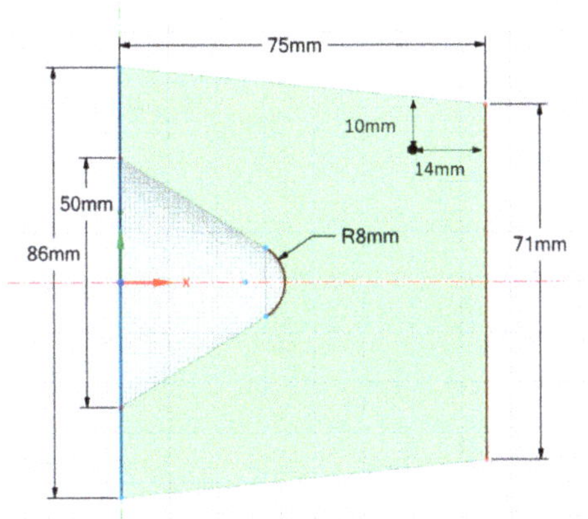

Figure 2. Location of the measuring point in the outlet nozzle. [own source].

Table 1. Boundary conditions for Fluent analysis.

Fuel Type	Rotation Speed [rpm]	Inlet and Outlet Temperature [K]	Gas Velocity at Inlet [m/s]	Heat Transfer Coefficient for Wall and Cone [W/(m^2· K)]
kerosene	31,630	1047	130	159.9
kerosene and hydrogen	31,630	1088	133	158.7
kerosene	47,110	1076	209	228.9
kerosene and hydrogen	47,110	1002	205	234.4
kerosene	64,200	1000	298	316.2
kerosene and hydrogen	65,830	978	306	327.1

To simulate the flow inside the nozzle, it was necessary to solve the basic equations of fluid motion. The first equation is the continuity equation:

$$\frac{\partial \rho}{\partial t} + (\rho \mathrm{v}_i)_{,i} = 0 \tag{1}$$

where ρ is the fluid density, kg/m^3, t is time, s, and v_i $(i = 1,2,3)$ are velocity vectors in the Cartesian coordinate system, m/s. In pointer notation, the expression $(\rho \mathrm{v}_i)_{,i}$ means $\mathrm{div}\left(\rho \vec{\mathrm{v}}\right)$.

The second equation is the conservation of momentum equation:

$$\rho\left(\frac{\partial \mathrm{v}_i}{\partial t} + \mathrm{v}_j \mathrm{v}_{i,j}\right) = \sigma_{ji,j} + \rho \mathrm{F}_i \tag{2}$$

where σ_{ji} $(i = 1,2,3)$, $j = (1,2,3)$ is the stress tensor $\sigma_{ji} = \sigma_{ij}$, F_i is the external force, N. The constitutive relations between the stress tensor and the strain rate for a Newtonian fluid are given by

$$\sigma_{ij} = -\left(p + \frac{2}{3}\mu v_{k,k}\right)\delta_{ij} + \mu\left(v_{i,j} + v_{j,i}\right) \tag{3}$$

where p is the pressure, Pa, μ is the dynamic viscosity coefficient, Pa·s, consistent with Satherland's law, δ_{ij} is the Kronecker symbol.

The third equation is the energy conservation equation:

$$\rho\left(\frac{\partial e}{\partial t} + \mathrm{v}_i e_{,i}\right) = \sigma_{ij}\mathrm{v}_{j,i} - q_{i,i} \quad (4)$$

where e is the internal energy, J, k is the thermal conductivity coefficient for air, W/(mK), and q is the heat flux determined from Fourier's law $q_i = -kT_{,i}$, W/m^2, T is the temperature, K.

Equations (1)–(4) were solved numerically using the finite volume method.

The above equations are valid for laminar flows. For real flow, the presence of vortex flows must be taken into account. Their behaviour is reflected in various turbulence models. The SST k–ω model was used for the described analysis due to its advantages in calculating parameters related to both free flows and boundary layers [25,26]. This model accurately simulates jet separation and is less susceptible to errors when boundary conditions change, which makes it numerically stable. Additionally, it is characterized by moderate computational requirements, making it a common choice for CFD analyses.

In the analysis of gas flow through the nozzle, the boundary conditions were temperature and gas velocity. The dynamic pressure and temperature were defined at the outlet. Heat transfer was determined by convection on the nozzle inner wall and turbine cone. The wall thickness was assumed to be 3 mm. Calculations were performed for an ambient pressure of 100,330 Pa. The boundary conditions are presented in Table 1. The gas velocities used in the table were estimated based on the dynamic pressure measured during the experiment. The heat transfer coefficient results assumed for the boundary condition are explained in the next step and are based on the data in Table 2.

Table 2. Parameter values used for calculations using Formula (5).

Inlet and Outlet Temperature [K]	Reynolds Number [-]	Nusselt Number [-]	Prandtl Number [-]
1047	85,920	179.9	0.733
1088	82,058	173.6	0.735
1076	131,005	252.3	0.734
1002	144,746	272.8	0.731
1000	210,796	368.5	0.731
978	224,561	387.4	0.730

In the second stage, the Steady-State Thermal module was used. Based on the calculations, the temperature distribution across the entire model was obtained. In this case, the temperature field on the inner wall of the outlet nozzle was mapped. This distribution constituted one of the boundary conditions used in the calculations. Convection was assumed to occur on the outer and inner walls of the outlet nozzle. The convection coefficient value varied as a function of temperature and was determined based on the empirical Dittus–Boelter correlation for turbulent flow in smooth tubes [27]:

$$Nu = 0.023Re^{0.8}Pr^{0.4} \quad (5)$$

where Nu is the Nusselt number, Re is the Reynolds number, and Pr is the Prandtl number.

This correlation is widely applied in engineering heat transfer calculations for estimating convective heat transfer coefficients in turbulent internal flows.

The results are presented in Table 2.

The same values for this parameter were assumed in the ANSYS Fluent analysis.

As described above, in the thermal analysis, heat transfer with the initial condition:

$$T = T_0 \tag{6}$$

In the three-dimensional model of the nozzle, it was calculated according to the following formula:

$$\rho c_p \frac{\partial T}{\partial t} = \nabla(\mathrm{k}\nabla T) \tag{7}$$

where k is the thermal conductivity coefficient changing under the considered direction in the Cartesian coordinate system, and $\frac{\partial T}{\partial t}$ is assumed to be $T = \text{const.}$

In the inner and outer walls, the heat transfer was calculated according to the boundary condition of the third type:

$$-k\nabla T = \alpha\left(T - T_f\right) \tag{8}$$

where α is the heat transfer coefficient, $\mathrm{W}/\left(\mathrm{m}^2{\cdot}\mathrm{K}\right)$ and T_f is the fluid temperature, K.

For the last nozzle wall (turbine side), the following condition was assumed:

$$\frac{\partial T}{\partial n} = 0 \tag{9}$$

The remaining air parameters were as shown in Table 3.

Table 3. Air parameters for tested rotational speeds.

Rotational Speed [rpm]	Temperature [K]	Density [kg/m^3]	Flow Velocity [m/s]	Dynamic Viscosity Coefficient [Pa· s]	Thermal Conductivity Coefficient [W/(m· K)]
31,630	1047	0.334	145.7	4.47×10^{-5}	0.0702
31,630 *	1088	0.321	148.5	4.58×10^{-5}	0.0722
47,110	1076	0.325	232.5	4.56×10^{-5}	0.0717
47,110 *	1002	0.349	228.2	4.35×10^{-5}	0.0679
64,200	1000	0.349	332.0	4.34×10^{-5}	0.0678
65,830 *	978	0.357	340.7	4.28×10^{-5}	0.0667

* a mixture of kerosene and hydrogen.

In the third stage of the analysis, the temperature distribution in the entire structure of the outlet nozzle calculated in the second stage was implemented and served as input data for calculations in ANSYS Static Structural, Figure 3.

In addition, a fixed support boundary condition was applied to the inner wall of the nozzle flange, and an average pressure acting on the inner wall was imposed, Figure 4. This condition was applied due to the attachment of the remaining part of the engine to the housing at this point.

This pressure was estimated based on flow analysis. The exact input data values are presented in Table 4. The mechanism of small quasi-static deformations of materials behaving according to Hooke's law is described by conservative laws, i.e., conservation of mass, momentum, and energy. In addition to conservative laws, a constitutive law is necessary to fully describe the solid-state case under consideration. Using Duhamel–Neumann's law, the relationship between temperature change and stress in a material can be expressed as follows:

$$\sigma_{ij} = 2\mu_L\varepsilon_{ij} + (\lambda_L e - \beta\Delta T)\delta_{ij} \tag{10}$$

where the Lame constant μ_L

$$\mu_L = \frac{E}{2(1+\nu)} \tag{11}$$

the Lame constant λ_L

$$\lambda_L = \frac{2\nu\mu_L}{1-2\nu} \quad (12)$$

thermoelastic constant β

$$\beta = \alpha(3\lambda_L + 2\mu_L) \quad (13)$$

temperature difference

$$\Delta T = T - T_{s-f} \quad (14)$$

where E is Young's modulus, Pa; ε_{ij} is the strain; e is expansion (the first strain invariant); T_{s-f} is stress-free temperature; ν is Poisson's ratio; and α is thermal expansion coefficient, 1/K.

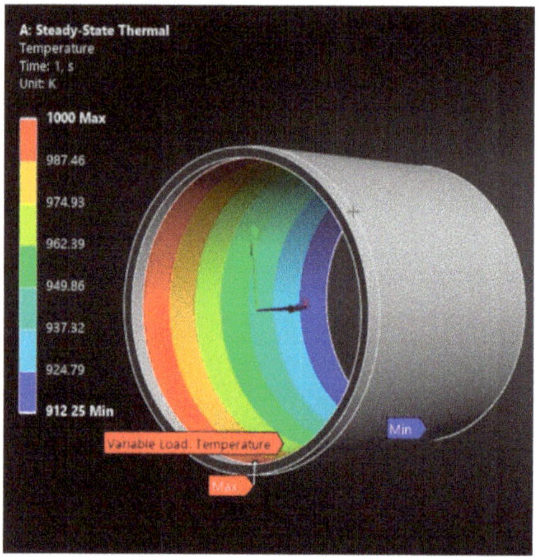

Figure 3. The given temperature distribution on the inner surface of the outlet nozzle model.

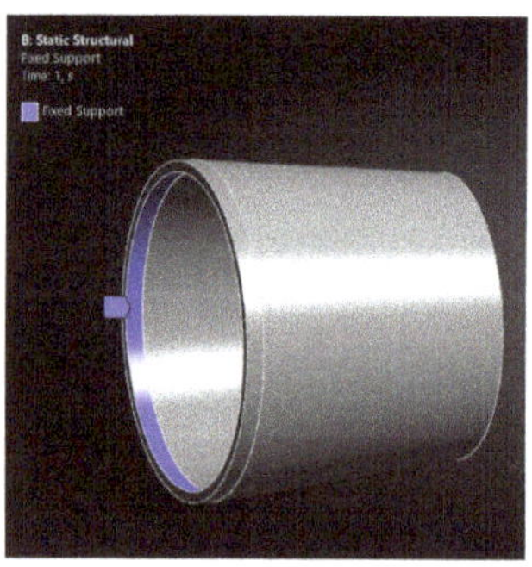

Figure 4. Fixed the support condition in the outlet nozzle.

Strength calculations were performed using the finite element method.

The remaining properties of the adopted material, i.e., 316 stainless steel, for the outlet nozzle model are presented below, Table 5. All described analyses were additionally simplified due to the stationary condition, which means that the parameter values did not change over time.

Table 4. Boundary conditions for strength analysis.

Fuel Type	Rotation Speed [rpm]	Absolute Pressure Inside the Nozzle [Pa]	Heat Transfer Coefficient for the Wall [W/(m^2· K)]
kerosene	31,630	113,330	159.9
kerosene and hydrogen	31,630	113,830	158.7
kerosene	47,110	133,430	228.9
kerosene and hydrogen	47,110	132,230	234.4
kerosene	64,200	167,830	316.2
kerosene and hydrogen	65,830	171,430	327.1

Table 5. Nozzle material properties.

Parameter	Value and Unit
Density	7990 [kg/m^3]
Modulus of elasticity	200 [GPa]
Specific heat	500 [J/(kg· K)]
Isotropic coefficient of thermal conductivity	16.3 [W/(m· K)]
Isotropic coefficient of thermal expansion	1.2×10^{-5} [1/K]

The basic analysis, described above, was extended with additional calculations and consideration of additional phenomena. Firstly, thermal radiation was included in the gas flow analysis. In ANSYS, the radiative transfer equation was solved using the Discrete Ordinates model. This model assumed a temperature-dependent thermal emissivity coefficient. Secondly, in the analysis of gas flow through the nozzle, the thermal conductivity coefficient was also dependent on temperature. Thirdly, in the strength analysis, the ther-mal expansion coefficient was dependent on temperature. All these coefficients are pre-sented in Table 6.

Table 6. Thermal emissivity, isotropic coefficient of thermal conductivity, and isotropic coefficient of thermal expansion dependent on temperature for extended analysis.

Temperature [K]	Thermal Emissivity [-]	Isotropic Coefficient of Thermal Conductivity [W/(m·K)]	Isotropic Coefficient of Thermal Expansion [1/K]
300	0.2	16	1.59×10^{-5}
400		17	$1.65 \times \cdot 10^{-5}$
500	0.3	18	
600		18.5	1.77×10^{-5}
700		19	
800	0.46	19.5	1.89×10^{-5}
900	0.52	20	
1000		20.5	2×10^{-5}
1100	0.61		2.05×10^{-5}

3. Flow Analysis Results in the Nozzle Model

The numerical analysis used the temperature measured during the experimental tests. The temperature was recorded using a thermocouple located near the nozzle outlet, Figure 5. The graph shows the temperature distribution for kerosene combustion as averaged. The average temperature value was determined based on tests conducted under various ambient conditions. Figure 5 also presents the values obtained during the experiment on which the numerical analysis was based. Verification of the operating parameters resulted from maintaining the engine speed for a certain period of time to achieve temperature measurement stabilization. For simplicity, this parameter was assumed constant across the entire nozzle outlet cross-section.

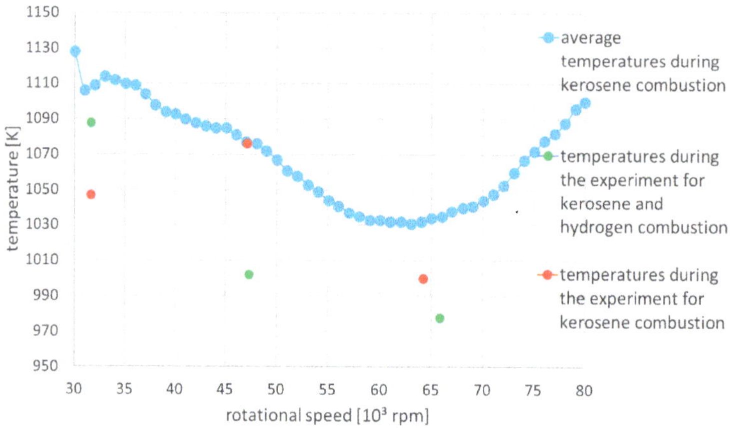

Figure 5. Results of local temperature measurement in the nozzle during experimental tests.

The analysis considered three engine operation cases for kerosene and kerosene with hydrogen combustion. The first case involved a rotational speed of 31,630 rpm in both cases. The second case involved a speed of 47,110 rpm, for which the engine also operated in both combustion modes considered. The third case involved two different rotational speeds, i.e., 64,200 rpm and 65,830 rpm. The lower value concerns kerosene combustion, while the higher value concerns kerosene and hydrogen co-combustion. In this situation, the engine produces almost the same thrust for both different speeds, i.e., 157.9 N for kerosene and 157.0 N for both fuels co-combustion. In the case of kerosene combustion for speeds 31,630 rpm and 47,110 rpm, thrust is 22.6 N and 64.7 N, respectively. In the case of kerosene and hydrogen co-combustion for speeds 31,630 rpm and 47,110 rpm, thrust is 26.5 N and 70,6 N, respectively. The dynamic pressure field for the considered cases is presented in Figures 6–8.

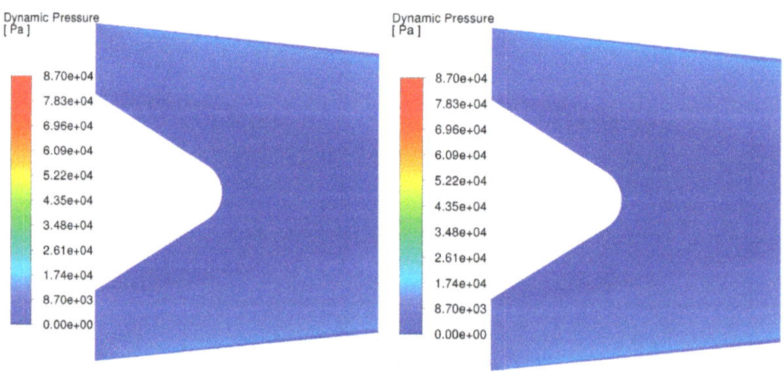

Figure 6. Dynamic pressure distribution in the outlet nozzle for a speed of 31,630 rpm during kerosene combustion (**left**) and kerosene and hydrogen co-combustion (**right**)—basic analysis.

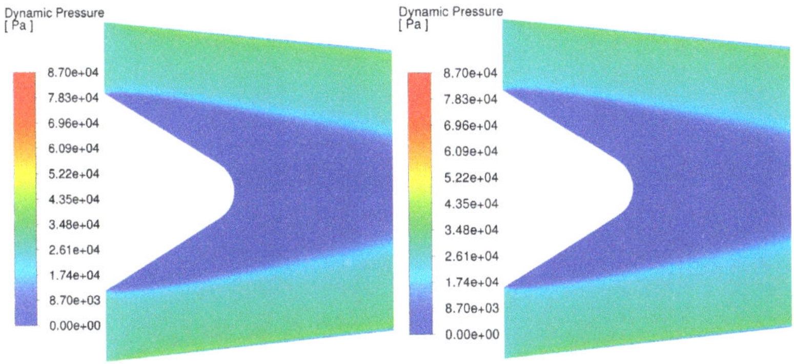

Figure 7. Dynamic pressure distribution in the outlet nozzle for a speed of 47,110 rpm during kerosene combustion (**left**) and kerosene and hydrogen co-combustion (**right**)—basic analysis.

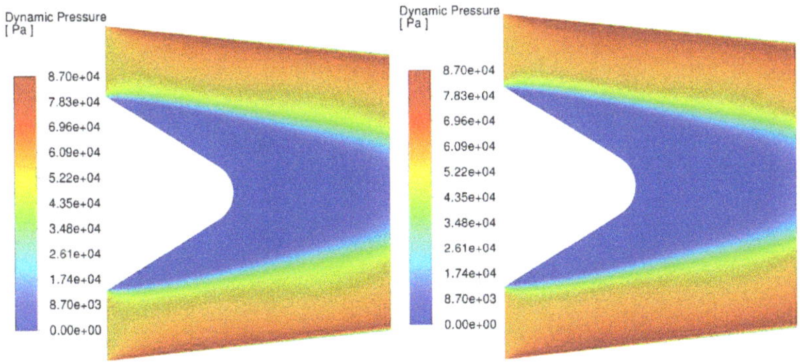

Figure 8. Dynamic pressure distribution in the outlet nozzle for a speed of 64,200 rpm during kerosene combustion (**left**) and for a speed of 65,830 rpm during co-combustion of kerosene and hydrogen (**right**)—basic analysis.

Numerical calculations showed that the dynamic pressure, and therefore the speed, increased for kerosene and hydrogen co-combustion at rotational speeds of 31,630 rpm and 65,830 rpm. For a speed of 47,110 rpm in this combustion mode, a reduction in the dynamic pressure was recorded, Table 7. This direction of change is in contradiction to the thrust, which increased for kerosene and hydrogen co-combustion compared to kerosene combustion alone. It should be remembered that there is a gradient in exhaust gas velocity in the exhaust cross-section, and during the experiment, the static and total pressures were measured at a single point. Adopting the simplification of the analysis, which involves assuming a point-measured value for the entire exhaust cross-section, may sometimes result in an unphysical change in the direction of the dynamic pressure drop due to local flow disturbances during the experiment.

A lower-velocity flow region forms in the central part. This is due to the cone located in the centre of the nozzle, which is swept by gas during engine operation. A lower-velocity region also occurs at the edge of the nozzle wall. Its thickness increases towards the engine's exhaust cross-section. This is related to the loss of exhaust gas energy, which increases with distance from the turbine section due to friction between fluid particles and the nozzle wall.

In the case of the extended analysis, adding the additional conditions described in the Methods section did not result in a significantly different dynamic pressure distribution, Table 7. These conditions are related to heat transfer and stresses in the nozzle material; therefore, their impact on the flow character analysis is limited. Due to the very similar results for the considered rotational speeds, the pressure distributions for this analysis are not presented.

Table 7. Maximum dynamic pressure in gas flow.

Fuel Type	Rotation Speed [rpm]	Maximum Dynamic Pressure [Pa] (Basic Analysis)	Maximum Dynamic Pressure [Pa] (Extended Analysis)
kerosene	31,630	1.56×10^4	1.58×10^4
kerosene and hydrogen	31,630	1.63×10^4	1.65×10^4
kerosene	47,110	4.05×10^4	4.10×10^4
kerosene and hydrogen	47,110	3.89×10^4	3.94×10^4
kerosene	64,200	8.25×10^4	8.36×10^4
kerosene and hydrogen	65,830	8.70×10^4	8.82×10^4

In each case considered, the highest temperature region is located near the turbine. The temperature field is presented in Figures 9–11. At higher engine speeds, co-combustion of kerosene and hydrogen resulted in a lower maximum temperature compared to combustion of kerosene alone. For the lowest engine speed, i.e., 31,630 rpm, the situation is reversed. This corresponds to the temperatures measured during the experiment (Figure 5). This change in the situation may be related to different engine operating settings at minimum engine speeds compared to higher engine speeds. It should be noted that there is a significant reduction in kerosene consumption compared to the situation where kerosene is the fuel source. The same phenomenon also occurs when the engine is fueled solely with kerosene. In this case, this deviates from the general trend of increasing kerosene consumption with decreasing engine speed. In the case of co-combustion, different control settings can be applied for both fuels. It is visible that hydrogen consumption increases significantly with decreasing engine speed.

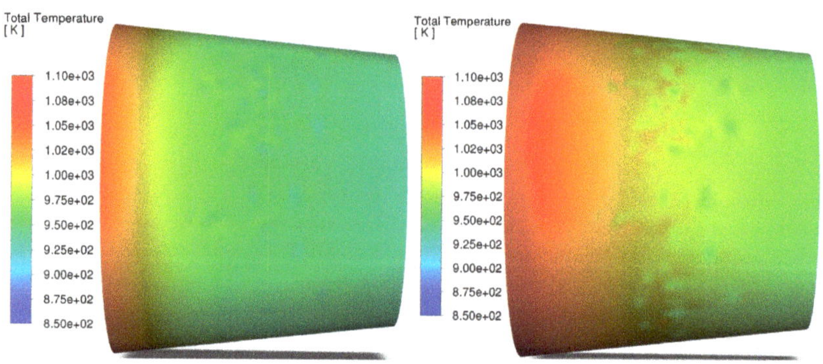

Figure 9. Temperature distribution in the outlet nozzle for a speed of 31,630 rpm during kerosene combustion (**left**) and kerosene and hydrogen co-combustion (**right**)—basic analysis.

The application of extended analysis, as with the pressure results, did not result in significant differences in the temperature distributions on the nozzle model wall (Table 8). The differences in this case reach several degrees Kelvin. This means that for these conditions, convection fully describes the temperature changes in the model domain under consideration. For this reason, the presentation of temperature distributions on the nozzle model wall was also omitted.

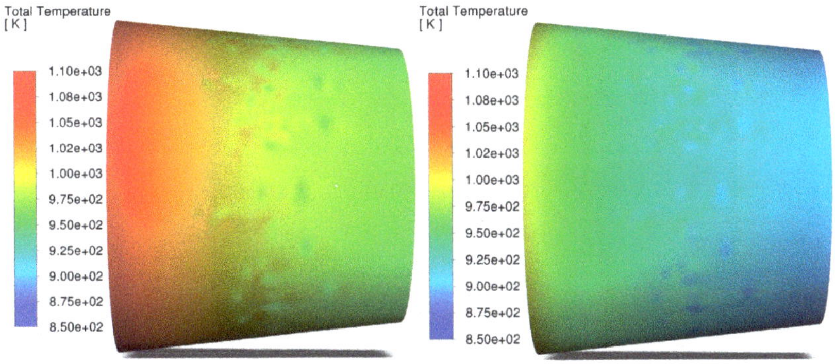

Figure 10. Temperature distribution in the outlet nozzle for a speed of 47,110 rpm during kerosene combustion (**left**) and kerosene and hydrogen co-combustion (**right**)—basic analysis.

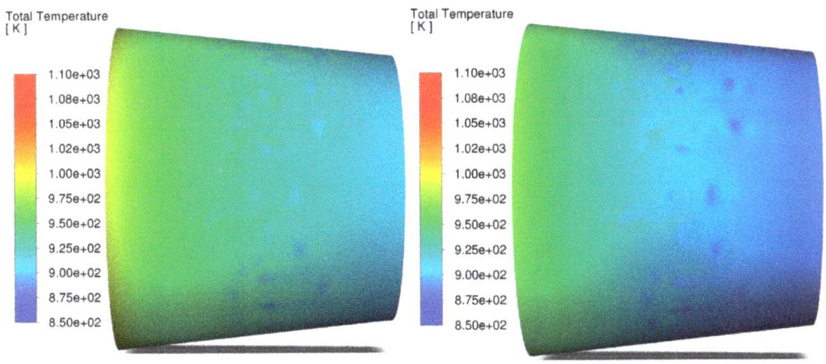

Figure 11. Temperature distribution in the outlet nozzle for a speed of 64,200 rpm during kerosene combustion (**left**) and for a speed of 65,830 rpm during co-combustion of kerosene and hydrogen (**right**)—basic analysis.

Table 8. Maximum wall temperature.

Fuel Type	Rotation Speed [rpm]	Maximum Temperature [K] (Basic Analysis)	Maximum Temperature [K] (Extended Analysis)
kerosene	31,630	1.05×10^3	1.05×10^3
kerosene and hydrogen	31,630	1.09×10^3	1.09×10^3
kerosene	47,110	1.08×10^3	1.08×10^3
kerosene and hydrogen	47,110	1.00×10^3	1.00×10^3
kerosene	64,200	1.00×10^3	1.00×10^3
kerosene and hydrogen	65,830	9.78×10^2	9.78×10^2

4. Results of Strength Analysis in the Nozzle

For the assumed rotational speeds, another strength analysis was performed in Ansys Mechanical. According to the assumptions described in the methods section, the temperature distribution in the nozzle was modelled, and strength calculations were performed. The temperature field was approximated based on the obtained distributions, Figures 9–11. Maximum temperature values are presented in Table 8.

Based on the assumed temperature distribution, the known coefficient of thermal expansion, and the given geometry dimensions, the stresses and strains of the exhaust nozzle model were calculated. The highest stresses in the solid occurred at the highest temperature points and are located near the turbine outlet. In the figures, stress is presented in the form of the equivalent von Mises stress, Figures 12–14.

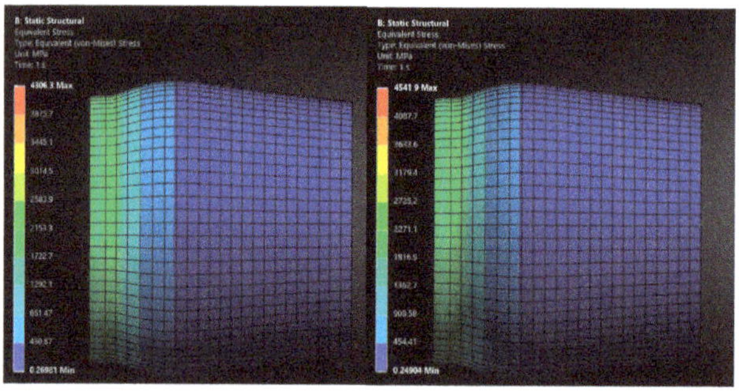

Figure 12. Stress distribution in the outlet nozzle at a speed of 31,630 rpm during kerosene combustion (**left**) and kerosene and hydrogen co-combustion (**right**)—basic analysis.

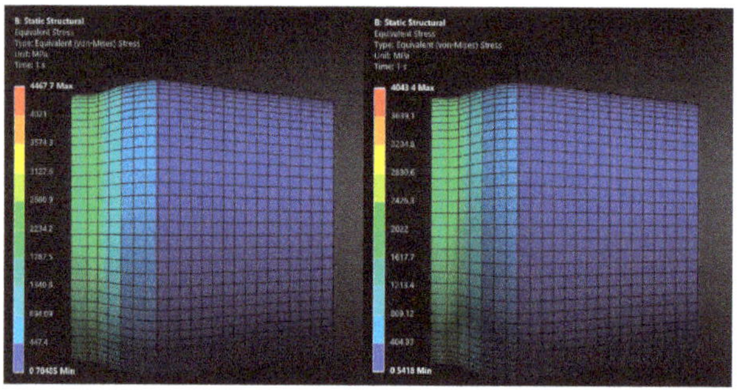

Figure 13. Stress distribution in the outlet nozzle at a speed of 47,110 rpm during kerosene combustion (**left**) and kerosene and hydrogen co-combustion (**right**)—basic analysis.

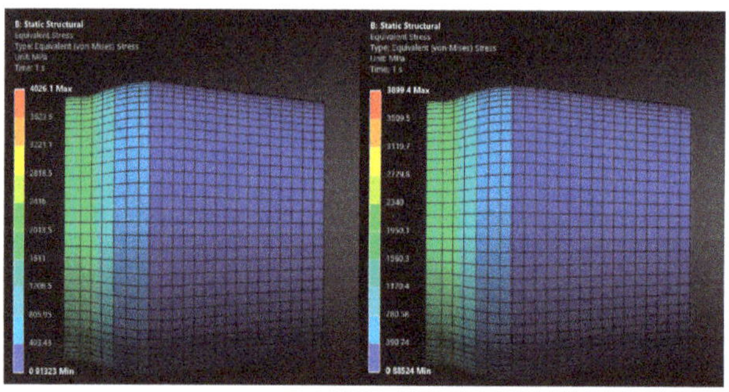

Figure 14. Stress distribution in the outlet nozzle for a speed of 64,200 rpm during kerosene combustion (**left**) and for a speed of 65,830 rpm during co-combustion of kerosene and hydrogen (**right**)—basic analysis.

In the nozzle model, the greatest deformation occurs near its outlet cross-section, Figures 15–17. As in the previous analyses, the nature of changes during hydrogen and kerosene co-combustion is the same as for kerosene combustion alone. The differences concern the values of the considered rotational speeds. Their magnitudes are not significant, and the deformation distribution is analogous to the stress distribution in the nozzle near the turbine. According to formula (10), the deformation in the unconstrained region changes proportionally to the change in stress at the constraint.

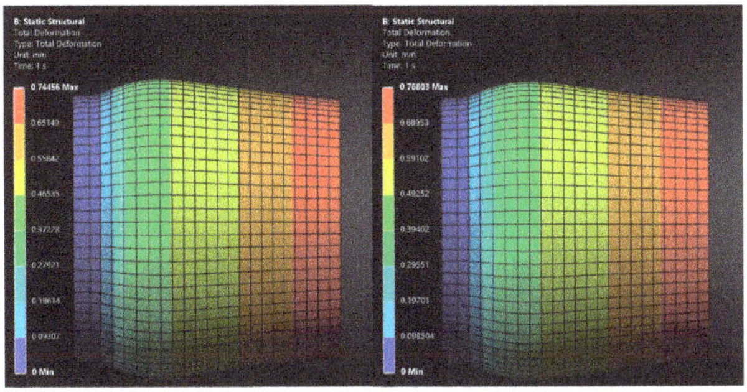

Figure 15. Deformation of the outlet nozzle at a speed of 31,630 rpm during kerosene combustion (**left**) and kerosene and hydrogen co-combustion (**right**)—basic analysis.

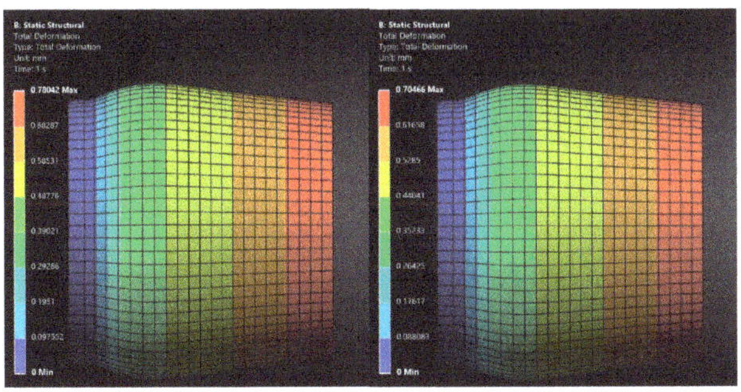

Figure 16. Deformation of the outlet nozzle at a speed of 47,110 rpm during kerosene combustion (**left**) and kerosene and hydrogen co-combustion (**right**)—basic analysis.

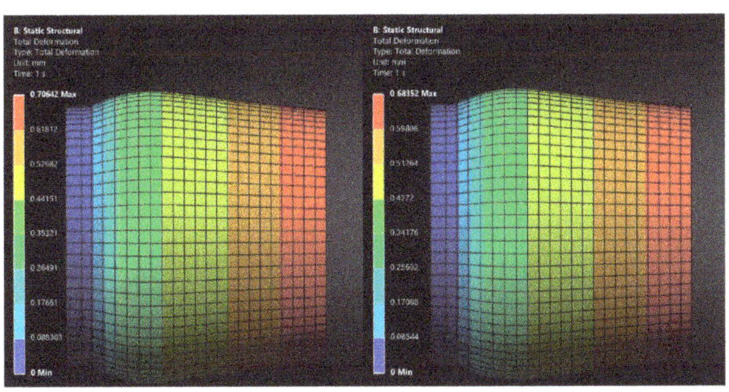

Figure 17. Deformation of the outlet nozzle at a speed of 64,200 rpm during kerosene combustion (**left**) and for a speed of 65,830 rpm during co-combustion of kerosene and hydrogen (**right**)—basic analysis.

The analysis showed that the maximum stresses in the nozzle model occurred at a rotational speed of 31,630 rpm for kerosene and hydrogen co-combustion and at a speed of 47,110 rpm for kerosene combustion. This stress was approximately 261 MPa. In these same cases, the greatest material deformation occurred, which was less than 0.8 mm. More detailed data on both parameters are provided in Tables 9 and 10.

Table 9. Maximum stress of the nozzle model.

Rotation Speed [rpm]	Maximum Stress on the Turbine Side [MPa] (Basic Analysis)	Maximum Stress on the Engine Outlet Side [MPa] (Basic Analysis)	Maximum Stress on the Turbine Side [MPa] (Extended Analysis)	Maximum Stress on the Engine Outlet Side [MPa] (Extended Analysis)
31,630	247.81	8.707	433.40	18.5
31,630 *	261.39	9.117	461.00	19.3
47,110	261.14	12.761	460.70	27.4
47,110 *	236.58	11.872	410.06	25.4
64,200	239.84	16.001	417.40	34.3
65,830 *	232.80	16.039	402.70	33.9

* a mixture of kerosene and hydrogen.

Table 10. Deformation of the nozzle model.

Rotation Speed [rpm]	Maximum Nozzle Deformation [mm] (Basic Analysis)	Maximum Nozzle Deformation [mm] (Extended Analysis)
31,630	0.744	1.34
31,630 *	0.788	1.41
47,110	0.780	1.40
47,110 *	0.704	1.25
64,200	0.706	1,26
65,830 *	0.684	1.21

* a mixture of kerosene and hydrogen.

The extended analysis showed that the maximum stresses that appeared in the nozzle model were 461 MPa. This represents 176.6% of the corresponding value for the basic analysis, Figure 18. This translated into an increase in deformation, which corresponds to 178.5% of the value obtained in the basic analysis, Figure 19. Because the maximum temperatures that appeared after the analysis did not exceed the maximum operating temperature, the obtained stress and deformation values are more unsatisfactory and unrealistic. This is primarily because the specified conditions are simplified. First, the set temperature for the flow is the same throughout the cross-section. When significant simplifications are applied, averaged values allow for obtaining results that are closer to those describing the actual phenomena. However, they will not enable a more differentiated presentation of parameter distributions, as would be the case with a larger number of measurement points from the experiment.

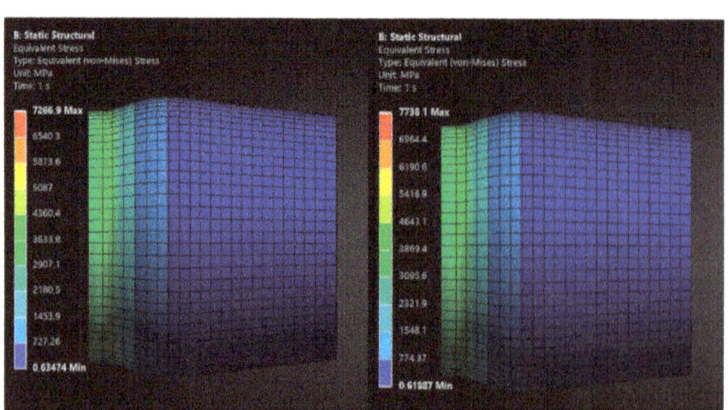

Figure 18. Stress distribution in the outlet nozzle at a speed of 31,630 rpm during kerosene combustion (**left**) and kerosene and hydrogen co-combustion (**right**)—extended analysis.

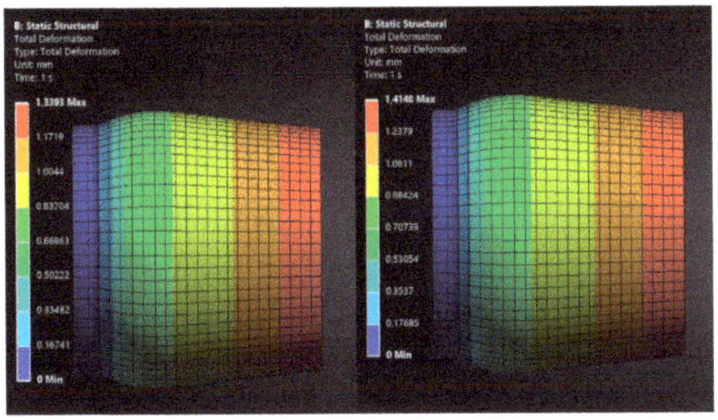

Figure 19. Deformation of the outlet nozzle at a speed of 31,630 rpm during kerosene combustion (**left**) and kerosene and hydrogen co-combustion (**right**)—extended analysis.

5. Conclusions

Based on the experimental measurements and numerical simulations presented in this study, the following conclusions can be drawn:

1. Thermomechanical loads remain within safe operational limits under kerosene and hydrogen co-combustion. The numerical analysis demonstrated that, for the examined engine rotational speeds (31,630 rpm to 65,830 rpm), the nozzle wall temperatures did not exceed the operational threshold of 920 °C (1193 K), ensuring thermal safety of the component. The overall distribution patterns of temperature, stress, and deformation remained similar regardless of the fuel type, indicating that co-combustion with hydrogen does not significantly alter the nozzle's thermomechanical behaviour compared to pure kerosene combustion.
2. For the basic analysis, the maximum stress values obtained in the nozzle reached approximately 261 MPa, located near the turbine outlet. For the extended analysis, the similarly located stress reached approximately 461 MPa. Given that the high-temperature yield strength of AISI 316 stainless steel decreases from ±150 MPa at 900 K to ±100 MPa at 1100 K [28], these stress levels suggest that local plastic deformation may occur under these thermal conditions. Despite the assumption of more accurate material properties, the obtained results, due to their magnitude, are less realistic. This means that calculations using more accurate material properties are more sensitive to the boundary conditions formulated for them.
3. Boundary condition simplifications lead to conservative stress overestimations. The application of a fully fixed support at the flange inner wall constrained the nozzle's natural thermal expansion, leading to an overestimation of axial stresses. In real operating conditions, the bolted flange connection allows for slight displacement, partially relieving thermally induced stresses. Additionally, the analysis was performed under stationary conditions with approximated temperature distributions and assumed heat transfer coefficients, which limits the precision of absolute stress values but provides a conservative estimation for comparative analysis.
4. Effect of hydrogen on nozzle loads is minor under tested conditions, but Measurement density is a limitation. The use of hydrogen affected the exhaust gas temperature nonlinearly across rotational speeds, increasing it at lower rpm (31,630 rpm) and slightly reducing it at higher rpm. However, due to the limited number of measurement points and nozzle geometry constraints, these effects appeared minor and localized in the numerical analysis. A more detailed experimental campaign with denser measurement grids would be required to capture subtle, localized differences in thermomechanical loads attributable to fuel type.

Author Contributions: Conceptualization, Ł.B. and B.C.; methodology, Ł.B. and B.C.; software, Ł.B. and B.C.; validation, Ł.B., B.C., A.F. and D.S.; formal analysis, Ł.B.; investigation, Ł.B.; resources, Ł.B.; data curation, Ł.B.; writing—original draft preparation, Ł.B. and B.C. and A.F.; writing—review and editing, Ł.B., B.C. and A.F.; visualization, Ł.B. and D.S.; supervision, Ł.B.; project administration, Ł.B. and B.C.; funding acquisition, Ł.B. and B.C. All authors have read and agreed to the published version of the manuscript.

Funding: This research was funded by the Polish Ministry of Science and Higher Education and the Poznan University of Technology's financial resources for statutory activity, grant numbers 0712/SBAD/5297 and 0712/SBAD/5298.

Data Availability Statement: The original contributions presented in this study are included in the article. Further inquiries can be directed to the corresponding authors.

Acknowledgments: We would like to sincerely thank Piotr W. Sielicki for his help in carrying out this experimental research.

Conflicts of Interest: The authors declare no conflicts of interest.

Nomenclature

CFD	Computational Fluid Dynamics
FEM	Finite Element Method
STJE	System Test and Joint Evaluation
UAV	Unmanned Aerial Vehicle

References

1. Wang, B.; Ting, Z.J.; Zhao, M. Sustainable aviation fuels: Key opportunities and challenges in lowering carbon emissions for the aviation industry. *Carbon Capture Sci. Technol.* **2024**, *13*, 100263. [CrossRef]
2. Xu, Z.; Fan, Y.; Zheng, Y.; Ding, S.; Zhu, M.; Li, G.; Wang, M.; Yu, Z.; Song, Y.; Chang, L.; et al. Emission reduction characteristics of heavy-fuel aircraft piston engine fueled with 100% HEFA sustainable aviation fuel. *Environ. Pollut.* **2025**, *368*, 125661. [CrossRef]
3. Brodzik, Ł.; Prokopowicz, W.; Ciupek, B.; Frąckowiak, A. Minimizing the Environmental Impact of Aircraft Engines with the Use of Sustainable Aviation Fuel (SAF) and Hydrogen. *Energies* **2025**, *18*, 472. [CrossRef]
4. Miniero, L.; Pandey, K.; De Falco, G.; D'Anna, A.; Noiray, N. Soot-free and low-NO combustion of Jet A-1 in a lean azimuthal flame (LEAF) combustor with hydrogen injection. *Proc. Combust. Inst.* **2023**, *39*, 4309–4318. [CrossRef]
5. Ciupek, B.; Brodzik, Ł.; Frąckowiak, A. Research on Carbon Footprint Reduction During Hydrogen Co-Combustion in a Turbojet Engine. *Energies* **2024**, *17*, 5397. [CrossRef]
6. Yan, W.; Li, T.; Xing, X.; Wang, X.; Liu, D. Experimental study on surface temperature and emissivity of rotating turbine blades of a micro turbojet engine. *Appl. Therm. Eng.* **2025**, *1248*, 25911. [CrossRef]
7. Li, H.; Zou, Z.; Chen, Y.; Du, P.; Fu, C.; Wang, Y. Experimental insights into thermal performance of a microtube precooler with drastic coolant properties variation and precooling impacts on turbojet engine operation. *Energy* **2023**, *278 Pt A*, 127916. [CrossRef]
8. Sogut, M.Z. Assessment of small-scale turbojet engine considering environmental and thermodynamics performance for flight processes. *Energy* **2020**, *200*, 117519. [CrossRef]
9. Beltrán, L.; Sandoval, J.; Llain, J.; Carmona, M.; Audivet, C.; Pugliese, V. Hydrogen combustion in micromix burners: Present stages, opportunities, and challenges. *Int. J. Hydrogen Energy* **2024**, *96*, 622–638. [CrossRef]
10. Sundararaj, R.H.; Sekar, T.C.; Arora, R.; Kushari, A. Effect of nozzle exit area on the performance of a turbojet engine. *Aerosp. Sci. Technol.* **2021**, *116*, 106844. [CrossRef]
11. Samal, S.; Tomášťík, J.; Václavek, L.; Chandra, M.; Kopeček, J.; Stachiv, I.; Šittner, P. Recovery of deformation surface of superelastic and shape memory NiTi alloy. *Appl. Surf. Sci. Adv.* **2025**, *25*, 100684. [CrossRef]
12. Yang, S.; Gao, S.; Xue, W.; Wu, B.; Duan, D. Phenomenological modeling of wear mechanisms between nickel-based superalloy blades and ceramic-based abradable coatings in turbomachines. *J. Mater. Res. Technol.* **2023**, *27*, 4191–4203. [CrossRef]
13. Kirubaharan, A.M.K.; Kuppusami, P.; Ghosh, C.; Priya, R.; Ningshen, S.; Kumar, D.D.; Divakar, R. Metal-ceramic diffusion barrier nanocomposite coatings on nickel based superalloys for corrosion and high temperature oxidation resistance. *Ceram. Int.* **2022**, *48*, 31281–31288. [CrossRef]
14. Ghahramani, Z.; Zareh, M.; Pourfarzaneh, H.; Pazooki, F. Optimization the TIT profile in an annular combustion of a turbojet engine based on smart modeling and CFD simulation. *J. Taiwan Inst. Chem. Eng.* **2023**, *148*, 104812. [CrossRef]

15. Xu, Y.; Deng, W.; Liu, X.; Xu, H.; Li, Z. Full engine 3D simulation scheme considering rotor motion for turbojet engine under crosswind conditions. *Appl. Therm. Eng.* **2025**, *269 Pt A*, 125951. [CrossRef]
16. Aygun, H. Effects of air to fuel ratio on parameters of combustor used for gas turbine engines: Applications of turbojet, turbofan, turboprop and turboshaft. *Energy* **2024**, *305*, 132346. [CrossRef]
17. Sekar, M. Gaseous fuel injection assisted with rich hydrogen content in turbojet engine for enhanced thrust and combustion efficiency. *Int. J. Hydrogen Energy* **2024**, *78*, 564–571. [CrossRef]
18. Aygun, H.; Kirmizi, M.; Kilic, U.; Turan, O. Multi-objective optimization of a small turbojet engine energetic performance. *Energy* **2023**, *271*, 126983. [CrossRef]
19. Wang, C.; Yu, X.; Ha, C.; Liu, Z.; Fang, J.; Qin, J.; Shao, J.; Huang, H. Thermodynamic analysis for a novel chemical precooling turbojet engine based on a multi-stage precooling-compression cycle. *Energy* **2023**, *262 Pt A*, 125352. [CrossRef]
20. Cican, G.; Silivestru, V.; Mirea, R.; Osman, S.; Popescu, F.; Sapunaru, O.V.; Ene, R. Performance and Emissions Assessment of a Micro-Turbojet Engine Fueled with Jet A and Blends of Propanol, Butanol, Pentanol, Hexanol, Heptanol, and Octanol. *Fire* **2025**, *8*, 150. [CrossRef]
21. Lee, D.; Chung, H.; Kang, Y.S.; Rhee, D.-H. A Study of an Integrated Analysis Model with Secondary Flow for Assessing the Performance of a Micro Turbojet Engine. *Appl. Sci.* **2024**, *14*, 7606. [CrossRef]
22. Xu, Z.; Wang, M.; Li, G.; Hu, X.; Yang, P.; Zhu, M.; Zhang, B.; Chang, L.; Chen, L. Experimental Investigation of Particulate Number Measurement Methodology for Micro-Turbojet Engine Emissions. *Aerospace* **2024**, *11*, 548. [CrossRef]
23. Cican, G.; Gall, M.; Bogoi, A.; Deaconu, M.; Crunțeanu, D.E. Experimental Investigation of a Micro Turbojet Engine Chevrons Nozzle by Means of the Schlieren Technique. *Inventions* **2023**, *8*, 145. [CrossRef]
24. Brodzik, Ł. Gas Temperature Distribution in the Combustion Chamber of a GTM400 MOD Turbojet Engine Powered by JET A-1 Fuel and Hydrogen. *Energies* **2024**, *17*, 745. [CrossRef]
25. Karim, M.M.; Rahman, M.M.; Alim, M.A. Performance of SST k-ω turbulence model for computation of viscous drag of axisymmetric underwater bodies. *Int. J. Eng.* **2011**, *24*, 139–146.
26. Costa Rocha, P.A.; Barbosa Rocha, H.H.; Moura Carneiro, F.O.; Vieira da Silva, M.E.; Valente Bueno, A. k-ω SST (shear stress transport) turbulence model calibration: A case study on a small-scale horizontal axis wind turbine. *Energy* **2014**, *65*, 412–418. [CrossRef]
27. Incropera, F.P.; DeWitt, D.P.; Bergman, T.L.; Lavine, A.S. *Fundamentals of Heat and Mass Transfer*, 7th ed.; Wiley: Hoboken, NJ, USA, 2011.
28. American Society of Mechanical Engineers. *ASME Boiler and Pressure Vessel Code, Section II, Part D—Properties (Metric)*, 2021st ed.; American Society of Mechanical Engineers: New York, NY, USA, 2021.

energies

MDPI

Article

Analysis of the Accuracy of the Inverse Marching Method Used to Determine Thermal Stresses in Cylindrical Pressure Components with Holes

Magdalena Jaremkiewicz

Faculty of Environmental and Energy Engineering, Cracow University of Technology, 31-155 Cracow, Poland; magdalena.jaremkiewicz@pk.edu.pl

Abstract

In the paper, the inverse solution of the heat conduction problem is analysed, which is applied to calculate transient thermal stresses on the internal surface of a thick-walled pipe weakened by a hole. The analysis considered a one-dimensional heat transfer problem when heat is transferred in a radial direction. In the inverse marching method, the measurement of the wall temperature at one point of a thermally insulated pipeline is used. The technique was verified regarding the distance between the point where the wall temperature is measured and the internal surface, the number of finite volumes in the inverse region, and the time step size are selected. The influence of these parameters on the accuracy of the calculated temperature, thermal stresses, heat transfer coefficient on the internal surface of the pipeline and thermal stresses at the hole edge was assessed. The reference values used to verify the technique were those calculated using the analytical method and the direct solution of the heat conduction problem, and the generated 'measurement data' were disturbed by random errors.

Keywords: thermal stresses; inverse heat conduction problem; finite volume method

1. Introduction

A literature review shows that many industries, including energy (nuclear, conventional, and renewable), metallurgy, semiconductors, automotive, aerospace, and even medicine, require correct determination of thermal stresses.

In recent years, the finite element method (FEM) has been the most widely described and used method for thermal stress analysis. Tools that also use computational fluid dynamics (CFD) are being improved for determining stresses, including thermal stresses, e.g., in research on additive manufacturing [1,2].

Monitoring thermal stress in conventional power generation is important for several reasons. The increasingly rapid development of renewable energy, primarily based on photovoltaics and wind power, characterised by unpredictability in electricity production, is resulting in the need to start up, shut down or change the load of power units more frequently. This, in turn, causes thermo-mechanical fatigue and creep in these units' equipment components, shortening their lifespan. In addition, older generating units often exceed their design service life. To ensure safe operation of the equipment, it is necessary to monitor the operating conditions of the power plant and assess the remaining service life. Knowledge of thermal stresses is also essential when determining the optimum heating or cooling rate of pressure components [3], where the condition of not exceeding the permissible stresses must be met.

Much of the work in the field of thermal stress determination concerns nuclear power plants [4–6], whose safe operation is particularly important. In [4,5], thermal stresses were determined in the corners of pressure vessel nozzles of nuclear reactors. In [4], this was calculated based on temperature gradients predicted in the cross-section and in [5], based on simple equations developed to predict the stress intensity factor. In both works, the methods developed were intended to replace FEM for determining thermal stresses due to the high computational costs of FEM in three-dimensional elements. Residual stresses resulting from thermal shocks in pressure components of nuclear power plants are also investigated. For example, in [6] the relationship between residual stresses and thermal stresses during thermal shock in a nuclear reactor pressure vessel was investigated.

Thermal stresses are also determined in steam turbines [7–9]. In [7], an algorithm was developed to determine stresses in critical turbine components (rotor, shut-off and control valves) and to optimise their start-up. In [8], thermal stresses were determined in the rotor of combined medium- and high-pressure turbine stages in a common case and compared to stresses in turbine rotors operating in separate cases. In [9], the existing procedures for starting and stopping steam turbines were evaluated regarding the thermal loads in the high-pressure turbine rotor. Ansys software was used in all studies.

In pressure components, the highest thermal stresses are on the internal surface of the component, being is washed by a working fluid at high pressure and temperature. European Standard EN 12952-3 [10] and TRD 301 [11] describe the procedures for determining stresses in thick-walled pressure components. Thermal stresses occurring in thick-walled pressure components not weakened by holes are determined based on the known temperature distribution across the wall thickness. In practice, thick-walled pressure elements have stubs, and the thermal stresses at the edge of the hole made in the shell are much greater. For this location, the thermal stresses calculated for an element not weakened by holes must be multiplied by the stress concentration factor determined based on the heat transfer coefficient on the inner surface [10], whereby the standard recommends using a constant and specified value for the heat transfer coefficient.

The unsteady temperature distribution and thermal stresses in a thick-walled cylindrical pressure element can be determined by solving a direct heat conduction problem using FEM. An example of such a solution, where the developed model uses the ambient temperature, the external surface temperature and the temperature of the working fluid inside the pipe, is presented in [12]. A second example, where, in turn, the working fluid temperature measured with a new design thermometer was used in the calculation algorithm and the pipeline was assumed to be thermally insulated, is presented in [13]. The newly designed thermometer allows for more accurate temperature measurements compared to the classical thermometers used in practice.

Another approach for calculating unsteady thermal stresses in thick-walled components is to determine the temperature distribution using the inverse solution of the heat conduction problem [14]. The method is based on measuring the temperature at one or more points inside the wall to be analysed. The determination of the temperature distribution in a thermally insulated cylindrical element based on the measurement of the wall temperature at the outer surface is presented by [15], and near the inner surface is shown by [16,17]. This method determines the temperature distribution in the inverse region (between the measurement point and the inner surface) using the finite volume method (FVM).

Inverse methods can also be used to assess the influence of material inhomogeneities on the temperature distribution and stresses occurring in the wall. For example, in [18], the problem of analysing the temperature and thermal stresses in a multilayered sphere made of a functionally graded material (FGM), when the temperature at the inner surface is unknown, was reduced to an inverse thermoelasticity problem and, using FEM, the temperature distribution in the wall was determined from the known temperature and circumferential strain at the outer surface of the element.

The disadvantage of inverse methods is their sensitivity to random errors in the input data. For example, their impact on the calculation results can be reduced by using regularisation methods such as the Tikhonov method, discrete Fourier transform, energy regularisation method, etc. Research on the stability of inverse problems using selected regularisation methods is presented in articles [19–21]. Another effective and simple way to reduce the impact of random errors on the solution of an inverse problem is to smooth the measurement data using digital filters [22].

The aim of this article is to evaluate the accuracy of the method for determining the unsteady temperature and thermal stresses in a thick-walled cylindrical pressure element weakened by an opening using the inverse method. This method is well known and has been described for cylindrical elements in [14–17], while this article investigates the best conditions for its application. It was assumed that the temperature measurement is performed inside the wall of the thermally insulated element; therefore, in the area from the temperature measurement point to the outer surface, the temperature field was determined based on the direct solution of the heat conduction problem, and from the inner surface to the temperature measurement point based on the inverse solution of the heat conduction problem. The inverse problem is solved using the finite volume method (FVM). The accuracy of this method was analysed by determining the most favourable distance of the temperature measurement point from the internal surface, the number of finite volumes (control volumes) in the inverse region, and the time step size. It was performed based on a computational test. For the assumed working fluid temperature rise and heat transfer coefficient on the inner surface of the pipeline with an opening of a specific geometry, the following values were determined: the exact temperature and thermal stress at the inner surface and the "measured data", i.e., the temperature at a specific distance from the inner surface, which was perturbed by random errors. Based on "measured data" and using the analysed algorithm, the temperature and thermal stresses at the edge of the opening of the inner surface of the element were determined again, and the results were compared with the exact data.

Determining thermal stresses using a tested method has many advantages. It does not require measuring the internal surface temperature, which would be impossible in the case of pressure elements. The actual temperature distribution is calculated across the wall thickness of a thick-walled element, allowing for accurate calculation of the average wall temperature and thermal stresses. The calculation of the heat transfer coefficient on the inner surface of the pressure component does not require the use of Nusselt numbers, which were developed for specific fluid flow conditions and for hydraulically developed flow (due to the fittings and valves used in the pipeline, this condition is sometimes difficult to achieve). The advantage of the described method over others is that it is simple and easy to apply in practice, allows for online calculations and is not computationally expensive (unlike FEM, for example). Although the application of the inverse problem using FVM to determine the temperature distribution in the wall is known [14–17], no analysis of the influence of the number of control volumes, the time step and the distance of the measuring point from the inner surface on the accuracy of the calculations has been carried out so far.

2. Determination of Thermal Stress in Pressure Components

The high operating pressure of the working medium used in power plants necessitates the use of thick-walled components. Fatigue analysis may be necessary if pressure parts are subjected to significant variable loads. Examples of variable loads include variable pressures, transient temperature conditions, restrictions on expansion and contraction during normal temperature changes, forced vibrations, or variable external loads. Therefore, one of the necessary steps in fatigue analysis may be determining the thermal stresses caused by temperature differences in the wall. Thermal stresses in pressure components reach their highest values during changes in the load on the device (especially during start-up and shutdown). They are caused by changes in the temperature of the working fluid and, consequently, by uneven temperature distribution across the entire wall thickness.

Calculation procedures for thick-walled pressure components have been standardised, resulting in the European standard EN 12952-3 [10] and the German standard TRD 301 [11]. They describe, among other things, the methodology for calculating thermal stresses. These procedures are limited to determining thermal stresses in quasi-steady temperature fields across the thickness of the element wall, which rarely occurs in practice. Furthermore, a parabolic temperature distribution in the wall is assumed, which does not give satisfying results in the case of sudden and rapid temperature changes over time.

The next part of this section describes the determination of total circumferential stresses on the inner surface of a pressure element weakened by an opening, including thermal stresses, using standard [10]. These equations are commonly used by boiler manufacturers due to their simplicity, despite their approximate nature. However, it is possible to use more complex models to calculate stresses in real time, thanks to the development of Distributed Control Systems (DCS) in power plants.

2.1. Circumferential Thermal and Total Stresses Assuming a Quasi-Steady Temperature Field

On the internal surface of the pressure element, the total circumferential stresses at the edge of the opening (at the P point) σ_P should not exceed the allowable circumferential stresses σ_{al} [10]:

$$\sigma_P \leq \sigma_{al}. \tag{1}$$

This condition forms the basis for determining the permissible heating and cooling rates for thick-walled pressure elements. The total circumferential stresses at the edge of the opening consist of stresses caused by pressure and thermal stresses [10]:

$$\sigma_P = \alpha_p \sigma_p + \alpha_T \sigma_T, \tag{2}$$

where α_p denotes the pressure stress concentration factor, σ_p is the stress caused by pressure, α_T denotes the thermal stress concentration factor, and σ_T is the thermal stress. Stress caused by both pressure and thermal stress, multiplied by the appropriate concentration factors, occurs at the edge of the opening on the inside of the pressure element. A schematic diagram of a thick-walled pressure component (drum wall) weakened by a hole with the position of point P indicated is shown in Figure 1.

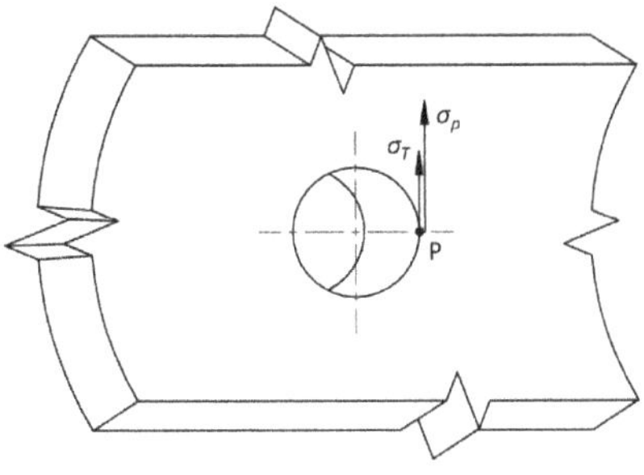

Figure 1. Fragment of a weakened drum wall with an opening.

Circumferential stresses caused by the pressure of the working fluid in a thick-walled element without holes are expressed by the following equation [10]:

$$\sigma_p = \frac{p_n r_m}{s}, \tag{3}$$

where p_n is the working fluid pressure, s is the wall thickness, and r_m is the average radius of the cylindrical pressure element. The radius r_m is calculated as the arithmetic mean of the inner radius r_{in} and the outer radius r_{out} of the wall.

Thermal stresses on the internal surface of a cylindrical component are determined by the following formula [10]:

$$\sigma_T = \frac{E\beta}{1-\nu}\left(\overline{T} - T|_{r=r_{in}}\right), \tag{4}$$

where E denotes Young's modulus, β is the coefficient of linear thermal expansion, ν is Poisson's ratio, $\overline{T}$ denotes the mean temperature across the wall thickness, T is the temperature, and r is the radius.

The mean temperature across the wall thickness of a cylindrical element is determined by the equation:

$$\overline{T} = \frac{2}{r_{out}^2 - r_{in}^2}\int_{r_{in}}^{r_{out}} rT(r,t)dr, \tag{5}$$

where t denotes the time variable and r denotes the radial variable.

A quasi-steady state in the wall of a pressure element occurs when the temperature of the working fluid changes at a constant rate and the temperature difference across the wall thickness is constant over time. This means that thermal stresses are also independent of time.

The mean temperature across the wall thickness can be determined by solving Fourier's heat conduction equation:

$$\frac{\partial T}{\partial t} = \kappa \nabla^2 T, \tag{6}$$

where κ denotes thermal diffusivity. In a quasi-steady state, where the wall temperature changes at a constant rate v_T over time, it can be written that:

$$\frac{\partial T}{\partial t} = v_T. \tag{7}$$

If it is additionally assumed that heat in the cylindrical wall is transferred only in the radial direction, Fourier's equation takes the form:

$$\frac{1}{r}\frac{d}{dr}\left(r\frac{dT}{dr}\right) = \frac{v_T}{\kappa}. \tag{8}$$

Equation (8) will be solved for a quasi-steady state and a thermally insulated pipeline; therefore, the boundary conditions take the following form:

$$T|_{r=r_{in}} = v_T t, \tag{9}$$

$$-k\frac{dT}{dr}\bigg|_{r=r_{out}} = 0, \tag{10}$$

where k denotes the thermal conductivity coefficient.

Substituting the solution of Equation (8):

$$T = v_T t + \frac{1}{4}\frac{v_T}{\kappa}\left(r^2 - r_{in}^2 - 2r_{out}^2 ln\frac{r}{r_{in}}\right) \tag{11}$$

into Equation (5) results in:

$$\overline{T} = \frac{2}{r_{out}^2 - r_{in}^2}\left\{\frac{1}{2}v_T t\left(r_{out}^2 - r_{in}^2\right) + \frac{1}{4}\frac{v_T}{\kappa}\left[\frac{1}{4}\left(r_{out}^4 - r_{in}^4\right) - \frac{1}{2}r_{in}^2\left(r_{out}^2 - r_{in}^2\right) - r_{out}^4 ln\frac{r_{out}}{r_{in}} + \frac{1}{2}r_{out}^2\left(r_{out}^2 - r_{in}^2\right)\right]\right\} \quad (12)$$

Next, substituting Equations (11) and (12) into Equation (4) gives [10]:

$$\sigma_T = \phi\frac{E\beta}{1-\nu}\frac{v_T s^2}{\kappa}, \quad (13)$$

where ϕ denotes the shape factor expressed by the equation:

$$\phi = \frac{1}{8}\frac{(u^2-1)(3u^2-1) - 4u^4 lnu}{(u^2-1)(u-1)^2}, \quad (14)$$

and $u = r_{out}/r_{in}$.

The pressure stress concentration factor for cylindrical shells is determined using the following formula [10]:

$$\alpha_p = 2.2 + e^A\zeta^B, \quad (15)$$

where

$$A = -1.14\left(\frac{s_b}{s}\right)^2 - 0.89\frac{s_b}{s} + 1.43, \quad (16)$$

$$B = 0.326\left(\frac{s_b}{s}\right)^2 - 0.59\frac{s_b}{s} + 1.08, \quad (17)$$

$$\zeta = \frac{r_{mb}}{r_m}\sqrt{\frac{r_m}{s}}. \quad (18)$$

In Equations (16)–(18), s_b is the wall thickness of the stub, s is the wall thickness of the shell, r_{mb} is the mean radius of the stub and r_m is the mean radius of the shell.

In turn, the thermal stress concentration factor is determined by the formula [10]:

$$\alpha_T = \left\{\left[2 - \frac{h+2700}{h+1700}z + \frac{h}{h+1700}\left(e^{-7z} - 1\right)\right]^2 + 0.81z^2\right\}^{1/2}, \quad (19)$$

where

$$z = \frac{r_{mb}}{r_m}, \quad (20)$$

and h denotes the heat transfer coefficient at the inner surface of the shell.

The analysed case assumes heat transfer in the wall of a cylindrical pressure element only in the radial direction and that the cylindrical element can freely elongate in the axial direction. If heat transfer also occurs in other directions, i.e., circumferential and/or axial, or if the support of the element has changed, the stress concentration factor must be determined using FEM.

The allowable stress σ_{al} in Equation (1) is determined based on the diagram showing the relationship between the values of stresses destroying a sample of a given material and the number of load cycles of this sample (Wöhler diagram) from [10]. The procedure described applies to an element that can freely extend and is not affected by significant external forces.

In a quasi-steady state, Equation (1) is sufficiently accurate for determining the permissible heating rates from a cold state. However, when the temperature of the working fluid varies over time, especially during rapid temperature changes, Equation (2) does not give satisfactory results. This occurs when hot water floods the evaporator at the start of the start-up process, in superheated steam temperature controllers when water is injected, or when there is a sudden drop in pressure during a boiler failure. Nevertheless, with time-varying heating or cooling rates of the pressure element, Equation (2) remains valid.

This article focuses on determining transient thermal stresses in a thick-walled element weakened by an opening.

2.2. Unsteady Thermal Stresses in a Cylindrical Element

Transient thermal stresses can be determined using Equation (4), where the temperature distribution as a function of time and space can be achieved by analytical methods or by numerical methods, e.g., FEM or FVM. Using numerical methods, the temperature of the wall is calculated only at discrete points, and the mean temperature is determined using a selected approximation method [15,23]. The integral in Equation (3) can be solved, for example, using the trapezoidal rule for M discrete points:

$$\overline{T} = \frac{1}{r_{out}^2 - r_{in}^2} \sum_{i=2}^{M} (r_{i-1}T_{i-1} + r_iT_i)\Delta r, \tag{21}$$

where r_i is the radius defining the position of node i, T_i is the temperature at node i, and Δr is the radial step.

3. Determination of a One-Dimensional Temperature Field in a Cylindrical Wall

In the case of thick-walled pressure elements, the wall temperature can only be measured inside the wall and/or on its outer surface. In this case, the pipe wall can be divided into a direct and an inverse region (Figure 2). In Figure 2, point N indicates the location of the temperature measurement inside the pipeline wall. The unsteady temperature field at the wall thickness is then determined from the solution of the direct and inverse heat conduction problem.

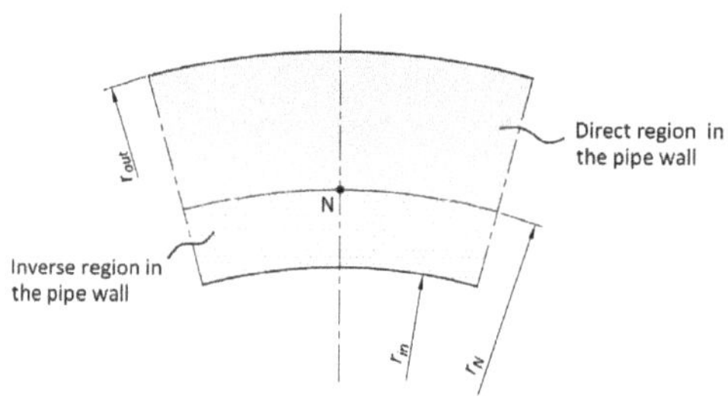

Figure 2. Division of the pipeline wall into direct $r_N \leq r \leq r_{out}$ and inverse $r_{in} \leq r \leq r_N$ areas.

The general formula of the heat conduction equation for anisotropic solids is presented as follows [24]:

$$c(T)\rho(T)\frac{\partial T}{\partial t} = \nabla(\mathbf{K}\nabla T) + \dot{q}_v, \tag{22}$$

where c denotes the specific heat capacity, ρ is the density, $\mathbf{K}$ is the thermal conductivity tensor, and $\dot{q}_v$ is energy generation rate per unit volume.

The solution to the direct heat conduction problem is well known and will not be described in detail here. To solve the inverse problem, the accuracy analysis of which is the subject of this manuscript, the FVM was used [24]. Assuming that the temperature field is two-dimensional, the physical properties and $\dot{q}_v$ are functions of temperature, Equation (22) can be transformed into the following form:

$$\Delta V_i c(T_i)\rho(T_i)\frac{\partial T_i}{\partial t} = \sum_{j=1}^{n_c} \dot{Q}_{i,j} + \Delta V_i \dot{q}_v(T_i). \tag{23}$$

It is assumed that node i is located in the centre of the analysed finite volume area surrounded by n_c adjacent finite volumes (in the centre of which node j is located). In Equation (22), $\dot{Q}_{i,j}$ denotes the heat flux rate transferred from node j to node i, while ΔV_i denotes the volume of the finite volume with node i. This equation allows the temperature distribution to be determined in the case of two-dimensional heat conduction, whereas in the case analysed in this article, it will be used to transfer heat in only one direction (radial).

The proposed solution to the inverse problem is stable and highly accurate if condition [25]

$$\Delta \text{Fo} \geq 0.05 \tag{24}$$

is satisfied. The Fourier number in Equation (23) is expressed by the formula:

$$\Delta \text{Fo} = \frac{\kappa \Delta t}{\left(r_N - r_{in}\right)^2}, \tag{25}$$

where r_N denotes the radius at which the temperature is measured inside the wall (at point N), and Δt denotes the time step.

Nevertheless, this method is sensitive to random temperature measurement errors. To reduce their impact on the calculation results, the temperature measured over time can be smoothed using a selected digital filter [22]. Digital filters also allow the determination of temperature derivatives over time based on the measured temperature, which is disturbed by random errors.

Detailed Description of the Calculation Algorithm

In the presented method, the temperature distribution in the wall of a cylindrical element is determined by a temperature measurement T_N taken inside the wall at point N (Figure 3). It is assumed that the pipe is thermally insulated.

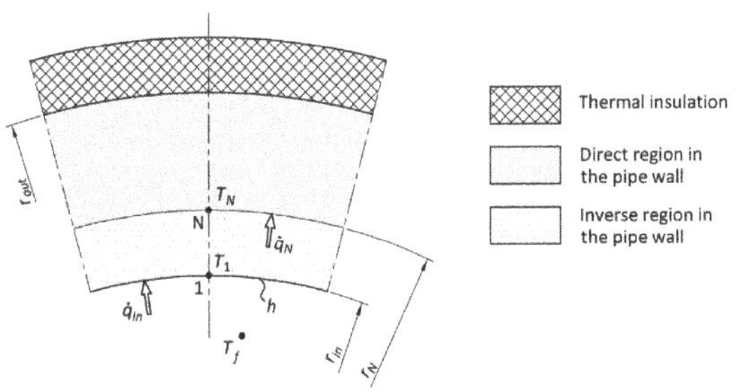

Figure 3. View of a fragment of the analysed thick-walled cylindrical element with the indicated temperature measurement point N.

The cross-section of the pipeline, as shown in Figure 3, is divided into a direct and an inverse region, with the boundary between them located at a radius of r_N.

In the analysed case, it was additionally assumed that the material of the cylindrical element is isotropic, there is no energy generation per unit volume ($\dot{q}_v = 0$), and heat is transferred only in the radial direction. Then, the heat conduction Equation (22) takes the following form [16,25]:

$$c(T)\rho(T)\frac{\partial T}{\partial t} = \frac{1}{r}\frac{\partial}{\partial r}\left[k(T) r \frac{\partial T}{\partial r}\right]. \tag{26}$$

First, in the presented method, the heat conduction Equation (26) is solved as a direct problem using boundary conditions:

$$T|_{r=r_N} = T_N, \tag{27}$$

$$-k(T)\left.\frac{\partial T}{\partial r}\right|_{r=r_{out}} = 0. \tag{28}$$

This allows the temperature distribution in the direct area ($r_N \leq r \leq r_{out}$) and the heat flux density $\dot{q}_N$ at the boundary between the direct and inverse areas (at point N) to be determined.

Next, it is possible to solve the heat conduction Equation (26) as an inverse problem with boundary conditions defined on the radius r_N, i.e.,

$$T|_{r=r_N} = T_N, \tag{29}$$

$$-k(T)\left.\frac{\partial T}{\partial r}\right|_{r=r_N} = \dot{q}_N. \tag{30}$$

This solution uses the FVM (Equation (23)), in which temperature derivatives are determined using differential quotients:

$$\left.\frac{\partial T}{\partial r}\right|_{r_{i+1}} = \frac{T_{i+1} - T_i}{\Delta r}, \quad \left.\frac{\partial T}{\partial r}\right|_{r_i} = \frac{T_i - T_{i-1}}{\Delta r}, \tag{31}$$

The solution to this problem makes it possible to determine the temperature distribution in the inverse region ($r_{in} \leq r \leq r_N$). Figure 4 shows the division of the inverse region into finite volumes (three cases with different numbers of finite volumes).

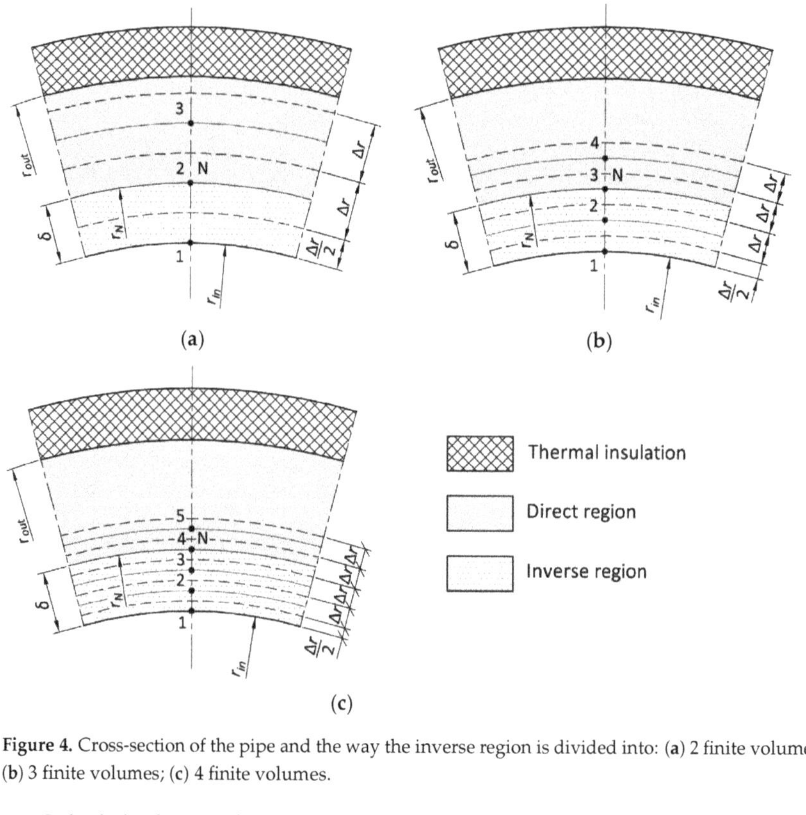

Figure 4. Cross-section of the pipe and the way the inverse region is divided into: (**a**) 2 finite volumes; (**b**) 3 finite volumes; (**c**) 4 finite volumes.

In both the direct and inverse solutions, it was assumed that physical properties, i.e., specific heat c, density ρ and thermal conductivity k are temperature-dependent.

In the described method, from the energy balance equation for the finite volume in which node N is located, which has the form:

$$\pi\left[{r_N}^2-\left(r_N-\frac{\Delta r}{2}\right)^2\right]c(T_N)\rho(T_N)\frac{dT_N}{dt}=2\pi\left(r_N-\frac{\Delta r}{2}\right)\frac{k(T_{N-1})+k(T_N)}{2}\frac{T_{N-1}-T_N}{\Delta r}+2\pi r_N\dot{q}_N. \quad (32)$$

an equation for the temperature at node $N-1$ is derived:

$$T_{N-1}=\frac{(\Delta r)^2\left(r_N-\frac{\Delta r}{4}\right)}{r_N-\frac{\Delta r}{2}}\frac{c(T_N)\rho(T_N)}{k(T_{N-1})+k(T_N)}\frac{dT_N}{dt}-\frac{2r_N\Delta r}{r_N-\frac{\Delta r}{2}}\frac{\dot{q}_N}{k(T_{N-1})+k(T_N)}+T_N \quad (33)$$

The energy balance equation for subsequent nodes (in descending order), i.e., from $N-1$ to 2, is as follows:

$$\begin{aligned}&\pi\left[\left(r_{in}+(2i-1)\tfrac{\Delta r}{2}\right)^2-\left(r_{in}+(2i-3)\tfrac{\Delta r}{2}\right)^2\right]c(T_i)\rho(T_i)\tfrac{dT_i}{dt}\\&=2\pi\left[r_{in}+(2i-3)\tfrac{\Delta r}{2}\right]\tfrac{k(T_{i-1})+k(T_i)}{2}\tfrac{T_{i-1}-T_i}{\Delta r}+2\pi\left[r_{in}+(2i-1)\tfrac{\Delta r}{2}\right]\tfrac{k(T_i)+k(T_{i+1})}{2}\tfrac{T_{i+1}-T_i}{\Delta r},\end{aligned} \quad (34)$$

where $i=2,\ldots,N-1$.

Based on this, the formula for the temperature at node T_{i-1} can be determined:

$$T_{i-1}=2(\Delta r)^2\frac{2r_{in}+(2i-2)\Delta r}{2r_{in}+(2i-3)\Delta r}\frac{c(T_i)\rho(T_i)}{k(T_{i-1})+k(T_i)}\frac{dT_i}{dt}-\frac{2r_{in}+(2i-1)\Delta r}{2r_{in}+(2i-3)\Delta r}\frac{k(T_i)+k(T_{i+1})}{k(T_i)+k(T_{i-1})}(T_{i+1}-T_i)+T_i \quad (35)$$

The equation for T_{i-1} (for $i=2,\ldots,N$) is non-linear, i.e., it contains a heat conduction coefficient $k(T_{i-1})$ which is unknown. For this reason, iterative calculations are performed, assuming in the first iteration ($n=0$) that $k\left(T_{i-1}^{(0)}\right)$ is equal to $k(T_i)$. The iterations are repeated until the condition:

$$\left|T_{i-1}^{(n+1)}-T_{i-1}^{(n)}\right|\le\varepsilon \quad (36)$$

is met. The tolerance ε in condition (36) is approximately 0.00001 K. Of course, the iterative process does not need to be carried out if constant values of physical properties are assumed.

The calculation algorithm is as follows. First, for a given time t, the direct problem is solved to determine the temperature distribution at discrete points on the wall thickness in the area $r_N\le r\le r_{out}$ and the heat flux density $\dot{q}_N$ at radius r_N. Then, marching towards the inner surface, the temperatures are calculated at successive nodes in the inverse area ($r_{in}\le r\le r_N$). Based on the calculated $\dot{q}_N$ and the measured temperature T_N, the temperature in node T_{N-1} is determined using Equation (33) in an iterative process until condition (36) is satisfied. Based on the calculated T_{N-1} temperature, the T_{N-2} temperature is calculated using Equation (35), again conducting the calculations in n iterations. The procedure for determining the temperatures in the subsequent nodes is repeated until the temperature in node 1 is determined. At this stage, the algorithm for time t ends and is then repeated for time $t+\Delta t$ and so on. A 9-point digital filter [22] was used in the calculation algorithm. First, the temperatures (including the temperature at node N, disturbed by random errors) in the direct area, necessary for calculating the heat flux $\dot{q}_N$, were smoothed. Then, the temperatures calculated in the subsequent nodes from $N-1$ to 1 in the inverse area were smoothed. The mean temperature across the entire wall thickness for successive time instants can be calculated using Equation (21), which for a wall divided into a direct and an inverse area takes the form:

$$\overline{T}=\frac{2}{r_{out}^2-r_{in}^2}\int_{r_{in}}^{r_{out}}rT(r,t)dr=\frac{2}{r_{out}^2-r_{in}^2}\left[\frac{r_{out}^2-r_N^2}{2}\overline{T}_{direct}+\frac{r_N^2-r_{in}^2}{2}\overline{T}_{inv}\right], \quad (37)$$

where $\overline{T}_{direct}$ and $\overline{T}_{inv}$ is the mean temperature of the inverse and direct area of the wall, respectively.

In order to calculate thermal stresses in a cylindrical element weakened by a hole, it is also necessary to determine the heat transfer coefficient h on its inner surface. In this case, the FVM can also be used. This can be carried out by determining the heat flux on the inner surface of the pipe $\dot{q}_{in}$ and measuring the temperature of the working fluid T_f. The heat flux density is determined from the energy balance equation for node 1:

$$\pi\left[\left(r_{in}+\frac{\Delta r}{2}\right)^2-r_{in}^2\right]c(T_1)\rho(T_1)\frac{dT_1}{dt}=2\pi r_{in}\dot{q}_{in}+2\pi\left(r_{in}+\frac{\Delta r}{2}\right)\frac{k(T_2)+k(T_1)}{2}\frac{T_2-T_1}{\Delta r}, \quad (38)$$

from which we obtain:

$$\dot{q}_{in}=\frac{\left(r_{in}+\frac{\Delta r}{2}\right)^2-r_{in}^2}{2r_{in}}c(T_1)\rho(T_1)\frac{dT_1}{dt}-\frac{k(T_2)+k(T_1)}{2}\frac{r_{in}+\frac{\Delta r}{2}}{r_{in}\Delta r}(T_2-T_1). \quad (39)$$

Then, from the boundary condition:

$$\dot{q}\big|_{r=r_{in}}=h\left(T_f-T\big|_{r=r_{in}}\right), \quad (40)$$

where

$$T\big|_{r=r_{in}}=T_1,\ \dot{q}\big|_{r=r_{in}}=\dot{q}_{in} \quad (41)$$

the heat transfer coefficient can be determined:

$$h=\frac{\dot{q}_{in}}{T_f-T_1}. \quad (42)$$

The heat transfer coefficient is determined as a function of time t. In practice, very accurate measurements of the working fluid temperature T_f are necessary to calculate the heat transfer coefficient in this way.

4. Analysis of Algorithm Accuracy Using Computational Tests

The computational validation of the method for determining thermal stresses for a thick-walled cylindrical element weakened by a hole was performed for a steam header with an external diameter of 355 mm and a wall thickness of 50 mm. The header has a stub with an external diameter of 42.4 mm and a wall thickness of 3.2 mm. The pipe is made of P91 steel. Properties of P91 steel as a function of temperature:

$$k(T)=-0.003\times10^{-10}T^5+4.741\times10^{-10}T^4-2.874\times10^{-7}T^3+6.438\times10^{-5}T^2-4.177\times10^{-4}T+28.676, \quad (43)$$

$$c(T)=1.41\times10^{-6}T^3-6.43\times10^{-4}T^2+4.88\times10^{-1}T+439.80 \quad (44)$$

The functions of the thermal conductivity coefficient and specific heat capacity with respect to temperature were determined by approximating data taken from [24]. The coefficient of determination for both determined functions is approximately equal to 1. The density of steel was assumed to be a constant value of $\varrho=7750\ \mathrm{kg/m^3}$ due to its small variation in the temperature range for which the calculation test was performed.

The calculation test was carried out in such a way that 'measurement data' was first generated analytically by solving the direct conduction problem. It was assumed that the pipeline was thermally insulated, the temperature of the working fluid T_f rose suddenly from 20 °C to 170 °C, and the heat transfer coefficient on the surface washed by the fluid h was 1500 $\mathrm{W/(m^2K)}$. For these conditions, temperature profiles over time were determined on the inner and outer surfaces of the pipe and at 49 points inside the wall for time steps of 1, 2, 3, 4 and 5 s. The distances between successive points are the same, i.e., 1 mm. The 'measurement data' is the temperature at point N located at a distance of 6, 12 or 18 mm from the inner surface, disturbed by random errors with a normal distribution, a mean of zero and a variance σ^2 of approx. 0.01 K^2 (the exact value depends on the time step and thus the amount of data). The relatively low variance of random errors disturbing the 'measurement data' results from the fact that random errors in the measurement of the temperature inside the wall of a thick-walled element are minimal due to the environment in which the thermometer is located and the high thermal inertia of the wall. Besides temperature, the exact thermal stresses on the inner surface of the wall without an opening and weakened by the opening were also calculated.

Next, following the algorithm described in Section Detailed Description of the Calculation Algorithm, the inner surface temperature is determined based on the 'measured' temperature at the point N in the wall of the thick-walled cylindrical element. In addition, the heat flux, heat transfer coefficient, thermal stresses on the inner surface of the pipe, and thermal stresses at the edge of the opening are determined.

As mentioned, calculations were performed for three different distances of the temperature measurement point N from the internal surface, i.e., 6, 12 and 18 mm. For each of these cases, the inverse region was first split into 2, then into 3, and then into 4 finite volumes. The time steps for which the calculations were carried out are 1, 2, 3, 4, and 5 s. Figure 4 shows how the inverse region of a cylindrical element is divided into 2, 3 and 4 finite volumes. Due to heat transfer only in the radial direction, the division into finite volumes is only made in the cross-section of the pipe.

The results of the research presented in this manuscript include an analysis of the influence of the number of finite volumes in the inverse area, the distance of the temperature measurement point N from the internal surface, and the time step size on the accuracy of the described algorithm and the determination of thermal stresses in elements weakened by an opening.

For the calculated values of temperature, thermal stresses and heat transfer coefficient on the internal surface, root mean square errors were determined, where the exact values of temperature and thermal stresses calculated from the direct heat conduction problem during the generation of 'measurement data' were taken as reference values. The equation from which the root mean square error was calculated is as follows:

$$s_n = \sqrt{\frac{S}{n-1}}, \tag{45}$$

where n denotes number of measurement points. The general formula for the sum S gives the equation:

$$S = \sum_{i=1}^{n} [y_{exact}(t_i) - y(t_i)]^2 \tag{46}$$

where $y_{exact}(t_i)$ denotes the exact value and $y(t_i)$ denotes the value calculated using the presented algorithm. The calculation results are presented in Tables 1 and 2.

The most accurate calculation results were obtained for the case where the measurement point is located at a distance δ = 6 mm from the inner surface, the time step is 1 s, and the inverse region is divided into two finite volumes. The root mean square error of the internal surface temperature calculation using the described algorithm $s_{n,T}$ is 0.365 K, and the error in determining the thermal stresses in the element not weakened by the opening $s_{n,\sigma}$ is 1.119 MPa. The root mean square error of thermal stresses at the edge of the opening $s_{n,\sigma\times\alpha}$ is also the smallest in this case and amounts to 1.688 MPa, even though for δ = 6 mm the heat transfer coefficient on the inner surface is determined with the lowest accuracy

($s_{n,h}$ = 208 W/m^{2}K). For a distance of δ = 12 mm, the smallest root mean square errors were obtained for a time step of 1 s and a division of the inverse region into 4 finite volumes. On the other hand, when the measuring point is located at a distance δ = 18 mm from the inner surface, the highest accuracy of calculations was obtained for a time step of 1 s and division into 4 finite volumes in the case of temperature, and for a time step of 2 s and division into 4 finite volumes in the case of thermal stresses. It is not possible to determine a rule for the most favourable division into finite volumes for a given time step or a given distance of point N from the inner surface.

Table 1. Root mean square errors of the calculated temperature on the inner surface $s_{n,T}$ and thermal stresses on the inner surface $s_{n,\sigma}$ of the pipe not weakened by the hole when the measuring point N is located at a distance δ from the internal surface.

Time Step Δt, s	Number of Finite Volumes	δ=6 mm		δ=12 mm		δ=18 mm	
		$s_{n,T}$, K	$s_{n,\sigma}$, MPa	$s_{n,T}$, K	$s_{n,\sigma}$, MPa	$s_{n,T}$, K	$s_{n,\sigma}$, MPa
1	2	0.365	1.119	0.841	2.577	1.834	5.509
	3	0.383	1.185	0.514	1.573	1.446	4.289
	4	0.379	1.177	0.482	1.487	1.240	3.752
2	2	1.014	2.431	1.094	2.179	1.965	4.834
	3	0.959	2.251	1.143	2.508	1.416	3.036
	4	0.946	2.201	1.152	2.581	1.379	3.011
3	2	1.091	3.067	1.126	2.897	1.562	4.168
	3	1.000	2.793	1.233	3.352	1.294	3.332
	4	0.985	2.745	1.241	3.403	1.318	3.474
4	2	1.221	3.589	1.445	4.043	1.360	3.821
	3	1.120	3.297	1.473	4.242	1.457	4.071
	4	1.116	3.288	1.460	4.231	1.507	4.267
5	2	1.304	3.963	1.704	4.972	1.342	4.158
	3	1.207	3.698	1.650	4.923	1.628	4.810
	4	1.222	3.750	1.617	4.855	1.687	4.999

For the smallest distance of the measuring point N from the inner surface, the results of the calculations using the presented algorithm are the most accurate. This is because the surface temperature is reproduced based on the temperature measurement and how it changes at a given time step. The closer the measuring point is to the inner surface, the faster the changes in the measured temperature are recorded and the more accurately it is reproduced on the surface using the solution of the inverse heat conduction problem. For a greater distance of the measuring point N from the surface of the element, the thermometer may indicate a change in temperature only after a few or several seconds, despite the change in surface temperature.

The larger the time step for which the calculations are performed, the smaller the root mean square errors of the calculated heat transfer coefficients. When calculating the temperature in successive finite volume nodes towards the inner surface of the inverse area, a random error propagates. The use of a digital filter partially, but not completely, eliminates its influence on the temperature calculation results. The heat transfer coefficient, on the other hand, is determined on the basis of the heat flux calculated from formula (39), where there is a temperature difference between adjacent nodes 2 and 1, which thus reduces the influence of random error. At the same time, in the case of a larger time step, the digital filter better eliminates temperature disturbances caused by random errors that have disturbed the 'measurement data'. The digital filter used in the algorithm is a 9-point filter, which means that the data is smoothed based on the next 9 temperature values over time, with the smoothed value located at the centre point of the 9-point interval.

Table 2. Root mean square errors of the heat transfer coefficient on the inner surface $s_{n,h}$ and thermal stresses at the edge of the hole on the inner surface $s_{n,\sigma\times\alpha}$ of the pipe when the measuring point N is located at a distance δ from the internal surface.

Time Step Δt, s	Number of Finite Volumes	δ=6 mm		δ=12 mm		δ=18 mm	
		$s_{n,h}$, W/(m^{2}K)	$s_{n,\sigma\times\alpha}$, MPa	$s_{n,h}$, W/(m^{2}K)	$s_{n,\sigma\times\alpha}$, MPa	$s_{n,h}$, W/(m^{2}K)	$s_{n,\sigma\times\alpha}$, MPa
1	2	208.0	1.688	1201.8	11.095	4561.9	27.606
	3	141.4	1.799	689.1	2.484	5508.6	19.690
	4	119.1	1.796	456.5	2.104	17491.0	46.140
2	2	126.6	3.663	380.6	3.168	1194.3	8.130
	3	109.8	3.391	232.8	3.707	766.9	5.942
	4	104.9	3.299	184.9	3.855	508.8	4.331
3	2	85.1	4.680	193.4	4.355	527.2	6.421
	3	78.3	4.248	135.6	5.132	306.6	4.968
	4	77.6	4.133	116.3	5.223	230.0	5.256
4	2	77.4	5.494	153.1	6.180	382.3	5.835
	3	74.6	5.004	113.7	6.543	222.2	6.209
	4	77.3	4.906	99.6	6.528	173.7	6.557
5	2	55.5	6.088	100.8	7.656	241.0	6.313
	3	60.9	5.601	70.5	7.622	123.7	7.411
	4	71.1	5.545	62.6	7.515	95.7	7.731

The least accurate results were obtained for δ = 18 mm, a time step of 1 s and division of the inverse area into two finite volumes. Increasing the number of finite volumes in this case increases the accuracy of the calculations of the internal surface temperature and thermal stresses in the pipe wall without holes. Nevertheless, the significant error in determining the heat transfer coefficient and thermal stresses in the element weakened by the hole means that the case where δ = 18 mm and Δt = 1 s should be rejected entirely. This is because for this distance of the measuring point from the inner surface, condition (24) for stability of the inverse problem solution (which includes the determination of the heat flux density used to calculate the heat transfer coefficient) is satisfied for time steps of 2 s and larger.

It can be seen that the most accurate results of temperature and thermal stress calculations on the inner surface, regardless of the time step, were obtained for a distance δ = 6 mm.

By analysing the root mean square errors of thermal stresses at the edge of the opening in Table 2, it can be concluded that slightly larger errors in determining the heat transfer coefficient are acceptable. The criterion for allowing larger errors in determining the heat transfer coefficient should be the accuracy of the calculated thermal stress concentration factor. The reference value of this factor for the analysed case is 1.5056. As already mentioned, Table 2 shows that the most accurate values of thermal stresses at the edge of the opening for δ = 6 mm are obtained for Δt = 1 s and 2 finite volumes. For this case, the root mean square error of the thermal stress concentration factor is $s_{n,\alpha}$ = 0.0197. For a distance δ of 12 mm, the most accurate calculations are for $\Delta t = 1$ s and 4 finite volumes, where $s_{n,\alpha}$ is 0.0461. In contrast, for $\delta = 18$ mm, the most favourable case is a division into 4 finite volumes and a time step Δt of 2 s, where $s_{n,\alpha}$ is 0.08932. Analysis of the remaining results summarised in Table 2 leads to the conclusion that the root mean square error of the stress concentration factor should not exceed 10% of the reference value.

The thermal stresses at the edge of the opening in the pressure element calculated using the presented algorithm were compared with the stresses obtained using the recommendations of EN 12952-3 [10]. This standard recommends assuming a constant value for the heat transfer coefficient on the inner surface of the pressure component according to the type of working fluid, i.e., $h = 1000$ W/(m^{2}K) for steam and $h = 3000$ W/(m^{2}K) for water. The comparison was made for the most favourable cases in terms of the accuracy of the calculated thermal stresses using a calculation algorithm for the three analysed distances δ of 6, 12 and 18 mm. For a distance δ of the measuring point N from the inner surface of the pipe of 6 mm, $\Delta t = 1$ s and division into two finite volumes, the root mean square error calculated for thermal stresses at the edge of the opening, where the stress concentration factor is determined in accordance with the standard, is: for steam $s_{n,h1000} = 4.619$ MPa, and for water $s_{n,h3000} = 7.497$ MPa. For a distance δ of 12 mm, $\Delta t = 1$ s and division into 4 finite volumes, these errors are: $s_{n,h1000} = 4.864$ MPa and $s_{n,h3000} = 7.625$ MPa. In contrast, for $\delta = 18$ mm, $\Delta t = 2$ s and division into 4 finite volumes: $s_{n,h1000} = 7.391$ MPa and $s_{n,h3000} = 6.895$ MPa. In all cases, regardless of the location of the measurement point, the calculations of thermal stresses in the element weakened by the opening are more accurate when using the algorithm presented in the manuscript than those performed in accordance with the recommendations of EN 12952-3.

Figures 5 and 6 present graphs of temperatures and thermal stresses on the inner surface of a thick-walled cylindrical element for selected cases. The most favourable cases regarding the accuracy of the calculated thermal stresses at the edge of the hole were selected for the smallest and largest distance of the measuring point from the inner surface of the pressure element, i.e., $\delta = 6$ mm and $\delta = 18$ mm. Figure 7 shows the heat transfer coefficient graphs for the case where the temperature measuring point is at a distance δ of 6 mm from the inner surface. The most accurate values of heat transfer coefficients were selected for the smallest and largest time step, i.e., $\Delta t = 1$ s and $\Delta t = 5$ s. Figures 5–7 show both graphs of values calculated using the described algorithm and reference values.

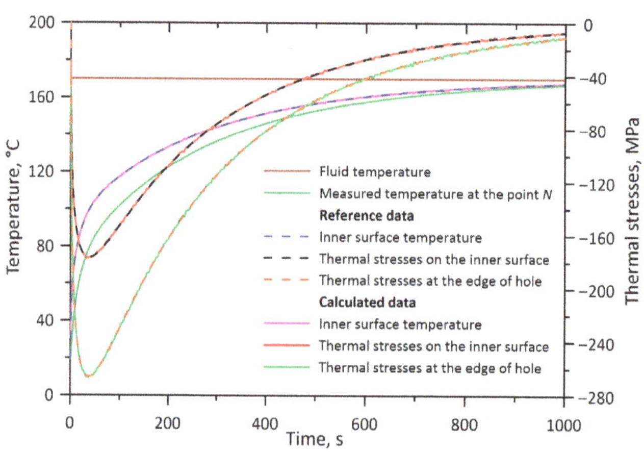

Figure 5. Comparison of reference and calculated temperatures and thermal stresses on the internal surface of the pipe for a case where the distance $\delta = 6$ mm, the time step size $\Delta t = 1$ s and the number of finite volumes is 2.

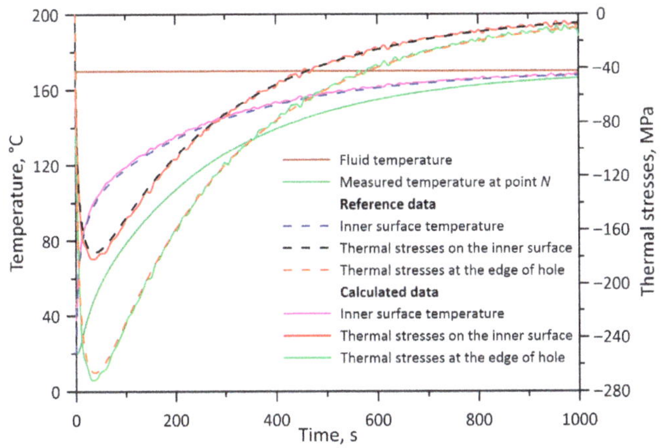

Figure 6. Comparison of reference and calculated temperatures and thermal stresses on the internal surface of the pipe for a case where the distance $\delta = 18$ mm, the time step size $\Delta t = 2$ s and the number of finite volumes is 4.

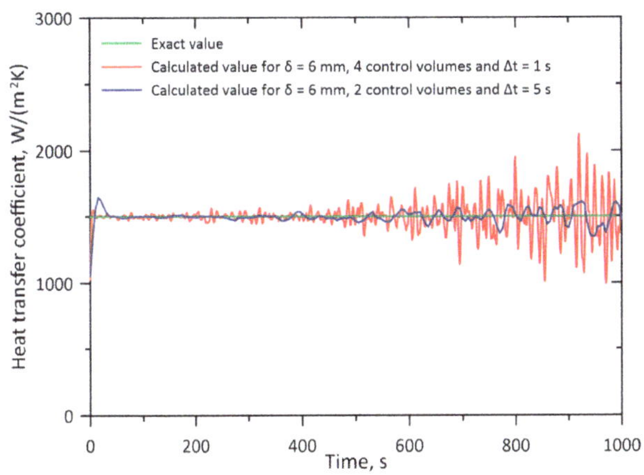

Figure 7. Assumed (exact) heat transfer coefficient at the pipe's internal surface and values calculated by the described algorithm for a measurement point N at a distance δ of 6 mm from the inner surface, for $\Delta t = 1$ s and division into 4 finite volumes and $\Delta t = 5$ s and division into 2 finite volumes.

5. Conclusions

The manuscript analyses the accuracy of a calculation method for determining thermal stresses in thick-walled cylindrical elements. This method is based on measuring the temperature at a single point inside the thermally insulated wall of a pipe and uses the solution of the direct and inverse heat conduction problem. The analysis considers the influence of the time step size, the number of finite volumes in the inverse region and the location of the measuring point. Based on the calculations performed, it can be concluded that

- The most optimal time step size and number of finite volumes depend on the location of the measurement point inside the pipe wall. Test calculation results indicate that the smaller the distance between the measurement point and the pipe's inner surface, the more accurate the results. In a situation where the position of the measuring point is fixed and cannot be changed, it is worth performing test calculations to help select the optimal time step size and number of finite volumes in the inverse area.

- The root mean square errors of the temperature calculated on the inner surface of the cylindrical element are small and range from 0.365 K to 1.965 K.
- The root mean square errors of thermal stresses on the inner surface of a cylindrical element that is not weakened by a hole in the most favourable cases for δ = 6, 12 and 18 mm are in the range from 1.119 MPa to 3.011 MPa, with the maximum value of these stresses being approx. −177 MPa. Similarly, for a cylindrical wall weakened by holes, the root mean square errors of thermal stresses at the edge of the hole range from 1.688 MPa to 4.331 MPa, with a maximum stress value of approx. −266 MPa. This demonstrates the importance of accurately determining the temperature distribution in the pipeline wall and selecting the best possible conditions (time step, distance and number of nodes) for performing calculations using the presented algorithm.
- The least accurate heat transfer coefficient values, regardless of the distance δ, are obtained for a time step of 1 s. The larger the time step, the smaller the root mean square error. It can also be noted that even slightly higher than acceptable errors in determining the heat transfer coefficient do not have a significant impact on the accuracy of determining thermal stresses in an element weakened by an opening. From the analysis of the results summarised in Table 2, it can be concluded that the criterion for obtaining accurate thermal stress values at the edge of the opening is the root mean square error of the stress concentration factor, which should not exceed 10% of the reference value. Despite this, the accuracy of the determination of the heat transfer coefficient is not insignificant. For example, if, for δ = 6 mm, Δt = 1 s and 2 finite volumes, the heat transfer coefficient h recommended by the standard [10] (1000 W/(m^{2}K) for steam and 3000 W/(m^{2}K) for water) is used to calculate the thermal stress at the edge of the hole, the root mean square error increases to 4.619 MPa and 7.497 MPa, respectively, where for h determined from the method presented was 1.688 MPa.
- Analysing the calculation results, it can be concluded that the method of determining the heat transfer coefficient described in the article is sensitive to random errors. It follows that a better way to determine the heat transfer coefficient is to calculate it from the correlation with the Nusselt number or, alternatively, as described in [16].

Funding: This work was funded by the National Science Centre in Poland within the framework of the research project no. 2021/43/B/ST8/01170.

Data Availability Statement: Data available in a publicly accessible repository. The original data presented in the study are openly available in RODBUK at https://doi.org/10.58099/PK/YFTBD4.

Conflicts of Interest: The authors declare no conflicts of interest. The funders had no role in the design of the study; in the collection, analyses, or interpretation of data; in the writing of the manuscript; or in the decision to publish the results.

References

1. Chen, F.; Yan, W. High-fidelity modelling of thermal stress for additive manufacturing by linking thermal-fluid and mechanical models. *Mater. Des.* **2020**, *196*, 109185. [CrossRef]
2. Xu, P.; Li, Q.; Wang, C.; Li, L.; Tan, D.; Wu, H. Interlayer healing mechanism of multipath deposition 3D printing models and interlayer strength regulation method. *J. Manuf. Process.* **2025**, *141*, 1031–1047. [CrossRef]
3. Dzierwa, P.; Taler, D.; Trojan, M.; Taler, J. Optimum Heating of Boiler Evaporator. *Heat Transf. Eng.* **2017**, *39*, 1217–1226. [CrossRef]
4. Oh, C.; Lee, S.; Jhung, M.J.; Huh, N.-S. Analytical approach to estimate the thermal stress distribution of reactor pressure vessel nozzle corners with a constant cooldown rate. *Int. J. Press. Vessel. Pip.* **2022**, *197*, 104608. [CrossRef]
5. Jeong, S.-H.; Chung, K.-S.; Ma, W.-J.; Yang, J.-S.; Choi, J.-B.; Kim, M.K. Thermal stress intensity factor solutions for reactor pressure vessel nozzles. *Nucl. Eng. Technol.* **2022**, *54*, 2188–2197. [CrossRef]
6. Olivera, S.J.; Mostafavia, M.; Hosseinzadehb, F.; Paviera, M.J. Redistribution of residual stress by thermal shock in reactor pressure vessel steel clad with nickel alloy. *Int. J. Press. Vessel. Pip.* **2019**, *169*, 37–47. [CrossRef]

7. Radin, Y.A.; Kontorovich, T.S.; Golov, P.V. Monitoring the Thermal Stress State in Steam Turbines. *Power Technol. Eng.* **2020**, *53*, 719–723. [CrossRef]
8. Radin, Y.A.; Kontorovich, T.S. Influence of the Arrangement of the Highand Intermediate-Pressure Cylinders of Steam Turbines with Different Bypass Circuits on Their Thermal Stress State During Start-Ups and Shutdowns. *Power Technol. Eng.* **2021**, *54*, 720–725. [CrossRef]
9. Radin, Y.A.; Kontorovich, T.S. Influence of Parameter Deviations Vis-À-Vis Assignment Schedule on Thermally Stressed State of Main Thermal Power Plant Equipment. *Power Technol. Eng.* **2024**, *57*, 918–921. [CrossRef]
10. *European Standard EN 12952-3*; Water-Tube Boilers and Auxiliary Installations. Part 3: Design and Calculation for Pressure Parts. European Committee for Standardization: Bruxelles, Belgium, 2001.
11. *TRD 301*; Zylinderschalen Unter Innerem Überdruck. Technische Regeln für Dampfkessel (TRD). Heymanns Beuth Köln-Berlin: Berlin, Germany, 2001.
12. Teixeira Júnior, M.; Zilio, G.; Mortean, M.V.V.; de Paiva, K.V.; Oliveira, J.L.G. Experimental and numerical analysis of transient thermal stresses on thick-walled cylinder. *Int. J. Press. Vessel. Pip.* **2023**, *202*, 104884. [CrossRef]
13. Jaremkiewicz, M.; Dzierwa, P.; Taler, D.; Taler, J. Monitoring of transient thermal stresses in pressure components of steam boilers using an innovative technique for measuring the fluid temperature. *Energy* **2019**, *175*, 139–150. [CrossRef]
14. Taler, J.; Duda, P. Experimental verification of space marching methods for solving inverse heat conduction problems. *Heat Mass Transf.* **2000**, *36*, 325–331. [CrossRef]
15. Taler, J.; Zima, W.; Jaremkiewicz, M. Simple method for monitoring transient thermal stresses in pipelines. *J. Therm. Stress.* **2016**, *39*, 386–397. [CrossRef]
16. Jaremkiewicz, M.; Taler, J. Measurement of Transient Fluid Temperature in a Pipeline. *Heat Transf. Eng.* **2017**, *39*, 1227–1234. [CrossRef]
17. Taler, D.; Taler, J.; Kaczmarski, K.; Jaremkiewicz, M.; Dzierwa, P.; Trojan, M. Monitoring of thick-walled pressure elements to determine transient temperature and stress distributions using the measured fluid's pressure and wall's temperature. *Energy* **2024**, *309*, 133121. [CrossRef]
18. Kushnir, R.M.; Yasinskyy, A.V.; Tokovyy, Y.V. Effect of Material Properties in the Direct and Inverse Thermomechanical Analyses of Multilayer Functionally Graded Solids. *Adv. Eng. Mater.* **2022**, *24*, 2100875. [CrossRef]
19. Ciałkowski, M.; Joachimiak, M.; Mierzwiczak, M.; Frąckowiak, A.; Olejnik, A.; Kozakiewicz, A. The analysis of the stability of the Cauchy problem in the cylindrical double-layer area. *Arch. Thermodyn.* **2023**, *44*, 563–579. [CrossRef]
20. Joachimiak, M.; Joachimiak, D. Stabilization of boundary conditions obtained from the solution of the inverse problem during the cooling process in a furnace for thermo-chemical treatment. *Int. J. Heat Mass Transf.* **2024**, *224*, 125274. [CrossRef]
21. Joachimiak, M.; Joachimiak, D.; Ciałkowski, M. Investigation on Thermal Loads in Steady-State Conditions with the Use of the Solution to the Inverse Problem. *Heat Transf. Eng.* **2022**, *44*, 963–969. [CrossRef]
22. Taler, J. *Theory and Practice of Identifying Heat Transfer Processes*; Zakład Narodowy imienia Ossolińskich: Wrocław, Poland, 1995. (In Polish)
23. Taler, J.; Zima, W. Solution of inverse heat conduction problems using control volume approach. *Int. J. Heat Mass Transf.* **1999**, *42*, 1123–1140. [CrossRef]
24. Taler, J.; Duda, P. *Solving Direct and Inverse Heat Conduction Problem*; Springer: Berlin/Heidelberg, Germany, 2006.
25. Taler, J. A new space marching method for solving inverse heat conduction problems. *Forsch. Ingenieurwesen* **1999**, *64*, 296–306. [CrossRef]

energies

MDPI

Article

In Situ Winter Performance and Annual Energy Assessment of an Ultra-Lightweight, Soil-Free Green Roof in Mediterranean Climate: Comparison with Traditional Roof Insulation

Luca Evangelisti *, Edoardo De Cristo and Roberto De Lieto Vollaro

Department of Industrial, Electronic and Mechanical Engineering, Roma Tre University, Via Vito Volterra 62, 00146 Rome, Italy; edoardo.decristo@uniroma3.it (E.D.C.); roberto.delietovollaro@uniroma3.it (R.D.L.V.)
* Correspondence: luca.evangelisti@uniroma3.it

Abstract

Green roofs are effective passive strategies for enhancing building energy efficiency and indoor thermal comfort, particularly in response to climate change. This study presents an experimental and numerical assessment of an ultra-lightweight, soil-free green roof system for Mediterranean climates. In situ thermal monitoring was carried out on two identical test rooms in Rome (Italy), comparing the green roof to a traditional tiled roof under winter conditions. Results revealed a 45% reduction in thermal transmittance. These data were used to calibrate a dynamic TRNSYS 18 model and then applied to annual simulations of energy demand and indoor comfort across different roof configurations, including expanded polystyrene-insulated reference roofs. The model was calibrated in accordance with ASHRAE Guideline 14, achieving an MBE within ±10% and a CV(RMSE) within ±30% for hourly data, ensuring the simulation's reliability. The green roof reduced cooling energy demand by up to 58.5% and heating demand by 11.6% relative to the uninsulated reference case. Compared to insulated roofs, it maintained similar winter performance while achieving summer operative temperature reductions up to 0.99 °C and PPD decreases up to 2.94%. By combining field measurements with calibrated simulations, this work provides evidence of the green roof's effectiveness as a passive retrofit solution for Mediterranean buildings.

Keywords: green roof; dynamic thermal simulation; TRNSYS calibration; in situ measurement; Mediterranean climate; thermal comfort assessment; soil-free substrate; urban heat island

1. Introduction

The building sector plays a critical role in achieving global decarbonization goals, accounting for approximately 36% of final energy consumption and nearly 40% of CO_2 emissions worldwide [1]. In response to this environmental challenge, the European Union has established ambitious targets through the 2030 Climate and Energy Framework [2] and the Renovation Wave strategy [3], promoting deep energy renovation as a primary lever to enhance building performance and climate resilience [4,5].

Within this framework, nature-based solutions are increasingly acknowledged for their dual potential to improve thermal performance while simultaneously mitigating the urban heat island effect and enhancing environmental quality in urban areas [6–9]. Among these, green roofs have gained particular attention due to their ability to reduce building energy demand, regulate indoor temperatures, and deliver ecosystem co-benefits [10–12].

The role of green roofs is particularly relevant in Mediterranean urban environments [13,14], characterized by hot summers, increasing climatic stress, and dense built fabrics [15,16]. In these contexts, lightweight green roofs represent a viable solution for retrofitting existing buildings that lack the structural capacity to support conventional green roof systems [17–19]. While the existing Mediterranean literature on green roof performance is extensive [16], studies focusing specifically on soil-free or ultra-lightweight systems remain scarce. Such configurations, often based on synthetic growing media or modular pre-vegetated mats, are particularly relevant for retrofitting buildings with limited structural capacity. Investigations have examined the performance of soil-free and ultra-lightweight green roofs in different climates [20–22], yet experimental evidence under real Mediterranean operating conditions remains limited, underscoring the relevance of the present study. However, the thermal and energy performance of such systems is highly dependent on roof design, climatic conditions, and simulation assumptions [23–25].

Although several studies have assessed green roof performance through numerical simulations, most rely on non-calibrated models, which limits predictive reliability. As documented in a recent systematic review [16], there is a clear need for studies that simultaneously combine in situ experimental validation, high-resolution urban climate data, and calibrated annual energy simulations to assess the performance of lightweight green roofs in Mediterranean environments.

Moreover, a critical and often overlooked issue concerns the meteorological input data used in simulations. As thoroughly discussed in a previous study [26], the widespread reliance on standardized Typical Meteorological Year (TMY) datasets, typically derived from airport stations, often fails to capture the different thermal dynamics of densely built urban areas, where microclimatic variations can be substantial. This mismatch may lead to considerable inaccuracies in estimating the passive potential of green roofs, undermining the reliability of simulation-based approaches. Furthermore, TMY datasets may fail to capture recent climate trends or extreme weather events, which could potentially compromise simulation accuracy [27,28]. Periodic updates and site-specific calibration are therefore strongly recommended.

To overcome these methodological limitations, this study adopts an integrated approach that combines high-resolution experimental validation, calibrated dynamic simulations, and updated urban climate datasets representative of Mediterranean conditions.

The investigated green roof system, designed within the framework of the "GRINN-S" research project, is a soil-free, extensive solution optimized for buildings with limited structural load capacity. Its performance was experimentally assessed through in situ thermal monitoring under real operating conditions. Various techniques can be employed to monitor the surface temperature of green roof layers with heterogeneous compositions, including advances in non-contact methods such as spectral pyrometry [29]. In this study, the choice of contact-based sensors was made in accordance with the recommendations and best practices discussed in our recent systematic review on the thermal and energy performance assessment of Mediterranean green roofs [16].

The resulting dataset was used to calibrate a building energy model developed in TRNSYS 18 [30], which was subsequently validated according to ASHRAE Guideline 14 [31]. Once validated, the model was applied to a simplified residential prototype to simulate year-round thermal performance and energy demand under the climatic conditions of Rome (Italy), using urban weather data. The analysis included a comparative assessment with conventional roof insulation strategies aimed at quantifying differences in energy demand, thermal behavior, and indoor thermal comfort. By integrating empirical evidence, numerical accuracy, and site-specific climatic forcing, this study delivers robust and transferable insights to support the deployment of lightweight green roofs as a scalable and climate-responsive retrofit strategy for the Mediterranean building stock.

This work distinguishes itself from previous studies by combining high-resolution in situ winter monitoring, a rigorously calibrated TRNSYS model driven by site-specific urban climate data, and a comparative analysis with varying EPS (Expanded Polystyrene) insulation levels, providing new evidence on the seasonal performance of an innovative ultra-lightweight green roof in Mediterranean conditions.

The paper is organized as follows: Section 2 defines the aim and scope of the study. Section 3 describes the methodological approach, including both the in situ experimental setup and the dynamic simulation procedures. Section 4 serves a dual function: it presents the results of the thermal characterization and dynamic simulations, and critically discusses the key findings, with an emphasis on their practical applicability and contribution to the scientific literature. Finally, Section 5 summarizes the key contributions and outlines directions for future research.

2. Aim and Scope

This study advances the current state of knowledge on the thermal and energy performance of green roofs in Mediterranean climates by addressing several critical research gaps identified in the literature. In contrast to the majority of existing studies that rely on uncalibrated simulation models, this research integrates high-resolution in situ experimental monitoring with a rigorously calibrated TRNSYS 18 model, validated according to ASHRAE Guideline 14 standards. Moreover, it incorporates updated, site-specific urban weather data instead of conventional airport-derived TMY datasets, thereby capturing the distinct microclimatic conditions of dense Mediterranean urban areas and improving predictive reliability. It focuses on an innovative ultra-lightweight, soil-free green roof system specifically designed for buildings with limited structural capacity, which has been scarcely investigated in real operating conditions. The study provides a direct, systematic comparison between the green roof and reference roofs equipped with different levels of EPS insulation, assessing not only heating and cooling energy demand but also indoor thermal comfort indicators over an annual cycle. By integrating empirical validation, climate-responsive modeling, and a comprehensive comparative framework, this work aims to provide novel and transferable insights to support the scalable adoption of lightweight green roofs as a climate-adaptive retrofit strategy for the Mediterranean building stock.

The research framework is structured into three sequential and interlinked phases: (i) the empirical thermal characterization of a novel lightweight green roof system; (ii) the development and validation of a calibrated simulation model based on real boundary conditions; (iii) the comparative assessment of annual energy performance across multiple roof configurations under site-specific Mediterranean climates.

This approach was adopted to fulfill the following key research objectives:

- to quantify the potential reduction in energy demand resulting from the installation of an ultra-light green roof system on conventional buildings' roofs;
- to assess the impact of the green roof on inner surface temperature profiles and indoor thermal conditions under real and simulated operating scenarios;
- to simulate how different roof insulation levels influence the thermal performance of a green roof-equipped building envelope.

This framework addresses a critical gap identified in the recent literature [16], specifically the lack of integrated approaches that combine empirical validation, site-specific urban climate data, and dynamic simulation.

3. Methodology

The green roof system analyzed in this study was developed within the "GRINN-S" project, a publicly funded initiative aimed at designing lightweight, nature-based solutions for energy retrofitting in Mediterranean climates. As illustrated in Figure 1, the prototype consists of a soil-free extensive green roof, featuring a synthetic substrate over a polyethylene root barrier, equipped with a subirrigation system and an automated control unit. Designed for buildings with limited structural capacity, it combines high thermal efficiency with minimal structural load impact. During the winter season, the vegetative layer enters a dormant phase, characterized by negligible metabolic activity and halted growth, thus eliminating the need for irrigation and allowing the system to function in fully passive mode. The full-scale installation enabled extended in situ thermal monitoring under real operating conditions, providing a robust experimental foundation for calibrating and validating a dynamic simulation model.

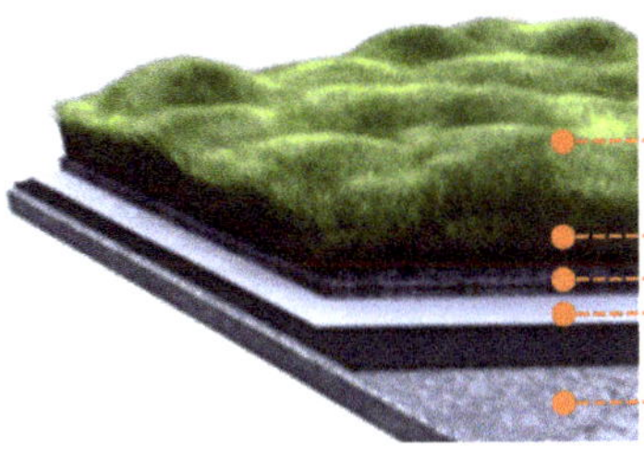

Figure 1. Green roof stratigraphy.

The methodological framework adopted in this study combines empirical monitoring and numerical simulation to evaluate the thermal and energy performance of an extensive ultra-lightweight green roof system. The approach is structured into two interrelated macro-phases described in the following sections.

3.1. Experimental Phase

The experimental campaign started during January 2025 near Rome (Italy), on two thermally conditioned test rooms located side by side (see Figure 2) and characterized by the same constructive technologies (solid bricks plastered on both sides, and a typical composite slab roof with hollow clay infill blocks and reinforced concrete ribs). The winter monitoring period was selected to meet ISO 9869-1 [32] requirements for U-value determination, ensuring a consistent indoor–outdoor temperature gradient above 10 °C, which minimizes the influence of variable solar gains and wind speed on measured heat flux. This stable thermal gradient allows for a more accurate estimation of intrinsic thermophysical properties. The two test rooms will be referred to below as P1 (the one characterized by a traditional clay-tile roof, serving as reference) and P2 (the one with the green roof).

Both test rooms were equipped with a controlled heating system based on infrared lamps regulated by thermostats set to maintain an indoor air temperature of 20 °C. Heat flux sensors were mounted on the inner side of the roofs, and thermocouples were installed to acquire surface and air temperature data at 10 min intervals. Figure 3 provides some pictures related to the installation phase.

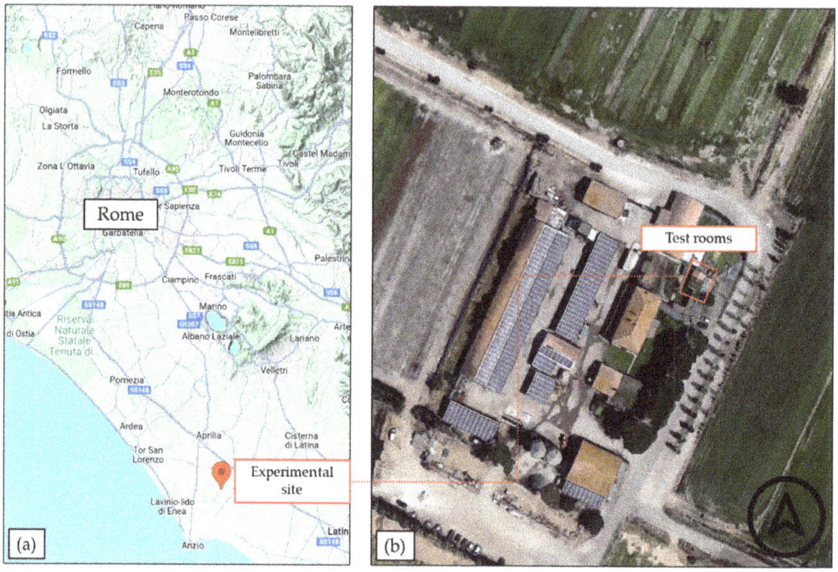

Figure 2. Geographical location of the test site, approximately 50 km from Rome, in central Italy (**a**); top view of the experimental site (**b**).

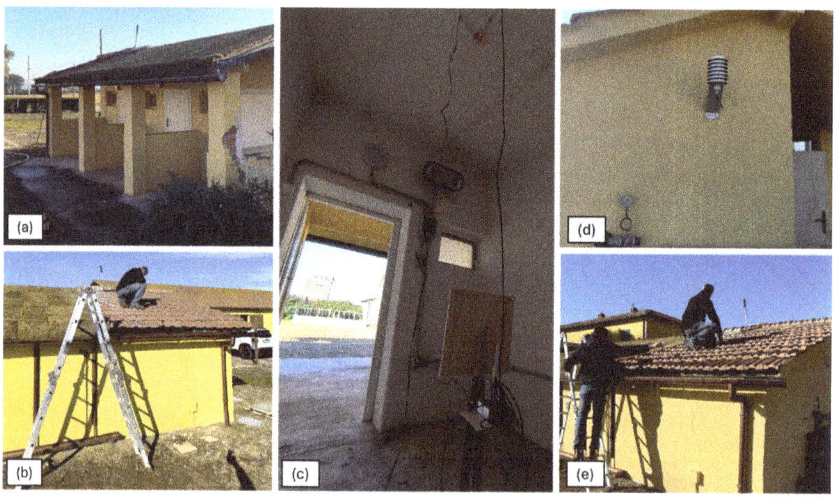

Figure 3. The test rooms (**a**,**b**); the heating system and the sensors within a test-room (**c**); external air temperature sensor with the radiation shield (**d**); sensor installation phase (**e**).

Figure 4 illustrates the overall sensor installation layout. Heat flux sensors (Hukseflux, model HFP01 [33]) and contact surface temperature sensors (LSI Lastem, model EST124 [34]) were installed on the inner surface of the roofs. Within the test rooms, air temperature sensors (LSI Lastem, model EST033 [35]) were installed and shielded to prevent direct radiation from the heating system. Moreover, EST124 sensors were used to measure the temperature on the external surface of the conventional roof (P1), and the temperature beneath the green roof system, at the interface between the green layer and the structural roof (P2). Finally, an EST033 sensor (equipped with a radiation shield) was installed for measuring the external air temperatures.

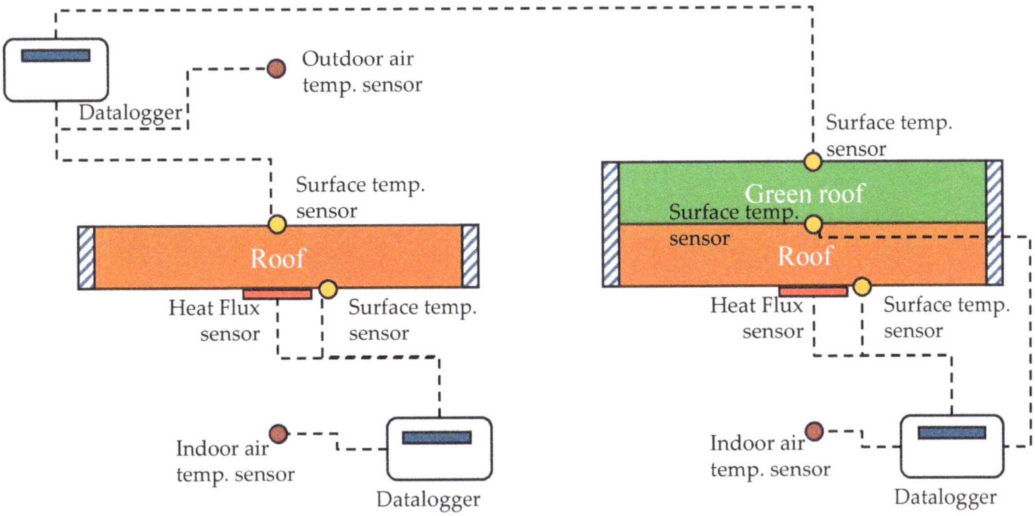

Figure 4. Schematic representation of the sensors' installation layout.

The collected data was post-processed to calculate the thermal transmittance (U-value) of both roof configurations. The analysis followed the ISO 9869-1 standard [32], applying the progressive average method, which allows for the estimation of thermal transmittance under real operating conditions:

$$U = \frac{\sum q}{\sum(T_{int} - T_{ext})} \tag{1}$$

where q is the heat flux density, and T_{int} and T_{ext} are the internal and external air temperatures, respectively.

The three convergence criteria defined by the standard were applied to validate the measurements. In particular: (i) the measurement duration must be at least 72 h; (ii) at the end of the measurement period, the calculated thermal transmittance value must not differ by more than ±5% from the value obtained 24 h earlier; (iii) the analysis of data from the initial period equal to INT(2DT/3) days must yield a result that does not differ by more than ±5% from the value obtained by analyzing the data from the final period of the same duration (where DT is the total duration of the test in days, and INT denotes the integer part of the expression).

The assessment of measurement uncertainty was carried out in accordance with the principles of the ISO Guide to the Expression of Uncertainty in Measurement. The analysis considered the statistical variability of the measurements, with the standard error of the mean used to quantify the influence of random fluctuations. The individual uncertainty contributions from the heat flux sensor and from the internal and external air temperature sensors were combined by applying the law of propagation of uncertainties, using the root-sum-of-squares method. The expanded uncertainty, corresponding to a 95% confidence level, was obtained by applying a coverage factor k = 2, in line with international metrological practice.

3.2. Simulation Phase

The experimental dataset was used to calibrate a dynamic simulation model in TRNSYS 18. The model was constructed using TRNSYS Build to define the building envelope and internal conditions, and the dedicated Type 785 (see the TESS library for more details [36]) was used to represent the thermal dynamics of the green roof system. Experimentally measured indoor and outdoor air temperatures, recorded from 16–23 January 2025, were imposed as thermal boundary conditions.

Although the calibration dataset refers to winter conditions, this study represents a preliminary stage of an extensive monitoring campaign, for which only winter in situ measurements were available. As mentioned before, the winter period was selected as it ensures stable indoor–outdoor temperature gradients, in line with standard recommendations, allowing accurate estimation of the roof system's thermophysical parameters. While certain properties may vary slightly with temperature and moisture content, the calibrated parameters provide a reliable basis for year-round simulations. The use of TRNSYS in this context remains robust, as the model explicitly incorporates dynamic processes relevant to summer conditions, such as solar radiation, evapotranspiration, and thermal inertia, ensuring that seasonal performance is realistically reproduced despite the winter-based calibration.

Model calibration was assessed using two statistical indexes recommended by ASHRAE Guideline 14: the Mean Bias Error (MBE) and the Coefficient of Variation of the Root Mean Square Error (CV(RMSE)). The equations of these indexes are reported below:

$$MBE = \frac{\sum_i (m_i - s_i)}{\sum_i m_i} (\times 100) \tag{2}$$

$$CV(RMSE) = \frac{\sqrt{\sum_i \frac{(m_i - s_i)^2}{N}}}{\overline{m}} (\times 100) \tag{3}$$

where m_i and s_i are the measured and simulated values, respectively. N is the number of data points acquired, and $\overline{m}$ is the mean value of the measured data. According to ASHRAE Guideline 14, a simulation model is calibrated when the MBE falls within ±10% and the CV(RMSE) falls within ±30% for hourly data. From the calibrated model, effective thermophysical properties (thermal conductivity, specific heat capacity, and mass density) can be derived.

Finally, the validated green roof model was implemented in a simplified building simulation to evaluate annual energy performance and comfort conditions. The building model was intentionally kept simple, as it directly represents the test rooms used for the experimental campaign. This approach ensures consistency between the numerical and experimental setups and allows us to isolate the effect of the roof configuration on the thermal response. In particular, the reference building consisted of a single-zone volume (6-by-6 m square floor plan structure), characterized by a height of 3 m, with envelope stratigraphy based on the typological data from the TABULA project [37]. In particular, the vertical walls are characterized by solid bricks plastered on both sides. The structural part of the roof is composed of hollow clay blocks and concrete. Finally, the basement is constructed with reinforced concrete. The stratigraphy is reported in Table 1, together with the thermophysical properties of each layer. These properties were selected to be representative of typical construction materials used in Mediterranean buildings and fall within the standard ranges reported in [38,39].

Table 1. Construction layers, listed from the inner to the outer side.

Component	Material	Thickness [m]	Thermal Conductivity [W/mK]	Specific Heat Capacity [J/kgK]	Mass Density [kg/m^3]
Walls	Plaster	0.020	0.870	1000	1600
	Solid brick	0.200	0.800	840	1600
	Plaster	0.020	0.870	1000	1600
Roof	Plaster	0.015	0.870	1000	1600
	Hollow clay block	0.120	0.400	840	800
	Concrete	0.040	1.400	1000	2200
Basement	Concrete	0.300	1.400	1000	2200

To explore different retrofit scenarios, the roof stratigraphy was modified by adding a thermal insulation layer of expanded polystyrene (EPS) with three thicknesses (0.02 m, 0.04 m, and 0.06 m), followed by an additional 0.08 m concrete layer on top. The selected EPS insulation thicknesses were chosen to represent typical low-to-moderate retrofit scenarios applicable to existing buildings with limited structural load capacity, in line with the design constraints of the ultra-lightweight green roof system. These values also reflect common practice in the Mediterranean context for cost-effective interventions where structural reinforcement is not feasible. Thicker insulation layers were not considered, as they would fall outside the scope of lightweight retrofit strategies investigated in this study. In particular, the EPS is characterized by a thermal conductivity equal to 0.045 W/mK, a specific heat capacity of 1300 J/kgK, and a mass density of 28 kg/m^3. In this new configuration, the green roof system was installed on top of the added concrete layer.

In all cases, the modeled building features a total glazed surface area of 12 m^2, equally distributed across the four façades. The windows are equipped with single-pane glass, 6 mm thick, characterized by a thermal transmittance of 5.69 W/m^{2}K.

The HVAC system simulation was carried out by setting the indoor temperature to 20 °C for heating and 26 °C for cooling, while maintaining a constant indoor relative humidity of 50%. Internal heat gains from occupants were implemented using the predefined TRNSYS profile ASHRAE_115W-Person_AIII_24C, assigned as absolute gains. According to the model output, each occupant contributed approximately 252 kJ/h (70 W), distributed as 151.2 kJ/h (42 W) radiative and 100.8 kJ/h (28W) convective heat, reflecting a metabolic activity level consistent with ASHRAE Class AIII. In the dynamic simulation, an air exchange rate of 0.5 1/h was assumed, representing typical natural ventilation conditions for residential buildings without mechanical ventilation systems [40].

The wind speed (v) values from the climatic files were used to compute the external convective coefficients for surfaces, setting the following equation in TRNSYS Build [41]:

$$h_c = 4v + 4 \tag{4}$$

In addition to assessing the thermal performance and energy impact of the green roof system, this study aimed to evaluate its influence on indoor thermal comfort conditions. To this end, the TRNSYS Build model was configured to compute several comfort-related variables, including Mean Radiant Temperature, Operative Temperature, Predicted Mean Vote (PMV), and Predicted Percentage of Dissatisfied (PPD). Throughout the annual simulation period, the clothing factor (clo) varied according to a simplified seasonal schedule, reflecting typical occupant adaptation to outdoor climate conditions. A value of 1.2 clo was assigned during the coldest months (January, February, and December), 0.9 clo during transitional periods (March, April and October, November), and 0.5 clo during the warmest months (from May to September). This time-dependent profile was implemented to improve the accuracy of PMV and PPD calculations. In addition, a metabolic rate of 1.2 met was assumed, corresponding to light sedentary activity, and a typical indoor air velocity of 0.1 m/s was applied in accordance with ISO 7730 [42] and ASHRAE 55 [43] recommendations.

Simulations were performed using urban weather data acquired from a meteorological station located in the city center of Rome (see Figure 5a). The area is characterized by mid-rise historical buildings (typically 4–6 stories), narrow streets, and limited open spaces. In such a dense urban fabric, wind speed is typically reduced by building-induced sheltering, while long-wave radiation exchange is affected by the high level of sky-view obstruction. As highlighted in [26], this approach enables a more accurate assessment of building thermal behavior under realistic urban heat stress conditions (Figure 5b–d illustrate the comparison between the weather conditions observed in the city center and at Fiumicino Airport (FCO)). By analyzing multiple roof stratigraphy, the study investigates how varying insulation levels affect the building's energy demand in a Mediterranean climate.

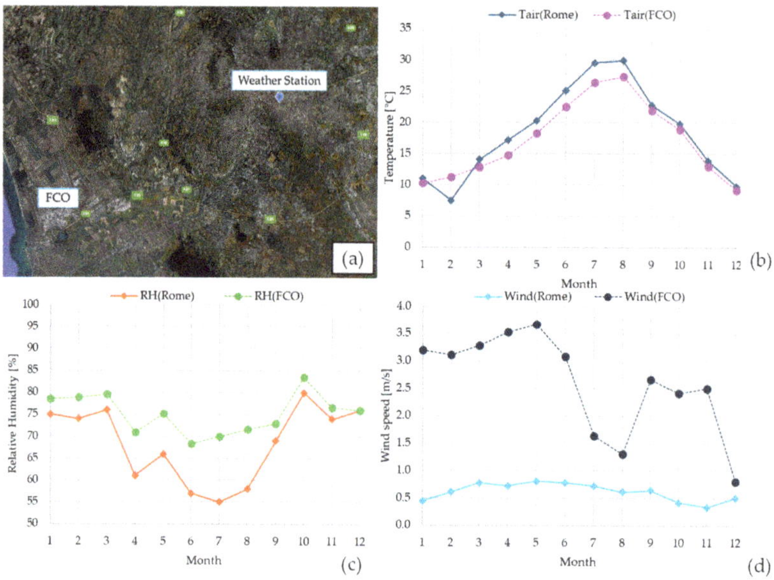

Figure 5. (**a**) Location of the weather station in Rome (urban area) and Fiumicino Airport (FCO, coastal area). Average weather conditions in the city center of Rome and Fiumicino airport (year 2024): (**b**) air temperature (Tair), (**c**) relative humidity (RH) and (**d**) wind speed (Wind).

Figure 6 illustrates the methodological flowchart, detailing the sequential steps and data exchange between the experimental phase and the simulation process.

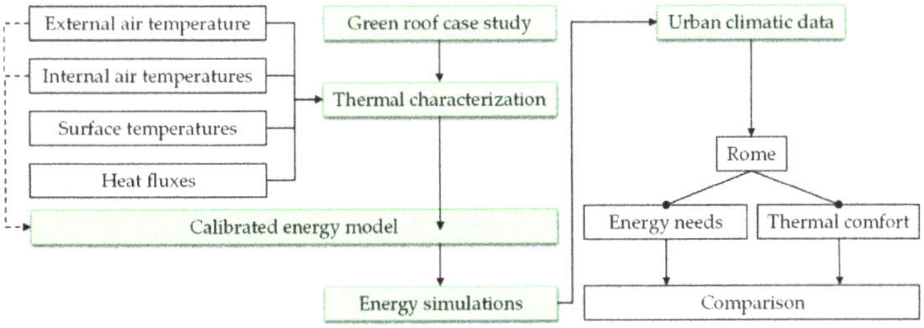

Figure 6. Flowchart of the methodological approach.

4. Results and Discussion

4.1. Experimental Results

The analysis of the data acquired during the monitoring campaign allowed for a clear assessment of the time evolution of the physical quantities involved in the determination of the U-value, following the average method outlined in ISO 9869-1 and reported in Equation (1). The experimental results focused on the most representative winter monitoring period, the week from 16–23 January 2025.

Figure 7a displays the indoor air temperatures recorded in the two test rooms, along with the outdoor air temperature. The indoor conditions remained stable throughout the monitoring period, indicating effective environmental control, while the outdoor temperature exhibited the expected diurnal fluctuations typical of Mediterranean winter conditions. A consistent thermal gradient between indoor and outdoor environments was maintained, satisfying a key requirement for in situ U-value estimation. As reported in the literature [44], a minimum temperature difference of 10 °C is recommended to ensure a reliable heat flux across the envelope (this condition was met for the majority of the monitoring period in both P1 and P2).

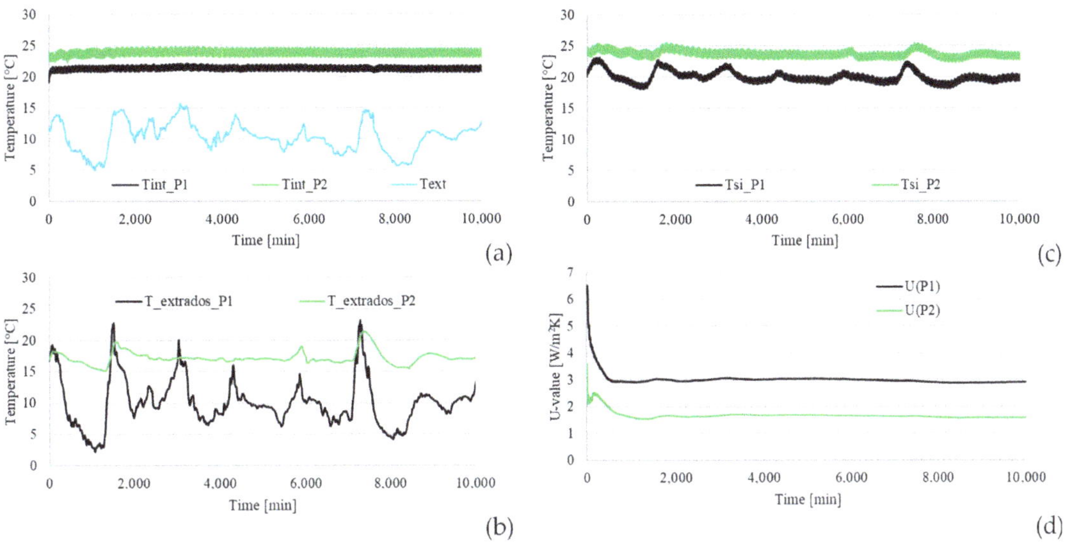

Figure 7. (**a**) Indoor air temperatures in test rooms P1 (black) and P2 (green), and outdoor air temperature (blue); (**b**) Temperatures measured at the external surface (extrados) of the structural roof element for P1 (black) and P2 (green); (**c**) Internal roof surface temperatures for P1 (black) and P2 (green); (**d**) Time evolution of thermal transmittance for P1 (black) and P2 (green), calculated using the progressive average method.

Figure 7b shows the evolution of external surface temperatures at the roof level. In room P2, the sensor was positioned below the vegetated layer, at the interface between the green roof system and the structural slab, thereby capturing the buffered thermal response of the system. In contrast, the traditional roof in P1, being directly exposed, exhibited strong diurnal fluctuations, with sharp daytime peaks and rapid cooling at night, indicative of low thermal inertia. The green roof in P2 showed a markedly more stable thermal profile, with reduced temperature swings and higher average values, particularly during the coldest hours, confirming its thermal damping capacity.

Figure 7c reports the internal surface temperatures of the roof assemblies. The green roof configuration consistently maintained higher surface temperatures and exhibited reduced fluctuations compared to the traditional roof. This behavior confirmed the thermal buffering effect of the green system, driven by the combined contribution of vegetation, substrate, and added mass. The result is an improved stability of internal conditions and enhanced thermal comfort, particularly relevant during winter in Mediterranean climates.

Finally, Figure 7d illustrates the time evolution of U-value, computed using the progressive average method. After an initial transient phase, values stabilized within approximately 33 h, fulfilling the convergence criteria defined by ISO 9869-1, with a variation within the range ±5%. The green roof achieved a U-value approximately 45% lower than that of the traditional tiled roof, confirming its superior insulating performance and overall contribution to improving the thermal characteristics of the building envelope. Specifically, the U-value was 2.897 ± 0.017 W/m^{2}K for the reference roof and 1.588 ± 0.010 W/m^{2}K for the green roof, highlighting the substantial improvement in thermal transmittance achieved by the latter. Corresponding numerical values and validation criteria are summarized in Table 2.

Table 2. Average thermal transmittance values and convergence criteria.

U-Value	P1	Criterion Satisfied	P2	Criterion Satisfied
U (last value)	2.897	☑	1.588	☑
U (24 h before)	2.867	☑(1.0%)	1.579	☑ (0.6%)
U (first2/3; last2/3)	2.957; 3.027	☑ (−2.3%)	1.654; 1.719	☑ (−3.8%)

To provide deeper insight into the thermal behavior and performance benefits of the green roof system, the data acquired over the entire month of January was analyzed. The comparison between the two configurations clearly highlights the green roof's effectiveness in mitigating surface temperature fluctuations and enhancing indoor thermal comfort throughout the monitoring period.

In terms of heat flux, the green roof significantly reduced thermal energy transfer through the roof structure. In January, the average heat flux measured in P2 was approximately 32% lower than in P1, confirming the insulating capacity of the green stratigraphy. Moreover, the indoor air temperatures in P2 were consistently higher, with an average difference of +2.3 °C, indicating improved thermal stability. A similar trend was observed for internal surface temperatures. In P2, the average surface temperature was 3.79 °C higher than in P1, further supporting the green roof's role in moderating indoor thermal conditions.

Overall, the empirical data demonstrate the green roof's capacity to attenuate heat fluxes and stabilize interior environments during winter, validating its effectiveness as a passive solution for improving both energy performance and occupant comfort in Mediterranean climates.

4.2. Simulation Results

The experimental data served as the basis for calibrating a dynamic simulation model developed in TRNSYS 18 (see Figure 8). The building geometry and internal conditions were defined using TRNSYS Build, while the thermal behavior of the green roof system was represented through the dedicated Type 785 component. The model was thermally driven by applying measured boundary conditions, specifically the indoor and outdoor air temperatures recorded during the monitoring campaign. In TRNSYS, Type 9 is a standard component used to import time-dependent data from external files and supply them as dynamic inputs to the simulation model. In this study, experimentally measured indoor and outdoor air temperatures, acquired from 16–23 January 2025, were employed as thermal boundary conditions. The comparison between the simulated and measured roof surface temperatures (extrados) for room P2 enabled the calibration of the green roof model. This calibration process allowed for the identification of equivalent thermo-physical properties (thermal conductivity, specific heat capacity, and mass density) characterizing the green roof system.

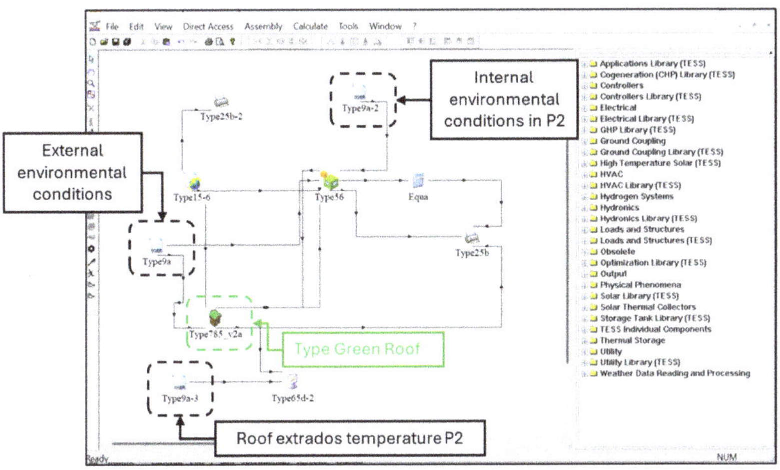

Figure 8. TRNSYS model created through Simulation Studio.

The experimental data allowed the following values to be obtained: a thermal conductivity of 0.265 W/mK, a specific heat capacity of 1380 J/kgK, and a density of 575 kg/m^3. The accuracy of the calibration procedure was confirmed by comparing the simulated and measured surface temperatures at the extrados of P2 (see Figure 9), as well as by the resulting values of the calibration indexes. The model achieved an MBE of 2.8% and a CV(RMSE) of 8.7%, both complying with the acceptable limits established by ASHRAE Guideline 14.

In this ultra-lightweight, soil-free green roof, seasonal variations in thermal behavior are primarily influenced by vegetation activity rather than substrate moisture content. During summer, active evapotranspiration from the vegetation canopy can enhance cooling and slightly reduce the thermal conductivity of the underlying layers due to lower retained moisture. In winter, vegetation enters a dormancy phase, evapotranspiration is minimal, and increased moisture retention within the drainage and filter layers may slightly increase effective thermal conductivity. These effects are implicitly accounted for in the TRNSYS simulations through the modeling of plant shading, evapotranspiration, and moisture-related thermal changes, although future monitoring covering both summer and winter would allow direct validation for this specific system.

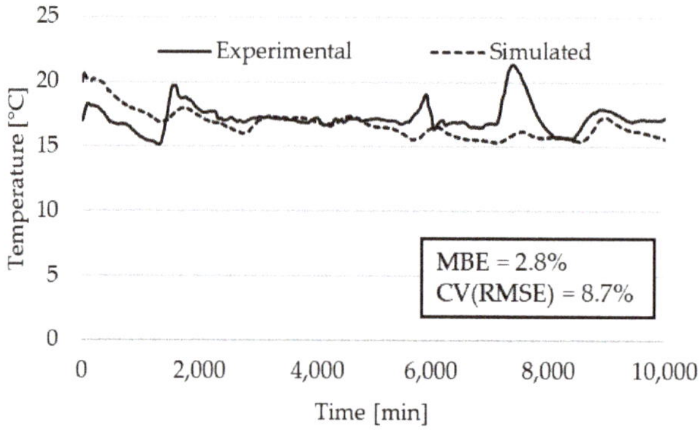

Figure 9. Comparison between experimental and simulated extrados temperatures, and calibration criteria.

As mentioned in the methodology section, the validated green roof model was implemented in a simplified building simulation to evaluate annual energy performance and comfort conditions. The dynamic simulations provided insights into the comparative energy performance of the ultra-lightweight green roof and the reference roof across different insulation levels (0 cm, 2 cm, 4 cm, and 6 cm). The results, summarized in Figure 10, highlight the seasonal impact of the green roof on both heating and cooling energy demand.

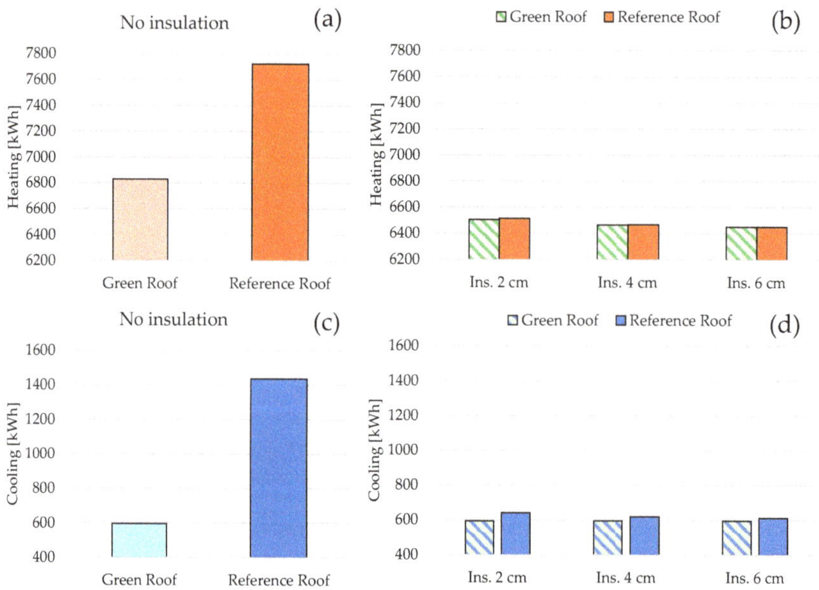

Figure 10. Annual heating and cooling energy demand for the green roof and the reference roof under different insulation scenarios: uninsulated conditions (**a**,**c**); EPS insulation thicknesses of 2 cm, 4 cm, and 6 cm (**b**,**d**).

In the absence of traditional insulation (Figure 10a), the green roof demonstrated a clear thermal advantage during the winter season, reducing heating energy demand by 11.6% compared to the reference roof. This reduction reflects the insulating effect of the multi-layer green roof system, which enhances thermal resistance and attenuates heat loss.

However, as conventional insulation is introduced (Figure 10b), the difference between the two solutions becomes negligible, indicating that adding an additional insulating layer within the roof stratigraphy offers limited improvements in terms of winter energy performance. However, it is worth noting that expanded polystyrene (EPS) is a petroleum-derived material, which raises concerns regarding its environmental sustainability and life cycle impact.

On the other hand, Figure 10c,d illustrate the outcomes in terms of cooling energy demands, documenting a contrasting trend where the green roof consistently outperforms the reference roof across all insulation levels. Without insulation (0 cm), the green roof achieves a 58.5% reduction in cooling demand, confirming its superior ability to mitigate solar heat gains through evapotranspiration and shading effects. Even with increasing insulation thickness, the green roof maintains a cooling advantage, though with decreasing percentage variations: −7.3% at 2 cm, −3.9% at 4 cm, and −2.7% at 6 cm. Similar percentage differences can be obtained by comparing the green roof without additional EPS to the reference roof equipped with insulating material.

To provide a more comprehensive and comparable assessment of the results, Tables 3 and 4 present the heating and cooling energy demands, normalized per unit roof area, for the green roof and reference roof configurations as a function of roof insulation thickness.

Table 3. Normalized heating energy demand for the green roof and reference roof configurations under different roof insulation thicknesses.

Heating	No Insulation [kWh/m^2]	Insulation 2 cm [kWh/m^2]	Insulation 4 cm [kWh/m^2]	Insulation 6 cm [kWh/m^2]
Green Roof	189.68	180.68	179.59	179.16
Reference Roof	214.50	180.93	179.62	179.15

Table 4. Normalized cooling energy demand for the green roof and reference roof configurations under different roof insulation thicknesses.

Cooling	No Insulation [kWh/m^2]	Insulation 2 cm [kWh/m^2]	Insulation 4 cm [kWh/m^2]	Insulation 6 cm [kWh/m^2]
Green Roof	16.55	16.52	16.54	16.55
Reference Roof	39.90	17.82	17.22	17.00

The calibrated model confirms that the thermal performance of green roofs is not only comparable to that of conventional insulation during winter but also superior in summer, thereby enhancing annual energy efficiency and indoor thermal comfort. The findings underline a seasonal complementarity between green roofs and conventional insulation. For poorly insulated buildings, the green roof offers dual benefits, reducing both heating and cooling demands. In well-insulated scenarios, its primary contribution shifts towards summer performance, where conventional materials cannot replicate the thermal inertia, evapotranspiration, and surface temperature damping provided by green roofs.

Table 5 summarizes the monthly differences between the green roof (GR) and the reference roof (REF) in terms of indoor thermal performance indicators, namely: Mean Radiant Temperature (ΔMRT), Operative Temperature (ΔTOP), Predicted Mean Vote (ΔPMV), and Predicted Percentage of Dissatisfied (ΔPPD), under the uninsulated roof scenario.

Table 5. Monthly differences between the green roof (GR) and reference roof (REF) in mean radiant temperature (ΔMRT), operative temperature (ΔTOP), predicted mean vote (ΔPMV), and percentage of dissatisfied occupants (ΔPPD), under the uninsulated scenario. Values calculated as GR–REF.

Month	ΔMRT [°C]	ΔTOP [°C]	ΔPMV [-]	ΔPPD [%]
January	0.64	0.32	0.06	−1.37
February	0.68	0.34	0.06	−1.61
March	0.12	0.02	0.00	−0.44
April	−0.40	−0.44	−0.10	1.30
May	−0.73	−0.66	−0.15	−1.17
June	−0.85	−0.57	−0.16	−0.94
July	−0.99	−0.52	−0.15	−2.94
August	−0.92	−0.50	−0.14	−2.32
September	−0.78	−0.75	−0.22	4.47
October	−0.29	−0.30	−0.07	1.63
November	0.39	0.20	0.03	−0.75
December	0.70	0.35	0.06	−1.56

The results highlight the seasonal responsiveness of the ultra-lightweight green roof system in the Mediterranean climate of Rome. During the colder months (January through March, and November to December), the green roof configuration consistently outperforms the reference roof, exhibiting higher mean radiant temperatures, ranging from +0.12 °C in March to +0.68 °C in February, and increased operative temperatures, from +0.02 °C to +0.34 °C in the same period. The highest mean radiant temperature of +0.70 °C was found in December. These temperature increases correspond to improved thermal comfort conditions, as evidenced by slightly higher PMV values (up to +0.06 in December) and reductions in PPD ranging from −1.61% (February) to −0.44% (March). These results suggest that the green roof enhances indoor thermal comfort during the heating season, even in the absence of conventional insulation. This performance is likely due to the thermal buffering effect of the green roof layers, which reduce heat losses by dampening temperature fluctuations and delaying heat exchange with the outdoor environment.

In the shoulder season (April), the green roof system shows a slight performance penalty. Both mean radiant and operative temperatures are lower than the reference case (ΔMRT = −0.40 °C, ΔTOP = −0.44 °C), resulting in decreased thermal comfort (ΔPMV = −0.10) and an increased share of dissatisfied occupants (ΔPPD = +1.30%). This behavior can be attributed to reduced solar gains combined with limited thermal insulation, which may lead to a cooling effect not always desirable in spring.

As temperatures rise (May), the green roof begins to regain its thermal moderation role. ΔMRT and ΔTOP remain negative (−0.73 °C and −0.66 °C, respectively), but this contributes to a perceptible improvement in summer comfort conditions, reflected in reduced PPD (−1.17%) and lower PMV (−0.15). This shift anticipates the favorable performance typically observed in green roofs during the cooling season. This trend continues and intensifies during the peak summer months (June through August), where the green roof consistently reduces indoor thermal loads. In July, the system achieves a maximum reduction in mean radiant temperature of −0.99 °C and a ΔPMV of −0.15, with a significant drop in ΔPPD (−2.94%), indicating a meaningful improvement in perceived comfort. Similarly, operative temperature is reduced by −0.50 °C in August, while PPD reductions range from −0.94% (June) to nearly −3% (July), confirming the capacity of the green roof to attenuate thermal stress during heat-intensive periods. Similarly to April, in September, a small comfort penalty was observed (ΔPPD = +4.47%), likely due to reduced solar gains during a period with still mild outdoor temperatures.

Overall, the ultra-lightweight green roof demonstrated a favorable impact on indoor thermal conditions across most of the year, particularly during the winter season, where it effectively reduced discomfort despite the absence of additional insulation. While performance during transitional months requires careful consideration, the observed cooling potential in May suggests promising behavior during the summer, which will be further investigated. These findings reinforce the role of lightweight, soil-free green roof systems as effective passive solutions for climate-adaptive retrofitting in Mediterranean regions. Their implementation can contribute to improved indoor comfort, reduced energy demand, and enhanced building resilience in a warming climate, especially when tailored to the local seasonal thermal dynamics.

Table 6 compares the indoor thermal performance of the green roof with three flat roof scenarios featuring different levels of EPS insulation (2 cm, 4 cm, and 6 cm).

Table 6. Monthly differences in indoor thermal comfort parameters between the green roof (GR) and reference roofs (REF) with three levels of EPS insulation (2 cm, 4 cm, 6 cm). Values refer to differences in mean radiant temperature (ΔMRT), operative temperature (ΔTOP), predicted mean vote (ΔPMV), and predicted percentage of dissatisfied occupants (ΔPPD), calculated as GR–REF.

Insulation	2 cm	2 cm	2 cm	2 cm	4 cm	4 cm	4 cm	4 cm	6 cm	6 cm	6 cm	6 cm
Month	**ΔMRT** [°C]	**ΔTOP** [°C]	**ΔPMV** [-]	**ΔPPD** [%]	**ΔMRT** [°C]	**ΔTOP** [°C]	**ΔPMV** [-]	**ΔPPD** [%]	**ΔMRT** [°C]	**ΔTOP** [°C]	**ΔPMV** [-]	**ΔPPD** [%]
January	0.03	0.01	0.00	−0.05	0.01	0.01	0.00	−0.02	0.01	0.00	0.00	−0.01
February	0.03	0.01	0.00	−0.06	0.01	0.01	0.00	−0.03	0.01	0.00	0.00	−0.02
March	−0.01	−0.01	0.00	0.01	−0.01	0.00	0.00	0.01	−0.01	0.00	0.00	0.01
April	−0.04	−0.03	−0.01	0.19	−0.02	−0.02	0.00	0.11	−0.02	−0.01	0.00	0.07
May	−0.09	−0.09	−0.02	0.15	−0.05	−0.05	−0.01	0.08	−0.03	−0.03	−0.01	0.06
June	−0.11	−0.09	−0.03	0.42	−0.06	−0.05	−0.01	0.23	−0.04	−0.03	−0.01	0.16
July	−0.11	−0.08	−0.02	−0.03	−0.06	−0.04	−0.01	−0.01	−0.04	−0.03	−0.01	0.00
August	−0.11	−0.08	−0.02	0.02	−0.06	−0.04	−0.01	0.02	−0.04	−0.03	−0.01	0.01
September	−0.08	−0.07	−0.02	0.81	−0.04	−0.04	−0.01	0.43	−0.03	−0.03	−0.01	0.29
October	−0.03	−0.02	0.00	0.12	−0.01	−0.01	0.00	0.07	−0.01	−0.01	0.00	0.04
November	0.01	0.01	0.00	−0.02	0.00	0.00	0.00	−0.01	0.00	0.00	0.00	0.00
December	0.03	0.01	0.00	−0.06	0.01	0.01	0.00	−0.03	0.01	0.00	0.00	−0.02

Across all indicators (ΔTMR, ΔTOP, ΔPMV, and ΔPPD), the differences between the green roof and the insulated reference roofs remain minimal and nearly constant regardless of the EPS thickness. This confirms that the green roof's contribution to indoor thermal comfort is not significantly influenced by the underlying insulation layer, and that increasing insulation levels does not enhance or compromise its performance. These findings suggest that the thermal behavior of the ultra-lightweight green roof is largely independent of additional roof insulation, reinforcing its applicability as a stand-alone passive solution, especially in Mediterranean area retrofitting scenarios.

In summary, the green roof performs comparably to a lightly insulated reference roof (EPS 2 cm) during winter and outperforms it during summer in terms of cooling effect and thermal comfort. Compared to well-insulated roofs (EPS 4–6 cm), the performance gap narrows significantly in both heating and cooling seasons. These findings reinforce the green roof's potential as a passive design strategy, particularly suitable for retrofits where insulation is limited or where summer overheating is a major concern.

5. Conclusions

This study investigated the thermal behavior and energy performance of an ultra-lightweight, soil-free green roof system specifically designed for the Mediterranean climate, through an integrated experimental and numerical approach. The work addressed a critical gap in existing literature, which often lacks combined empirical validation and dynamic simulation calibrated with real boundary conditions. By merging high-resolution in situ monitoring data, urban climate datasets, and a validated TRNSYS simulation model, this research offers insights into the effectiveness of green roofs as passive systems for building energy retrofitting through comparative analysis with traditional insulation strategies applied to existing buildings.

The experimental campaign, conducted during the winter season, revealed that the green roof reduced thermal transmittance by approximately 45% compared to a traditional tiled, non-insulated roof. Surface and indoor air temperatures were consistently higher in the green roof test room, confirming the system's thermal buffering capacity and its contribution to improved comfort conditions in cold weather. These empirical findings provided the basis for calibrating a dynamic thermal model in TRNSYS 18, which reproduced the measured data with high accuracy, achieving an MBE of 2.8% and a CV(RMSE) of 8.7%, in full compliance with ASHRAE Guideline 14 standards.

Once validated, the calibrated model was used to simulate annual building energy performance and indoor thermal comfort for different roof configurations (characterized by different insulation levels). The simulations confirmed the seasonal effectiveness of the green roof. In winter, under uninsulated conditions, it reduced heating demand by 11.6% compared to the reference case. More significantly, in summer, it led to a cooling demand reduction of 58.5%, thanks to its combined shading, evapotranspiration, and thermal inertia effects. When compared to insulated reference roofs (EPS layers of 2 cm, 4 cm, and 6 cm), the green roof maintained comparable performance in winter and continued to offer an advantage in summer, with cooling energy savings ranging from −7.3% to −2.7%, depending on insulation thickness.

Thermal comfort analysis further supported these findings. During the colder months, the green roof ensured higher mean radiant and operative temperatures, improving perceived comfort even in the absence of conventional insulation. In the warm season, it significantly reduced indoor thermal stress, with operative temperatures reduced by up to 0.99 °C and PPD values lowered by nearly 3% in peak summer conditions. Notably, the performance of the green roof was found to be largely unaffected by the presence or thickness of EPS insulation layers. The comparative analysis demonstrated that adding more insulation did not significantly alter the indoor comfort outcomes associated with the green roof, highlighting its robustness and potential to function effectively as a standalone passive solution.

The ultra-lightweight green roof system presented in this study proved to be a climate-responsive, structurally compatible, and energetically effective solution for improving both winter and summer performance in Mediterranean buildings. Its capacity to offer thermal benefits without relying on petroleum-derived insulation materials reinforces its potential role in sustainable retrofit strategies.

The absence of summer in situ data represents a limitation of this preliminary stage of the work. Future developments will include summer monitoring, which will allow both the integration of warm-season boundary conditions into the calibration process and a direct assessment of the simulation model's accuracy when only winter data are available.

Furthermore, future research should incorporate a life cycle assessment of the green roof compared to conventional insulation strategies to quantify long-term environmental impacts. Moreover, exploring synergies between green roofs and other passive systems (such as natural ventilation or solar control elements) could unlock further potential in climate-adaptive building design. Lastly, long-term evaluations of system durability, vegetation dynamics, and maintenance requirements will be essential to ensure reliable and scalable deployment across the Mediterranean building stock.

Author Contributions: Conceptualization, L.E. and E.D.C.; methodology, L.E. and E.D.C.; software, E.D.C.; validation, L.E. and R.D.L.V.; investigation, L.E. and E.D.C.; resources, R.D.L.V.; data curation, L.E. and E.D.C.; writing—original draft preparation, E.D.C.; writing—review and editing, L.E. and R.D.L.V.; supervision, L.E. and R.D.L.V. All authors have read and agreed to the published version of the manuscript.

Funding: This research was funded by the European Regional Development Fund (ERDF) 2021–2027 under the "Riposizionamento Competitivo RSI" program, Project "GRINN-S—Green Roof INNovativo Sensorizzato per la sostenibilità degli edifici," grant number CUP F19J23000510007.

Data Availability Statement: The data that support the findings of this study are available from the corresponding author upon reasonable request.

Conflicts of Interest: This study was conducted within the framework of an ongoing collaborative project involving Bindi Secondo Srl, iComfort Srl, and the Department of Industrial, Electronic and Mechanical Engineering of Roma Tre University, which is scheduled for completion in November 2025. The present paper reports only a preliminary and independent portion of the research, specifically the analysis of experimental thermal data acquired during the winter monitoring phase, which was carried out exclusively by Roma Tre University. The authors declare no conflicts of interest. The industrial partners had no involvement in the scientific analysis, interpretation of the data, or the writing of the manuscript. Details on project funding are reported in the Funding section.

References

1. IEA Global Status Report for Buildings and Construction 2019. Available online: https://www.iea.org/reports/global-status-report-for-buildings-and-construction-2019 (accessed on 20 June 2025).
2. European Council. The 2030 Climate and Energy Framework. In *Climate Change: What the EU is Doing*; European Council: Brussels, Belgium, 2025.
3. European Commission. Renovation Wave. In *Energy, Climate Change, Environment*; European Commission: Brussels, Belgium, 2025.
4. Guattari, C.; De Cristo, E.; Evangelisti, L.; Gori, P.; Cureau, R.J.; Fabiani, C.; Pisello, A.L. Thermal Characterization of Building Walls Using an Equivalent Modeling Approach. *Energy Build.* **2025**, *329*, 115226. [CrossRef]
5. De Cristo, E.; Evangelisti, L.; Guattari, C.; De Lieto Vollaro, R. An Experimental Direct Model for the Sky Temperature Evaluation in the Mediterranean Area: A Preliminary Investigation. *Energies* **2024**, *17*, 2228. [CrossRef]
6. Mihalakakou, G.; Souliotis, M.; Papadaki, M.; Menounou, P.; Dimopoulos, P.; Kolokotsa, D.; Paravantis, J.A.; Tsangrassoulis, A.; Panaras, G.; Giannakopoulos, E.; et al. Green Roofs as a Nature-Based Solution for Improving Urban Sustainability: Progress and Perspectives. *Renew. Sustain. Energy Rev.* **2023**, *180*, 113306. [CrossRef]
7. Cuce, P.M.; Cuce, E.; Santamouris, M. Towards Sustainable and Climate-Resilient Cities: Mitigating Urban Heat Islands Through Green Infrastructure. *Sustainability* **2025**, *17*, 1303. [CrossRef]
8. Bovo, M.; Santolini, E.; Barbaresi, A. An Alternative Modular Wooden System for Fast Assembly/Disassembly of Buildings. *Buildings* **2025**, *15*, 1196. [CrossRef]
9. Gholami, M.; Barbaresi, A.; Tassinari, P.; Bovo, M.; Torreggiani, D. A Comparison of Energy and Thermal Performance of Rooftop Greenhouses and Green Roofs in Mediterranean Climate: A Hygrothermal Assessment in WuFi. *Energies* **2020**, *13*, 2030. [CrossRef]
10. Bevilacqua, P. The Effectiveness of Green Roofs in Reducing Building Energy Consumptions across Different Climates. A Summary of Literature Results. *Renew. Sustain. Energy Rev.* **2021**, *151*, 111523. [CrossRef]
11. Bellazzi, A.; Barozzi, B.; Pollastro, M.C.; Meroni, I. Thermal Resistance of Growing Media for Green Roofs: To What Extent Does the Absence of Specific Reference Values Potentially Affect the Global Thermal Resistance of the Green Roof? An Experimental Example. *J. Build. Eng.* **2020**, *28*, 101076. [CrossRef]
12. Kaboré, M.; Bozonnet, E.; Salagnac, P. Building and Urban Cooling Performance Indexes of Wetted and Green Roofs—A Case Study under Current and Future Climates. *Energies* **2020**, *13*, 6192. [CrossRef]
13. Pumo, D.; Alongi, F.; Cannarozzo, M.; Noto, L.V. Climate Adaptive Urban Measures in Mediterranean Areas: Thermal Effectiveness of an Advanced Multilayer Green Roof Installed in Palermo (Italy). *Build. Environ.* **2023**, *243*, 110731. [CrossRef]
14. Maiolo, M.; Pirouz, B.; Bruno, R.; Palermo, S.A.; Arcuri, N.; Piro, P. The Role of the Extensive Green Roofs on Decreasing Building Energy Consumption in the Mediterranean Climate. *Sustainability* **2020**, *12*, 359. [CrossRef]
15. Bevilacqua, P.; Mazzeo, D.; Bruno, R.; Arcuri, N. Experimental Investigation of the Thermal Performances of an Extensive Green Roof in the Mediterranean Area. *Energy Build.* **2016**, *122*, 63–79. [CrossRef]

16. De Cristo, E.; Evangelisti, L.; Barbaro, L.; De Lieto Vollaro, R.; Asdrubali, F. A Systematic Review of Green Roofs' Thermal and Energy Performance in the Mediterranean Region. *Energies* **2025**, *18*, 2517. [CrossRef]
17. Abu Qadourah, J. Energy Efficiency Evaluation of Green Roofs as a Passive Strategy in the Mediterranean Climate. *Results Eng.* **2024**, *23*, 102519. [CrossRef]
18. Coma, J.; Pérez, G.; Solé, C.; Castell, A.; Cabeza, L.F. Thermal Assessment of Extensive Green Roofs as Passive Tool for Energy Savings in Buildings. *Renew Energy* **2016**, *85*, 1106–1115. [CrossRef]
19. Gomes, M.G.; Silva, C.M.; Valadas, A.S.; Silva, M. Impact of Vegetation, Substrate, and Irrigation on the Energy Performance of Green Roofs in a Mediterranean Climate. *Water* **2019**, *11*, 2016. [CrossRef]
20. Fei, Y.; Fu, D.; Xu, C.; Singh, R.P. Component Design Optimization of Green Roof Substrate Layer Based on the Assessment of Multifunctional Performance. *Environ. Res.* **2023**, *238*, 117190. [CrossRef]
21. Tachibana, D.; Naoki, S.; Kikuchi, S.; Maki, T.; Sato, Y.; Umazume, D.; Imai, K. Trial Application of Factory Rooftop Greening System with Ultra-Lightweight Substrate. *AIJ J. Technol. Des.* **2010**, *16*, 411–414. [CrossRef]
22. Muscas, D.; De Albuquerque Landi, F.F.; Fabiani, C.; Grohmann, D.; Rocchi, L. Zoysia Soil-Less Green Roof's Performance: A Life Cycle Assessment. *Environ. Clim. Technol.* **2022**, *26*, 955–967. [CrossRef]
23. Cascone, S. Green Roof Design: State of the Art on Technology and Materials. *Sustainability* **2019**, *11*, 3020. [CrossRef]
24. Gagliano, A.; Detommaso, M.; Nocera, F.; Berardi, U. The Adoption of Green Roofs for the Retrofitting of Existing Buildings in the Mediterranean Climate. *Int. J. Sustain. Build. Technol. Urban Dev.* **2016**, *7*, 116–129. [CrossRef]
25. Morakinyo, T.E.; Kalani, K.W.D.; Dahanayake, C.; Ng, E.; Chow, C.L. Temperature and Cooling Demand Reduction by Green-Roof Types in Different Climates and Urban Densities: A Co-Simulation Parametric Study. *Energy Build.* **2017**, *145*, 226–237. [CrossRef]
26. De Cristo, E.; Evangelisti, L.; Battista, G.; Guattari, C.; De Lieto Vollaro, R.; Asdrubali, F. Annual Comparison of the Atmospheric Urban Heat Island in Rome (Italy): An Assessment in Space and Time. *Buildings* **2023**, *13*, 2792. [CrossRef]
27. Lou, S.; Li, D.H.W.; Huang, Y.; Zhou, X.; Xia, D.; Zhao, Y. Change of Climate Data over 37 Years in Hong Kong and the Implications on the Simulation-Based Building Energy Evaluations. *Energy Build.* **2020**, *222*, 110062. [CrossRef]
28. Rady, M.; Muhammad, M.K.I.; Shahid, S. Evolving Typical Meteorological Year (TMY) Data for Building Energy Simulation: A Comprehensive Review of Methods, Challenges, and Future Directions. *Adv. Build. Energy Res.* **2025**, *19*, 269–299. [CrossRef]
29. Magunov, A.N.; Pylnev, M.A.; Lapshinov, B.A. Spectral Pyrometry of Objects with Unknown Emissivities in a Temperature Range of 400–1200 K. *Instrum. Exp. Tech.* **2014**, *57*, 86–90. [CrossRef]
30. TRNSYS 18. Available online: https://www.trnsys.com/ (accessed on 20 June 2025).
31. *ASHRAE Guideline 14*; Measurement of Energy and Demand Savings. ASHRAE: Peachtree Corners, GA, USA, 2002.
32. ISO 9869-1. *Thermal Insulation—Building Elements—In Situ Measurement of Thermal Resistance and Thermal Transmittance.* Available online: https://www.en-standard.eu/une-iso-9869-1-2023-thermal-insulation-building-elements-in-situ-measurement-of-thermal-resistance-and-thermal-transmittance-part-1-heat-flow-meter-method/?gad_source=1&gad_campaignid=22489671069&gbraid=0AAAAAD6CNv-YT_UJBIOFJrPbxsnPJMf4S&gclid=CjwKCAjw49vEBhAVEiwADnMbbOISzN-hq-PFoltpNyaGQ1NZ7B3Rul5Xa4x1EeU7n6gRoC-KXMcZExoCUKsQAvD_BwE (accessed on 9 August 2025).
33. Hukseflux Thermal Sensors HFP01 Heat Flux Sensor. Available online: https://www.hukseflux.com/products/heat-flux-sensors/heat-flux-sensors/hfp01-heat-flux-sensor (accessed on 26 November 2024).
34. LSI Lastem Sensori per La Misura Della Temperatura Superficiale. Available online: https://lsi-lastem.com/it/prodotti/temperatura-a-contatto/ (accessed on 26 November 2024).
35. LSI LASTEM Environmental Monitoring Solutions—Air Temperature. Available online: https://www.lsi-lastem.com/it/prodotti/temperatura-aria-indoor/ (accessed on 30 January 2025).
36. Thermal Energy System Specialists, LLC (TESS). *TRNSYS Type 785—Green Roof Model Documentation*; Thermal Energy System Specialists, LLC (TESS): Madison, WI, USA. Available online: https://www.trnsys.com/tess-libraries/individual-components.php.html (accessed on 12 August 2025).
37. Loga, T.; Stein, B.; Diefenbach, N. TABULA Building Typologies in 20 European Countries—Making Energy-Related Features of Residential Building Stocks Comparable. *Energy Build.* **2016**, *132*, 4–12. [CrossRef]
38. American Society of Heating, Refrigerating and Air-Conditioning Engineers (ASHRAE) (Ed.) *ASHRAE Handbook—Fundamentals*; SI Edition; ASHRAE: Peachtree Corners, GA, USA, 2021.
39. Chartered Institution of Building Services Engineers (CISBE) (Ed.) *Environmental Design (CIBSE Guide A)*, 7th ed.; Chartered Institution of Building Services Engineers (CISBE): London, UK, 2006; ISBN 1-903287-66-9.
40. *EN 15242:2007*; Ventilation for Buildings—Calculation Methods for the Determination of Air Flow Rates in Buildings Including Infiltration. The European Committee for Standardization: Brussels, Belgium, 2007. Available online: https://store.uni.com/en-15242-2007 (accessed on 12 August 2025).
41. *ISO 6946:2017*; Building Components and Building Elements Thermal Resistance and Thermal Transmittance Calculation Methods. The International Organization for Standardization: Geneva, Switzerland, 2017.

42. *ISO 7730*; Ergonomics of the Thermal Environment—Analytical Determination and Interpretation of Thermal Comfort Using Calculation of the PMV and PPD Indices and Local Thermal Comfort Criteria. The International Organization for Standardization: Geneva, Switzerland, 2005.
43. *ASHRAE Standard 55*; Thermal Environmental Conditions for Human Occupancy. ASHRAE: Peachtree Corners, GA, USA, 2023. Available online: https://www.ashrae.org/technical-resources/bookstore/standard-55-thermal-environmental-conditions-for-human-occupancy (accessed on 27 July 2025).
44. Bienvenido-Huertas, D.; Moyano, J.; Marín, D.; Fresco-Contreras, R. Review of in Situ Methods for Assessing the Thermal Transmittance of Walls. *Renew. Sustain. Energy Rev.* **2019**, *102*, 356–371. [CrossRef]

energies

MDPI

Article

Performance of Double Pipe Heat Exchanger—Partially Occupied by Metal Foam—Is Better Enhanced Using Robust Adaptive Barrier Function-Based Sliding Mode Control

Luma F. Ali [1], Shibly A. AL-Samarraie [2] and Amjad J. Humaidi [2,*]

[1] Mechanical Engineering Department, College of Engineering, University of Baghdad, Baghdad 10071, Iraq; luma.f@coeng.uobaghdad.edu.iq

[2] College of Control and Systems Engineering, University of Technology, Baghdad 10066, Iraq; shibly.a.alsamarraie@uotechnology.edu.iq

* Correspondence: amjad.j.humaidi@uotechnology.edu.iq

Abstract

Numerous thermal practical applications utilize shell and tube heat exchanger appliances to transfer heat energy between hot and cold working fluids. Incorporating metal foam to the outer periphery of inner tube improves the heat transfer process from hot water in the tube side to cold water in the shell side and consequently improves heat exchanger performance. In this study, the integration of use of a porous material together with designing a robust adaptive controller could efficiently regulate the outlet cold water temperature to the desired value. This is achieved with respect to the time required for cold water to reach the desired temperature (settling time) and the amount of hot water volume flow during a certain time span. A barrier function-based adaptive sliding mode controller (BF-based adaptive SMC) is proposed, which requires only the information of temperature measurement of cold water. The stability of BF-based adaptive SMC is proved utilizing Lyapunov function analysis. The effectiveness of proposed controller is verified via numerical results, which showed that the proposed controller could achieve considerable accuracy of cold water temperature using suitable design parameters. In addition, the robustness of controller against variation in inlet temperature is also verified. Another improvement to performance of heat exchanger system is achieved by adding the metal foam of aluminum material on inner pipe perimeter with wide range of metal foam to outer inner pipe diameters ratio ($1 \leq s \leq 1.8$). The results showed that the settling time is significantly reduced which enables outlet cold water to reach the required temperature faster. With respect of the case of non-adding metal foam on inner pipe outer circumference, when $s = 1.2$, the settling time and hot water temperature are reduced by $1/2$ and 17.3%, respectively, while for $s = 1.8$, they are decreased by $\leq 1/20$ and 35.3% correspondingly. Accordingly, the required volume flow for hot water is reduced considerably.

Keywords: double-pipe heat exchanger; metal foam; heat transfer; adaptive sliding mode control; barrier function

1. Introduction

Frequent applications include heat transfer operations; however, conversion, employment, and energy recovery in every manufacturing, commercial, and domestic application comprise a heat transmission process. In most of these demands, heat is transported through heat exchanger devices which are designed to effectively transmit heat between two fluids without pending into direct interaction. Nowadays, heat exchangers find extensive utilization across diverse industrial and engineering applications; power plants, air conditioning, thermal heating, refrigeration, manufacturing industries, etc. [1,2]. Consequently, improving thermal operation of heat exchange has an instant influence on the energy, material, and cost economy. Accordingly, augmenting heat transmission above that in traditional or normal practice can considerably enhance thermal efficiency in such implementations in addition to their design and operation [2]. There are widespread types of heat exchangers which can be simply factory-made, such as double-pipe or so-called shell and tube heat exchanger type. This type becomes the greatest noteworthy fragment in small and large engineering and technical applications. Also, it has attracted important attention from researchers, engineers, and industries due to numerous compensations, such as compact design, flexibility, versatility, modularity, easy cleaning and maintenance, and cost-efficacy [3,4].

Heat transmission in heat exchangers including the double-pipe heat exchanger can be enhanced by various techniques, such as heat sink appliances that can be combined with heat exchangers to improve heat transmission. These heat sink mechanisms comprise metal wires, disks, fins, rings, porous media, supercritical CO_2 with circular tetrahedral lattice structures, and other complex assemblies [5–8]. Metal foam which represents one of the porous media types can be utilized for supplementing heat transmission because of its small volume and low production cost. Additionally, metal foam has combinations of physical, structural, and mechanical properties that cannot be attained in other materials such as elevated mechanical strength, light weight, raised electrical and thermal conductivity, strong flow-mixing capability, and high specific surface area [9–12]. Augmentation of employing metal foam in flow and heat transfer appliances is due to its unique thermo-physical properties such as high thermal conductivity, porosity, and fluid flow mixing in addition to the increase in the heat transfer surface area which raises the heat transmission rate as compared with components or surfaces without metal foam insertion [13–20].

Performance of double-pipe heat exchangers can be enhanced by inserting metal foam of different geometries on the inner and/or outer cylindrical periphery of outer tube (shell side) and/or inner tube (pipe side). Metal foam insertion can be accomplished fully or partially filled across required position according to the type of working fluids, shell- and tube-side dimensions, working fluids velocity, type of heat exchanger application, maintenance requirements, and many other factors that affect heat exchanger performance and efficiency. Recently, numerous studies have mainly concentrated on the heat transfer process in fully and partially foam-filled heat exchangers with different geometries such as metal foam fins, foam blocks, foam heat sinks, and foam wrapped tubes [12,21–28].

Increased efforts have been spent improving the quality of control in the chemical process industry, mainly for the temperature control systems in heat exchanger appliances. The designer is frequently faced with the problem of maintaining control system stability and performance (robustness) in the presence of significant plant model mismatch, nonlinearity, and external disturbances [29]. The Proportional–Integral–Derivative (PID) controller was utilized by many authors to design temperature control considering the linear model of heat exchanger [30–32]. Also, the fuzzy Proportional–Derivative (FPD) controller and PID controller were implemented by [33] and compared with the traditional PID controller. On the other hand, refs. [29,34] applied the PID controller for the feedback-linearized heat exchanger. Consequently, the PID controller is effective for linear model plant with constant perturbation, and so, for the case of a nonlinear model with non-constant perturbation, the controller efficiency degrades.

Nonlinear control design techniques were also applied to nonlinear models of heat exchanger and also for addressing the uncertainty in the models. The H_∞ robust controller design theory is applied to the heat exchanger control system with defined uncertainties, like parametric uncertainty and performance, as specified in [35]. By utilizing the dynamic state feedback in [34], the controller was designed by linearizing the heat exchanger model and then linear control theory can be used to regulate temperature to the desired value. Moreover, the sliding mode control technique is a well-known robust control method which is used to control different types of systems. The SMC has several advantages, such as robustness against external disturbances and uncertainties in parameters. Thus, a first-order SMC with integral sliding variable was employed by [36], while a time-varying integral sliding variable was utilized by [37] to combine the benefit of control system robustness and convergence rate. Additionally, in [38], an adaptive fuzzy sliding mode controller was designed for strong robustness and high control precision. Afterwards, for first-order SMC, the convergence is asymptotic; however, for finite time stability, higher order SMCs have been utilized by many authors. Ref. [39] proposed three different terminal sliding mode controllers and was verified through numerical simulations and implemented using an experimental setup. Also, in [40], the super-twisting control (STC) was employed for the temperature control of the heat exchanger. They showed that the STC can be practically implemented for process control using mechanical positioning actuators in real-world applications. Furthermore, for a precise control for the outlet temperature of cold water, a Terminal Synergetic Control (TSC) was proposed in [41], where, in their work, it was shown that synergetic control-based techniques offer superior potential solutions for nonlinear feedback control problems. Finally, a Higher-Order Sliding Mode (HOSM) controller for a heat exchanger connected via a data communication network was proposed by [42]. Besides its ability for chattering attenuation, the HOSM controller compensates for the random communication network and process delays in the model uncertainties present in the heat exchanger.

Model predictive control (MPC) is a control method based on periodically solving a constrained optimal control problem in every time step to evaluate the optimal input signal. The MPC was modified by [43] for a constraint removal approach which achieves the robustness required for practical application to a laboratory-scaled heat exchanger. They analyzed the control performance of the heat exchanger from the industrial perspective considering computational time and energy consumption. Additionally, ref. [44] proposed modified single layer economic model predictive control which integrates the dynamic economic optimization with the objective function of conventional tracking model predictive control. Their results showed that the economic model predictive control provides good quality control at a lower operational cost. Moreover, two control strategies were performed by [45] to identify the best-performing strategy for a countercurrent flow-plate heat exchanger in a virtual environment. The first controller is based on an inverse model of the plant, with linear algebra techniques and numerical methods; the second controller is an MPC. They showed that the MPC controller has the shortest settling time and lowest steady-state error.

Sliding mode control is a robust design methodology based on a systematic scheme that ensures the attractiveness of sliding manifold [46]. During sliding motion, the system becomes invariant to system uncertainties and external disturbances. This is known as the invariance property, which represents the main advantage of sliding mode control [47]. Conversely, the main disadvantage is the chattering problem [48]. The chattering problem can be overcome by suitable selection of the control gain. The barrier function has been augmented with the SMC formula, and it represents an adaptive control gain [49] and also with ISMC [50,51]. With the aid of using the barrier function in SMC, there is no need for either the precise system model knowledge or the ultimate bounds on its uncertainty and disturbances [52]. Hence, an adaptive SMC is obtained and additionally the chattering is eliminated where the combination of the barrier function with the SMC makes the control law continuous [53].

The aim of the present work is to explore the effect and enhancement of adding metal foam to the outer perimeter of the inner pipe for a parallel flow double-pipe heat exchanger. The heat exchanger performance will be measured by fixing the cold outlet temperature via a robust controller. An adaptive SMC using the barrier function will be designed to regulate robustly the outlet cold water to the desired temperature. Then, performance of the controlled output heat exchanger will be measured via the time required to reach the required outlet cold water temperature and additionally the amount of hot water volume flow through the inner pipe during certain time span. The main contributions of the present work can be summarized in the following points:

- The double-pipe heat exchanger mathematical model has been derived from the first principles in the presence of metal foam insertion at the outer perimeter of the inner pipe (tube side). This also includes the derivation of overall thermal conductance;
- A robust barrier function-based sliding mode controller has been designed to enforce the outlet cold water temperature to follow a desired value;
- The insertion of metal foam on the outer periphery of double-pipe heat exchanger tube side could reduce both the settling time and hot water volume flow and hence improve the performance of the system;
- Improvement of the sustainability metric in terms of energy and consumed water, where both the volume and temperature of hot water have been decreased. By virtue of adding metal foam and fusing the proposed robust BF-based adaptive SMC, one can keep low consumption of hot water flow and, simultaneously, maintain lower temperature of the outlet hot water.

2. Double-Pipe Heat Exchanger Mathematical Model

A common double-pipe heat exchanger (shell and tube heat exchanger), shown in Figure 1, is composed of two concentric pipes with different diameters; the inner and outer pipes are so-called tube and shell sides, respectively. Two working fluids are flowing in the heat exchanger and heat transmission between them through the solid pipe wall is taking place. One of these fluids runs inside the tube side and the other fluid flows through the shell side (annular space between the two pipes). Two types of flow arrangement are probable for these working fluids, parallel flow and counter flow. In parallel flow, both hot and cold fluids enter the heat exchanger at the same end and move in a similar direction while working fluids in counter flow arrangement run in the opposite direction. In the present work, parallel flow arrangement is performed extensively.

To derive the mathematical model, the following assumptions are taken into consideration:

- The thermophysical properties of both cold and hot fluids under consideration are constant;
- The variation in fluid velocity and temperature radially is negligible, and thus the kinetic and potential energy changes are negligible;
- The outer surface of the heat exchanger is assumed to be perfectly insulated, so that there is no heat loss to the surrounding medium, and any heat transfer occurs between the two fluids only;
- Axial heat conduction along the tube is usually insignificant and can be considered negligible.

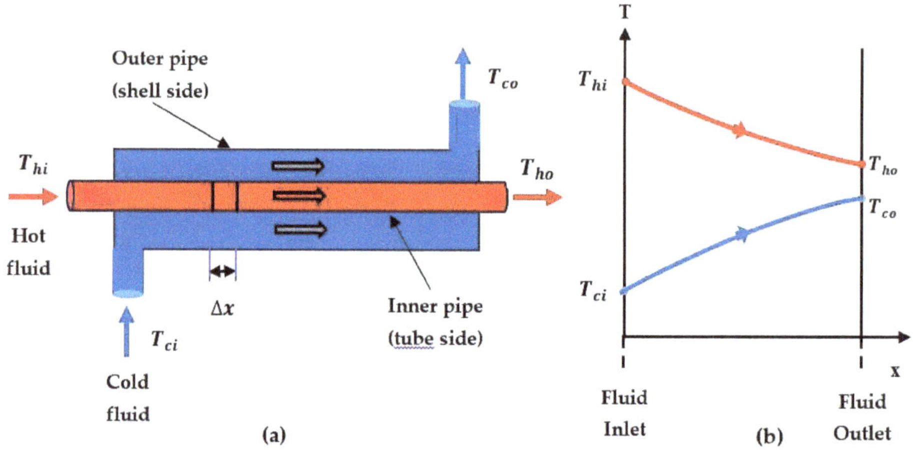

Figure 1. Schematic diagram of a double-pipe heat exchanger. (**a**) Parallel flow heat exchanger; (**b**) Temperature profile for parallel flow.

Referring to Figure 1, consider an incremental element Δx and along x to which the principle of energy conservation is applied. Energy balance is applied to differential element on tube side (either shell or inner tube). In the element at a particular distance $x - \Delta x$ and time t, the heat balance equation is given by [54,55] the following:

$$\begin{pmatrix}\text{Rate of change of}\\ \text{energy in the}\\ \text{element}\Delta\text{x}\end{pmatrix} = \begin{pmatrix}\text{convective flow of}\\ \text{energy into the}\\ \text{element}\Delta\text{x}\end{pmatrix} - \begin{pmatrix}\text{convective flow of}\\ \text{energy out of the}\\ \text{element}\Delta\text{x}\end{pmatrix} + \begin{pmatrix}\text{heat transfer}\\ \text{to the}\\ \text{element}\Delta\text{x}\end{pmatrix}, \tag{1}$$

and it can be written as follows:

$$Q_{store,\Delta x} = Q_x - Q_{x+\Delta x} + Q_{radial,\ \Delta x},$$

If the velocity of fluid averaged across the tube is constant, i.e., independent of x, then unsteady-state lumped energy balance is given by [34] the following:

$$\frac{d(\rho \forall C p T)}{dt} = \rho C p \dot{V}(T_{x-\Delta x} - T_x) + UA\Delta T_{LMTD}, \tag{2}$$

where ρ is fluid density; $\forall$ is volume of fluid; Cp is fluid specific heat; T is temperature; t is time duration; $\dot{V}$ is fluid volume flow rate; U is the overall heat transfer coefficient; A is cross section area; and ΔT_{LMTD} is the logarithmic mean temperature difference.

Equation (2) can be utilized to derive the following equation for the shell side (cold fluid) as follows:

$$\frac{dT_c}{dt} = \frac{\dot{V}_c}{\forall_c}(T_{x-\Delta x} - T_x) + \frac{UA}{\rho_c \forall_c C p_c}\Delta T_{LMTD}, \tag{3}$$

And the tube side (hot fluid) is casted as follows:

$$\frac{dT_h}{dt} = \frac{\dot{V}_h}{\forall_h}(T_{x-\Delta x} - T_x) - \frac{UA}{\rho_h \forall_h C p_h}\Delta T_{LMTD}, \tag{4}$$

where subscripts c and h refer to cold and hot working fluid, respectively.

It must be noticed that the negative sign for the second term in the right side of Equation (4) is because heat transfer is transmitted from the element in tube side (hot fluid) to that in shell side (cold fluid).

Cold T_c and hot T_h fluid temperature in the left side of Equations (3) and (4), respectively, can be possessed as a bulk mean temperature of inlet and outlet temperature, $T_c = \frac{T_{ci}+T_{co}}{2}$ and $T_h = \frac{T_{hi}+T_{ho}}{2}$. Thus, Equations (3) and (4) become the following:

$$\frac{d\left(\frac{T_{ci}+T_{co}}{2}\right)}{dt} = \frac{\dot{V}_c}{\forall_c}(T_{ci} - T_{co}) + \frac{UA}{\rho_c \forall_c Cp_c}\Delta T_{LMTD}, \tag{5}$$

$$\frac{d\left(\frac{T_{hi}+T_{ho}}{2}\right)}{dt} = \frac{\dot{V}_h}{\forall_h}(T_{hi} - T_{ho}) - \frac{UA}{\rho_h \forall_h Cp_h}\Delta T_{LMTD}, \tag{6}$$

In the present work, T_{ci} and T_{hi} are considered constant. Thus, $\frac{dT_{ci}}{dt} = 0$ and $\frac{dT_{hi}}{dt} = 0$ and Equations (5) and (6) are presented as follows:

$$\frac{dT_{co}}{dt} = \frac{2}{\forall_c}\left[\dot{V}_c(T_{ci} - T_{co}) + \frac{UA}{\rho_c Cp_c}\Delta T_{LMTD}\right], \tag{7}$$

$$\frac{dT_{ho}}{dt} = \frac{2}{\forall_h}\left[\dot{V}_h(T_{hi} - T_{ho}) - \frac{UA}{\rho_h Cp_h}\Delta T_{LMTD}\right], \tag{8}$$

Meanwhile, if cold T_c and hot T_h fluid temperature in the left side of Equations (3) and (4) are taken equal to outlet temperature, $T_c = T_{co}$ and $T_h = T_{ho}$, then Equations (3) and (4) become the following:

$$\frac{dT_{co}}{dt} = \frac{\dot{V}_c}{\forall_c}(T_{ci} - T_{co}) + \frac{UA}{\rho_c \forall_c Cp_c}\Delta T_{LMTD}, \tag{9}$$

$$\frac{dT_{ho}}{dt} = \frac{\dot{V}_h}{\forall_h}(T_{hi} - T_{ho}) - \frac{UA}{\rho_h \forall_h Cp_h}\Delta T_{LMTD}, \tag{10}$$

Thus, Equations (9) and (10) are represented as follows:

$$\frac{dT_{co}}{dt} = \frac{1}{\forall_c}\left[\dot{V}_c(T_{ci} - T_{co}) + \frac{UA}{\rho_c Cp_c}\Delta T_{LMTD}\right], \tag{11}$$

$$\frac{dT_{ho}}{dt} = \frac{1}{\forall_h}\left[\dot{V}_h(T_{hi} - T_{ho}) - \frac{UA}{\rho_h Cp_h}\Delta T_{LMTD}\right], \tag{12}$$

In general form, Equations (7), (8), (11) and (12) can be casted as follows:

$$\frac{dT_{co}(t)}{dt} = \frac{a}{\forall_c}\left[\dot{V}_c(t)(T_{ci} - T_{co}(t)) + \frac{UA}{\rho_c Cp_c}\Delta T_{LMTD}(t)\right], \tag{13}$$

$$\frac{dT_{ho}(t)}{dt} = \frac{a}{\forall_h}\left[\dot{V}_h(t)(T_{hi} - T_{ho}(t)) - \frac{UA}{\rho_h Cp_h}\Delta T_{LMTD}(t)\right], \tag{14}$$

where a may be either equal 1 or 2. In the present work, a is possessed equal to 1. Additionally, $\Delta T_{LMTD}(t)$ is determined using the following equation:

$$\Delta T_{LMTD}(t) = \frac{(T_{hi} - T_{ci}) - (T_{ho}(t) - T_{co}(t))}{ln[(T_{hi} - T_{ci})/(T_{ho}(t) - T_{co}(t))]}, \tag{15}$$

2.1. Overall Thermal Conductance

The overall heat transfer coefficient multiplied by surface area through which heat is transferred (UA) is known as overall thermal conductance. Generally, heat transfer rate in double-pipe heat exchanger can be assessed using the following equation:

$$Q = \frac{\Delta T}{R} = UA_s \Delta T_{LMTD} = U_i A_i \Delta T_{LMTD} = U_o A_o \Delta T_{LMTD}, \quad (16)$$

where R is the overall thermal resistance; U_i and U_o are inner and outer overall heat transfer coefficient, respectively; A_i and A_o are inner and outer surface area correspondingly; and A_s is the surface area.

By re-writing Equation (16), the total thermal resistance for inner tube with non-negligible wall thickness can be formulated as follows (shown in Figure 2):

$$\frac{1}{UA_s} = \frac{1}{U_i A_i} = \frac{1}{U_o A_o} = R = \frac{1}{h_i A_i} + \frac{ln(D_o/D_i)}{2\pi k L} + \frac{1}{h_o A_o}, \quad (17)$$

where k is the inner pipe thermal conductivity; h_i and h_o are heat transfer coefficient inside inner pipe and on outer periphery of inner pipe, respectively; D_o and D_i are inner and outer diameter of inner pipe correspondingly; and L is the length of inner pipe.

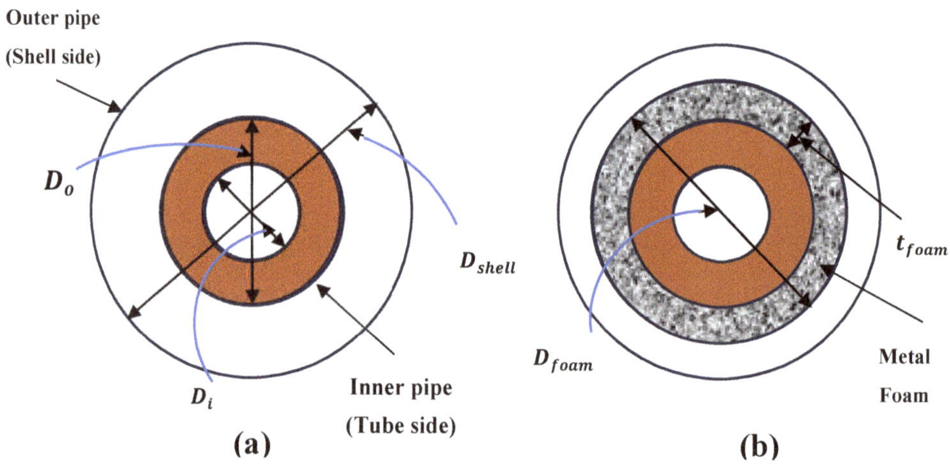

Figure 2. Heat exchanger cross section (**a**) without adding metal foam; (**b**) metal foam is added on outer periphery of iner pipe.

As mentioned previously, metal foam can be added adjacent to the solid wall to enhance heat transmission. In the present work, a metal foam layer of different thicknesses t_{foam} is supplemented on the outer perimeter of inner pipe (exposed in Figure 2) and its diameter D_{foam} can be stated as follows:

$$D_{foam} = D_o + \left(2 \times t_{foam}\right), \quad (18)$$

Consequently, Equation (17) can be presented as follows for the case of adding metal foam on the outer perimeter of inner tube by appending metal foam conduction thermal resistance ($R_{cond,foam} = \frac{ln\left(D_{foam}/D_o\right)}{2\pi k_{eff}L}$) [54,55]:

$$\frac{1}{UA} = \frac{1}{U_iA_i} = \frac{1}{U_oA_o} = R = \frac{1}{h_iA_i} + \frac{ln(D_o/D_i)}{2\pi kL} + \frac{ln\left(D_{foam}/D_o\right)}{2\pi k_{eff}L} + \frac{1}{h_oA_o}, \quad (19)$$

2.2. Calculation of Heat Transfer Coefficients

In order to estimate the overall heat transfer coefficient, inner heat transfer coefficient h_i and outer heat transfer coefficient h_o can be calculated for the two cases of inner pipe. These cases include without and with adding metal foam on the outer perimeter of inner pipe.

1. The inner heat transfer coefficient h_i for internal side of inner pipe (hot water) can be determined by employing the following equations [2,5,6,55,56]:

$$\text{For } Re_i \leq 2100\text{:} \ Nu = 1.86\left(\frac{Re_i\ Pr_i\ D_i}{L}\right)^{1/3}\left(\frac{\mu_b}{\mu_s}\right)^{0.14}, \quad (20)$$

$$\text{For } 2100 < Re_i < 10000\text{:} \ Nu = 1.86\left(\frac{Re_i\ Pr_i\ D_i}{L}\right)^{1/3}\left(\frac{\mu_b}{\mu_s}\right)^{0.14}, \quad (21)$$

$$\text{For } Re_i \geq 10000\text{:} \ Nu = 0.023Re_i^{0.8}Pr_i^n, \quad (22)$$

where $Re_i = \frac{V_hD_i}{\nu_i}$ is inner Reynolds number; $V_h = \frac{\dot{m}_h}{\rho_iA_c} = \frac{\dot{m}_h}{\rho_i\left(\frac{1}{4}\pi D_i^2\right)}$ is fluid velocity inside tube side; $Nu = \frac{h_iD_i}{k_i}$ is Nusselt number; k_i is tube-side fluid thermal conductivity; Pr_i is tube-side Prandtl number; μ_b and μ_s are dynamic viscosity at bulk and surface temperature, respectively; $\dot{m}_i$ is tube-side fluid mass flow rate; ρ_i is tube-side fluid density; A_c is inner tube cross-section area; ν_i is tube-side fluid kinematic viscosity; and n is a constant and it is taken as $n = 0.4$ for heating and 0.3 for cooling of fluid flowing through tube during heat exchanger operation.

2. The outer heat transfer coefficient h_o for the outer side of the inner pipe (cold water in annulus region) can be assessed by utilizing the following equations [5,56]:

$$V_c = \frac{\dot{V}_c}{\rho_oA_o} = \frac{\dot{V}_c}{\rho_o\left[\frac{1}{4}\pi\left(D_{s,i}^2 - D_{t,o}^2\right)\right]}, \quad (23)$$

Instead of using $D_{i,h}$ in the tube Equations (20)–(22), equivalent diameter equation D_e can employed as given below:

$$D_e = \frac{4A_{s,c}}{P} = \frac{4\pi\left(D_{s,i}^2 - D_{t,o}^2\right)}{4\pi D_{t,o}} = \frac{D_{s,i}^2 - D_{t,o}^2}{D_{t,o}}, \quad (24)$$

where V_c is cold fluid velocity inside shell side; $A_{s,c}$ is cross section area of annulus region (between outer diameter of pipe side and inner diameter of shell); P is perimeter of annulus region; $D_{s,i}$ is inner diameter of outer heat exchanger pipe (shell side); and $D_{t,o}$ is outer diameter of inner pipe (tube side).

2.3. Thermally Steady Outlet Temperature

In this section, the thermally steady-state outlet temperature is derived by equating the steady-state heat transfer rate equations. These heat rate equations include the equation of heat transmission to cold water (shell side), given as follows:

$$Q_c = \dot{m}_c C_{pc}(T_{c\_out} - T_{c\_in}), \tag{25}$$

The equation of heat transmission from hot water (tube side) is stated as follows:

$$Q_h = \dot{m}_h C_{ph}(T_{h\_in} - T_{h\_out}), \tag{26}$$

The average heat transfer rate, which is represented as follows:

$$Q = UA\,\frac{(T_{hi} - T_{ci}) - (T_{ho} - T_{co})}{ln[(T_{hi} - T_{ci})/(T_{ho} - T_{co})]}, \tag{27}$$

As the steady-state condition is applied, the above three heat transfer rate Equations (25)–(27) can be equated because heat is transmitted from the hot fluid through inner pipe wall towards cold fluid. Thus,

$$Q = Q_c = Q_h, \tag{28}$$

By solving Equation (28) with respect to T_{co} and T_{ho}, the outlet cold and hot temperature is obtained as function of UA, mass flow rate of cold and hot water, specific heat of water, and inlet cold and hot water temperature. An interesting point that can be deduced from heat balance Equation (28) for T_{co} is that the maximum allowable outlet cold water can be estimated for a certain hot and cold input water temperature and also for specific cold and hot water mass flow rate. Accordingly, this is stated in the following lemma.

Lemma 1. *Using the heat balance Equation (28) for certain cold and hot water inlet temperature and cold and hot water volumetric flow rates, the steady-state outlet hot water temperature is bounded by the following:*

$$T_{co} < \frac{\alpha T_{hi} + T_{ci}}{(1+\alpha)}, \tag{29}$$

where $\alpha = \dot{V}_h/\dot{V}_c$.

Proof. The two equations which are obtained from Equation (28) are given by the following:

$$0 = \dot{V}_c(T_{ci} - T_{co}) + \frac{UA}{\rho_c C p_c}\Delta T_{LMTD}, \tag{30}$$

$$0 = \dot{V}_h(T_{hi} - T_{ho}) - \frac{UA}{\rho_h C p_h}\Delta T_{LMTD}, \tag{31}$$

From which, the following equation can be attained:

$$\dot{V}_c(T_{ci} - T_{co}) + \dot{V}_h(T_{hi} - T_{ho}) = 0, \tag{32}$$

This leads to the following:

$$T_{co} = \frac{\dot{V}_h}{\dot{V}_c}(T_{hi} - T_{ho}) + T_{ci}, \tag{33}$$

Let $\alpha = \dot{V}_h/\dot{V}_c$ be the ratio of inlet hot water flow rate to inlet cold water flow rate, then,

$$T_{co} = -\alpha T_{ho} + \alpha T_{hi} + T_{ci}, \tag{34}$$

with the assumption of no heat generation, the following equation is casted:

$$T_{co} < T_{ho}, \tag{35}$$

Then, from Equation (34), the following is obtained:

$$T_{co} < -\alpha T_{co} + \alpha T_{hi} + T_{ci} \tag{36}$$

or it can be expressed as follows:

$$T_{co} < \frac{\alpha T_{hi} + T_{ci}}{(1+\alpha)}, \tag{37}$$

□

From Lemma 1, it is clear that the bound on T_{co} is function to α in addition to inlet cold and hot water temperature.

Remark 1. *For a certain $\alpha = \dot{V}_h/\dot{V}_c, T_{hi}$, and T_{ci}, the outlet cold water temperature for which the heat exchanger is designed must be selected such that inequality Equation (37) does not violate.*

Remark 2. *For anyα, the time history of outlet cold temperature from the first instant to steady-state condition is included in the following set $\Sigma = \left\{ T_{co} \middle| T_{ci} < T_{co} < \frac{\alpha T_{hi}+T_{ci}}{(1+\alpha)} \right\}$.*

Remark 3. *An interesting estimation for the outlet cold water from inequality Equation (37) can be obtained for $\alpha = 1$ which shows that T_{co} will be less than the average temperature of inlet cold- and hot water temperature. Meanwhile, for $\alpha >> 1$, T_{co} approaches the inlet hot water temperature T_{hi}.*

2.4. State Space Model

The double-pipe heat exchanger mathematical model given in Equations (13) and (14) with $a = 1$ is re-written in the state space model by defining the state variables x_1 and x_2 as follows:

$$\left.\begin{aligned} x_1 &= T_{co}(t) \\ x_2 &= T_{ho}(t) \end{aligned}\right\}, \tag{38}$$

Hence, the double-pipe heat exchanger dynamics, in terms of state variables $x = (x_1, x_2)$, is expressed by the following:

$$\frac{dx_1}{dt} = f_1(x), \tag{39}$$

$$\frac{dx_2}{dt} = f_2(x) + g_2(x)u, \tag{40}$$

where $x = (x_1, x_2)$, $f_1(x) = \frac{1}{\forall_c}\left[\dot{V}_c(T_{ci} - x_1) + \frac{UA}{\rho_c Cp_c}\Delta T_{LMTD}\right]$, $f_2(x) = -\frac{1}{\forall_h}\frac{UA}{\rho_h Cp_h}\Delta T_{LMTD}$, $g_2(x) = \frac{1}{\forall_h}(T_{hi} - x_2)$, $\Delta T_{LMTD} = \frac{(T_{hi}-T_{ci})-(x_2-x_1)}{\ln\left(\frac{T_{hi}-T_{ci}}{x_2-x_1}\right)}$, and finally $u = \dot{V}_h$ is the volumetric flow rate of hot fluid which presents the control input.

The state space model can be put also in a general form as follows:

$$\frac{dx}{dt} = f(x) + g(x)u, \tag{41}$$

where $f(x) = [f_1(x)\ f_2(x)]^T$ and $g(x) = [0\ g_2(x)]^T$. The heat exchanger state model is state feedback linearizable system as stated in the following Lemma.

Lemma 2. *The state space model of the double-pipe heat exchanger as given by Equations (39) and (40) is state feedback linearizable which can be transformed to a second-order canonical form via the state transformation* $x \to y$:

$$\left.\begin{array}{l} y_1 = x_1 \\ y_2 = \dot{x}_1 \end{array}\right\}, \tag{42}$$

where y_2 *is assumed to be measured or estimated.*

Proof. By following the procedure of deriving the linearizing output $y = h(x)$ in [57], firstly the dimension of the matrix $\{g, [f, g]\}(x)$ must be two, as shown below:

$$im\{g(x), [f,g](x)\} = dim\begin{bmatrix} 0 & \frac{\partial f_1}{\partial x_2} g_2 \\ g_2 & * \end{bmatrix}(x) = 2, \tag{43}$$

where $[f, g]$ is the Lie bracket and $\frac{\partial f_1}{\partial x_2}(g_2)^2 \neq 0\ \forall\ x \neq 0$.

Secondly, since $span\{g\}$ is involutive, the double-pipe heat exchanger is a linearizable system. Finally, the linearizing output $h(x)$ must satisfy the following condition:

$$\frac{\partial h}{\partial x} g = 0; \qquad \frac{\partial \left(L_f h\right)}{\partial x} g \neq 0, \ and \qquad h(0) = 0, \tag{44}$$

where $L_f h(x)$ is the Lee derivative of $h(x)$ with respect to f. So, $\frac{\partial h}{\partial x} g = \frac{\partial h}{\partial x_2} g_2 = 0$, this leads to $\frac{\partial h}{\partial x_2} = 0$, which means that $h = h(x_1)$. Eventually, let $h(x) = x_1$, which also satisfies the condition $\frac{\partial (L_f h)}{\partial x} g \neq 0$ because $L_f h(x) = f_1(x)$ then $\frac{\partial (L_f h)}{\partial x} = \frac{\partial f_1(x)}{\partial x_2} g_2 \neq 0\ \forall x$. Hence, the double-pipe heat exchanger state space model is linearizable with the linearizing output $h(x) = x_1$. Consequently, the change in variables is $y_1 = h(x)$ and $y_2 = L_f h(x) = f_1(x)$ which ends the proof. □

The linearized double-pipe heat exchanger state space model is specified by the following:

$$\left.\begin{array}{l} \dot{y}_1 = y_2 \\ \dot{y}_2 = F(x) + G(x)u \end{array}\right\}, \tag{45}$$

where $F(x) = \frac{\partial f_1(x)}{\partial x}\begin{bmatrix} f_1(x) \\ f_2(x) \end{bmatrix}$, and $G(x) = \frac{\partial f_1(x)}{\partial x_2} g_2(x)$. Also, it is assumed that $G(x) > 0, \forall x$.

Note that it does not need to transform the control u to a new control v (using $u = -\frac{1}{G(x)}\left(-F(x) + v\right)$) in order to write Equation (42) as $\dot{y}_1 = y_2$ and $\dot{y}_2 = v$. This is because $F(x)$ and $G(x)$ are considered as uncertain functions and accordingly the controller needs to be robust and adaptive, as is stated in the next section.

3. Barrier Function-Based Sliding Mode Control Law

One challenging problem in control engineering is the design of controllers for uncertain systems. The model inaccuracies, due to un-modeled or neglected system dynamics, uncertainty in model parameters, and external disturbances, are the sources of uncertainties. One of the most efficient robust control methodologies that can deal with uncertain systems is the sliding mode control (SMC) [48].

In the present work, the proposed controller employs barrier function (BF) instead of the discontinuous control term. The barrier function is defined as follows:

Definition 1. *([49]) For some $\epsilon > 0$, which is known and fixed, the BF can be defined as an even continuous function $k_{bf} : z \in (-\epsilon, \epsilon) \rightarrow k_{bf}(z) \in [b, \infty]$ strictly increasing on, $[0, \epsilon)$.*

- $\lim_{|x| \rightarrow \epsilon} k_{bf}(z) = +\infty$;
- $k_{bf}(z)$ has a unique minimum at zero and $k_{bf}(0) = b \geq 0$.

In the present study, a class of semi-definite BFs is considered as $k_{bf}(z) = \frac{|z|}{\epsilon - |z|}$. The SMC gain k is used as a function of the sliding variable σ via barrier function, i.e.,

$$k = \frac{|\sigma|}{\epsilon - |\sigma|}, \tag{46}$$

By using the gain in Equation (46), the SMC law becomes continuous, adaptive, and with attenuating or eliminating chattering.

To present our proposed controller, we need first to define the sliding variable. Thus, the sliding variable s, with respect to Equation (45), is defined by the following:

$$\sigma = e_2 + \lambda e_1, \qquad \lambda > 0, \tag{47}$$

where e_1 and e_2 are the error functions which are defined as follows:

$$\left.\begin{array}{r} e_1 = y_1 - y_r = T_{co}(t) - T_{cor}(t) \\ e_2 = \dot{e}_1 = y_2 - \dot{y}_r = \dot{T}_{co}(t) - \dot{T}_{cor}(t) \end{array}\right\}, \tag{48}$$

Also, the time rate of change in σ is given by the following:

$$\dot{\sigma} = \dot{y}_2 - \ddot{y}_r + \lambda(y_2 - \dot{y}_r) = F(x, y) + G(x)u, \tag{49}$$

In the present work, we propose the use of a variable structure controller that consists of three controllers and the switching between them depends on the state position in state space. The controllers are presented as follows:

1. The first controller uses the maximum hot water flow-rate as the control input when the state lies in the following region:

$$\Omega_I = \{x(t) | \sigma(t) \leq -\epsilon\}, \tag{50}$$

where ϵ is a small positive number. That is if $x(t) \in \Omega_I$, then

$$u = u_{max}, \tag{51}$$

2. The second controller utilizes the barrier function as the adaptive gain law for the sliding mode controller. The control law for this controller is given by the following:

$$u = -k(\sigma) sign(\sigma), \tag{52}$$

where, as in Equation (48), $k(t, s)$ can be defined as follows:

$$k(\sigma) = k_o \frac{|\sigma|}{\epsilon - |\sigma|}, \; k_o > 0, \tag{53}$$

It is used when $x(t) \in \Omega_{II}$ and $u \leq u_{max}$ where

$$\Omega_{II} = \{x(t)|-\epsilon < \sigma(t) < 0\}, \tag{54}$$

3. The third controller is simply justifying the positive control input nature of the system. If $x(t) \in \Omega_{III}$, where $\Omega_{III} = \{x(t)|\sigma(t) \geq 0\}$, then the controller is given by the following:

$$u = 0, \tag{55}$$

The three above regions Ω_I, Ω_{II}, and Ω_{III} are shown in Figure 3 and the above variable structure controller is stated in the following theorem.

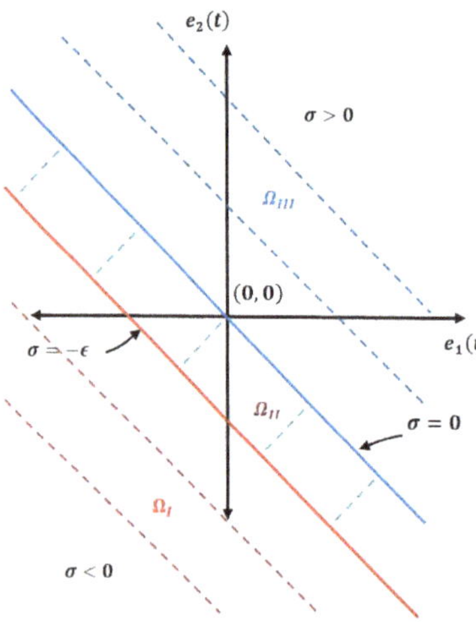

Figure 3. Control regions.

Theorem 1. *For the double-pipe heat exchanger which is defined by Equations (39) and (40), the proposed variable structure controller in Equations (52)–(57) enforces output cold water to follow the desired temperature with ultimate error bound given by the following:*

$$|e_1| \leq \frac{\epsilon}{\lambda}, \tag{56}$$

Proof. Let us assume that the state is initiated in Ω_{II}, then the second controllers, Equations (54) and (55), are used. Accordingly, we need to show that the error e_1 between the outlet cold water and desired outlet temperature is ultimately bounded by (58). To derive the inequality Equation (58), the following candidate Lyapunov function is employed:

$$V(\sigma) = \frac{1}{2}\sigma^2, \tag{57}$$

Its time rate of change is given by the following:

$$\dot{V}(\sigma) = \sigma\dot{\sigma} = \sigma(e_2 + \lambda\dot{e}_2), \tag{58}$$

Then for constant desired outlet cold temperature and the control law in Equations (52) and (53) we have the following:

$$\dot{V}(\sigma) = \sigma(\dot{y}_2 + \lambda y_2) = \sigma(F(x) + G(x)u + \lambda y_2),$$
$$= \sigma(F(x) - G(x)k(t,s)sign(s) + \lambda y_2),$$
$$\leq -G(x)k(\sigma)|\sigma| + G(x)|H(x,y)||\sigma|,$$
$$= -G(x)k_o\frac{|\sigma|^2}{\epsilon - |\sigma|}|\sigma| + G(x)|H(x,y)||\sigma|, \tag{59}$$

where $H(x,y) = \frac{F(x)+\lambda y_2}{G(x)}$. Therefore,

$$\dot{V}(\sigma) < -(1-\theta)G(x)k_o\frac{|\sigma|^2}{\epsilon - |\sigma|},\ 0 < \theta < 1, \tag{60}$$

$\forall|\sigma|$ such that

$$-\theta k_o\frac{|\sigma|^2}{\epsilon - |\sigma|} + |F(x,y)||\sigma| < 0, \tag{61}$$

The last inequality is solved for $|\sigma|$

$$|\sigma| > \frac{|F(x,y)|}{(\theta k_o + |F(x,y)|)}\epsilon, \tag{62}$$

Hence, $\dot{V}(\sigma) < 0$ for all state where s satisfies this inequality. Accordingly, the ultimate bound is presented as follows:

$$|\sigma| \leq b = \frac{|F(x,y)|}{(\theta k_o + |F(x,y)|)}\epsilon < \epsilon, \tag{63}$$

Which proves that when the state in Ω_{II}, the sliding variable s is bounded by ϵ. The ultimate bound with respect to the error $e_1 = T_{co}(t) - T_{cor}(t)$ can be derived from Equation (9),

$$e_2 + \lambda e_1 = \sigma, \tag{64}$$

by solving for e_1, we obtain

$$e_1(t) = e_1(0)\exp(-\lambda t) + \exp(-\lambda t)\int_0^t exp(\lambda\tau)\sigma(\tau)d\tau, \tag{65}$$

This leads to the following:

$$|e_1(t)| \leq |e_1(0)|\exp(-\lambda t) + \exp(-\lambda t)\int_0^t exp(\lambda\tau)|\sigma(\tau)|d\tau,$$
$$\leq |e_1(0)|\exp(-\lambda t) + \epsilon\exp(-\lambda t)\int_0^t exp(\lambda\tau)d\tau,$$
$$= |e_1(0)|\exp(-\lambda t) + \left(\frac{\epsilon}{\lambda}\right)(1 - exp(-\lambda t)), \tag{66}$$

As $t \to \infty$,

$$\lim_{t\to\infty}|e_1(t)| \leq \left(\frac{\epsilon}{\lambda}\right), \tag{67}$$

This proves that the error function $e_1(t)$ is asymptotically approaching the ultimate bound $\left(\frac{\epsilon}{\lambda}\right)$.

To this end, it must be shown that Ω_{II} is attractive if the state is initiated outside it. So, if the state is started in Ω_I with $u = u_{max}$, $T_{co}(t) \in \Sigma$ according to Remark 2. That means from Lemma 1, if the desired outlet cold water $T_{cor}(t)$ lies in Σ then with $u = u_{max}$, $T_{co}(t)$ will enter Ω_{II} in finite time and this proves the attractiveness Ω_{II} when the state is initiated in Ω_I.

Finally, it is required to show the attractiveness of Ω_{II} when the state is initiated in the region where $s(t) \geq 0$. In this case, $u = 0$, accordingly, Equation (34) with $\alpha = 0$, the steady-state outlet cold water temperature becomes the following:

$$T_{co} = T_{ci}, \tag{68}$$

Therefore, after a certain finite period of time, the state returns to enter Ω_{II} since $T_{cor}(t) > T_{ci}$. This ends the proof where via switching between the tree control laws according to the specified region, the outlet cold water temperature is eventually forced to follow the desired value. □

Remark 4. *In the proposed control law, u_{max} is not necessary to be the maximum available hot water flow rate.The operator can use an appropriate flow rate value and it is assigned as u_{max} but it is necessary to check that the condition $T_{cor}(t) \in \Sigma$ is satisfied.*

Remark 5. *The control law in Ω_{II} can be put in a more compact from as follows:*

$$u = Sat_{u_{max}}(k(\sigma)), \tag{69}$$

where

$$Sat_{u_{max}}(k(\sigma)) = \begin{cases} u_{max} & if\ \ k(\sigma) \geq u_{max} \\ k(\sigma) & if\ \ k(\sigma) < u_{max} \end{cases}, \tag{70}$$

Corollary 1. *The proposed controller in theorem 1 is a continuous controller.*

Proof. If the state is initiated in Ω_{II}, then the control law is given by $u = k(\sigma) = k_0 \frac{|\sigma|}{\epsilon - |\sigma|}$. The control formula in this region is a continuous function of s. But, if the state is initiated in Ω_I, then $u = u_{max}$ until the state enter Ω_{II} where during a certain period of time after entering Ω_{II}, the computed control u is greater than u_{max} as stated in Remark 5. This is because it is initially very near to the boundary of barrier function and according to Equation (70), the control u is fixed at u_{max}. After this period of time, the control u becomes equal to u_{max} and that is natural, since s goes away from the barrier function boundary. Then, due to the continuity of control law in Ω_{II}, control effort starts decreasing until it reaches a certain value such that the thermal steady outlet temperature equation is satisfied based on the desired outlet cold water temperature. This proves the continuity of the proposed control law. □

Remark 6. *The proposed control law in the above theorem is adaptive and works without the knowledge of system parameters or upper bound on their values. In fact, the structure of the mathematical model is the only thing that needs to be known, as given in Equations (11) and (12), in addition to the inlet and outlet cold and hot temperatures.*

Figure 4 illustrates the mechanism of integrating the BF-based adaptive sliding mode controller to the heat exchanger.

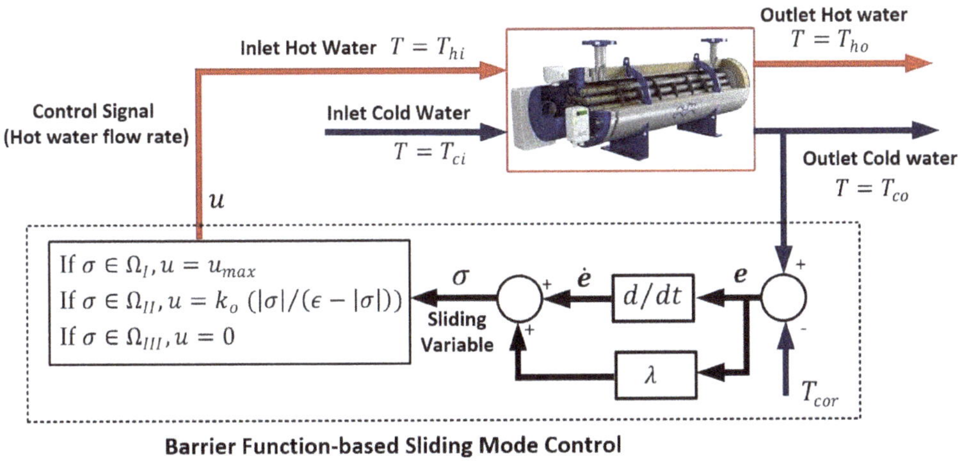

Figure 4. Schematic diagram of controlled heat exchanger based on BF-based SMC.

4. Results and Discussions

This section is devoted to presenting the numerical simulations for the double-pipe heat exchanger utilizing the proposed controller using the barrier function based on adaptive SMC. In the first part of this section, the heat exchanger dynamic system is simulated for fixed hot water volume flowrate and for different metal foam diameter. Then, in the second part which is devoted to test control system performance, the heat exchanger model is simulated for different desired outlet cold water temperatures. The only information required is the measurements of the inlet and outlet cold and hot water temperature. Next, in the third part of the simulation experiments, double-pipe heat exchanger performance enhancement is examined through the results of numerical simulations after adding metal foam with different diameters.

The heat exchanger mathematical model parameters that are used in the simulation are listed in Table 1 below, including the geometrical and the materials information required to calculate the overall thermal conductance UA and the other state space model parameters in Equations (49) and (40).

Table 1. Heat exchanger model parameter values [2,21,55]. * Effective thermal conductivity for water-saturated metal foam of 10 PPI thermal [58].

Parameter	Value	Parameter	Value
T_{hi}	85 °C	D_{si}	0.108 m
T_{ci}	20 °C	μ	855×10^{-6} N.s/m^2
$\forall_c$	0.0029 m^3	L	1.92 m
$\forall_h$	0.0043 m^3	k	0.671 W/m^2.K
$\dot{V}_c$	2.5096×10^{-6} m^3/s	k_{eff} *	7.6 W/m^2.K
ρ_c	966 kg/m^3	D_{to}	0.0548 m
ρ_h	966 kg/m^3	D_{ti}	0.0536 m
Cp_c	4204 J/kg.K	u_{max}	1.6667×10^{-5} m^3/s
Cp_h	4204 J/kg.K		

4.1. Effect of Metal Foam Insertion on Outlet Cold Water Temperature for Fixed Cold and Hot Water Flow Rates

The effect of inserting metal foam layer on the outer periphery of inner pipe in a double-pipe heat exchanger is examined in the present part of the results. The results are based on simulating the heat exchanger with the parameters listed in Table 1.

The only variable parameter in the heat exchanger system is the diameter of inserted metal foam and for simplicity it was taken as a percent from the outlet diameter of the inner pipe (tube side) D_{to}, i.e., the metal foam diameter D_{foam} is related to D_{to} by the following relation:

$$D_{foam} = s.D_{to}, \tag{71}$$

where $s = 1$ refers to the heat exchanger without metal foam, while when $s = D_{si}/D_{to}$, the metal foam fills totally the gap between outer pipe D_{to} and inner shell D_{si} diameters.

For feasibility in engineering applications, it can be mentioned that if the annulus is filled completely with water without metal foam ($s = 1$), the annulus mass is 13 kg and if the annulus is fully filled with metal foam ($s = 2$) the annulus mass becomes 15.25 kg. Therefore, the mass increase is about 2.25 kg ($\approx 17\%$) and this amplification can be neglected with respect to the overall mass of heat exchanger and can be integrated with the design consideration of heat exchanger.

The effect of adding metal foam is examined for the range $1 \le s \le 1.8 < 1.97 = D_{si}/D_{to}$ with inlet hot water volume flow rate equal to u_{max}. Figure 5 reveals that the overall thermal conductance UA is an increasing function with the increasing in the metal foam diameter D_{foam}. This behavior can be attributed to the reduction in thermal resistance as a result of increasing in effective thermal conductivity of metal foam. Note that in this paper, the results which are related to the metal foam diameter are referred to by their corresponding value of s.

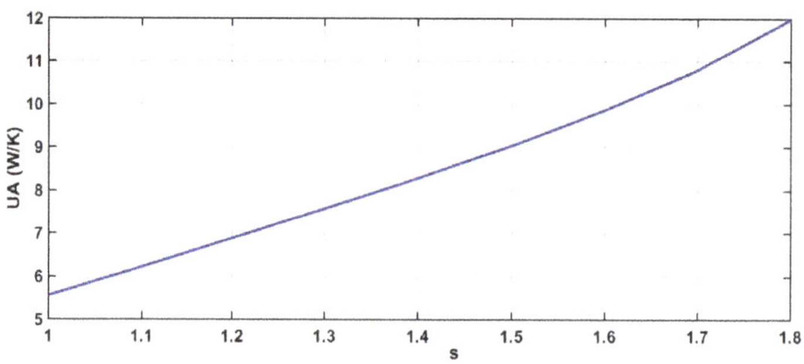

Figure 5. Overall thermal conductance UA vs. metal foam diameter ($D_{foam} = s.D_{to}$).

With the same inlet hot water volume flow rate, the numerical simulation results for different metal foam diameters are plotted in Figure 6. This figure reveals that the effect of adding metal foam to the heat exchanger, where the outlet cold water temperature is at steady state, is increased with the increase in the metal foam diameter. As the thickness of inserted metal foam is increased, this tends to raise the heat transmissions from hot water in the tube side to cold water in the shell side. Consequently, this is a direct result of increasing UA where a larger amount of heat energy is transformed from the hot water to the cold water.

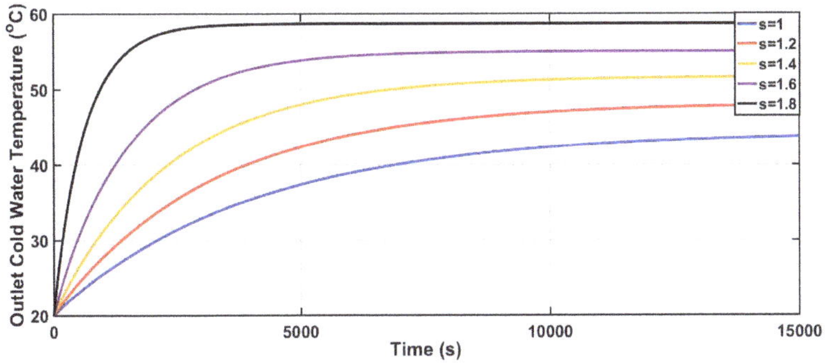

Figure 6. Outlet cold water temperature for different metal foam.

4.2. Testing the SMC Performance

As mentioned above, the proposed barrier function-based SMC is first tested for the double-pipe heat exchanger using selected control design parameter values of $k_o = 5u_{max}$, $\epsilon = 1$, and $\lambda = 2$. The results in this part are obtained for the double heat exchanger with the addition of metal foam where $s = 1.25$. Figure 7 shows the simulation results for three different, desired outlet cold water temperature where all the selected desired outlet cold temperatures are within the set Σ. It is observed that the control performance is well clarified where the outlet cold water converges to the desired temperature with a steady-state error less than $\frac{\epsilon}{\lambda} = 0.5\ ^\circ\mathrm{C}$ (inequality Equation (69)). Also, it can be noticed from Figure 7 that the transient period for all required cold water temperature coincides. This is because the state is always initiated in Ω_I and subsequently the control u is u_{max}.

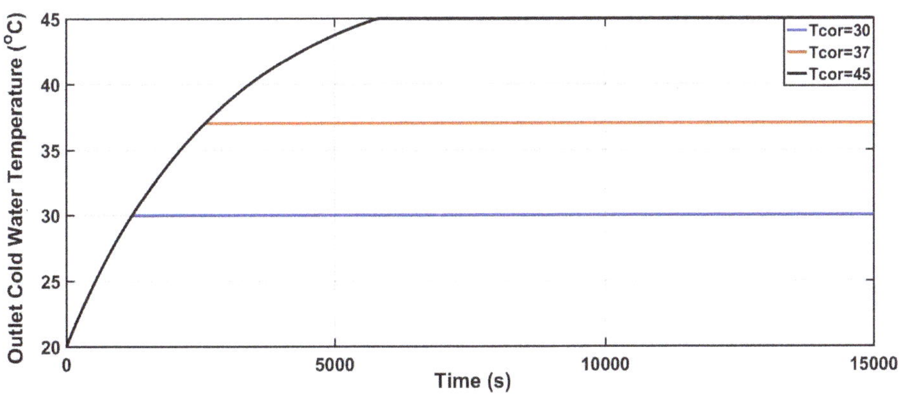

Figure 7. Outlet cold water temperature for different required temperature.

Also, in order to examine the control robustness simulation test, firstly it is demonstrated with different inlet cold and hot water temperatures, secondly through the different cold water inlet volume flow rate, and finally with different effective metal foam thermal conductivity. In Figure 8, the plot shows that the cold water converges to the desired temperature ($T_{cor} = 45$) and satisfies inequality Equation (71) irrespective of the change in the inlet cold water temperature.

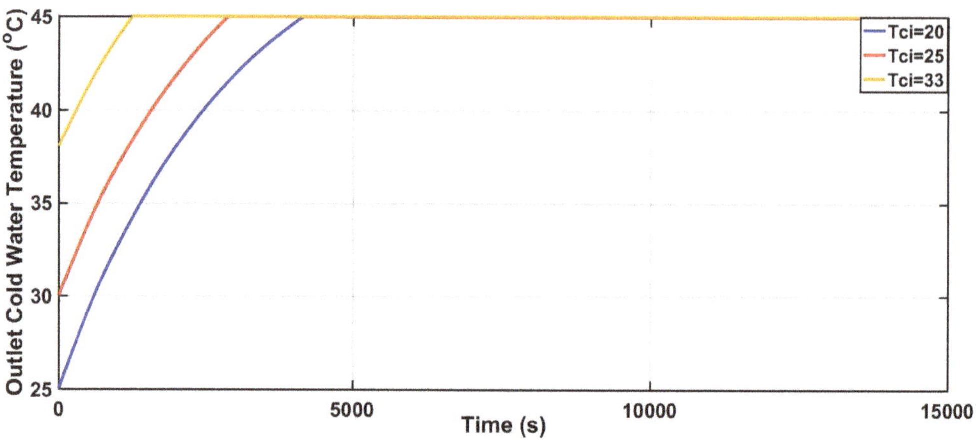

Figure 8. Outlet cold water temperature for different inlet cold water temperature.

Meanwhile, in Figure 9, the outlet cold water temperature is plotted when the inlet cold water flow rate is varied ($\pm 10\%$ of the nominal cold water volume flow rate $\dot{V}_c = 2.5096 * 10^{-6} \mathrm{m}^3/\mathrm{s}$) in order to accommodate the change in the cold-water volume flow rate due to metal foam insertion. Again, the proposed controller forces cold water to follow the desired temperature with a small variation in settling time.

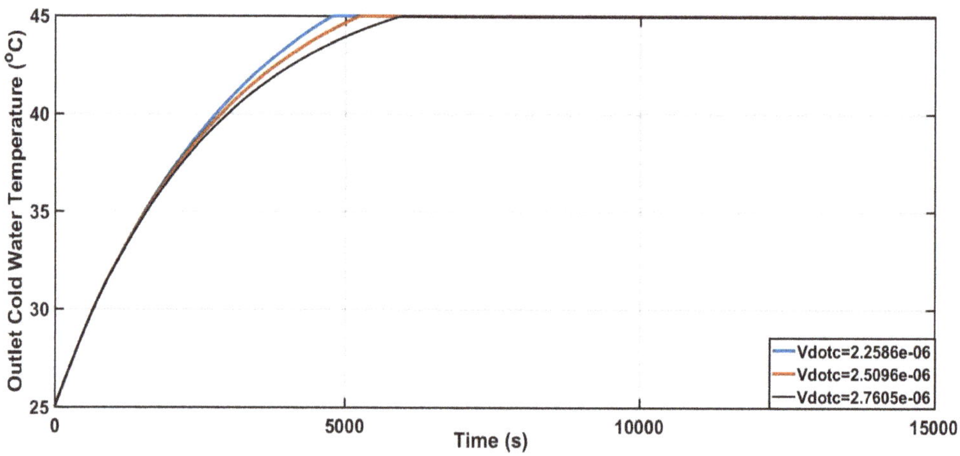

Figure 9. Outlet cold water temperature for different inlet cold water flow rate.

For the case of different metal foam porosity (0.909, 0.937, and 0.971 [58]) and consequently different metal foam effective thermal conductivity, the proposed controller against this type of uncertainty is robust, as revealed in Figure 10.

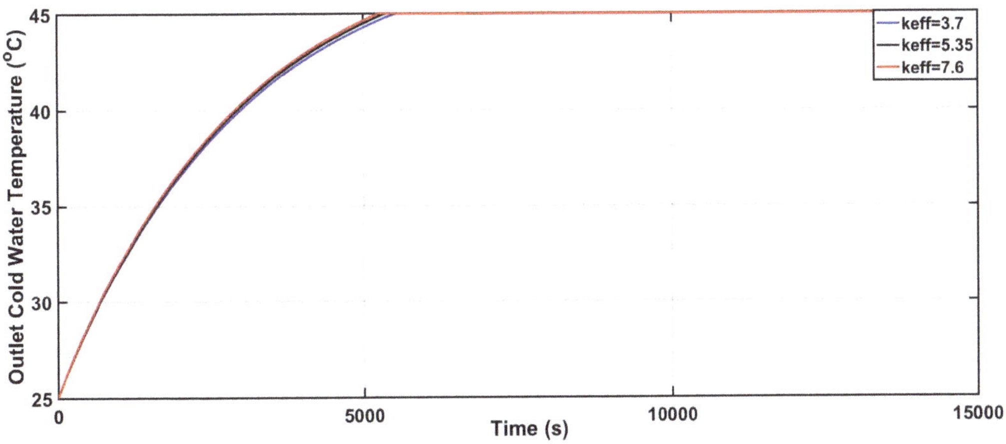

Figure 10. Outlet cold water temperature for different effective thermal conductivity.

For a stepwise desired outlet cold temperature, Figure 11 demonstrates the ability and performance of the proposed controller where the outlet cold water temperature follows the desired reference with the specified accuracy. Later, it is shown that by inserting metal foam, the settling time is reduced and consequently, the outlet cold water follows the required temperature quickly.

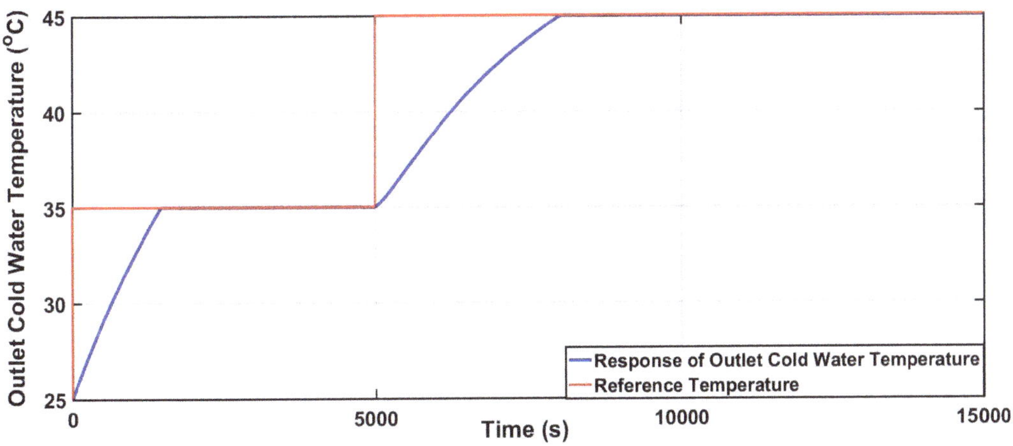

Figure 11. Outlet cold water temperature for stepwise required temperature ($s = 1.25$).

Finally, for the 45 °C as a reference outlet cold water temperature, the hot water volume flow rate (the control input) is continuous, as can be seen from Figure 12 below where this result is proved in Corollary 1.

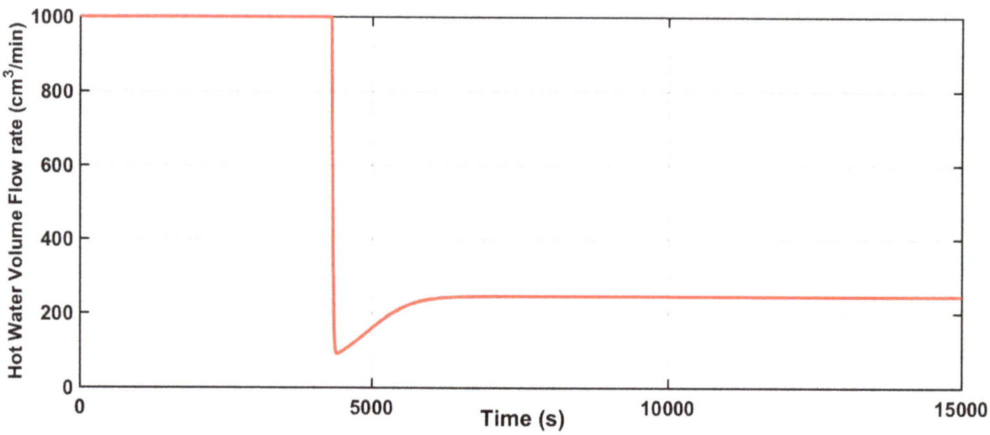

Figure 12. Hot water volume flow rate $\left(\mathrm{cm}^3/\mathrm{min}\right)$.

4.3. Testing the Enhancement of Adding Porous Material to the Heat Exchanger

In this part, the simulation results can answer the question about the evidence of adding porous material to the double-pipe heat exchanger with respect of the heat exchanger control system performance. Two factors are considered in evaluating the performance enhancement. The first factor is the settling time which is the time required to enter the positively invariant set Ω that is a set where $|T_{co}(t) - T_{cor}(t)| \leq \frac{\epsilon}{\lambda}$. Meanwhile, the second factor is the hot water volume flow during a time span including the transient period and certain time interval throughout steady-state condition.

In Figure 13, the cold-water temperature state is plotted for different metal foam diameters. This figure clarifies that the settling time is reduced significantly with the increase in the metal foam diameter. The settling time is also shown in Figure 14 for different foam diameter where for $s = 1$, the settling time is 10,800 s while for $s = 1.2$, the settling time is 4870 s which means that the cold water with $s = 1.2$ reaches the required temperature less than half the time spend for the case without metal foam. Additionally, when $s = 1.8$, the settling time reduces greater than 20 times the case of without adding metal foam ($s = 1$), which proves the significance of adding the metal foam to the heat exchanger.

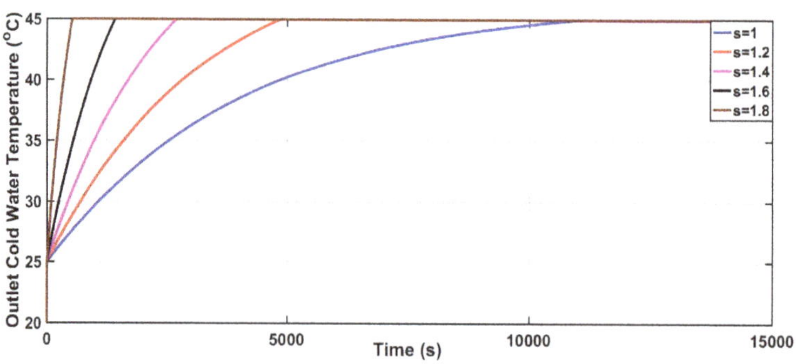

Figure 13. Outlet cold water temperature for different metal foam diameter.

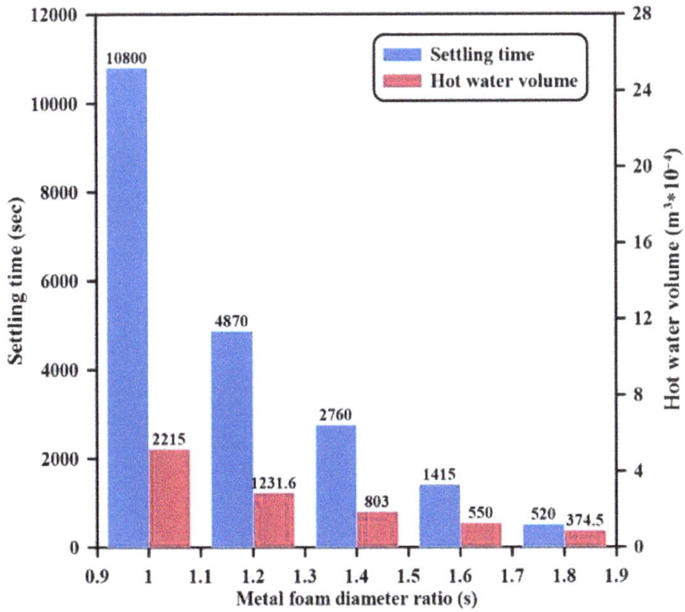

Figure 14. Settling time and hot water volume for different metal foam diameter ratio.

The reduction in the hot water volume (the second factor) is also shown in Figure 14. The addition of metal foam not only reduces significantly the settling time but also the required hot water volume, where it is measured here for a time span of 15,000 s. The settling time for different metal foam diameter ratio s is replotted in Figure 15 where the significance of the addition of metal foam on the heat exchanger control system response is clarified. Finally, the performance enhancement via adding metal foam for a stepwise required temperature is clarified in Figure 16. The enhancement is clear when the result in this figure with $s = 1.8$ is compared with those in Figure 11 where $s = 1.25$.

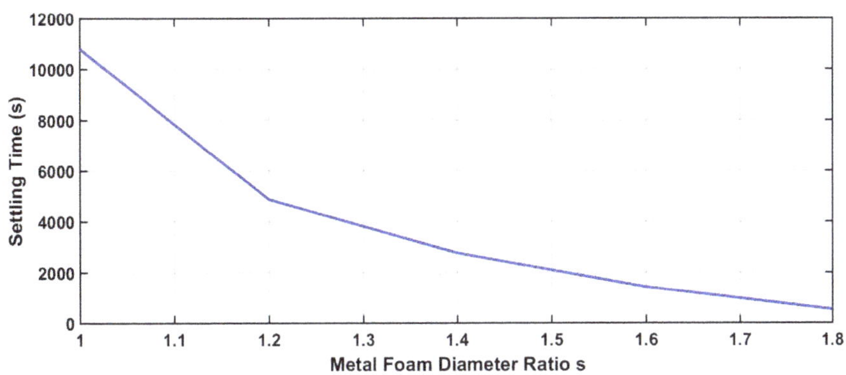

Figure 15. Settling time vs. different metal foam diameter ratio s.

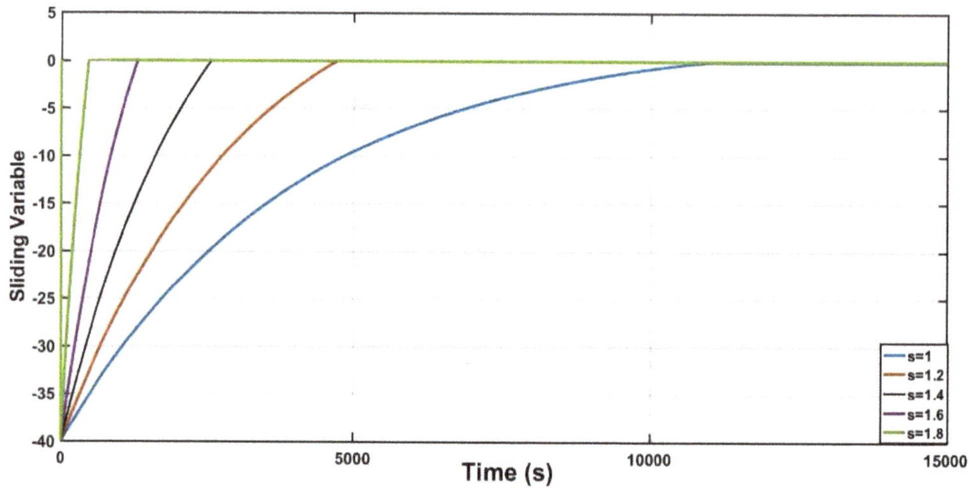

Figure 16. Sliding variable plot vs. time for different metal foam diameter ratio.

Additionally, the effect of adding metal foam for various diameters on the sliding variable is shown in Figure 16, where the reaching time is decreased significantly. After that, the cold-water temperature asymptotically reaches the desired value during sliding motion according to the sliding variable Equation (49) with a time constant equal to 1/2 as stated previously. As a result, the settling time which consists of reaching time and time spent during sliding phase is reduced and is illustrated in Figure 13.

An important contribution of adding metal foam, where large hot water volume flow rate reduction is obtained with increasing metal foam ratio, is proved in Figure 17. From this figure, it can be deduced that during the reaching phase, the hot water volume flow rate is constant and equal u_{max} but after that it is reduced during sliding motion phase. The reaching time is decreased with respect of the metal foam diameter; therefore, the period of time during which $u = u_{max}$ is reduced and consequently less control effort is required. Moreover, this figure shows that the steady-state hot water volume flow rate is also reduced with increasing metal foam diameter. In context to the reduction in steady-state hot water volume flow rate, the steady-state outlet hot water temperature is reduced with rising metal foam diameter as depicted in Figure 18. For steady-state condition and from Figures 17 and 18, both outlet hot water temperature and volume flow rate values are decreased with metal foam diameter increasing. Basically, according to this result, with both the outlet cold water temperature and volume flow rate values fixed, the thermal steady outlet temperature is satisfied and specifically Equation (32) is held. Accordingly, sustainable energy and consuming water requirements are attained as volume and temperature of hot water are decreased, which are a result of utilizing the current proposed control system and adding metal foam.

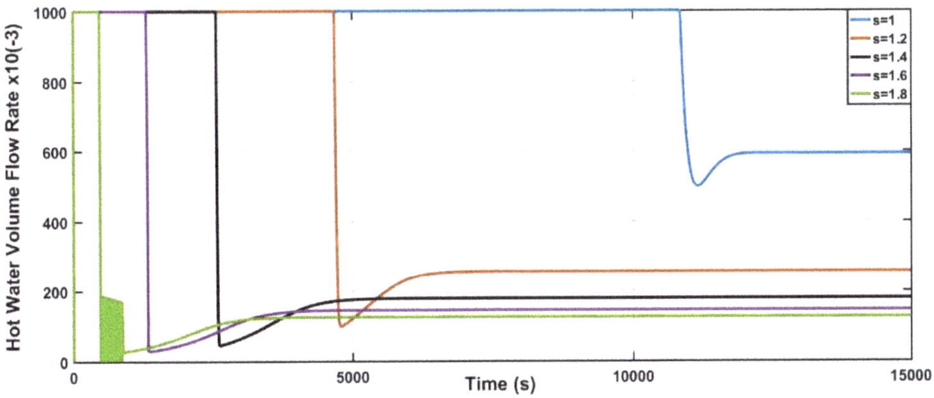

Figure 17. Hot water volume flow rate (the controller u) for different metal foam diameter ratio.

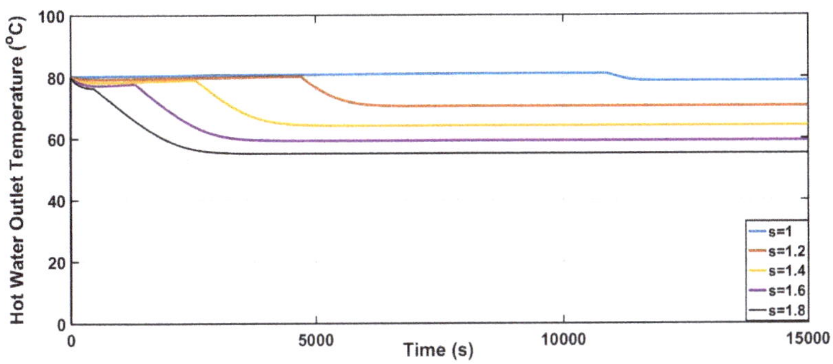

Figure 18. Outlet hot water temperature for different metal foam diameter ratio.

Finally, the performance enhancement via adding metal foam for a stepwise required temperature is clarified in Figure 19. The enhancement is clear when the result in this figure with $s = 1.8$ is compared with those in Figure 11 where $s = 1.25$.

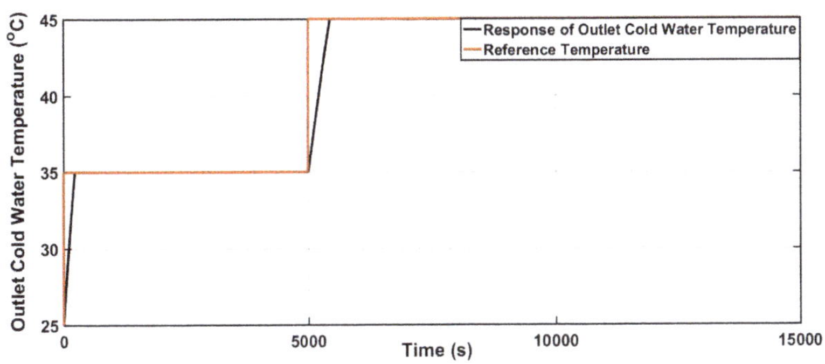

Figure 19. Outlet cold water temperature for stepwise required temperature ($s = 1.8$).

5. Conclusions

The present work addresses the performance enhancement for the double-pipe heat exchanger results from adding the metal foam to the outer diameter. The thermal conductance UA has been derived where Equation (19) showed that its value is increased with increasing metal foam diameter. The simulation results demonstrated the effect of the increase in in the thermal conductance UA, where it can be seen that the heat transfer from hot to cold water increased as in Figure 6. In order to study the effect of adding the metal foam, the adaptive and robust SMC has been designed to enforce the cold water to follow a certain desired value with the hot water volume flow rate play the role of the control input. The control stability and performance has been proved analytically through the use of Lyapunov function and also the simulation results reveal this fact. By using the designed controller, the simulation results reveal that a significant reduction occurred in the settling time and amount of hot water volume flow. Also, these results demonstrate that the enhancement in heat exchanger performance is achieved by inserting metal foam in addition to controlling the outlet cold water temperature. For $s = 1.8$, it was found that the reduction in settling time reaches $1/20$ times the case of non-adding metal foam ($s = 1$). Finally, from these results, the insertion of the metal foam to the double-pipe heat exchanger control system is recommended.

Author Contributions: Conceptualization, L.F.A., A.J.H. and S.A.A.-S.; methodology, L.F.A., A.J.H. and S.A.A.-S.; validation, A.J.H. and S.A.A.-S.; formal analysis, L.F.A., A.J.H. and S.A.A.-S.; investigation, L.F.A. and S.A.A.-S.; writing—review and editing, L.F.A. and A.J.H., writing—original draft preparation, L.F.A. and S.A.A.-S.; supervision, A.J.H. and S.A.A.-S.; funding acquisition, S.A.A.-S. and L.F.A. All authors have read and agreed to the published version of the manuscript.

Funding: This work is not financially supported by any organization and the fees were paid by the authors.

Data Availability Statement: The data presented in this study are available on request from the corresponding author.

Acknowledgments: The authors gratefully acknowledge all their colleagues for their co-operation.

Conflicts of Interest: The authors declare no conflicts of interest.

References

1. Alam, T.; Kim, M.-H. A Comprehensive Review on Single Phase Heat Transfer Enhancement Techniques in Heat Exchanger Applications. *Renew. Sustain. Energy Rev.* **2018**, *81*, 813–839. [CrossRef]
2. Bejan, A.; Kraus, A.D. *Heat Transfer Handbook*; John Wiley: Hoboken, NJ, USA, 2003.
3. Omidi, M.; Farhadi, M.; Jafari, M. A Comprehensive Review on Double Pipe Heat Exchangers. *Appl. Therm. Eng.* **2017**, *110*, 1075–1090. [CrossRef]
4. Li, W.; Zhang, W.; Li, Z.; Yao, H.; Cui, P.; Zhang, F. Investigation of the Heat Transfer Performance of Multi-Borehole Double-Pipe Heat Exchangers in Medium-Shallow Strata. *Energies* **2022**, *15*, 4798. [CrossRef]
5. Thulukkanam, K. *Heat Exchanger Design Handbook*; CRC Press: Boca Raton, FL, USA, 2013. [CrossRef]
6. Sekulić, D.P.; Shah, R.K. *Fundamentals of Heat Exchanger Design*; John Wiley & Sons, Inc.: Hoboken, NJ, USA, 2023. [CrossRef]
7. Liu, J.; Guo, W.; Yin, M.; Xi, W.; Sunden, B. Flow and Heat Transfer Characteristic of Regenerative Cooling Channels Using Supercritical CO_2 with Circular Tetrahedral Lattice Structures. *Case Stud. Therm. Eng.* **2025**, *71*, 106204. [CrossRef]
8. Zachi, F.J.; Ali, L.F. Experimental Study of Natural Convection Heat Transfer on an Enclosure Partially Filled Porous Medium Heated from below by Constant Heat Flux. *AIP Conf. Proc.* **2023**, *2651*, 050002. [CrossRef]
9. Mahmoudi, Y.; Hooman, K.; Vafai, K. *Convective Heat Transfer in Porous Media*; CRC Press: Boca Raton, FL, USA, 2019. [CrossRef]
10. Nield, D.A.; Bejan, A. *Convection in Porous Media*; Springer International Publishing: Cham, Switzerland, 2017. [CrossRef]
11. Kaviany, M. *Principles of Heat Transfer in Porous Media*; Springer: New York, NY, USA, 1995. [CrossRef]
12. Fiedler, T.; Movahedi, N. Compact Aluminium Foam Heat Exchangers. *Metals* **2023**, *13*, 1440. [CrossRef]
13. Alkinani, I.H.; Ali, L.F. Natural Convection in Annulus between Two Concentric Cylinders Partially Filled with Metal Foam Distributed with New Suggested Design. *IOP Conf. Ser. Earth Environ. Sci.* **2022**, *961*, 012032. [CrossRef]
14. Kuruneru, S.T.W.; Vafai, K.; Sauret, E.; Gu, Y. Application of Porous Metal Foam Heat Exchangers and the Implications of Particulate Fouling for Energy-Intensive Industries. *Chem. Eng. Sci.* **2020**, *228*, 115968. [CrossRef]
15. Chen, X.; Sun, C.; Xia, X.; Liu, R.; Wang, F. Conjugated Heat Transfer Analysis of a Foam Filled Double-Pipe Heat Exchanger for High-Temperature Application. *Int. J. Heat Mass Transf.* **2019**, *134*, 1003–1013. [CrossRef]

16. Lu, W.; Zhao, C.; Tassou, S. Thermal Analysis on Metal-Foam Filled Heat Exchangers. Part I: Metal-Foam Filled Pipes. *Int. J. Heat Mass Transf.* **2006**, *49*, 2751–2761. [CrossRef]
17. Alomar, O.R.; Hamdoon, O.M.; Salim, B.M. Analysis of Two-Phase Flow in a Double-Pipe Heat Exchanger Filled with Porous Media. *Int. J. Heat Mass Transf.* **2020**, *156*, 119799. [CrossRef]
18. Arasteh, H.; Salimpour, M.R.; Tavakoli, M.R. Optimal Distribution of Metal Foam Inserts in a Double-Pipe Heat Exchanger. *Int. J. Numer. Methods Heat Fluid Flow* **2019**, *29*, 1322–3142. [CrossRef]
19. Abdulwahed, A.S.; Ali, L.F. Numerical Investigation of Natural Convection in a Square Enclosure Partially Filled with Horizontal Layers of a Porous Medium. *Heat Transf.* **2023**, *52*, 874–889. [CrossRef]
20. Ali, L.F.; Humaidi, A.J. Offset Temperature and Amplitude–Frequency Effect on Convection Heat Transfer in Partially Gradient Porous Cavity with Different Outlet Port Locations. *Processes* **2025**, *13*, 2279. [CrossRef]
21. Hamzah, J.A.; Nima, M.A. Experimental Study of Heat Transfer Enhancement in Double-Pipe Heat Exchanger Integrated with Metal Foam Fins. *Arab. J. Sci. Eng.* **2020**, *45*, 5153–5167. [CrossRef]
22. Buonomo, B.; di Pasqua, A.; Manca, O.; Nappo, S. Entropy Generation Analysis on Heat Exchanger in Aluminum Foam. *Tec. Ital. J. Eng. Sci.* **2021**, *65*, 166–173. [CrossRef]
23. Shirvan, K.M.; Mirzakhanlari, S.; Kalogirou, S.A.; Öztop, H.F.; Mamourian, M. Heat Transfer and Sensitivity Analysis in a Double Pipe Heat Exchanger Filled with Porous Medium. *Int. J. Therm. Sci.* **2017**, *121*, 124–137. [CrossRef]
24. Tian, H.; Zhao, T.; Shi, L.; Chen, T.; Ma, X.; Zhang, H.; Shu, G. Assessment and Optimization of Exhaust Gas Heat Exchanger with Porous Baffles and Porous Fins. *Appl. Therm. Eng.* **2020**, *178*, 115446. [CrossRef]
25. Fiedler, T.; Moore, R.; Movahedi, N. Manufacturing and Characterization of Tube-Filled ZA27 Metal Foam Heat Exchangers. *Metals* **2021**, *11*, 1277. [CrossRef]
26. Alhusseny, A.; Turan, A.; Nasser, A. Rotating Metal Foam Structures for Performance Enhancement of Double-Pipe Heat Exchangers. *Int. J. Heat Mass Transf.* **2017**, *105*, 124–139. [CrossRef]
27. Abadi, G.B.; Kim, K.C. Experimental Heat Transfer and Pressure Drop in a Metal-Foam-Filled Tube Heat Exchanger. *Exp. Therm. Fluid Sci.* **2017**, *82*, 42–49. [CrossRef]
28. Ahmad, F.; Al-Kayiem, H.H.; Soon, W.P.K. *ICPER 2020, Proceedings of the 7th International Conference on Production, Energy and Reliability*; Springer: Berlin/Heidelberg, Germany, 2022. [CrossRef]
29. Alsop, A.W.; Edgar, T.F. Nonlinear Heat Exchanger Control through the Use of Partially Linearized Control Variables. *Chem. Eng. Commun.* **1989**, *75*, 155–170. [CrossRef]
30. Reddy, V.S.; Subhadra, H.; Prananvanand, S.; Juliet, A.V.; Ramesh, G.; Lakshmi, G.S.; Reddy, C.L.; Reddy, K.S. Controller Design for Temperature Regulation in a Nonlinear Industrial Heat Exchanger System. *E3S Web Conf.* **2025**, *616*, 10. [CrossRef]
31. Pallavi, P.; Vankunavath, P.; Ilaiah, S.; Reddy, G.P.; Bandi, A.; Hossain, M.; Jin, Y. Real-Time Temperature Control of a Shell and Tube Heat Exchanger by IMC Based PID Controller. *Epic. Ser. Comput.* **2023**, *91*, 155–163.
32. Markowski, M.; Trafczynski, M.; Pavlovičová, E.; Oravec, J.; Alabrudzinski, S.; Kisielewski, P.; Urbaniec, K.; Elwertowski, K.; Gostynski, D. Impact of Industrial Constraints on the Dynamic Performance of a PID-Controlled Hybrid Heat-Integrated Distillation System with a Plate Heat and Mass Exchanger. *Int. J. Heat Mass Transf.* **2025**, *252*, 127445. [CrossRef]
33. A.A.EMhemed, A.; Alsseid, A.; Hanafi, D. Modelling and Controller Design for Temperature Control of Power Plant Heat Exchanger. *Univers. J. Control. Autom.* **2017**, *5*, 49–53. [CrossRef]
34. Rahman, M.H.R.F.; Devanathan, R. Modelling and Dynamic Feedback Linearisation of a Heat Exchanger Model. In Proceedings of the IEEE Conference on Control Applications, Glasgow, UK, 24–26 August 1994; IEEE: New York, NY, USA; pp. 1801–1806. [CrossRef]
35. Vasičkaninová, A.; Bakošová, M.; Čirka, L.; Kalúz, M. Robust Controller Design for a Heat Exchanger. *Chem. Eng. Trans.* **2016**, *52*, 247–252. [CrossRef]
36. Pirela, M.P.; Sandoval, J.P.G.; Camacho, O. Discontinuous Feedback Control Strategies for a Heat Exchanger. NOVASINERGIA REVISTA DIGITAL DE CIENCIA, INGENIERÍA Y TECNOLOGÍA. *Novasinergia* **2019**, *2*, 80–87. [CrossRef]
37. Boonyaprapasorn, A.; Kuntanapreeda, S.; Ngiamsunthorn, P.S.; Kumsaen, T.; Sethaput, T. Time-Varying Sliding Mode Controller for Heat Exchanger with Dragonfly Algorithm. *Int. J. Electr. Comput. Eng.* **2023**, *13*, 3958–3968. [CrossRef]
38. Sun, H.-X.; Zhang, J.-T. Application of Adaptive Fuzzy Sliding-Mode Controller for Heat Exchanger System in District Heating. In Proceedings of the Proceedings-International Conference on Intelligent Computation Technology and Automation, ICICTA 2008, Changsha, China, 20–22 October 2008; pp. 850–854. [CrossRef]
39. Almutairi, N.B.; Zribi, M. Control of a Plate Heat Exchanger Using the Terminal Sliding Mode Technique. *Ind. Eng. Chem. Res.* **2012**, *51*, 4610–4623. [CrossRef]
40. Khimani, D.; Patil, M.; Godse, P.; Barai, R. A Super-Twisting Control Design for Shell and Tube Heat Exchanger. *J. Electr. Syst.* **2024**, *20*, 8191–8200.
41. Boonyaprapasorn, A.; Simatrang, S.; Kuntanapreeda, S.; Ngiamsunthorn, P.S.; Kumsaen, T.; Sethaput, T. Terminal Synergetic Control for Plate Heat Exchanger. *J. Adv. Res. Fluid Mech. Therm. Sci.* **2024**, *117*, 189–202. [CrossRef]

42. Shah, D.; Shah, A.; Mehta, A. Higher Order Networked Sliding Mode Controller for Heat Exchanger Connected via Data Communication Network. *Eur. J. Control.* **2021**, *58*, 301–314. [CrossRef]
43. Dyrska, R.; Horváthová, M.; Bakaráč, P.; Mönnigmann, M.; Oravec, J. Heat Exchanger Control Using Model Predictive Control with Constraint Removal. *Appl. Therm. Eng.* **2023**, *227*, 120366. [CrossRef]
44. Seban, L.; Boruah, N.; Roy, B. Modified Single Layer Economic Model Predictive Control and Application to Shell and Tube Heat Exchanger. *IFAC-PapersOnLine* **2016**, *49*, 754–759. [CrossRef]
45. Siza, J.; Llanos, J.; Velasco, P.; Moya, A.P.; Sumba, H. Model Predictive Control (MPC) of a Countercurrent Flow Plate Heat Exchanger in a Virtual Environment. *Sensors* **2024**, *24*, 4511. [CrossRef] [PubMed]
46. Al-Samarrai, S.A.; Al-Nadawi, Y.K.; Hama, T.G.; Al-Gadery, T.A. Robust Adaptive Sliding Mode Controllers Design for a Non-Holonomic Mobile Robot. In *Studies in Computational Intelligence*; Springer Science and Business Media Deutschland GmbH: Berlin/Heidelberg, Germany, 2023; pp. 489–556. [CrossRef]
47. Al-Samarraie, S.A.; Gorial, I.I.; Mshari, M.H. An Integral Sliding Mode Control for the Magnetic Levitation System Based on Backstepping Approach. *IOP Conf. Ser. Mater. Sci. Eng.* **2020**, *881*, 012136. [CrossRef]
48. Utkin, V.; Guldner, J.; Shi, J. *Sliding Mode Control in Electro-Mechanical Systems*; CRC Press: Boca Raton, FL, USA, 2009. [CrossRef]
49. Obeid, H.; Fridman, L.M.; Laghrouche, S.; Harmouche, M. Barrier Function-Based Adaptive Sliding Mode Control. *Automatica* **2018**, *93*, 540–544. [CrossRef]
50. Abd, A.F.; Al-Samarraie, S.A. Integral Sliding Mode Control Based on Barrier Function for Servo Actuator with Friction. *Eng. Technol. J.* **2021**, *39*, 248–259. [CrossRef]
51. MohammadRidha, T.; Al-Samarraie, S.A. A Barrier Function-Based Integral Sliding Mode Control of Heart Rate During Treadmill Exercise. *Math. Model. Eng. Probl.* **2023**, *10*, 179–188. [CrossRef]
52. Hassan, M.R.; Al-Samarraie, S.A. Optimal Feedback Control for HVAC Systems: An Integral Sliding Mode Control Approach Based on Barrier Function. *Math. Model. Eng. Probl.* **2023**, *10*, 1053–1062. [CrossRef]
53. Mohammad, A.M.; Al-Samarraie, S.A.; Jaber, A.A. Barrier Function-Based Integral Sliding Mode Controller Design for a Single-Link Rotary Flexible Joint Robot. *Int. J. Smart Sens. Intell. Syst.* **2024**, *17*, 1–16. [CrossRef]
54. Cengel, Y.; Ghajar, A. *Heat and Mass Transfer: Fundamentals and Applications*; McGraw-Hill Science/Engineering/Math: Columbus, OH, USA, 2015.
55. Bergman, T.L.; Lavine, A.S.; Incropera, F.P.; DeWitt, D.P. *Fundamentals of Heat and Mass Transfer*; Wiley-Interscience: Hoboken, NJ, USA, 2011.
56. Eduardo, C. *Heat Transfer in Process Engineering*; McGraw-Hill Education: Columbus, OH, USA, 2010.
57. Khalil, H.K. *Nonlinear Systems*; Prentice Hall: Hoboken, NJ, USA, 2001.
58. Calmidi, V.V.; Mahajan, R.L. The Effective Thermal Conductivity of High Porosity Fibrous Metal Foams. *J. Heat Transf.* **1999**, *121*, 466–471. [CrossRef]

energies

MDPI

Article

Trefftz Method for Time-Dependent Boiling Heat Transfer Calculations in a Mini-Channel Utilising Various Spatial Orientations of the Flow

Magdalena Piasecka [1], Sylwia Hożejowska [2], Artur Maciąg [2,*] and Anna Pawińska [2]

[1] Faculty of Mechatronics and Mechanical Engineering, Kielce University of Technology, Al. Tysiaclecia Panstwa Polskiego 7, 25-314 Kielce, Poland; tmpmj@tu.kielce.pl

[2] Faculty of Management and Computer Modelling, Kielce University of Technology, Al. Tysiaclecia Panstwa Polskiego 7, 25-314 Kielce, Poland; ztpsf@tu.kielce.pl (S.H.); a.pawinska@tu.kielce.pl (A.P.)

* Correspondence: matam@tu.kielce.pl

Abstract

The main objective of this study was to investigate boiling heat transfer during refrigerant flow in a mini-channel heat sink. The test section consisted of multiple parallel mini-channels, each with a depth of 1 mm. The working fluid was heated by a thin layer of Haynes-230 alloy with a thickness of 0.1 mm. The outer surface temperature of the heater was measured using infrared thermography, while other thermal and flow-based parameters were recorded via a dedicated data acquisition system. The mini-channel heat sink was tested in seven different spatial orientations, with inclination angles relative to the horizontal plane of 45°, 60°, 75°, 90°, 105°, 120°, and 135°. The analysis focused on the early stage of the experiment, corresponding to the forced convection, boiling incipience, and subcooled boiling region. A time-dependent, two-dimensional model of heat transfer during flow boiling of a refrigerant in asymmetrically heated mini-channels was developed. The temperatures of both the heating foil and the working fluid (Fluorinert FC-770) were described using appropriate forms of the Fourier–Kirchhoff equation, subject to relevant boundary conditions. Two sets of time-dependent Trefftz functions were employed to solve the governing equations: one set corresponding to the two-dimensional Fourier equation and another, newly derived, for the energy equation in the fluid. The results include thermographic images of the heated surface, temperature distributions, fluid temperatures, local heat-transfer coefficients, and boiling curves. A comparison of the heat-transfer coefficients obtained using the Trefftz-based approach and those calculated using Fourier's law demonstrated satisfactory agreement.

Keywords: flow boiling; heat transfer coefficient; mini-channel; inverse problem; time-dependent; Trefftz method

1. Introduction

Miniaturised industrial and domestic devices require efficient cooling systems due to the high heat fluxes generated during operation. This is especially important for power electronics and microprocessors, which emit significant amounts of heat. One solution involves mini-channels with flow boiling, which can be directly integrated into heat-generating structures. This approach enables effective heat dissipation, with a relatively small temperature difference between the heating surface and the saturated liquid. The high efficiency of heat exchange in such systems results from a large heat-transfer-area-to-volume ratio and a high heat-transfer coefficient (HTC). In addition, some cooling systems focus on minimising pumping power requirements, leading to the use of flows with Reynolds numbers below 2000.

Flow boiling in mini-channels has emerged as a highly effective mechanism for thermal management in compact and high-power-density systems, including microelectronics, avionics, and renewable energy modules. As device miniaturisation continues and heat fluxes surpass conventional cooling limits, researchers have turned to microscale channel configurations, where boiling regimes can offer superior heat removal capabilities. However, challenges such as flow instability, early dryout, and limited critical heat flux have highlighted the need for innovative enhancement strategies to ensure reliable and efficient operation. The physical behaviour of two-phase mini-channel flow boiling in mini-channels is fundamentally different from that in conventionally sized channels. The increased influence of surface tension, capillary forces, and microscale confinement alters bubble dynamics, pressure drop characteristics, and the distribution of boiling regimes.

Recent research has explored a variety of techniques aimed at intensifying boiling heat transfer while maintaining flow stability and structural simplicity. These include surface engineering methods (e.g., porous and coated surfaces), geometric channel modifications (e.g., grooves, fins), and integrated diagnostic techniques (e.g., infrared thermography, high-speed flow visualisation). Studies have also addressed the roles of working fluid properties and temporal–spatial flow behaviour in local and overall HTC and boiling heat flux limits. The presented review of the literature, based on selected works, synthesises and analyses the findings of several research studies [1–5], offering a comprehensive perspective on the strategies currently used to analyse boiling heat transfer in mini-channel systems. These works provide insight into the mechanisms of heat transfer in mini-channels and microscale heat exchangers.

Bian et al. [6] designed and experimentally investigated a mini-channel heat sink with inclined bottom grooves (MC-BG) used to enhance the two-phase flow boiling performance. The heat sink, with channel dimensions of 200 mm length and 2 mm × 2 mm cross-section, incorporated grooves 0.5 mm deep, inclined 45° to the flow direction. Experiments were carried out with deionised water at two inlet temperatures (70 °C and 80 °C) and mass fluxes of 138.8, 230.3, and 331.9 kg/(m^2·s). The results were benchmarked against a smooth mini-channel configuration (SMC). The study demonstrated that the inclined grooves enhanced nucleate boiling by increasing the density of the active nucleation sites and suppressing excessive bubble growth and coalescence. This effect delayed the transition from bubbly to annular flow, thus improving boiling stability. Compared to the smooth channel, the MC-BG showed earlier onset of nucleate boiling and required lower levels of wall superheating and effective heat flux to initiate boiling. At an inlet temperature of 80 ° C and mass flux of 138.8 kg/(m^2·s), the maximum average heat-transfer coefficient in the two-phase region for MC-BG reached 30.70 kW/(m^2·K), representing an improvement of 18.31% over the SMC. Furthermore, MC-BG exhibited a lower pressure drop across most test conditions, confirming superior net heat-transfer performance and reduced boiling-induced instability. Flow instability analysis showed that groove structures mitigated fluctuation amplitudes. Instability increased with increasing heat flux and decreased with higher mass flux but remained largely unaffected by inlet temperature. The authors stated that, overall, the use of inclined grooves in mini-channel heat sinks presents a viable thermal management enhancement strategy, one with potential for further improvement through geometric optimisation of groove angle, height, and channel layout. In their experimental study, He et al. [7] developed a new interconnected biporous mini-channel (IBPM) to enhance both heat-transfer performance and flow stability in flow boiling applications. The design featured a biporous coating on the channel base and periodically distributed interconnections between channels. Flow boiling tests were performed at mass fluxes of 161.2, 255.2, and 349.2 kg/(m^2·s). High-speed visualisation revealed that confined elongated bubbles in the IBPM expanded and partially transferred vapour into adjacent channels at interconnection sites, promoting heat and mass transfer. The onset of nucleate boiling occurred at lower wall superheats in IBPM (from 1.1 to 2.7 °C), compared to biporous mini-channels without interconnections (from 2.3 to 3.4 °C), due to the modified flow field. The two-phase heat-transfer coefficient of IBPM was significantly higher across all mass fluxes, up to 1.84 times higher than BPM in the subcooled regime; this was attributed to an increase in the number of nucleation sites. Unlike BPM, IBPM exhibited strong single-phase heat-transfer sensitivity to mass flux. Importantly, no inlet backflow was observed in IBPM, and the pressure deviation remained between 0.10 and 0.34 kPa, confirming the improved flow stability. The study demonstrates that combining interconnected structures with biporous surfaces was effective in mitigating flow instabilities while enhancing boiling heat transfer, making IBPM a promising design for advanced thermal management systems.

Kumar and Kothadia [8] conducted a comparative thermal analysis of subcooled flow boiling in mini and conventional channels, with the use of water as a working fluid. The experiments were carried out in tubes of 2 mm (a mini-channel), 4 mm, and 11.7 mm diameter (conventional channels), maintaining a constant length-to-diameter ratio of 150. The study evaluated the wall temperature distribution, the local heat-transfer coefficient, and the temporal fluctuations, utilising mass fluxes of 150 to 2400 kg/(m^2·s) and heat fluxes from 109 to 1080 kW/m^2. In the subcooled boiling region, HTC was found to be strongly dependent on heat flux but not on mass flux in conventional channels. On the contrary, saturated flow boiling in these channels showed an increase in HTC with increasing mass flux. In mini-channels, significant wall temperature fluctuations emerged at boiling numbers exceeding 1.76×10^{-4}; this was associated with abrupt disturbances caused by the growth affecting the narrow flow passage. At higher boiling numbers, HTC in mini-channels increased but also became more unstable. Maximum HTC was observed in the 2 mm mini-channel up to Bo = 2.24×10^{-4}, beyond which the risk of dryout increased. On the contrary, 4 mm channels maintained circumferential temperature uniformity and stability across all boiling regimes. The study indicated the critical role of boiling number in determining the thermal stability and operational limits of mini-channel flow boiling. The need for geometry-specific models and better predictive methods tailored to small diameter channels was highlighted. Shang et al., in [9], investigated flow boiling heat transfer in smooth (SPMC) and porous (PPMC) parallel mini-channel heat sinks fabricated from 6061 aluminium alloy, targeting server chip cooling applications. Experiments with HFE-7100 were conducted under low-to-moderate mass fluxes in the range 121.0–241.9 kg/(m^2·s), and effective heat fluxes up to 9.1 W/cm^2. The PPMC structure, produced by surface etching, provided improved nucleation due to additional surface cavities, reducing wall temperatures by up to 2.39% (1.7 K) at 181.4 kg/(m^2·s) and 7.3 W/cm^2. Average wall temperatures remained below 75 °C under all tested conditions. Compared to SPMC, the PPMC also showed slightly higher local heat-transfer coefficients (HTCs), with the difference decreasing along the flow direction. Visualisation of flow revealed that slug and churn flow dominate the middle and downstream regions; no dryout occurred, up to 9.1 W/cm^2. These results offer practical insights for the optimization of mini-channel heat sink performance in electronics cooling under varying operating conditions.

In their study [10], Charnay et al. examined the flow boiling of R-245fa in a 3 mm inner-diameter tube at saturation temperatures in the range of 100–120 °C. The heat-transfer coefficient was analysed with respect to vapour quality, heat flux, and mass flux. At 60 °C, during intermittent flow, the coefficient was independent of the vapour quality and the mass flux but increased with the heat flux, indicating dominant nucleate boiling. In annular flow, it rose with both vapour quality and mass flux, suggesting combined boiling mechanisms. At 120 °C, the coefficient decreased in both regimes, reflecting reduced nucleate boiling activity. The study also compared its results with existing predictive models. Wang et al., in [11], proposed a counter-flow interconnected mini-channel (CFIM) heat sink and compared its performance with a conventional co-current configuration (CCM). Experiments using R1233zd(E) under varying thermal conditions demonstrated that the CFIM effectively suppressed backflow and dryout, improving flow stability and wall temperature uniformity. The design resulted in a 51.2% increase in the heat-transfer coefficient, a 56% improvement in the coefficient of performance (COP), and a 48.5% reduction in pressure drop, achieving heat fluxes up to 230.4 W/cm^2. These findings underscore the potential for high performance in two-phase thermal management applications.

The studies highlight that modifications to channel geometry (e.g., grooves, interconnections), surface enhancements, and the modification of flow configurations significantly influence both the heat-transfer performance and the hydrodynamic stability of mini-channel heat sinks. The selection of working fluid, inlet parameters, and thermal boundary conditions further impacts boiling dynamics, bubble behaviour, and flow regimes. At the same time, it must be emphasised that the choice of a computational method for analysing experimental or simulation results plays a crucial role in ensuring the accuracy and reliability of the findings. A properly selected and validated modelling approach enables a confident interpretation of the observed thermal and flow-related phenomena. These insights offer valuable guidance for the future design and optimisation of compact thermal management systems, particularly in high-heat-flux applications such as electronic device cooling or renewable energy systems. This study focusses on developing and solving a two-dimensional, and this is worth emphasising, time-dependent, model of heat transfer during boiling in asymmetrically heated mini-channels in different spatial orientations. The governing energy equations with their boundary conditions result in two inverse Cauchy-type problems, one concerning the solid heating foil and the other addressing the mini-channel with flowing fluid. Inverse problems are inherently ill-posed and highly sensitive to input data, often leading to unstable numerical solutions [12]. To counteract these challenges, it is crucial to use computational techniques that prioritise accuracy and stability, such as the Trefftz function-based approach.

In 1926, Erik Trefftz published [13]. The Ritz method belongs to the class of internal methods for solving partial differential equations, i.e., those in which the solution satisfies the initial and boundary conditions exactly and the equation approximately. The Trefftz method belongs to the class of external methods, in which the equation is strictly satisfied and the initial-boundary conditions approximated. From a numerical point of view, the Trefftz method has an advantage over the Ritz approach, because the latter requires the minimization of an n-dimensional integral for an n-dimensional differential equation, whereas the Trefftz method requires only an n-1-dimensional integral. The dynamic development of the method began in the 1970s. The works of Herrera, Jirousek, Sabina, and Zieliński [14–18] are worth mentioning. The shared aim of these works was to develop methods for obtaining the Trefftz function and to investigate the completeness of the resulting systems. In 1956, ref [19] was published, in which one-dimensional thermal polynomials were derived that strictly satisfy the non-stationary heat-conduction equation. It should be emphasized that the variable describing time is treated as continuous spatial variables.

The Trefftz method offers several significant advantages for solving both direct and inverse engineering problems. It is a meshless semi-analytical technique that approximates solutions to the governing differential equations by representing them as linear combinations of Trefftz functions (T-functions). The coefficients for linear combinations are determined based on known boundary conditions, ensuring stability and precision. Its primary strength lies in its ability to provide solutions that strictly satisfy the governing differential equations, thus ensuring high precision. Additionally, the method simplifies computations, as it typically employs polynomial T-functions. It also exhibits considerable flexibility, accommodating various types of boundary conditions, whether related to temperature distributions, fluid flow, or a combination of discrete and continuous conditions.

In [1–4], the Trefftz method was used to determine time-dependent solutions of partial differential equations, which include equations of the parabolic, hyperbolic, and parabolic–hyperbolic types. The classical Trefftz method is also used in [1] to solve time-dependent problems of the parabolic type. In [2], the authors, using Laplace and Laguerre transforms, reduce time-dependent partial differential equations to the Helmholtz equation, which they solve by combining the Trefftz method with the method of fundamental solutions. In [3], the heat equation is first discretised with respect to time and then the resulting set of elliptic equations is solved using the appropriate time-independent hybrid Trefftz-element approach. The spacetime collocation Trefftz method was adopted in [4] to solve the inverse heat-conduction problem by approximating numerical solutions using Trefftz base functions. In [1–4], the validity of the methods proposed was established by using a number of test problems to demonstrate the accuracy and effectiveness of the computational techniques based on T-functions. In these papers, the methods employing T-functions allowed for the obtaining of highly accurate semi-numerical and numerical solutions, with the maximum error in solving the differential equation not exceeding a value of one at any point.

A mathematical model of time-dependent heat transfer during the flow boiling of ecological refrigerants in mini-channels is presented in [5]. A hybrid combination of T-functions with FEM and the iterative Picard method allowed the determinations of the temperature distribution of the heating surface, the heat flux transferred to the fluid, and the heat-transfer coefficients at the heating wall surface–fluid interface. The model and calculation methods with T-functions were verified based on the experimental data. The results of the numerical calculation were compared with the results obtained from known correlations in the literature, giving satisfactory results. Hybrid calculation techniques using T-functions are also discussed in [1,20–22].

It is well established that numerous studies in scientific research focus on CFD modelling. For example, the study reported in [23] proposed a CFD–DEM-based strategy to investigate multi-field coupled particle flows in microreactors. Ultrasonic excitation was applied to control particle clustering, while fractal analysis was used to characterize distribution irregularities within the channels. An experimental observation platform was developed to validate the simulations. The results indicated that ultrasound significantly enhanced flow uniformity and particle dispersion, with inlet velocity and excitation frequency exerting strong influences on distribution patterns.

This paper proposes a two-dimensional approach to analysing time-dependent heat transfer during the flow boiling of a working fluid, Fluorinert FC-770, utilising asymmetrically heated mini-channels with different spatial orientations. The novelty of the study is in its introduction of new T-functions, which allow one to obtain a semi-analytical solution of the fluid energy equation under the assumption of a fixed form of the velocity vector. These functions, used alongside the classical T-functions for the two-dimensional Fourier equation, provide a basis for solving inverse heat-transfer problems and reconstructing the thermal-boundary conditions from transient temperature measurements. The calculations use experimental data, and the results are verified based on solutions obtained using a simplified approach based on Fourier's law.

It should be emphasised that this study has two main objectives. The first is to experimentally investigate the effect of channel inclination on boiling heat transfer during refrigerant flow in a mini-channel heat sink. The time-dependent measurements include the temperatures of the heated foil and the working fluid, electrical input parameters, and mass flow rate. The second objective is to demonstrate the applicability of the Trefftz method as a reliable semi-analytical tool for solving time-dependent direct and inverse heat-conduction problems in both the heating foil and the refrigerant. The resulting temperature fields and local heat-transfer coefficients are compared with those obtained from simplified models. By combining experiments with Trefftz-based analysis, the study provides a validation of the computational approach that cannot be achieved by CFD simulations alone. This methodological integration is rarely applied in mini-channel flow boiling research, which highlights the novelty and significance of the contribution.

2. Materials and Methods: Experimental Stand, Methodology, and Raw Data

2.1. Experimental Stand and Methods

A schematic diagram of the circulating loop for the working fluid (Fluorinert FC-770) implemented in the experimental setup is shown in Figure 1.

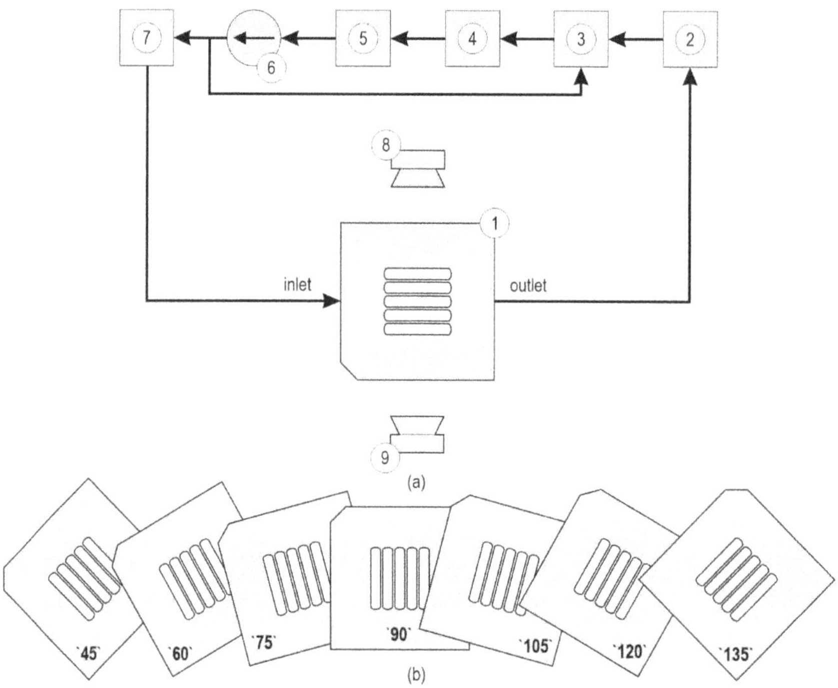

Figure 1. Schematic diagrams: (**a**) the circulating loop of the working fluid and the camera setup on the experimental stand (1—test section, 2—heat exchanger, 3—compensation tank, 4—deaerator, 5—filter, 6—gear pump, 7—Coriolis mass flow meter, 8—infrared camera, and 9—high-speed video camera); (**b**) spatial orientations of the test section (45°, 60°, 75°, 90°, 105°, 120°, and 135°).

The main components of the flow loop include the following: the test section with five parallel mini-channels, a gear pump, a compensation tank, a heat exchanger, and a

Coriolis mass flow meter (Figure 1). The core component of the experimental setup is the test section, which contains a group of five parallel mini-channels with rectangular cross-sections. Each channel has a fixed depth of 1 mm, a width of 6 mm, and a length of 43 mm. The working fluid flows through the mini-channels in a laminar regime and is heated by a thin heating foil made of Haynes-230 alloy, which is tensioned between two metallic frames. The temperature distribution on the outer surface of the foil is monitored using infrared thermography. The opposite side of the foil is observed through a glass plate to visually identify the flow structures. A measurement is recorded every second, for a duration of one minute. A detailed schematic of the test section is presented in Figure 2.

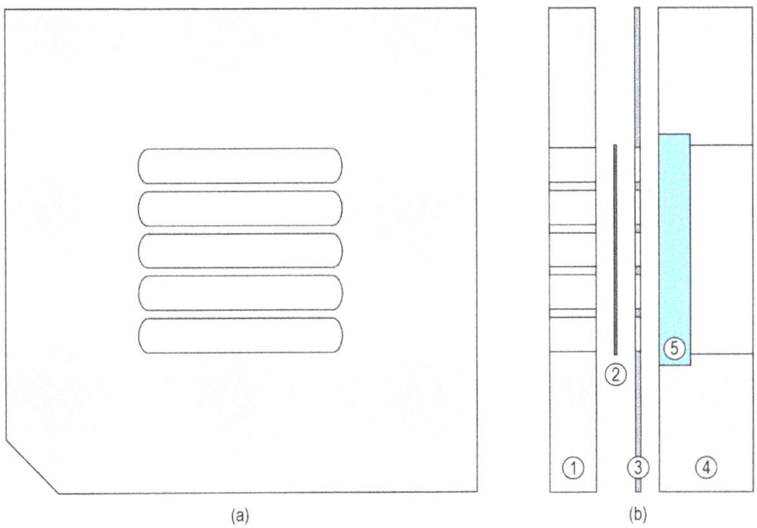

Figure 2. Schematic diagram of the test section: (**a**) view of the cover, with inspection windows for infrared thermographic measurement of foil temperature; (**b**) cross-sectional view of the main components (1—cover with inspection windows for IR thermography of the foil, 2—heating foil, 3—Teflon body with mini-channels, 4—cover with inspection windows for flow structure observation, and 5—glass plate).

2.2. Direct Experimental Data

The experimental dataset comprises measurements of the fluid temperature at the inlet and outlet of the mini-channel, fluid pressure, temperature distribution on the external surface of the heating foil, and mass flow rate. The principal experimental parameters, including their respective measurement ranges and absolute uncertainties, are summarised in Table 1. Additionally, the electric current and voltage drop across the heating foil were used in the calculation of the heat flux. The resulting mean relative errors, which were on the order of a few percent under subcooled boiling conditions, are discussed in detail in [24].

It should be emphasised that the early stage of the experiment was analysed in detail (the first 60 s of a 300 s test in this experimental series); this section corresponds to the forced convection, boiling incipience, and subcooled boiling region. Figure 3 presents the raw data obtained from the experiment, including the temperature of the heating foil, the fluid temperature at the inlet and outlet of the mini-channel, and the heat flux, for a selected inclination angle of the mini-channel relative to the horizontal plane (135°). Heat flux was calculated on the basis of the measured current and voltage drop across the heating foil and the known dimensions of the foil.

Table 1. Measurement ranges of key experimental parameters and the corresponding absolute measurement errors.

Measured Parameter	Measuring Device	Measuring Range	Absolute Error	Additional Information
Fluid temperature at the inlet, [K]	K-type Thermocouple, type K 221 b, Czaki Thermo-Product (Raszyn-Rybie, Poland)	286.05–295.45	0.34 K	The details associated with the calculation of the absolute error of the fluid temperature are described in [25]
Fluid temperature at the outlet, [K]		290.05–309.25		
Absolute pressure at the inlet, [kPa]	Gauge pressure: Cerabar S PMP71 m type, manufactured by Endress + Hauser; Atmospheric pressure: A-10 m type, manufactured by WIKA Polska (Wloclawek, Poland)	93–115	1 285 Pa	(1) A maximum measurement error of ±0.05% of reading (2) A maximum measurement error of 0.5% of full scale Details associated with the calculation of the absolute error for the fluid temperature are presented in [25]
Absolute pressure at the outlet, [kPa]		85–106		
Temperature of the heating foil, [K]	Infrared camera A655sc FLIR (resolution 640 × 480)	307.59–390.04	2 K	±2 K or ±2% in the range of 273.15 ÷ 393.15 K
Mass flow rate [kg/s]	Coriolis mass flowmeter Proline Promass A 100, Endress + Hauser (Wroclaw, Poland)	4.05×10^{-3}–4.53×10^{-3} kg/s	4×10^{-6} kg/s	±0.1% of the reading

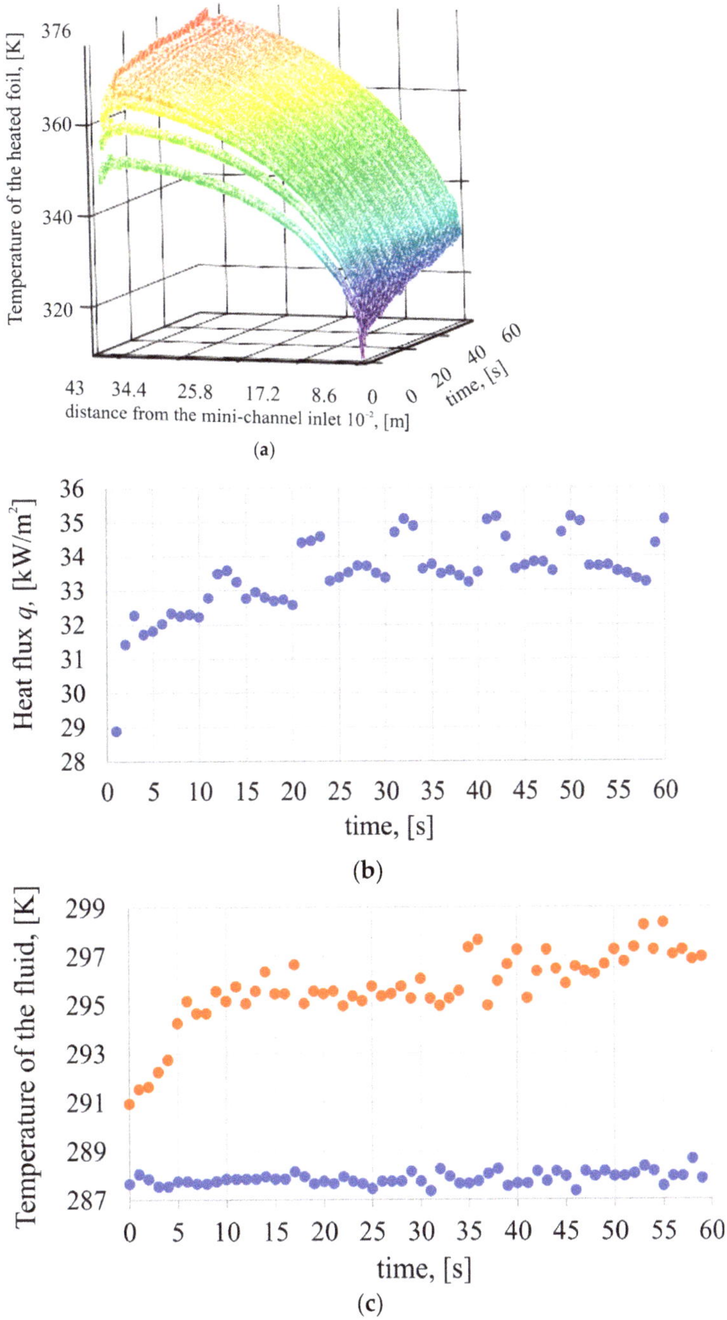

Figure 3. (**a**) Temperature of the outer surface of the heating foil, measured by infrared camera, in relation to time and the distance from the mini-channel inlet; (**b**) heat flux as a function of time; (**c**) bulk fluid temperature at the inlet (●●●) and outlet (●●●) of the mini-channel as function of time. The data presented correspond to the test section being inclined at an angle of 135°.

3. Mathematical Model

The mathematical model presented in the following is a modification of the model presented in [5]. All further considerations and calculations concern only one selected central mini-channel, for which two dimensions were taken into account: one in the flow direction (x), and one perpendicular to the flow (y). These relate to the thickness of the heating foil thickness δ_h and the mini-channel depth δ_M. In addition, it was assumed that the physical parameters of the module elements do not depend on the temperature, heat loss to the surroundings through the outer walls of the module, which are negligible—the entire measurement module is insulated, convective heat exchange takes place in the mini-channel, and the fluid flow is laminar with a known mass flow rate and known temperatures at the inlet and outlet that extend to and from the mini-channel. The temperatures of the heating foil T_h and the working fluid T_f satisfy the appropriate Fourier–Kirchhoff equation:

$$\lambda_h \nabla^2 T_h = \rho_h c_{p,h} \frac{\partial T_h}{\partial t} - \frac{q(t)}{\delta_h} \tag{1}$$

$$\lambda_f \nabla^2 T_f = \rho_f c_{p,f} \frac{\partial T_f}{\partial t} + c_{p,f} \rho_f v(y,t) \frac{\partial T_f}{\partial x} - g \rho_f v(y,t) sin\omega \tag{2}$$

where differential operator $\nabla^2 = \frac{\partial^2}{\partial x^2} + \frac{\partial^2}{\partial y^2}$, $q(t)$ denotes heat flux supplied to the heater and $v(y,t)$ means the velocity of the fluid in a single mini-channel. The velocity is determined based on the mass flow rate known from the measurements.

For the heating foil, it was assumed that the surface temperature of the heater not in contact with the fluid (i.e., for $y = 0$), determined from infrared camera measurements as T_{ij}^m, is prescribed, while the heater walls perpendicular to the fluid-contacting surface are considered insulated.

By analogy to [5], for the fluid energy equation, the following boundary conditions were adopted:

- The fluid temperatures at the inlet and outlet of the mini-channel are known as

$$T_f(0, y, t_j) = T_{f,in}(y, t_j) \tag{3}$$

$$T_f(L, y, t_j) = T_{f,out}(y, t_j) \tag{4}$$

- The temperatures of the fluid and the heating foil are equal at the contact surface, i.e.,

$$T_h(x, \delta_h, t) = T_f(x, \delta_h, t) \tag{5}$$

In addition, the boundary conditions for Equations (1) and (2) are shown in Figure 4.

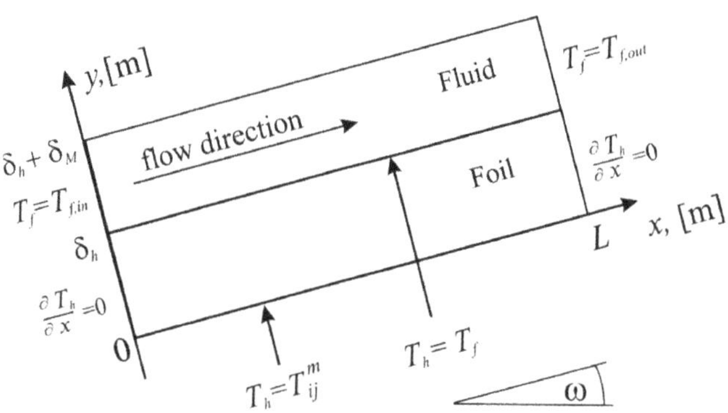

Figure 4. Scheme of the mini-channel and boundary conditions (illustrative figure, not to scale).

The effect of the assumptions made is the existence of two inverse problems relating to the heat transfer in the heating foil and the mini-channel. In the first step, the temperatures of the heating foil and the fluid were determined using the Trefftz method, similar to [26]. In the next step, using knowledge of the temperature distributions of the heating foil and the working fluid, the HTC at the contact surface was determined from the Robin condition:

$$\alpha_{2D}(x,t) = \frac{-\lambda_h \frac{\partial T_h}{\partial y}(x,\delta_h,t)}{T_h(x,\delta_h,t) - T_{f,ave}(x,\delta_h,t)} \tag{6}$$

where the values for the reference fluid temperature $T_{f,ave}$ are calculated by analogy to [5].

4. Calculations Method

4.1. Trefftz Functions for the Fourier–Kirchhoff Equations

Let us consider a one-dimensional Fourier equation of the form

$$\lambda \frac{\partial^2 T}{\partial x^2} = \rho c_p \frac{\partial T}{\partial t} \tag{7}$$

for which we make the substitution $\tau = \frac{\lambda t}{\rho c_p}$ and obtain

$$\frac{\partial^2 T}{\partial x^2} = \frac{\partial T}{\partial \tau} \tag{8}$$

In [19], for Equation (8), the Trefftz functions are given in the form

$$u_m(x,\tau) = \sum_{k=0}^{\left[\frac{m}{2}\right]} \frac{x^{m-2k}\tau^k}{(m-2k)!k!} \text{ for } m = 0,1,\ldots \tag{9}$$

where [.] means the floor function. As shown in [27], the products of the form

$$V_{k,0}(x,y,\tau) = u_m(x,\tau)u_n(y,\tau) \tag{10}$$

where $k = 0.5(1+(m+n))(m+n)+m$ for $m,n = 0,1,\ldots$, are the Trefftz functions for the equation

$$\nabla^2 T = \frac{\partial T}{\partial \tau} \tag{11}$$

Table 2 presents the properties of the function described in (10).

Table 2. Properties of the Trefftz functions.

$$\frac{\partial}{\partial x}(u_m(x,\tau)u_n(y,\tau)) = \begin{cases} m u_{m-1}(x,\tau)u_n(y,\tau) & \text{for } m = 1,2,\ldots,\ n = 0,1,\ldots \\ 0 & \text{for } m = 0,\ n = 0,1,\ldots \end{cases} \tag{12}$$

$$\frac{\partial}{\partial y}(u_m(x,\tau)u_n(y,\tau)) = \begin{cases} n u_m(x,\tau)u_{n-1}(y,\tau) & \text{for } m = 0,1,\ldots,\ n = 1,2,\ldots \\ 0 & \text{for } m = 0,1,\ldots,\ ,\ n = 0 \end{cases} \tag{13}$$

$$\frac{\partial}{\partial t}(u_m(x,\tau)u_n(y,\tau)) = \begin{cases} m(m-1)u_{m-2}(x,\tau)u_n(y,\tau) + n(n-1)u_m(x,\tau)u_{n-2}(y,\tau) & \text{for } m,n = 2,3\ldots \\ 0 & \text{for } m,n = 0,1 \end{cases} \tag{14}$$

These functions will be used to define the Trefftz function for the Fourier–Kirchhoff equation in the following form:

$$\mathcal{L}T = v(y,\tau)\frac{\partial T}{\partial x} \tag{15}$$

where $\mathcal{L}T = \nabla^2 T - \frac{\partial T}{\partial t}$.

In the further transformations we assume that the velocity $v(y,\tau)$ is a polynomial. First, we define the inverse operator of the operator $\mathcal{L}$ for a function of the form $x^n y^m \tau^k$ where n, m, and k are natural numbers, i.e.,

$$\mathcal{L}^{-1}\left(x^n y^m \tau^k\right) = \frac{1}{(m+2)(m+1)} x^n y^{m+2}\tau^k - \frac{n(n-1)}{(m+2)(m+1)}\mathcal{L}^{-1}\left(x^{n-2}y^{m+2}\tau^k\right) + \frac{k}{(m+2)(m+1)}\mathcal{L}^{-1}\left(x^n y^{m+2}\tau^{k-1}\right) \tag{16}$$

Let us define the new functions $V_n(x,y,\tau)$ as follows:

$$V_n(x,y,\tau) = \sum_{k=0}^{m} V_{n,k}(x,y,\tau) \tag{17}$$

where

$$V_{n,k} = \begin{cases} V_{n,0} \text{ for } k = 0 \\ \mathcal{L}^{-1}\left(v(y,\tau)\,\frac{\partial V_{n,k-1}}{\partial x}\right) \text{ for } k = 1,2,\ldots,m \end{cases} \tag{18}$$

In (18), $V_{n,0}$ is a T-function of the form (10), and m is the degree of the polynomial $V_{n,0}$ with respect to the variable x. Note that the function $V_{n,m}$ depends only on the variables y and τ. Then, it is easy to show that the functions $V_n(x,y,\tau)$ satisfy Equation (15), which means that they are Trefftz functions for this equation. The presented method for defining the Trefftz function for Equation (15) can be generalised to any form of velocity $v(y,\tau)$. One necessary condition is then to define the inverse operator $\mathcal{L}^{-1}$ for all summands in $v(y,\tau)x^n y^m \tau^k$.

4.2. Trefftz Method

The idea of the Trefftz method is to present the solution of the governing differential equation as a linear combination of functions that exactly satisfy this equation. To determine the solutions of Equations (1) and (2), two sets of the Trefftz functions defined by formula (10) and formula (17) will be used. Similarly to [5], the temperatures of the heating foil T_h and refrigerant T_f are approximated by the sum of the linear combination of the Trefftz functions defined by formulas (10) and (17), respectively, and the corresponding particular solutions of Equations (1) and (2), i.e.,

$$T_h(x,y,t) = V_{par,h}(x,y,t) + \sum_{n=1}^{N_h} f_n V_{n,0}(x,y,t) \tag{19}$$

$$T_f(x,y,t) = V_{par,f}(x,y,t) + \sum_{n=1}^{N_f} g_n V_n(x,y,t) \tag{20}$$

where the particular solutions are defined as follows:

$$V_{par,h}(x,y,t) = -\frac{q(t)}{2\lambda_h\delta_h}\,y^2 \tag{21}$$

$$V_{par,f}(x,y,t) = \mathcal{L}^{-1}\left(g\rho_f v(y,t)\sin\omega\right) \tag{22}$$

The linear combination coefficients f_n and g_n are determined based on the minimisation of the functional describing the mean square error for which the functions T_h and T_f satisfy known initial and boundary conditions. The Trefftz method can be used to solve both direct and inverse problems, whether time-dependent or time-independent, yielding a differentiable solution that exactly satisfies the governing differential equation and approximately satisfies the boundary conditions. It imposes no limitations on the number or type of the boundary conditions (temperature-related, flow-related, continuous, or discrete), and any number of T-functions can be used in the construction of the solution.

4.3. Simplified Approach

The simplifications adopted below allow us to determine the HTC based on Fourier's law, thereby verifying the calculation results obtained using the Trefftz method. It was assumed that the temperature of the heating foil, T_h, at each measurement point (x_i, t_j) satisfies the Fourier equation in the form

$$\lambda_h \frac{dT_h}{dy} = -q(t_j) \tag{23}$$

For $y = 0$, the temperature of the heater surface is known from the measurements of the infrared camera T_{ij}^m, i.e.,

$$T_h(x_i, 0, t_j) = T_{ij}^m \tag{24}$$

The fluid temperature is calculated using the following relationship:

$$T_f(x_i, \delta_h, t_j) = \begin{cases} T_{lin}(x_i, t_j) \ if \ T_h(x_i, \delta_h, t_j) \leq T_{sat}(x_i, t_j) \\ T_{sat}(x_i, t_j) \ if \ T_h(x_i, \delta_h, t_j) > T_{sat}(x_i, t_j) \end{cases} \tag{25}$$

where T_{lin} is a function that changes linearly from the temperature of the fluid at the inlet of the mini-channel to the temperature of the fluid at the outlet. The local HTC can be determined using the equation

$$\alpha_{1D}(x_i, t_j) = \frac{q(t_j)}{T_{ij}^m - \frac{q(t_j)}{\lambda_h}\delta_h - T_f(x_i, \delta_h, t_j)} \tag{26}$$

5. Results

Numerical calculations were performed for the heat flux q, ranging from 26.8 kW/m^2 to 42.6 kW/m^2, and the mass flow rate of the working medium, ranging from 4.05×10^{-3} kg/s to 4. $\times 10^{-3}$ kg/s. The remaining experimental parameters, including their measurement uncertainties, are listed in Table 1. The HTC was determined through a three-step process. First, the two-dimensional temperature of the heating foil was calculated using the T-functions defined by Equation (10) as shown in Figure 5. Next, based on the known constant fluid velocity and the temperature of the heating foil, the two-dimensional temperature of the fluid was determined using the Trefftz method, with new T-functions defined by formula (17). Finally, the HTC was calculated using Equation (6).

The results are illustrated through the HTC as shown in Figures 6–9:

- As a function of time and the distance from the inlet to the mini-channel for selected inclination angles, Figures 6 and 9;
- Versus distance to the mini-channel inlet for selected times and selected inclination angles, Figure 7;
- For all inclination angles, as a function of time, for two distances from the inlet to the mini-channel, Figure 8.

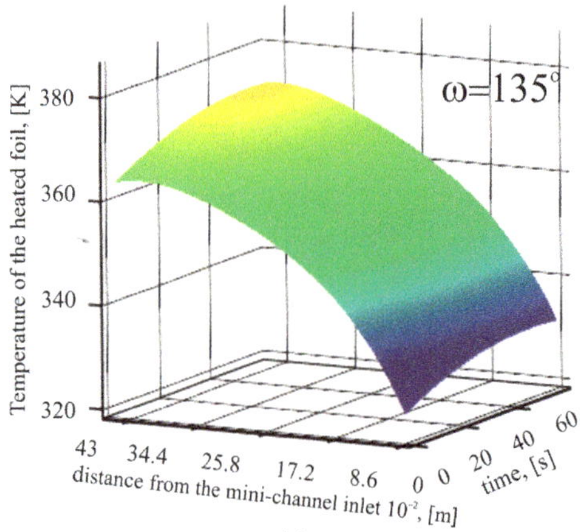

(a)

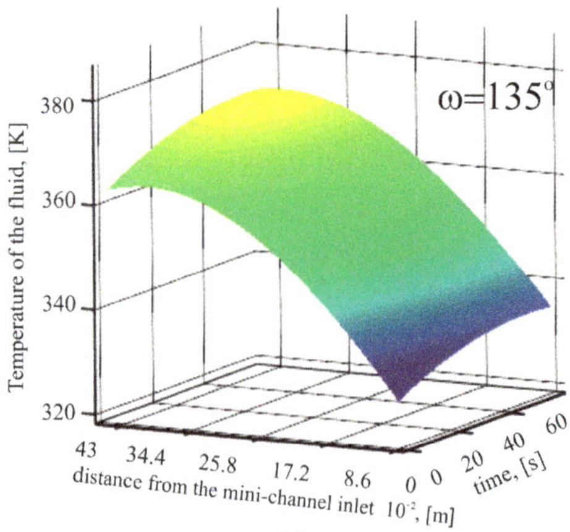

(b)

Figure 5. The two-dimensional temperature distributions of: the heating foil (**a**) and the working fluid (**b**), on the contact surface, as a function of time and the distance from the inlet to the mini-channel, for inclination angle $\omega = 135°$.

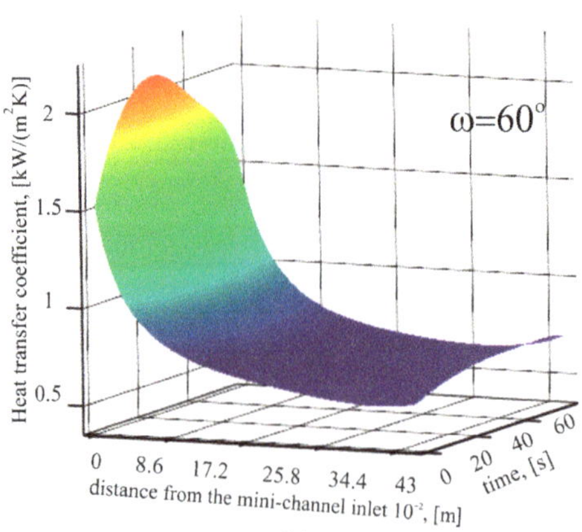

(a)

Figure 6. *Cont.*

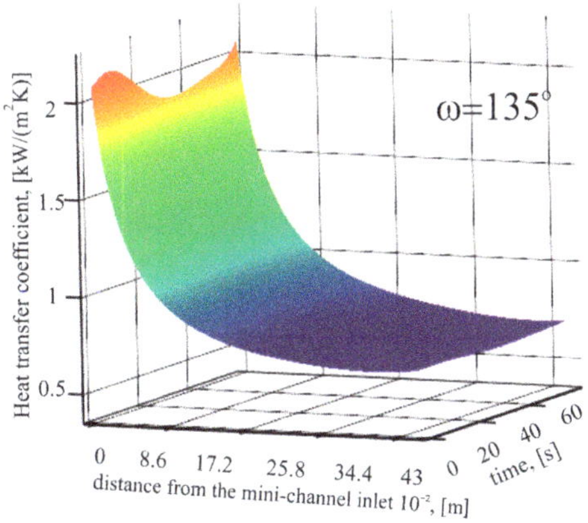

(**b**)

Figure 6. Heat-transfer coefficient $\alpha_{2D}(x,t)$, as a function of time and the distance from the mini-channel inlet, for inclination angles $\omega = 60°$ (**a**) and $\omega = 135°$ (**b**).

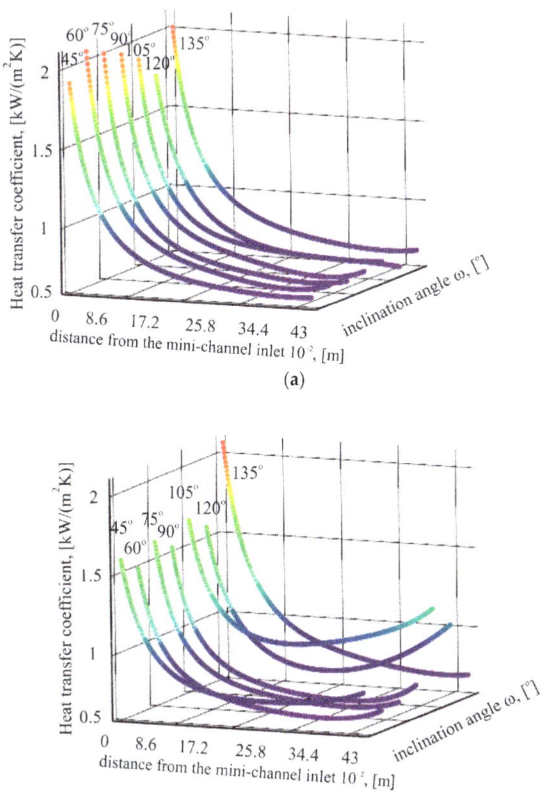

(**b**)

Figure 7. Heat-transfer coefficient $\alpha_{2D}(x,t)$ for successive inclination angles, as a function of distance from the mini-channel inlet, for the following times: t = 20 s (**a**) and t = 60 s (**b**).

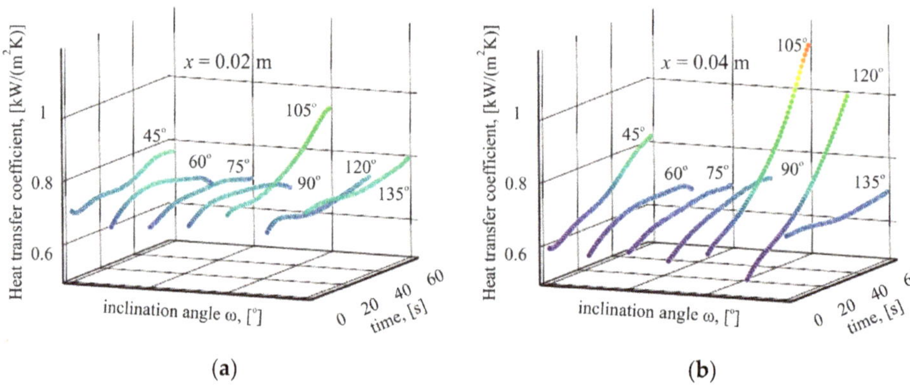

Figure 8. Heat-transfer coefficient $\alpha_{2D}(x,t)$ at two selected distances from the mini-channel inlet: (**a**,**b**) variation with time for successive inclination angles at x = 0.02 m (**a**) and x = 0.04 m (**b**).

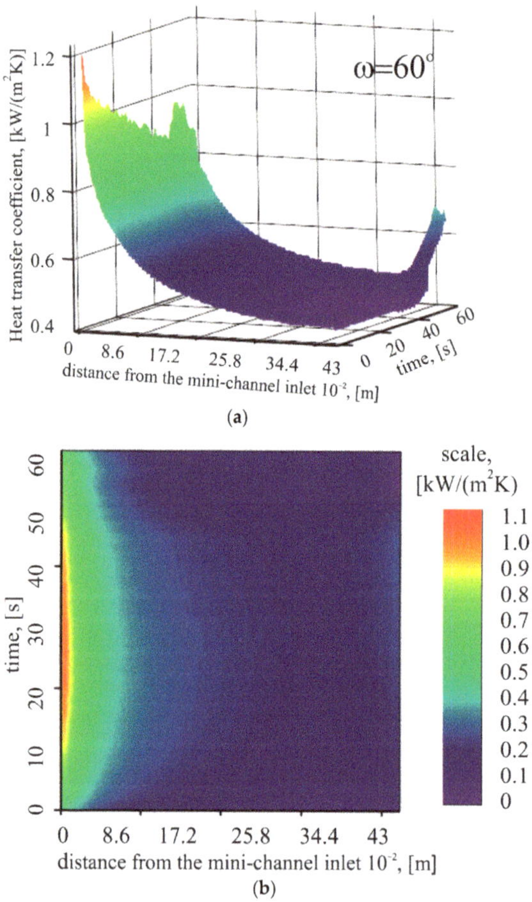

Figure 9. (**a**) The heat-transfer coefficient $\alpha_{1D}(x,t)$ as a function of time and the distance from the mini-channel inlet; (**b**) the difference $\alpha_{2D}(x,t) - \alpha_{1D}(x,t)$ as a function of time and the distance from the mini-channel inlet. The inclination angle is 60°.

5.1. The Trefftz Method with New T-Functions

Figure 5 show the two-dimensional temperature distributions of the heating foil and the working fluid, respectively, at the contact surface as a function of time and the distance from the inlet to the mini-channel for a selected inclination angle.

The new T-functions, given by formula (17), made it possible to obtain a solution to the Fourier–Kirchhoff equation for the fluid that satisfies the adopted boundary conditions with high accuracy. The mean differences between the fluid temperature T_f and the assumed boundary conditions (3)–(5) are presented in Table 3. The largest mean differences 7.10 K (2.5%) and 8.37 K (2.86%) were obtained for angle of 75° and for boundary conditions (3) and (4), respectively. Condition (5) was fulfilled with the greatest accuracy for each inclination angle.

Table 3. The mean differences between the calculated fluid temperature T_f and the assumed boundary conditions (3)–(5).

	Mean Differences, [K]		
Inclination Angle ω	**Conditions (3)**	**Conditions (4)**	**Conditions (5)**
45°	6.74	8.32	1.23
60°	6.78	8.36	1.05
75°	7.10	8.37	1.19
90°	6.22	7.86	0.99
105°	6.41	7.26	1.49
120°	6.73	7.57	1.31
135°	6.31	7.39	0.98

5.2. The HTC Analysis

Figures 6 and 7 show the heat-transfer coefficient $\alpha_{2D}(x,t)$, which is calculated using formula (6), as a function of time and the distance from the mini-channel inlet, for two selected inclination angles, 60° (Figure 6a) and 135° (Figure 6b), and as a function of distance from the inlet for two selected times (Figure 7), taking into account all seven inclination angles.

In Figure 6, a decreasing trend in HTCs is observed with increasing distance from the mini-channel inlet. This behaviour is consistent across all inclination angles considered. The HTC values range from approximately 0.5 kW/(m^2·K) to 3 kW/(m^2·K), with the highest values consistently recorded near the channel inlet, regardless of time and inclination angle. The profiles of the heat-transfer coefficient associated with the early times (e.g., t = 20 s) show a negligible dependence on the inclination angle (Figure 7a). However, more pronounced differences are observed toward the end of the heating period, as represented by t = 60 s (Figure 7b). Analysis of the results presented in Figures 6 and 7 indicates that, in general, the highest heat-transfer coefficients are achieved in both time intervals for the inclination angle of 120°.

The heat-transfer coefficient values $\alpha_{2D}(x,t)$ for all selected inclination angles are illustrated in Figure 8, which shows the continuous variation of $\alpha_{2D}(x,t)$ over time at two selected distances from the mini-channel inlet x = 0.02 m (Figure 8a) and x = 0.04 m (Figure 8b).

When analysing the results presented in Figure 8a, it can be observed that at the location x = 0.02 m, the heat-transfer coefficients for the mini-channel inclination angles of 60°, 75°, and 90° exhibit only minor differences throughout the entire time interval. In each case, the temporal evolution of the HTC is characterised by an initial increase followed by a gradual decline. This behaviour becomes more pronounced at x = 0.4 m (Figure 8b), where a distinct effect is observed in temperature increase over time (and hence heat flux) and the influence of channel inclination becomes more apparent. At the downstream location $x = 0.4$ m, which corresponds to the outlet region, the highest HTC values are once again recorded with an inclination angle of 105°, particularly during the later stages of the heating process. Generally, higher HTCs are obtained at $x = 0.4$ m, compared to $x = 0.2$ m, with the exception of the inclined position of 135°. Furthermore, for the two orientations of 45° and of 135°, the heat-transfer behaviour exhibits a clear reversal: at $x = 0.2$ m, higher HTC values are observed for 135° than for 45°, while at $x = 0.4$ m, the opposite trend is seen, and the position of 45° yields higher HTC values than the position of 135°. These variations are most evident in further increase in heat flux, corresponding to the advancing time.

The overall trends indicate that the inclination angle of the mini-channel significantly influences surface-heat-transfer performance and the flow pattern, even in an asymmetrically heated mini-channel, in which only one wall is heated and the working fluid flows above it. Higher HTC values are obtained at steeper inclination angles approaching the vertical, namely 105° and 135°, at which more effective vapour detachment from the heating surface occurs at the incipience of boiling, primarily due to gravitational forces.

This trend becomes more pronounced as the heat flux supplied by the heating foil increases, leading to the formation of vapour agglomerates within the liquid–vapour mixture; this is characteristic of the vertical position (the position of 90°, with fluid upward flow) and higher inclination angles (e.g., 105°, 120°) of the mini-channel. The gravitational component, acting in the direction of vapour buoyancy, facilitates a more rapid removal of vapour from the heated surface. This, in turn, reduces the residence time, lowers thermal resistance at the liquid–solid interface, and maintains the wettability of the heated wall, which are conditions beneficial to efficient nucleate boiling heat transfer. Furthermore, such spatial orientations of the mini-channel improve surface rewetting and promote liquid backflow, enabling continuous replenishment of liquid at the heated interface.

The angle of the mini-channel's inclination influences the overall heat-transfer behaviour. The observed intensification in heat transfer at specific inclination angles, particularly in downstream regions, is the result of a synergistic combination of improved vapour removal, reliable liquid supply, and favourable flow-regime evolution. These phenomena are fundamentally governed by gravity-driven effects acting within the geometrically confined and asymmetrically heated mini-channel specification.

In order to verify the calculations performed using the Trefftz method with newly defined T-functions, the HTC was determined from a simplified model based on Fourier's law. Figure 9a shows the HTC, calculated by formula (26), as a function of the time and distance from the mini-channel inlet (Figure 9a), and the differences between the HTCs calculated from formulas (6) and (26), i.e., $\alpha_{2D}(x,t) - \alpha_{1D}(x,t)$ (Figure 9b), which are also functions of time and distance. The average differences between the HTCs $\alpha_{2D}(x,t)$ and $\alpha_{1D}(x,t)$ do not exceed 0.3 kW/(m^{2}K) for all inclination angles. Figure 9b shows that the HTC for the two-dimensional approach achieves higher values than the HTC for the one-dimensional approach.

5.3. Boiling Curves

The boiling curves presented in this article illustrate the relationship between the heat flux and the temperature difference between the heated wall and the bulk fluid, as evaluated at selected positions along the mini-channel wall. These curves are based on the complete set of experimental data obtained during a gradual increase in heat flux. Boiling curves were generated at four axial locations relative to the mini-channel inlet (0.01 m, 0.02 m, 0.03 m, and 0.04 m), with results corresponding to the following inclination angles of the mini-channel: $\omega = 60°$ (Figure 10a), $\omega = 90°$ (Figure 10b), and $\omega = 135°$ (Figure 10c).

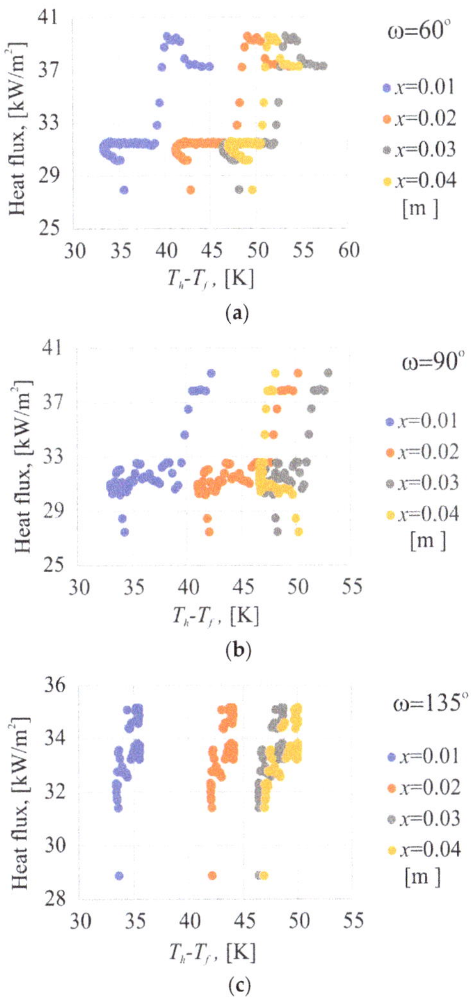

Figure 10. Boiling curves, constructed at four selected points from the mini-channel inlet; results obtained for the following inclination angles: (**a**) $\omega = 60°$, (**b**) $\omega = 90°$, and (**c**) $\omega = 135°$.

The course of the boiling curves reveals several important observations. As a subcooled liquid enters the asymmetrically heated mini-channel, heat transfer initially proceeds through single-phase forced convection. With increasing heat flux, the liquid near the heated wall becomes superheated, whereas the bulk of the fluid remains subcooled. The inception of spontaneous vapour bubble formation results in a sudden drop in wall temperature during ONB (onset of boiling). These vapour bubbles act as internal heat sinks, absorbing significant amounts of thermal energy from the heated surface. As the heat flux continues to increase, fully developed nucleate boiling occurs.

Analysis of the boiling curves obtained for ω = 60° (Figure 10a) reveals a distinct temperature drop corresponding to the onset of nucleate boiling (ONB), which shifts toward higher values for the temperature difference between the heating foil and the bulk fluid as the distance from the mini-channel inlet increases. The boiling curves constructed for ω = 90° (Figure 10b) exhibit a slightly smaller temperature drop at ONB compared to those observed for ω = 60°. Although the temperature difference between the heated wall and the bulk fluid remains of comparable magnitude, the data points show significantly greater scatter. On the contrary, for $\omega = 135°$ (Figure 10c), the temperature drop typically associated with ONB is not observed in the course of the boiling curves.

The differences in boiling curve profiles and the characteristics of the ONB region observed at various inclination angles of the mini-channel can also be attributed to gravity-driven effects influencing vapour bubble behaviour and liquid replenishment near the asymmetrically heated wall.

At a lower angle of the mini-channel ($\omega = 60°$), due to relatively stable bubble dynamics and efficient vapour evacuation, the temperature drop typically associated with ONB is distinct. As the distance from the inlet increases, development of the thermal boundary layer leads to a gradual shift of the boiling curve toward higher wall-to-fluid temperature differences. For $\omega = 90°$, where the mini-channel is in vertical orientation and the heated surface is at the bottom, buoyancy acts symmetrically with respect to gravity and the geometry of the channel. Continuous upward removal of the vapour is promoted, but increases in bubble interactions and vertical coalescence may result in a more chaotic and fluctuating detachment. As a consequence, the ONB remains observable, but is less sharply defined, due to temporal instability in the local bubble dynamics. However, at $\omega = 135°$, at which the heated surface is positioned above the liquid and orientated more horizontally, gravitational forces act more strongly on the liquid phase, significantly influencing the dynamics of the two-phase flow. In this configuration, the vapour bubbles generated on the heated wall tend to accumulate and coalesce beneath the surface because of limited buoyancy-driven detachment. As a result, larger and more oval-shaped vapour agglomerates are observed, which adhere for longer durations to the heated surface. This vapour accumulation inhibits the prompt departure of bubbles and delays the onset of nucleate boiling (ONB). Consequently, the boiling curves exhibit a smoother and more gradual transition into the nucleate boiling regime, without a clearly defined ONB point. Moreover, such spatial orientation of the heated surface reduces gravitational support for liquid backflow and rewetting of the wall, thereby limiting the replenishment of cooler liquid to the heated interface. This not only suppresses bubble nucleation due to insufficient wall wetting but also enhances the formation of a quasi-stable vapour layer that acts as a thermal barrier. The combined effects of impaired vapour detachment and weakened liquid renewal reduce the intensity of local heat transfer and mask the thermal signature of the ONB. As a result, boiling heat transfer under this orientation is less efficient, with poorer surface wetting and delayed establishment of fully developed nucleate boiling.

6. Conclusions

This study presents a time-dependent two-dimensional model for analysing boiling heat transfer during refrigerant flow in asymmetrically heated mini-channels. Particular attention is given to the results obtained in the early stage of the experiment that correspond to the forced convection, boiling incipience, and subcooled boiling region.

The mathematical formulation included two inverse Cauchy-type problems. The solution uses two sets of Trefftz functions, classical for the heating foil domain and newly developed for the working fluid domain. The application of new T-functions for the fluid domain marks a key innovation, enabling a semi-analytical solution under defined flow conditions.

It should be emphasised that the study pursues two intertwined objectives:

- Experimental analysis—this aim was to cover the investigation of the influence of channel inclination on boiling heat transfer during Fluorinert FC-770 flow in an asymmetrically heated mini-channel heat sink. The measurements focused on time-dependent data, including local foil temperature, inlet and outlet fluid temperatures, electrical parameters (current and voltage) of the supplied power, and mass flux. The strength of this approach lies in its ability to directly verify and validate the proposed computational model—an aspect that conventional CFD simulations alone cannot provide.

- Computational analysis—the Trefftz method was applied and validated for analysing coupled, time-dependent heat conduction and fluid flow. This analytical–numerical approach was used to solve both direct and inverse heat-conduction problems in the heated foil–mini-channel system. It enabled the determination of two-dimensional, transient temperature distributions in the heater and refrigerant, as well as local heat-transfer coefficients. The obtained results were subsequently compared with those derived from a simplified approach.

On the basis of these results and the associated analysis, the following insights have been derived:

1. The mathematical model of time-dependent heat transfer allowed the effective determination of (i) the temperature distributions of the heating foil and the fluid flowing through the mini-channel, (ii) the temperature gradient of the heating foil, and, subsequently, (iii) the heat-transfer coefficient (HTC).
2. Using the Trefftz method, two time-dependent inverse Cauchy-type problems were solved in two contact areas with different geometries and physical properties. The newly defined Trefftz functions were applied to solve the Fourier–Kirchhoff equation relative to the fluid.
3. The inclination angle of the mini-channel has a substantial impact on local heat-transfer coefficients and two-phase flow development. Although early-stage HTC values remain comparable across tested angles of the mini-channel, differences become more pronounced with increasing distance from the inlet and higher heat flux. Steeper inclinations (such as 105° and 120°) promote enhanced vapour detachment, improved surface rewetting, and liquid backflow, leading to higher HTCs. The highest HTC values occur closer to the outlet of the mini-channel, and at an angle of 105°.
4. The HTCs obtained from the two-dimensional and simplified approaches were similar. The two-dimensional model gave higher HTC values than the one-dimensional model, and the differences do not exceed 0.3 kW/(m^2 K).
5. The inclination angle of the mini-channel notably affects the boiling curve profile and the onset of nucleate boiling (ONB), mainly through gravity-driven influences on vapour bubble dynamics and liquid replenishment. At lower mini-channel inclination angles (e.g., $\omega = 60°$), stable bubble detachment and efficient vapour removal produce a distinct ONB point. At $\omega = 90°$, buoyancy aids vapour escape but introduces greater detachment fluctuations. Furthermore, at $\omega = 135°$, the heated surface facing upward delays the release of the vapour and limits wall rewetting, leading to the agglomeration of the vapour and a smoother and more gradual transition to nucleate boiling, without a clearly defined ONB point.

Author Contributions: Conceptualization, S.H. and M.P.; methodology, A.M., S.H., M.P. and A.P.; software, A.P. and A.M.; validation, M.P., A.P. and S.H.; formal analysis, M.P., S.H., A.P. and AM; investigation, M.P.; resources, M.P.; data curation, M.P.; writing—original draft preparation, M.P., S.H., A.P. and A.M; writing—review and editing, M.P. and S.H.; visualization, S.H. and A.P.; supervision, M.P.; project administration, M.P.; funding acquisition, M.P. All authors have read and agreed to the published version of the manuscript.

Funding: This research received no external funding.

Data Availability Statement: The original contributions presented in this study are included in the article.

Conflicts of Interest: The authors declare no conflict of interest.

Nomenclature

a, b, c	Constants
c_p	Specific heat capacity, J/(kg K)
f, g	Coefficient
g	Gravitational acceleration, m/s^2
N	Number of the Trefftz function
q	Heat flux (density), W/m^2
T	Temperature, K
t	Time coordinate, s
u	Trefftz function
v	Velocity, m/s
V	Trefftz function, particular solution
x	Coordinate in the direction of flow, m
y	Coordinate in the direction perpendicular to the flow and width of the test section partitions, m
Differential operators:	
$\nabla^2 = \frac{\partial^2}{\partial x^2} + \frac{\partial^2}{\partial y^2}$	
$\mathcal{L} = \nabla^2 - \frac{\partial}{\partial t}$	
$\mathcal{L}^{-1}$	Inverse operator
Greek letters:	
α	Heat-transfer coefficient, W/(m^2 K)
δ	Thickness, depth, m
λ	Thermal conductivity, W/(m K)
ρ	Density, kg/m^3
τ	Variable, m^2
ω	Angle of the test section inclination
Subscripts:	
ave	Average
f	FC-770 fluid
h	Heating foil
in	Inlet
lin	Linear
M	Mini-channel
out	Outlet
par	Particular solution
sat	Saturation
1D	Refers to one-dimensional approach
2D	Refers to two-dimensional approach
Superscript	
m	Measurement

References

1. Reutskiy, S.Y. A Trefftz type method for time-dependent problems. *Eng. Anal. Bound. Elem.* **2004**, *28*, 13–21. [CrossRef]
2. Cho, H.A.; Golberg, M.A.; Muleshkov, A.S.; Li, X. Trefftz Methods for Time Dependent Partial Differential Equations. *CMC* **2004**, *1*, 1–38.
3. Jirousek, J.; Qin, Q.H. Application of hybrid-Trefftz element approach to transient heat conduction analysis. *Comput. Struct.* **1996**, *8*, 195–201. [CrossRef]
4. Ku, C.Y.; Liu, C.Y.; Xiao, J.E.; Huang, W.P.; Su, Y. A spacetime collocation Trefftz method for solving the inverse heat conduction problem. *Adv. Mech. Eng.* **2019**, *11*, 1687814019861271. [CrossRef]
5. Piasecka, M.; Hożejowska, S.; Maciejewska, B.; Pawińska, A. Time-dependent heat transfer calculations with Trefftz and Picard methods for flow boiling in a mini-channel heat sink. *Energies* **2021**, *14*, 1832. [CrossRef]

6. Bian, Y.; Chen, Z.; Li, Z.; Liang, Y.; Li, Y.; Lu, X.; Yuan, D.; Feng, Z. Experimental investigation on the effects of inclined grooves on flow boiling heat transfer and instability in a minichannel heat sink. *Int. J. Heat Mass Transf.* **2025**, *236*, 126333. [CrossRef]
7. He, B.; Luo, X.; Yu, F.; Li, T.; Feng, Z.; Zhou, J. Enhanced flow boiling performance of interconnected bi-porous minichannel. *Int. Commun. Heat Mass Transf.* **2024**, *157*, 107770. [CrossRef]
8. Kumar, A.; Kothadia, H.B. Thermal analysis of flow boiling of highly subcooled water in mini and conventional channels. *Int. J. Heat Mass Transf.* **2024**, *223*, 125275. [CrossRef]
9. Shang, H.; Xia, G.; Li, R.; Miao, S. Experimental study on flow boiling heat transfer of HFE-7100 in minichannel heat sinks for professional-grade server chips cooling. *Int. Commun. Heat Mass Transf.* **2025**, *164*, 108825. [CrossRef]
10. Charnay, R.; Revellin, R.; Bonjour, J. Flow boiling heat transfer in minichannels at high saturation temperatures: Part I—Experimental investigation and analysis of the heat transfer mechanisms. *Int. J. Heat Mass Transf.* **2015**, *87*, 636–652. [CrossRef]
11. Wang, D.; Wang, D.; Hong, F.; Xu, J.; Zhang, C. Experimental study on flow boiling characteristics of R-1233zd(E) of counter-flow interconnected minichannel heat sink. *Int. J. Heat Mass Transf.* **2023**, *215*, 124481. [CrossRef]
12. Hadamard, J. Sur les problèmes aux dérivées partielles et leur signification physique. *Princet. Univ. Bull.* **1902**, *13*, 49–52.
13. Trefftz, E. Ein gegenstuck zum ritzschen verfahren. In Proceedings of the 2nd International Congress for Applied Mechanics, Zürich, Switzerland, 12–17 September 1926; pp. 131–137.
14. Herrera, I. Trefftz Method. In *Topics in Boundary Element Research*; Brebbia, C.A., Ed.; Springer: New York, NY, USA, 1984; Volume 1.
15. Herrera, I.; Sabina, F.J. Connectivity as an alternative to boundary integral equations: Construction of bases. *APMS* **1978**, *75*, 2059–2063. [CrossRef] [PubMed]
16. Herrera, I. Boundary methods: A criterion for completeness. *AMPS* **1980**, *77*, 4395–4398. [CrossRef] [PubMed]
17. Jirousek, J. Basis for development of large finite elements locally satisfying all field equations. *Comput. Methods Appl. Mech. Eng.* **1978**, *14*, 65–92. [CrossRef]
18. Jirousek, J.; Zieliński, A.P. Dual hybrid-Trefftz element formulation based on independent boundary traction frame. *Int. J. Numer. Methods Eng.* **1993**, *36*, 2955–2980. [CrossRef]
19. Rosenbloom, P.C.; Widder, D.V. Expansion in terms of heat polynomials and associated functions. *Trans. Am. Math. Soc.* **1956**, *92*, 220–266. [CrossRef]
20. Kołodziej, J.A.; Grabski, J.K. Many names of the Trefftz method. *Eng. Anal. Bound. Elem.* **2018**, *96*, 169–178. [CrossRef]
21. Li, Z.C.; Lu, T.T.; Huang, H.T.; Cheng, A.H.D. Trefftz, collocation, and other boundary methods—A comparison. *Numer. Methods Partial. Differ. Equ.* **2007**, *23*, 93–144. [CrossRef]
22. Qin, Q.H. *The Trefftz Finite and Boundary Element Method*; WIT Press: Southampton, UK; Boston, MA, USA, 2000.
23. Li, L.; Xu, P.; Li, Q.; Yin, Z.; Zheng, R.; Wu, J.; Bao, J.J.; Bai, W.Y.; Qi, H.; Tan, D.P. Multi-field coupling particle flow dynamic behaviors of the microreactor and ultrasonic control method. *Powder Technol.* **2025**, *454*, 120731. [CrossRef]
24. Piasecka, M.; Strąk, K. Boiling Heat Transfer during Flow in Vertical Mini-Channels with a Modified Heated Surface. *Energies* **2022**, *15*, 7050. [CrossRef]
25. Piasecka, M.; Strąk, K.; Maciejewska, B. Heat transfer characteristics during flow along horizontal and vertical minichannels. *Int. J. Multiph. Flow* **2021**, *137*, 103559. [CrossRef]
26. Hożejowski, L.; Hożejowska, S. Trefftz method in an inverse problem of two-phase flow boiling in a minichannel. *Eng. Anal. Bound. Elem.* **2019**, *98*, 27–34. [CrossRef]
27. Grysa, K.; Maciejewska, B. Trefftz Functions for Non-Stationary Problems. *J. Theor. Appl. Mech.* **2013**, *51*, 251–264.

energies

MDPI

Article

Experimental-Numerical Method for Determining Heat Transfer Correlations in the Plate-and-Frame Heat Exchanger

Dawid Taler [1], Ewelina Ziółkowska [2], Jan Taler [3,*], Tomasz Sobota [1], Magdalena Jaremkiewicz [1], Mateusz Marcinkowski [1] and Tomasz Cieślik [1]

[1] Department of Thermal Processes, Air Protection, and Waste Utilisation, Cracow University of Technology, ul. Warszawska 24, 31-155 Cracow, Poland; dawid.taler@pk.edu.pl (D.T.); tomasz.sobota@pk.edu.pl (T.S.); magdalena.jaremkiewicz@pk.edu.pl (M.J.); mateusz.marcinkowski@pk.edu.pl (M.M.); tomasz.cieslik@pk.edu.pl (T.C.)

[2] Department of Energy, CUT Doctoral School, Cracow University of Technology, al. Jana Pawła II 37, 31-864 Cracow, Poland; ewelina.ziolkowska@doktorant.pk.edu.pl

[3] Department of Energy, Cracow University of Technology, al. Jana Pawła II 37, 31-864 Cracow, Poland

* Correspondence: jan.taler@pk.edu.pl

Abstract

Plate heat exchangers are used in heat substations for domestic hot water preparation and building heating in municipal central heating systems. Water from the municipal water supply is heated by hot water from a district heating network. This paper presents a numerical method for simultaneously determining heat transfer correlations on the cold and hot water sides based on flow-thermal measurements of the plate heat exchanger. The unknown parameters in the functions approximating the Nusselt numbers, which depend on the Reynolds and Prandtl numbers, are determined using the least-squares method, so the sum of the squares of the differences in the calculated and measured temperatures at the heat exchanger outlet reaches a minimum. One or two correlations were sought for a plate heat exchanger, and the total number of parameters sought is between three and six. The limits of the 95% confidence intervals for all estimated parameters were also determined. Correlations for Nusselt numbers determined experimentally for a clean plate heat exchanger can be used in the online monitoring of the degree of fouling of plate heat exchangers installed in the substations of a large urban district heating network.

Keywords: plate-and-frame heat exchanger; thermal substation; heat transfer correlations; experimental testing; numerical method; scale deposits

1. Introduction

Plate and frame (gasketed) heat exchangers are widely used in heating, air-conditioning, the food industry and many other applications [1]. Their main advantage is their high heat output with a small heat exchanger size.

Both in design and performance calculations, it is necessary to know the heat transfer correlation for calculating the Nusselt numbers (Nu), which allow for calculating the mean heat transfer coefficients (HTCs) on the side of each fluid [2].

The Wilson method [3] is a popular method used for experimentally determining correlations for Nusselt numbers on both the hot and cold fluid sides. Sekulić and Shah [4] present various methods for experimentally determining the HTC and correlations for Nusselt numbers on the side of one or both working fluids. They also present the practical application of Wilson's plot method for determining correlations for Nusselt numbers on the gas and liquid sides in plate-fin and tube heat exchangers (PFTHE).

The Wilson method is also discussed by Taler [5] in the book on heat exchangers' modelling and testing [4]. The Wilson method is labour-intensive because the determination of correlations for Nusselt numbers is iterative. Correlations are determined sequentially. First, the correlation for the Nusselt number on the side of one fluid, for example the hot fluid, is determined, while on the side of the other fluid, i.e., the cold fluid, the mass flow rate is constant so that the HTC is constant. In the second iteration, the HTC on the cold fluid side is determined, while the mass flow rate on the hot fluid side is kept constant. The iterative process is then repeated until the coefficients in the Nusselt number correlations do not change. When one or both working fluids are liquids, it is difficult to maintain a constant HTC on one side of the partition when the flow rate and fluid temperature on the other side change. Despite the constancy of the mass flow rate, the HTC changes because the Prandtl number changes as a result of changes in fluid temperature, and therefore, the HTC changes despite the constant mass flow rate of the fluid. Thus, the basic condition in the iterative process of determining the HTC, proposed by Wilson, is not maintained. This disadvantage of Wilson's method is illustrated in [5] by determining the correlation for Nusselt numbers in a PFTHE. Another weakness of Wilson's method is linearising the nonlinear correlations of the Nusselt number on the Reynolds (Re) and Prandtl (Pr) numbers. By taking the logarithm of this nonlinear power-type heat transfer correlation $Nu = f(\mathrm{Re}, \mathrm{Pr})$ and introducing new variables, the determination of unknown coefficients is reduced to a linear least squares problem, usually linear regression. As a result of this operation, the unknown parameters in the correlation for the Nusselt number have different values than those obtained using the non-linear least squares method.

A commonly used technique for determining correlations on one side of a heat exchanger involves first estimating the overall HTC from experimental tests conducted on the entire heat exchanger. The HTC on the inner surface of the tubes is then calculated using well-established correlations for the Nusselt number in straight tubes, such as the Dittus–Boelter [6] or Gnielinski [7] equations. If transitional or turbulent flow occurs inside the exchanger tubes during experimental testing, Taler's correlation [8] can be used to calculate the HTC on the inner surface of the tubes.

Knowing the HTC, the internal HTC, and the thermal resistance of the tube wall, the HTC on the outer surface of the tubes can be determined. Subsequently, an appropriate function is identified to approximate the outer surface Nusselt numbers as a function of the Reynolds and Prandtl numbers, or other relevant parameters influencing this coefficient.

Nasrfard et al. [9] provide an example of such an approach, presenting experimental results on the condensation heat transfer of R141b in an intermittent flow regime on a smooth horizontal tube. Their study proposed a power-law correlation for calculating the Nusselt number as a function of the equivalent Reynolds and Prandtl numbers. A similar methodology to determine the Nusselt number correlation on one side of the exchanger can be found in many other publications. Wilson's method is used to derive correlations for the Nusselt number on the outer tube surfaces. Fu et al. [10] developed a tubular cross-flow serpentine tube heat exchanger for aero-engine cooling. A correlation was established for the Nusselt number on the cooling air side based on thermal flow tests of three different heat exchangers with different tube outer diameters: 2.2, 1.8, and 1.4 mm. The HTC from the flowing RP-3 kerosene to the inner surface of small-diameter tubes was calculated using Gnielinski's equation. The Wilson method was used to determine the unknown parameters in the power correlation for the air side Nusselt number. Shah et al. [11] carried out an experimental test to find power-type heat transfer correlations on the inner surface of the tubes through which the water/glycol solution flowed. Ammonia was expanding in the space between the tubes of the shell-and-tube heat exchanger. The tubes with a 3-D structured outside surface enhanced condensation heat transfer. The heat transfer correlation for the tube side HTC was determined by the modified Wilson plot method. Nguyen et al. [12] experimentally studied the condensation of R-513a refrigerant in a vertical plate heat exchanger in which the plate surfaces were electrochemically etched. The correlation for the Nusselt number on the cooling water side was found using the modified Wilson plot method. The inverse HTC on the condensing side of R-513a was calculated by subtracting the thermal resistance of the wall and the inverse HTC on the water side from the inverse overall HTC. Next, a power correlation was determined to estimate the Nusselt number on the R-513a side. An experimental study by Li et al. [13] investigated the condensation of R134a in a horizontal shell-and-tube heat exchanger. Micro-fins on the outer surface of the tubes were used to increase the HTC on the condensing R134a side. The HTC on the side of the hot water flowing inside the tubes was calculated using Gnielinski's equation [7], and the correlation for the outer HTC was established using the modified Wilson plot method. Shokouhmand et al. [14] investigated experimentally shell and coiled tube heat exchangers. The Wilson plot method was used to estimate the HTC on the outer surface of the coiled tube. The direct method was applied by Fronk and Garimella [15] to measure the HTC on the inner tube surface during condensation of ammonia and ammonia/water mixtures in minichannels. The HTC was calculated using its definition based on the measurement of the heat flux, wall and fluid temperatures.

Currently, instead of experimental research, flow and heat transfer modelling in heat exchangers is increasingly being carried out using various commercial Computational Fluid Dynamics (CFD) software. Based on computer simulations conducted at different mass flow rates and temperatures of both fluids, correlations are determined for the Nusselt number, usually on the side of one fluid. Taler D. et al. [16] established correlations for the air side Nusselt number on individual tube rows in plate-fin and tube heat exchangers (PFTHE). The HTC inside the tubes was calculated using the correlation available in the literature. The correlation proposed in [8] was used in [16] to estimate the HTC for water on the inner surface of the tubes. A similar procedure to that in [16] was used by Yu et al. [17] to determine the correlation for the Nusselt number on the flue gas side in a finned-tube heat exchanger in a gas-fired water boiler. The HTC on the water side was determined using Gnielinski's equation [7], and the correlation for the Nusselt number on the gas side was determined based on CFD modelling. The Nusselt number determined based on CFD simulation closely approximates the Nusselt number determined on the experimental stand. Calculations of the HTC on the internal surfaces of tubes using experimental correlations available in the literature can be avoided in PFTHEs by assuming a constant external tube surface temperature or a constant tube and fin surface temperature [18]. A constant temperature of the finned tube surface can be assumed because, in the case of air or other gases, the HTC depends mainly on the gas flow velocity, and the influence of the tube and fin temperatures is negligible. CFD modelling allows for a simple and inexpensive way to determine correlations for the Nusselt number on the gas side of PFTHEs, as well as in plate heat exchangers. Zhu [19] investigated the influence of the chevron angle in plate heat exchangers on the thermal performance of plate heat exchangers using CFD simulation. New correlations for calculating the Nusselt number in plate heat exchangers, considering the chevron angle value, were proposed [19]. However, it is important to note the large discrepancies in Nusselt numbers determined using CFD simulations with different turbulence models. This is due to the lack of suitable turbulence models, despite the fact that there are several dozens of them. However, the results obtained using CFD modelling require experimental verification.

Taler D. [20] proposed a method for simultaneously determining correlations for Nusselt numbers on the air and water sides in PFTHE. Unknown parameters in Nusselt number correlations were selected so that the sum of squares of differences between calculated and measured water and air temperatures at the heat exchanger outlet was minimum. The minimised sum of squares took into account the sums of squares of the differences between the measured and calculated temperatures at the heat exchanger outlet, taking into account the measured water and air temperatures but with different weights. The weighting factors in the sum of squares are smaller for air, due to the lower accuracy of measurements on the air side compared to the accuracy of measurements on the water side. An analytical model was used to calculate the water and air temperatures at the outlet of the tested PFTHE.

An overview of methods for determining HTC on the inner surface of tubes in condensation flow is provided in the paper by Marchetto et al. [21]. The discussed works are divided into three groups devoted to the direct method, the Wilson plot method and the boundary layer thickness method.

Artificial neural networks or other data-driven methods can also be used to calculate HTCs in heat exchangers. However, methods based on artificial intelligence require a huge database of HTCs determined experimentally using other methods to predict HTCs with sufficient accuracy.

A literature review shows that in most experimental studies on heat exchangers, the correlation for the Nusselt number is determined only on one fluid's side. The correlations available in the literature are usually used to determine the HTC on the side of the other fluid, for example, for the medium flowing in the tubes. Considering that the overall HTC is determined experimentally, the uncertainty of determining the average HTC using the formulas available in the literature may cause large errors in the correlations determined for the second medium using the Wilson method. It should be emphasised that the HTCs available in the literature were derived for straight tubes, while heat exchangers usually have multiple passes, which means that the direction of fluid flow in the tubes or manifolds is reversed. The fluid flow conditions inside the heat exchanger tubes differ from those in straight tubes.

The least squares method is used in the paper to determine unknown coefficients in correlations for Nusselt numbers on the hot and cold liquid sides. The Nusselt numbers are determined as nonlinear functions of the Reynolds and Prandtl numbers without transforming heat transfer correlations to obtain a linear least squares problem, as, for example, in Wilson's method. This ensures high accuracy in determining unknown coefficients in both correlations for hot and cold fluids. In the method presented in this paper, heat transfer correlations can even be complex functions of Reynolds and Prandtl numbers. Correlations for the Nusselt numbers do not have to be power functions as in Wilson's method.

2. Numerical-Experimental Method for Simultaneous Determination of the Heat Transfer Correlations on the Hot and Cold Water Side

The proposed method for determining heat transfer correlations is general and can be used to determine correlations for the Nusselt number on the hot and cold sides in various types of heat exchangers. For the determined correlations to be reliable, the measurement data must meet the following conditions:

- measurements of mass flow rates and temperatures of both working fluids should be carried out during steady-state operation of the heat exchanger,
- the range of inlet temperature changes of the hot and cold fluids should be large so that the range of Prandtl number changes for each fluid is large,

- the range of changes in the mass flow rates of the hot and cold fluids should be large so that the range of changes in the Reynolds number for each fluid is large,
- the uncertainties in the measurement of the temperature and mass flow rates of both working fluids should be small, i.e., the measuring instruments should be of high accuracy,
- the heat flow rates transferred from the hot liquid to the cold liquid, calculated based on measurement data, should not differ too much,
- the mathematical model of the heat exchanger should be highly accurate and closely approximate the measurement data,
- the number of measurement series should be large, in the order of several dozen measurement series with significantly different temperatures of the working fluids at the inlet to the heat exchanger and different mass flows of the working fluids,
- unknown parameters in correlations for the Nusselt number for hot and cold fluids should be selected so that the sum of the squares of the differences between the measured and calculated temperatures for all measurement series is as small as possible.

The plate heat exchanger under study is a counter-current heat exchanger. In the proposed method for determining the correlation for Nusselt number on the hot and cold water side, it is necessary to calculate the heat exchanger's cold and hot water outlet temperatures multiple times for each measurement data set. This section presents a procedure for calculating the cold and hot water outlet temperatures of a heat exchanger based on the P-NTU (Effectiveness- Number of Transfer Units) method.

2.1. Determination of Hot and Cold Water Temperatures at the Outlet of the Heat Exchanger

The P-NTU method [22] was used to determine the cold and hot water temperatures at the outlet of the heat exchanger. Effectiveness P_h is defined as follows (Figure 1)

$$P_h = \frac{\dot{Q}_h}{\dot{Q}_{h,\max}} = \frac{\dot{m}_h c_h (T_{h1} - T_{h2})}{\dot{m}_h c_h (T_{h1} - T_{c2})} = \frac{(T_{h1} - T_{h2})}{(T_{h1} - T_{c2})} \tag{1}$$

where P_h—effectiveness of the heat exchanger calculated for hot water; $\dot{Q}_h$—rate of heat flow in the heat exchanger, W; $\dot{Q}_{h,\max}$—maximum rate of heat flow in the heat exchanger, W; $\dot{m}_h$—mass flow rate of hot water, kg/s; c_h—specific heat of hot water, J/(kgK); T_{h1}, T_{h2}—temperature of hot fluid at the inlet and outlet of the heat exchanger, °C; T_{c2}, T_{c1}—temperature of cold fluid at inlet and outlet of the heat exchanger, °C.

The equation for the effectiveness of a counter-flow heat exchanger has the following form [5]

$$P_h = \frac{1 - \exp\left[-U_A A\left(\frac{1}{\dot{m}_h c_h} - \frac{1}{\dot{m}_c c_c}\right)\right]}{1 - \frac{\dot{m}_h c_h}{\dot{m}_c c_c}\exp\left[-U_A A\left(\frac{1}{\dot{m}_h c_h} - \frac{1}{\dot{m}_c c_c}\right)\right]} = \frac{1 - \exp[-(NTU_h - NTU_c)]}{1 - \frac{NTU_c}{NTU_h}\exp[-(NTU_h - NTU_c)]} \tag{2}$$

where U_A—overall HTC related to the area A, m^2; NTU_c, NTU_h—number of heat transfer units for cold and hot water; $\dot{m}_c$—mass flow rate of cold water, kg/s; c_c—specific heat of cold water, J/(kgK).

The numbers of heat transfer units for cold and hot water are given by the following formulas

$$NTU_c = \frac{U_A A}{\dot{m}_c c_c}\ NTU_h = \frac{U_A A}{\dot{m}_h c_h} \tag{3}$$

After calculating the effectiveness P_h for hot water using Equation (2), the hot water temperature T_{h2} at the outlet of the heat exchanger is determined from Equation (1)

$$T_{h2} = T_{h1} - P_h(T_{h1} - T_{c2}) \tag{4}$$

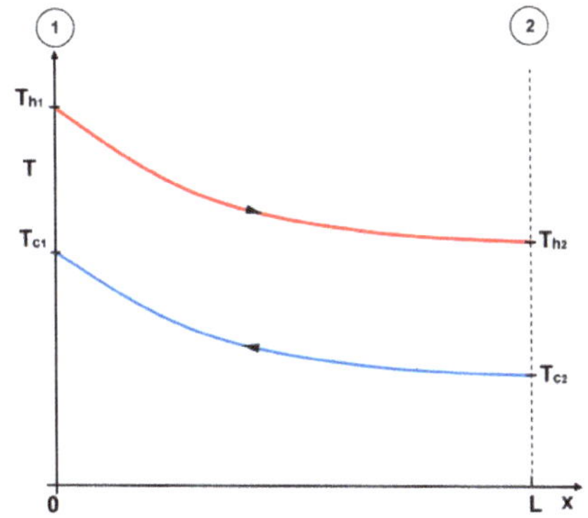

Figure 1. Temperature distribution of hot and cold fluid in the counterflow heat exchanger; T_{h1}, T_{h2} temperature of hot fluid at the inlet and outlet of the heat exchanger, T_{c2}, T_{c1} temperature of cold fluid at the inlet and outlet of the heat exchanger, ①-left side of the heat exchanger ($x = 0$), ②-right side of the heat exchanger ($x = L$).

By substituting Equation (2) into Formula (3), one obtains

$$\begin{aligned} T_{h2} &= T_{h1} - \frac{(T_{h1}-T_{c2})\left\{1-\exp\left[-U_A A\left(\frac{1}{\dot{m}_h c_h}-\frac{1}{\dot{m}_c c_c}\right)\right]\right\}}{1-\frac{\dot{m}_h c_h}{\dot{m}_c c_c}\exp\left[-U_A A\left(\frac{1}{\dot{m}_h c_h}-\frac{1}{\dot{m}_c c_c}\right)\right]} \\ &= T_{h1} - \frac{(T_{h1}-T_{c2})\{1-\exp[-(NTU_h-NTU_c)]\}}{1-\frac{NTU_c}{NTU_h}\exp[-(NTU_h-NTU_c)]} \end{aligned} \tag{5}$$

The heat flow rate transferred from the hot water $\dot{Q}_h$ is equal to the heat flow rate absorbed by the cold water $\dot{Q}_c$

$$\dot{m}_h c_h(T_{h1} - T_{h2}) = \dot{m}_c c_c(T_{c1} - T_{c2}) \tag{6}$$

From Equation (4) we obtain

$$T_{h1} - T_{h2} = P_h(T_{h1} - T_{c2}) \tag{7}$$

$$T_{c1} - T_{c2} = P_c(T_{h1} - T_{c2}) \tag{8}$$

where P_c—effectiveness of the heat exchanger for cold water.

Substituting expressions (7) and (8) into Equation (6) gives

$$\dot{m}_h c_h P_h(T_{h1} - T_{c2}) = \dot{m}_c c_c P_c(T_{h1} - T_{c2}) \tag{9}$$

$$\frac{\dot{m}_h c_h}{\dot{m}_c c_c} = \frac{P_c}{P_h} \tag{10}$$

After simple transformations, Equation (10) gives

$$P_c = \frac{\dot{m}_h c_h}{\dot{m}_c c_c} P_h = \frac{NTU_c}{NTU_h} P_h \tag{11}$$

The cold water temperature T_{c1} at the outlet of the heat exchanger, determined from Equation (6) is given by the formula

$$T_{c1} = T_{c2} + \frac{\dot{m}_h c_h}{\dot{m}_c c_c}(T_{h1} - T_{h2}) = T_{c2} + \frac{NTU_c}{NTU_h}(T_{h1} - T_{h2}) \tag{12}$$

Equation (8) can also be used to determine the temperature T_{c1}

$$T_{c1} = T_{c2} + P_c(T_{h1} - T_{c2}) \tag{13}$$

Using the P-NTU [22] or ε-NTU (Effectiveness-Number of transfer units) [23] method to determine hot and cold medium outlet temperatures is advantageous, especially for heat exchangers with complex flow systems. Formulas for calculating effectiveness P can be found in [22] and for ε in [23] for many heat exchangers of different designs. The respective arithmetic averages of the inlet and outlet temperatures were used to calculate all physical properties of the hot and cold water.

2.2. Method for Determining Unknown Coefficients in Correlations for Nusselt Numbers for Hot and Cold Water

Knowledge of the HTCs on both sides of a wall, for example, a plate, plain or finned tube, is essential for design or performance calculations of heat exchangers as well as for online monitoring systems for heat transfer surface fouling.

The overall HTC for a clean plate and frame heat exchanger is determined using the following equation:

$$\frac{1}{U} = \frac{1}{h_c} + \frac{\delta}{k_p} + \frac{1}{h_h} \tag{14}$$

where h_c and h_h—HTC for cold and hot water, respectively, $W/(m^2K)$; k_p—thermal conductivity of the plate, $W/(mK)$; δ—plate thickness, m.

Knowing the surface area A of the heat exchanger, the overall HTC U and the inlet temperatures of the hot T_{h1} and cold T_{c2} fluid, the temperature of the hot T_{h2} and cold fluid at the outlet of the heat exchanger can be calculated.

The HTCs h_c and h_h are calculated using the correlations for the Nusselt number on the cold and hot water side, which are determined based on experimental testing. The Nusselt number Nu_c on the cold water side is given by the following equation:

$$Nu_c = \frac{h_c D_h}{k_c} \tag{15}$$

The hydraulic diameter D_h of the channel is defined as follows:

$$D_h = \frac{4A_{ch}}{P_w} \tag{16}$$

where A_{ch}—channel flow area, P_w—wetted perimeter.

The Nusselt number on the hot water side is defined similarly to the cold water side

$$Nu_h = \frac{h_h D_h}{k_h} \tag{17}$$

The symbols k_c and k_h in Equations (15) and (17) represent the thermal conductivity of the cold and hot water.

The correlation for the Nusselt number on the hot water side was applied as follows

$$Nu_h = x_{1,h} \mathrm{Re}_h^{x_{2,h}} \mathrm{Pr}_h^{x_{3,h}} \tag{18}$$

where the Reynolds number Re_h and Prandtl number Pr_h are defined as follows

$$\mathrm{Re}_h = \frac{w_h D_h}{\nu_h} \tag{19}$$

The following correlation was assumed for the Nusselt number on the cold water side:

$$Nu_c = x_{1,c} \mathrm{Re}_h^{x_{2,c}} \mathrm{Pr}_h^{x_{3,c}} \tag{20}$$

where the Reynolds number Re_c and Prandtl number Pr_c are defined as follows

$$\mathrm{Re}_c = \frac{w_c D_c}{\nu_c}\ \mathrm{Pr}_c = \frac{c_c \mu_c}{k_c} \tag{21}$$

In Equations (19)–(21), the following designations are adopted: w_c, w_h average velocity of cold and hot water in the channel cross-section; ν_c, ν_h kinematic viscosity of cold and hot water.

Unknown coefficients $x_{1,h}$ and power exponents $x_{2,h}$, $x_{3,h}$ in correlation (18) for hot water and unknown coefficients $x_{1,c}$ power exponents $x_{2,c}$, $x_{3,c}$ in correlation (20) for cold water were determined based on experimental studies.

First, the number n of coefficients required for the correlations per Nusselt number for hot and cold water is determined.

Three cases were considered:

(a) the total number of unknown parameters in the correlation for cold water and for hot water is $n = n_h + n_c$, where the symbol n_h indicates a number of unknown parameters in correlation for the Nusselt number for hot water, n_c number of unknown parameters for cold water;

(b) the total number of unknown parameters in the correlation for cold water and for hot water is $n = 4$. There are two unknown parameters in each of the correlations for hot and cold water: $n_h = 2$ and $n_c = 2$;

(c) in both correlations for the Nusselt numbers, on the hot and cold sides, there is the same number of unknown parameters, i.e., $n_h = n_c = n$. The total number n of unknown coefficients and power exponents on the cold and hot water side is $n = 3$. It was assumed that: $x_{1,h} = x_{1,c}$, $x_{2,h} = x_{2,c}$ and $x_{3,h} = x_{3,c}$.

In the present study, $n_h = 3$ and $n_c = 3$. When different parameters are assumed in the correlations for the Nusselt number for hot and cold water, the total number of unknown parameters is $n = 4$ or $n = 6$.

The unknown coefficients (parameters) were determined from the condition of the minimum of the sum S of the differences of squares between the calculated and measured hot and cold water temperatures at the outlet of the heat exchanger

$$S = \sum_{i=1}^{m}\left[\left(T_{h2,i}^{cal} - T_{h2,i}^{meas}\right)^2 + \left(T_{c1,i}^{cal} - T_{c1,i}^{meas}\right)^2\right] \to \min \tag{22}$$

In Equation (22), the following designations are used, m—number of measuring series; $T_{h2,i}^{cal}$, $T_{c1,i}^{cal}$— calculated hot and cold water outlet temperatures of the exchanger for the i-th measuring series, respectively; $T_{h2,i}^{meas}$, $T_{c1,i}^{meas}$—the measured temperature of the hot and cold water at the exchanger outlet for the i-th measuring series, respectively.

The values of the unknown parameters $x_1, \ldots, x_n$ were determined using the Levenberg–Marquardt method [24,25]. Temperatures $T_{h2,i}^{cal}$, $T_{c1,i}^{cal}$ are functions of the parameters looked for $x_1, \ldots, x_n$.

The 95% confidence intervals of the determined parameters $x_1, \ldots, x_n$ were calculated using Gauss's law of transfer of variance formulated for indirectly determined quantities [8,26]. The mean square deviation was determined on the basis of the minimum sum of squares (22).

A detailed derivation of the equations used to determine the 95% confidence intervals for the determined parameters can be found in [8].

2.3. Uncertainty Analysis

The uncertainties for the estimated parameters were determined using the Gauss variance propagation rule. Confidence intervals of the determined parameters in the correlations for the heat transfer coefficients at the sides of the air and water. The real values of the determined parameters $\tilde{x}_1, \ldots, \tilde{x}_n$ are found with the probability of $P = (1 - \alpha) \cdot 100\%$ in the following intervals:

$$x_i - t_{2m-n}^{\alpha/2}\, s_t\, \sqrt{c_{ii}} \le \tilde{x}_i \le x_i + t_{2m-n}^{\alpha/2}\, s_t\, \sqrt{c_{ii}} \tag{23}$$

where x_i—parameter determined using the least squares method; $t_{2m-n}^{\alpha/2}$—quantile of the t-Student distribution for the confidence level $100(1-\alpha)\%$ and $2m-n$ degrees of freedom.

The least squares sum is characterized by the variance of the fit s_t^2, which is an estimate of the variance of the data σ^2 and is calculated according to

$$s_t = \sqrt{\frac{S_{\min}}{2m - n}} \tag{24}$$

where $2m$ denotes the number of measurement points and n stands for the number of searched parameters.

If the Levenberg–Marquardt iterative method [24–26] is used to solve the nonlinear least-squares problem, then the estimated variance-covariance matrix from the final iteration is

$$\mathbf{D}_x^{(s)} = s_t \mathbf{C}_x^{(s)} = s_t \left[\left(\mathbf{J}^{(s)} \right)^T \mathbf{J}^{(s)} \right]^{-1} \tag{25}$$

where the matrix $\mathbf{C}_x^{(s)}$ is

$$\mathbf{C}_x^{(s)} = \left[\left(\mathbf{J}^{(s)} \right)^T \mathbf{J}^{(s)} \right]^{-1} \tag{26}$$

The superscript (s) denotes the number of the last iteration while $\mathbf{J}$ is the Jacobian matrix.

The Jacobian matrix $\mathbf{J}$ is given by

$$\mathbf{J} = \frac{\partial \mathbf{T}^{cal}(\mathbf{x})}{\partial \mathbf{x}^T} = \left[\left(\frac{\partial T_i^{cal}(\mathbf{x})}{\partial x_j} \right) \right]_{2m \times n}, \; i = 1, \ldots, 2m, \; j = 1, \ldots, n \tag{27}$$

For the issue analyzed in this paper, the Jacobian matrix has the following form:

$$\mathbf{J} = \begin{bmatrix} \frac{\partial T_{h2,1}^{cal}}{\partial x_{1,h}} & \frac{\partial T_{h2,1}^{cal}}{\partial x_{2,h}} & \cdots & \frac{\partial T_{h2,1}^{cal}}{\partial x_{n,h}} \\ \vdots & \vdots & \vdots & \vdots \\ \frac{\partial T_{h2,m}^{cal}}{\partial x_{1,h}} & \frac{\partial T_{h2,m}^{cal}}{\partial x_{2,h}} & \cdots & \frac{\partial T_{h2,m}^{cal}}{\partial x_{n,h}} \\ \frac{\partial T_{c1,1}^{cal}}{\partial x_{1,c}} & \frac{\partial T_{c1,1}^{cal}}{\partial x_{2,c}} & \cdots & \frac{\partial T_{c1,1}^{cal}}{\partial x_{n,c}} \\ \vdots & \vdots & \vdots & \vdots \\ \frac{\partial T_{c1,m}^{cal}}{\partial x_{1,c}} & \frac{\partial T_{c1,m}^{cal}}{\partial x_{2,c}} & \cdots & \frac{\partial T_{c1,m}^{cal}}{\partial x_{n,c}} \end{bmatrix}_{2m \times n} \tag{28}$$

The partial derivatives in the Jacobian matrix are determined for the calculated for m hot $T_{h2,i}^{cal}$ and for m cold $T_{c1,i}^{cal}$ water outlet temperatures of the heat exchanger were calculated using central differential quotients. The symbol c_{ii} in Equation (23) denotes the diagonal element c_{ii} of the matrix $\mathbf{C}_x^{(s)}$.

Considering that the amount of measurement data is large and equals $2m = 68$ then the quantiles $t_{2m-n}^{\alpha/2}$ are equal to two. Having solved the non-linear least squares problem, the temperature differences of the calculated and measured outlet temperatures are known. Next, the minimum sum S_{min} of the squared temperature differences given by Equation (22) and the 95% confidence intervals can be calculated from Equation (23).

3. Thermal-Fluid Measurements of a Plate and Frame Heat Exchanger

Thirty-four measurement series were carried out. The following parameters were measured: hot and cold water volume flow rate at the inlet to the heat exchanger, and hot and cold water temperatures at the inlet and outlet of the heat exchanger. The station is equipped with two tanks, each with a capacity of 800 litres, whose task is to provide a constant temperature of hot and cold water at the inlet to the exchanger (Figure 2). Maintaining a constant temperature of hot and cold water at the exchanger inlet allows for testing of the plate heat exchanger under steady-state conditions.

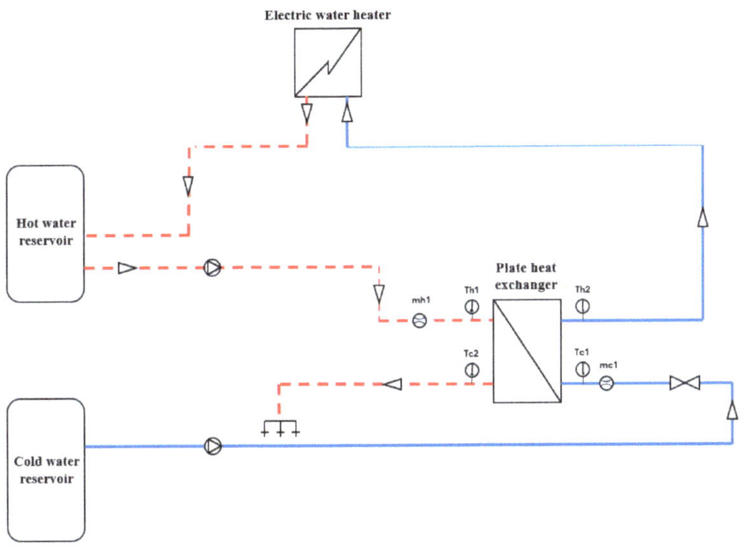

Figure 2. Laboratory setup for flow and thermal testing of plate and frame heat exchangers: red line—hot water; blue line—cold water.

A thermal flow study of the XB12M-1-16 plate heat exchanger (Figure 3), consisting of 16 chevron plates manufactured by Danfoss, Nordborg, Denmark, was carried out. Volume flow rates and hot and cold water temperatures at the inlet and outlet of the exchanger were measured in $m = 34$ measurement series. Hot water flows counter-current to cold water. During the tests, the hot water mass flow rates varied from 7.86×10^{-2} kg/s to 8.15×10^{-1} kg/s, and the cold water from 8.16×10^{-2} kg/s to 6.61×10^{-1} kg/s. The volume flow rate of hot and cold media was measured using axial turbine flow meters with a measuring range of 4 to 160 L/min, with a measurement accuracy of $\pm 2\%$ of the measured value. A new plate heat exchanger with clean plate surfaces was installed at the station. Thermal flow investigations of the exchanger were carried out over two days, so it was unnecessary to clean the exchanger plates during the tests. The cold and hot water flow rates and the temperature of the hot water at the inlet to the exchanger were varied. The cold water temperature at the inlet to the heat exchanger varied from 11.0 to 13.0 °C. The hot water temperature at the inlet to the heat exchanger varied over a wider range than for cold water, from 53.9 to 75.6 °C.

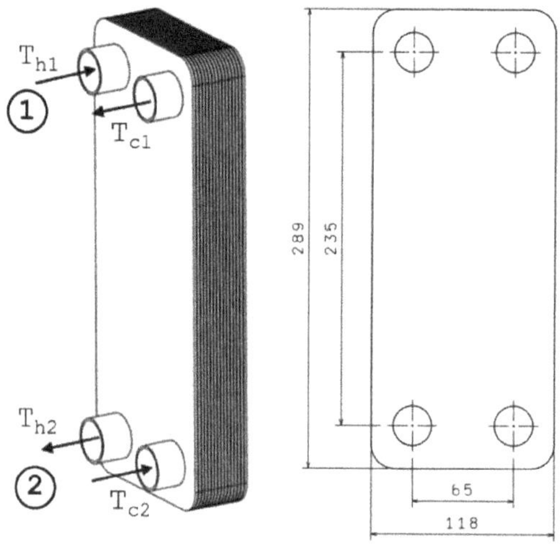

(a) (b)

Figure 3. Plate-and-frame heat exchanger, (**a**) heat exchanger with marked inlets and outlets, (**b**) single plate of Danfoss XB12M-1-16 heat exchanger with dimensions.

The temperature of cold and hot water was measured using K-type (NiCr-Ni) sheathed thermocouples with an outer diameter of 1.5 mm. The thermocouples were pre-calibrated. The uncertainty of water temperature measurement was ±0.5 K.

The hot water temperature T_{h1} at the exchanger inlet varied from 53.9 °C to 75.6 °C, and the cold water temperature from 11 °C to 13 °C. The measurements were carried out under steady-state conditions. After changing the operating parameters of the exchanger, for example, the flow rate of hot or cold water, it was necessary to wait until the operating parameters of the heat exchanger became independent of time.

The measurement data from the 34 measurement series are presented in Table 1.

Table 1. Measurement data for the studied plate-and-frame heat exchanger.

i	$\dot{V}_h$, L/min	T_{h1}, °C	T_{h2}, °C	$\dot{V}_c$, L/min	T_{c1}, °C	T_{c1}, °C
1	20.1	65.1	40.3	10.4	12.5	60.3
2	20.2	64.6	34.1	15.0	12.5	53.4
3	20.1	63.8	29.3	20.0	12.3	46.7
4	20.1	63.6	26.6	24.9	12.7	42.4
5	20.0	62.7	23.4	29.9	12.3	38.4
6	20.1	62.5	22.9	34.8	12.3	35.1
7	20.1	61.6	21.1	39.7	12.4	32.8
8	40.1	63.7	57.4	4.9	12.6	63.6
9	40.0	63.6	51.1	10.1	12.7	62.1
10	39.6	61.4	43.8	15.1	12.0	57.3
11	39.8	60.1	40.2	19.2	12.1	53.3
12	39.8	57.6	35.0	24.9	11.6	47.3
13	39.9	56.0	31.8	30.0	11.5	43.6
14	39.7	54.8	29.6	34.8	11.4	40.0
15	39.8	53.9	28.0	39.7	11.7	37.6

Table 1. *Cont.*

i	$\dot{V}_h$, L/min	T_{h1}, °C	T_{h2}, °C	$\dot{V}_c$, L/min	T_{c1}, °C	T_{c1}, °C
16	4.8	61.6	13.0	20.0	12.3	23.9
17	10.1	62.6	18.7	20.0	12.3	34.4
18	15.0	62.6	24.3	20.0	12.3	40.8
19	20.0	61.6	28.3	20.0	12.3	45.5
20	25.0	61.1	33.4	19.9	13.0	47.7
21	30.0	60.3	35.2	20.2	12.2	49.3
22	34.9	59.6	37.3	20.0	12.2	50.9
23	39.9	58.5	38.7	20.0	12.2	51.2
24	45.0	57.6	39.7	20.2	12.2	51.1
25	5.0	61.8	11.8	25.0	11.2	21.2
26	9.9	62.2	15.2	25.1	11.2	29.5
27	15.0	61.8	20.7	25.1	11.1	35.7
28	20.1	71.2	28.1	25.0	12.5	46.8
29	25.0	72.6	31.4	25.0	12.5	53.3
30	30.0	59.3	31.2	25.0	11.0	44.4
31	35.1	75.6	41.4	25.0	12.9	60.7
32	39.9	70.3	36.5	29.6	12.1	57.4
33	44.6	75.2	44.5	25.1	12.1	64.4
34	50.2	75.0	46.7	26.3	12.1	62.5

3.1. Correlations for Calculating Nusselt Numbers on the Hot and Cold Water Sides of a Plate Heat Exchanger

Heat transfer correlations were derived based on the measurement data presented in Table 1.

First, heat transfer correlations were determined with six unknown parameters: x_{1h}, x_{2h}, x_{3h} on the hot water side and x_{1c}, x_{2c}, x_{3c} on the cold water side.

3.1.1. Six Unknown Parameters (Three on the Hot Water Side and Three on the Cold Water Side)

The Nusselt numbers were approximated by the following power-type correlations:

$$Nu_h = x_{1,h}\mathrm{Re}_h^{x_{2,h}}\mathrm{Pr}_h^{x_{3,h}} \quad 55.44 \le \mathrm{Re_h} \le 852.96 \quad 2.95 \le \mathrm{Pr_h} \le 4.6 \tag{29}$$

$$Nu_c = x_{1,c}\mathrm{Re}_c^{x_{2,c}}\mathrm{Pr}_c^{x_{3,c}} \quad 62.38 \le \mathrm{Re}_c \le 378.89 \quad 4.46 \le \mathrm{Pr}_c \le 7.82 \tag{30}$$

From the minimum sum-of-squares condition (24), the following parameter values were obtained:

- Hot water

$$x_{1,,h} = 0.1902 \quad x_{2,h} = 0.6353 \quad x_{3,h} = 0.2990$$

- Cold water

$$x_{1,c} = 0.0817 \quad x_{2,c} = 0.8732 \quad x_{3,c} = 0.3300$$

The minimum sum of squares is $S_{\min} = 24.61\mathrm{K}^2$, and the root mean square error (RMSE)

$$s_t = \sqrt{S_{\min}/(m-n)} = \sqrt{24.61/(68-6)} = 0.67\mathrm{K}$$

The 95% confidence intervals for the determined parameters calculated according to the Gaussian principle of variance transfer [8] are as follows

$$0.1808 \le x_{1,h} \le 0.1996 \quad 0.5790 \le x_{2,h} \le 0.6917 \quad 0.2246 \le x_{3,h} \le 0.3734$$

$$0.0386 \leq x_{1,c} \leq 0.1248 \quad 0.8353 \leq x_{2,c} \leq 0.9111 \quad 0.2451 \leq x_{3,c} \leq 0.4150$$

The determined correlations for the Nusselt numbers on the hot and cold water sides have good accuracy. Table 2 summarises the calculated and measured hot and cold water temperatures at the heat exchanger outlet. The relative differences between the measured and calculated hot and cold water temperatures are also given.

Table 2. Calculated and measured cold and hot water temperatures at the outlet of the exchanger and the relative differences between the calculated and measured temperatures at the outlet of the exchanger.

i	T_{c1}^{cal}, °C	T_{c1}^{meas}, °C	T_{h2}^{cal}, °C	T_{h2}^{meas}, °C	ε_{T_c}, %	ε_{T_h}, %
1	59.16	60.30	40.51	40.30	1.89	−0.52
2	53.19	53.40	33.83	34.10	0.40	0.80
3	46.85	46.70	28.79	29.30	−0.32	1.75
4	42.43	42.40	26.30	26.60	−0.07	1.92
5	38.01	38.40	23.56	23.40	1.02	−0.69
6	35.17	35.10	22.17	22.90	−0.20	2.16
7	32.54	32.80	19.87	20.45	0.78	0.02
8	63.32	63.60	57.40	57.4	0.44	0.00
9	61.67	62.10	51.02	51.10	0.70	0.15
10	56.83	57.30	44.02	43.80	0.83	−0.51
11	53.16	53.30	39.97	40.20	0.26	0.57
12	47.39	47.30	34.87	35.00	−0.18	0.38
13	43.30	43.60	31.74	31.80	0.69	0.19
14	39.97	40.00	29.39	29.60	0.07	0.70
15	37.45	37.60	27.86	28.00	0.41	0.50
16	23.60	23.90	13.65	13.00	1.27	−4.98
17	34.16	34.40	18.52	18.70	0.71	0.96
18	41.00	40.80	23.64	24.30	−0.50	2.16
19	45.21	45.50	27.90	28.30	0.63	0.65
20	48.50	47.70	32.37	33.40	−1.67	2.16
21	49.72	49.30	34.62	35.20	−0.86	2.16
22	50.97	50.90	37.03	37.30	−0.14	0.73
23	51.26	51.20	38.62	38.70	−0.12	0.21
24	51.30	51.10	39.79	39.70	−0.39	−0.22
25	20.90	21.20	17.00	18.20	1.42	−4.87
26	29.09	29.50	16.00	15.20	1.40	−5.26
27	35.46	35.70	20.30	20.70	0.68	1.93
28	46.94	46.80	27.39	27.90	−0.31	1.92
29	52.21	53.30	31.97	31.40	2.04	−1.81
30	44.97	44.40	30.53	31.20	−1.28	2.16
31	60.87	60.70	40.61	41.40	−0.27	1.92
32	54.90	57.40	37.86	36.50	4.35	−3.73
33	63.87	64.40	45.36	44.50	0.82	−1.94
34	64.33	62.50	46.99	46.70	−2.92	−0.62

The relative differences ε_{T_c} and ε_{T_h} between the measured and calculated temperatures shown in Table 2 were calculated from the following equations:

$$\varepsilon_{T_c} = 100\frac{T_{c1,i}^{meas} - T_{c1,i}^{cal}}{T_{c1,i}^{meas}} \quad \varepsilon_{T_h} = 100\frac{T_{h2,i}^{meas} - T_{h2,i}^{cal}}{T_{h2,i}^{meas}} \tag{31}$$

From the analysis of the results shown in Table 2, the agreement between the calculated and measured temperatures at the heat exchanger outlet is very good. The maximum absolute value of the difference ε_{T_c} is 2.92% for cold water, and the difference ε_{T_h} for hot water is 5.26%. The Root Mean Square Error (RMSE) for the cold water is 2.09% and for hot water, 1.24%.

Table 3 compares the heat flow rate calculated from the hot water $\dot{Q}_h^{meas}$ and cold water sides $\dot{Q}_c^{meas}$, the arithmetic mean of both fluxes $\dot{Q}_m^{meas}$, and the relative difference $\varepsilon_{m,i}^{\dot{Q}}$ between the measured mean flux and the calculated flux.

Table 3. Measured and calculated heat flow rates transferred from hot to cold water, and the relative differences between the average measured and calculated heat flow rates.

i	$\dot{Q}_c^{meas}$, W	$\dot{Q}_h^{meas}$, W	$\dot{Q}_m^{meas}$, W	$\dot{Q}_m^{cal}$, W	ε_c^{meas}, %	$\varepsilon_{m,i}^{\dot{Q}}$, %
1	34,601.10	34,064.14	34,332.62	33,778.23	0.78	1.61
2	42,704.33	42,103.43	42,403.88	42,481.25	0.71	−0.18
3	47,898.54	47,402.77	47,650.66	48,108.81	0.52	−0.96
4	51,489.25	50,839.94	51,164.60	51,542.44	0.64	−0.74
5	54,346.77	53,753.79	54,050.28	53,534.17	0.55	0.95
6	55,264.24	54,440.22	54,852.23	55,437.32	0.75	−1.07
7	56,415.15	55,702.34	56,058.75	55,706.57	0.64	0.63
8	17,393.47	17,290.14	17,341.80	17,298.04	0.30	0.25
9	34,726.56	34,210.44	34,468.50	34,423.41	0.75	0.13
10	47,615.24	47,722.65	47,668.95	47,118.21	−0.11	1.16
11	55,066.15	54,258.92	54,662.54	54,880.80	0.74	−0.40
12	61,893.69	61,685.74	61,789.71	62,044.95	0.17	−0.41
13	67,059.88	66,264.81	66,662.34	66,428.02	0.60	0.35
14	69,318.64	68,693.64	69,006.14	69,253.81	0.45	−0.36
15	71,617.23	70,808.16	71,212.7	71,187.84	0.57	0.03
16	16,170.89	15,961.85	16,066.37	15,749.70	0.65	1.97
17	30,787.06	30,322.9	30,554.98	30,447.45	0.76	0.35
18	39,691.14	39,292.11	39,491.63	39,974.13	0.51	−1.22
19	46,229.25	45,576.95	45,903.10	45,829.58	0.71	0.16
20	48,067.50	47,408.06	47,737.78	49,169.80	0.69	−3.00
21	52,172.09	51,572.84	51,872.46	52,769.28	0.58	−1.73
22	53,881.41	53,325.05	53,603.23	53,978.85	0.52	−0.70
23	54,298.77	54,161.11	54,229.94	54,382.84	0.13	−0.28
24	54,701.24	55,247.63	54,974.44	54,982.70	−0.50	−0.02
25	17,433.93	17,104.11	17,269.02	16,907.62	0.96	2.09
26	32,010.68	31,827.39	31,919.04	31,286.44	0.29	1.98
27	43,015.63	42,180.19	42,597.91	42,590.11	0.98	0.02
28	59,696.88	58,979.68	59,338.28	59,946.27	0.60	−1.02
29	70,999.97	70,076.44	70,538.20	69,111.17	0.66	2.02
30	58,149.81	57,759.76	57,954.79	59,142.13	0.34	−2.05
31	83,170.48	81,567.99	82,369.23	83,458.74	0.97	−1.32
32	93,336.96	91,890.50	92,613.73	88,184.59	0.78	4.78
33	91,375.08	93,074.73	92,224.91	90,455.05	−0.92	1.92
34	92,265.31	96,594.41	94,429.86	95,609.80	−2.29	−1.25

The values of the heat flow rates transferred from hot to cold water for the $m = 34$ measurement series shown in Table 3 were calculated from the following expressions

$$\begin{aligned} \dot{Q}_{h,i}^{meas} &= \dot{m}_{h,i} c_{h,i} \left(T_{h1,i}^{meas} - T_{h2,i}^{meas}\right) \\ \dot{Q}_{c,i}^{meas} &= \dot{m}_{c,i} c_{c,i} \left(T_{c1,i}^{meas} - T_{c2,i}^{meas}\right) \\ \dot{Q}_{m,i}^{meas} &= \left(\dot{Q}_{c,i}^{meas} + \dot{Q}_{h,i}^{meas}\right)/2 \quad i = 1, \ldots, m \end{aligned} \tag{32}$$

The relative differences between the heat flow rates calculated from the hot water $\dot{Q}_{h,i}^{meas}$ or cold water side $\dot{Q}_{c,i}^{meas}$ and the average heat flow rates $\dot{Q}_{m,i}^{meas}$ were calculated from the following formulas

$$\begin{aligned} \varepsilon_{c,i}^{\dot{Q}} &= 100\left(\dot{Q}_{c,i}^{meas} - \dot{Q}_{m,i}^{meas}\right)/\dot{Q}_{m,i}^{meas} \\ \varepsilon_{h,i}^{\dot{Q}} &= 100\left(\dot{Q}_{h,i}^{meas} - \dot{Q}_{m,i}^{meas}\right)/\dot{Q}_{m,i}^{meas} \quad i = 1, \ldots, m \end{aligned} \tag{33}$$

Between the differences, there is a relationship $\varepsilon^{\dot{Q}}_{c,i} = -\varepsilon^{\dot{Q}}_{h,i}$.

The calculated heat flow rate from hot and cold water are equal to each other

$$\dot{Q}_i^{cal} = \dot{m}_{h,i}c_{h,i}(T^{meas}_{h1,i} - T^{cal}_{h2,i}) = \dot{m}_{c,i}c_{c,i}(T^{meas}_{c1,i} - T^{cal}_{c2,i}) \tag{34}$$

The differences between the average heat flow rate determined experimentally $\dot{Q}^{meas}_{m,i}$ and the calculated heat flow rates $\dot{Q}_i^{cal}$ were calculated from the equation

$$\varepsilon^{\dot{Q}}_{m,i} = 100(\dot{Q}^{meas}_{m,i} - \dot{Q}_i^{cal})/\dot{Q}^{meas}_{m,i} \quad i = 1, \ldots, m \tag{35}$$

In Equations (32)–(35) the following designations are used: $\dot{Q}^{meas}_{c,i}$, $\dot{Q}^{meas}_{h,i}$, $\dot{Q}^{meas}_{m,i}$—cold, hot and average heat flow rates, respectively, calculated for the i-th measurement series; $\dot{Q}_i^{cal}$—heat flow rate for the i-th measuring series calculated from the cold or hot water side; $\varepsilon^{\dot{Q}}_{c,i}$, $\varepsilon^{\dot{Q}}_{h,i}$—the difference between the experimentally determined heat flow rate; $\dot{Q}^{meas}_{c,i}$, $\dot{Q}^{meas}_{h,i}$ and the average value $\dot{Q}^{meas}_{m,i}$ for the i-th measurement series; $\varepsilon^{\dot{Q}}_{m,i}$—the difference between the average heat flow rates measured $\dot{Q}^{meas}_{m,i}$ and calculated $\dot{Q}_i^{cal}$.

An analysis of the values presented in Table 3 shows that the heat flow rate calculated from the temperature measurements on the cold and hot water sides show very good agreement. The differences between the average flow rate and the flow rate on the cold or hot water side for most points do not exceed ±1%. Only for measurement number 34 is the difference 2.29%. The calculated heat flow rate from hot to cold water also differs little from the average heat flow rate determined experimentally. The maximum difference is 4.78%.

Based on thirty-four measurement series in which the above-mentioned variables were measured, i.e., hot and cold water mass flow rates and inlet and outlet temperatures from the heat exchanger, unknown parameters were determined, i.e., coefficients and power exponents in correlations for the Nusselt number for hot and cold water. The values of parameters determined in correlations for Nusselt numbers clearly depend on the values of measured quantities, which means that the inverse problem is well-posed. Thus, the sensitivity coefficients determined for the Nusselt number in relation to the measured values should not be too small. A change in a given measured value should cause changes in the sought parameters appearing in the correlation for the Nusselt number and a change in the value of the Nusselt number. The sensitivity coefficients for the Nusselt number for the seventh measurement series (Table 1) are calculated below.

$$\frac{\partial Nu}{\partial \dot{V}_h} = \frac{Nu(\dot{V}_h+\Delta\dot{V}_h)-Nu(\dot{V}_h-\Delta\dot{V}_h)}{2\Delta\dot{V}_h} = \frac{Nu(20.1+2.01)-Nu(20.1-2.01)}{2\cdot 2.01} = \frac{9.252048-8.818098}{2\cdot 2.01} = 0.107948\,\frac{\text{min}}{\text{l}}$$

$$\frac{\partial Nu}{\partial T_{h1}} = \frac{Nu(T_{h1}+\Delta T_{h1})-Nu(T_{h1}-\Delta T_{h1})}{2\Delta T_{h1}} = \frac{Nu(61.1+1.0)-Nu(61.1-1.0)}{2\cdot 1.0} = \frac{9.619821-9.633703}{2\cdot 1.0} = -6.941\cdot 10^{-3}\,\frac{1}{\text{K}}$$

$$\frac{\partial Nu}{\partial T_{h2}} = \frac{Nu(T_{h2}+\Delta T_{h2})-Nu(T_{h2}-\Delta T_{h2})}{2\Delta T_{h2}} = \frac{Nu(21.1+1.0)-Nu(21.1-1.0)}{2\cdot 1.0} = \frac{9.262340-10.129780}{2\cdot 1.0} = -0.43372\,\frac{1}{\text{K}}$$

$$\frac{\partial Nu}{\partial \dot{V}_c} = \frac{Nu(\dot{V}_c+\Delta\dot{V}_c)-Nu(\dot{V}_c-\Delta\dot{V}_c)}{2\Delta\dot{V}_c} = \frac{Nu(39.7+2.0)-Nu(39.7-2.0)}{2\cdot 2.0} = \frac{27.938780-25.471890}{2\cdot 2.0} = 0.6167225\,\frac{\text{min}}{\text{l}}$$

$$\frac{\partial Nu}{\partial T_{c1}} = \frac{Nu(T_{c1}+\Delta T_{c1})-Nu(T_{c1}-\Delta T_{c1})}{2\Delta T_{c1}} = \frac{Nu(12.4+1.0)-Nu(12.4-1.0)}{2\cdot 1.0} = \frac{25.406170-27.587310}{2\cdot 1.0} = -1.09057\,\frac{1}{\text{K}}$$

$$\frac{\partial Nu}{\partial T_{c2}} = \frac{Nu(T_{c2}+\Delta T_{c2})-Nu(T_{c2}-\Delta T_{c2})}{2\Delta T_{c2}} = \frac{Nu(32.8+1.0)-Nu(32.8-1.0)}{2\cdot 1.0}$$
$$= \frac{25.896690-27.438820}{2\cdot 1.0} = -0.771065\frac{1}{\mathrm{K}}$$

The determined sensitivity coefficient values are high, which is beneficial for the accuracy of the determined correlations for Nusselt numbers for cold and hot water.

Next, the determination of correlations for Nusselt numbers on the hot and cold water sides for two unknown parameters on each side of the plate will be presented.

3.1.2. Four Unknown Parameters (Two on the Hot Water Side and Two on the Cold Water Side)

Heat transfer correlations were also determined, assuming two unknown parameters in the correlation for hot water (n_h = 2) and two unknown parameters on the cold water side (n_c = 2).

The Nusselt numbers were approximated by the following power-type correlations

$$Nu_h = x_{1,h}\mathrm{Re}_h^{x_{2,h}}\mathrm{Pr}_h^{0.29} \quad 55.44 \le \mathrm{Re}_h \le 852.96 \quad 2.95 \le \mathrm{Pr}_h \le 4.6 \tag{36}$$

$$Nu_c = x_{1,c}\mathrm{Re}_c^{x_{2,c}}\mathrm{Pr}_c^{0.41} \quad 62.38 \le \mathrm{Re}_c \le 378.89 \quad 4.46 \le \mathrm{Pr}_c \le 7.82 \tag{37}$$

The minimum of the sum of squares defined by Equation (24)

- Hot water

$$x_{1,h} = 0.2016 \quad x_{2,h} = 0.6202$$

- Cold water

$$x_{1,c} = 0.0622 \quad x_{2,c} = 0.9098$$

The minimum sum of squares is $S_{\min} = 25.03\mathrm{K}^2$, and the mean square error is

$$s_t = \sqrt{S_{\min}/(m-n)} = \sqrt{25.03/(68-4)} = 0.63\mathrm{K}$$

The 95% confidence intervals for the determined parameters calculated according to the variance transfer principle [8] proposed by Gauss are as follows:

$$0.1266 \le x_{1,h} \le 0.2765 \quad 0.5213 \le x_{2,h} \le 0.7191$$

$$0.0107 \le x_{1,c} \le 0.1137 \quad 0.8782 \le x_{2,c} \le 0.9413$$

Heat transfer correlations were then determined assuming 3 unknown parameters x_1, x_2, x_3, the same on the hot and cold water sides.

3.1.3. Three Unknown Parameters (n = 3)

$$Nu_h = x_1\mathrm{Re}_h^{x_2}\mathrm{Pr}_h^{x_3} \quad 55.44 \le \mathrm{Re}_h \le 852.96 \quad 2.95 \le \mathrm{Pr}_h \le 4.6 \tag{38}$$

$$Nu_c = x_1\mathrm{Re}_c^{x_2}\mathrm{Pr}_c^{x_3} \quad 62.38 \le \mathrm{Re}_c \le 378.89 \quad 4.46 \le \mathrm{Pr}_c \le 7.82 \tag{39}$$

From the minimum sum-of-squares condition (24), the following parameter values were obtained

$$x_1 = 0.115374 \quad x_2 = 0.757967 \quad x_3 = 0.3334$$

The minimum sum of squares is $S_{\min} = 26.81\text{K}^2$, and the mean square error is

$$s_t = \sqrt{S_{\min}/(m-n)} = \sqrt{26.81/(68-3)} = 0.64\text{K}$$

The 95% confidence intervals for the determined parameters, calculated according to the variance transfer principle [8] proposed by Gauss are as follows:

$$0.1127 \leq x_1 \leq 0.1180 \quad 0.7532 \leq x_2 \leq 0.7628 \quad 0.3220 \leq x_3 \leq 0.3448$$

It can be seen that the 95% confidence intervals for all three parameters are narrow. This demonstrates the good accuracy of the mathematical model of the heat exchanger as well as being a good indication of the quality of the measurement data.

4. Discussion

This paper presents a method for simultaneously determining the correlation between the hot and cold water sides of the Nusselt numbers as a function of the Reynolds number and Prandtl number. Two approaches were used to determine the correlations on the hot and cold water sides. Firstly, separate correlations per Nusselt number for hot and cold water were proposed. Three unknown parameters were determined for the correlation on the hot water side, and three parameters on the cold water side.

The determined correlations differ significantly in the values of the power exponents at the Reynolds numbers if we assume two different correlations for hot and cold water. In the case of the six parameters determined, the exponents at the Reynolds number differ significantly and are $x_{2,h} = 0.6353$ and $x_{2,c} = 0.8732$. Slightly smaller differences are found in the exponents at Prandtl numbers $x_{3,h} = 0.2990$ and $x_{3,c} = 0.3300$.

The number of unknown parameters in correlations for the Nusselt number was reduced to four to check whether correct results could be obtained with fewer than six parameters. As in the case of the six determined parameters, the exponents for the Reynolds numbers differ significantly for the four determined parameters when the correlations on the hot and cold water sides differ. The values of the exponents for the Reynolds numbers are $x_{2,h} = 0.6202$ and $x_{2,c} = 0.9098$ for hot and cold water, respectively.

The exponents for the Prandtl numbers were selected by a trial and error method, so the sum of the squares of the calculated and measured temperature differences was the smallest. The exponent for the Prandtl number for hot water, equal to 0.29, and the exponent for cold water, equal to 0.41, are very close to the corresponding values of 0.3 and 0.4 adopted by Dittus and Boelter [2–8].

The third approach proposed a common correlation for cold and hot water with three unknown parameters. The following parameter values were obtained $x_1 = 0.115374$, $x_2 = 0.757967$ and $x_3 = 0.3334$. The value of the parameter x_3 is close to 1/3 of the values found in correlations for the Nusselt number based on Chilton-Colburn analogies [2–8].

All proposed correlations are valid in the following ranges of Reynolds and Prandtl number changes, namely $55.44 \leq \text{Re}_h \leq 852.96$, $2.95 \leq \text{Pr}_h \leq 4.6$ for hot water and $62.38 \leq \text{Re}_c \leq 378.89$, $4.46 \leq \text{Pr}_c \leq 7.82$ for cold water.

Tables 4–6 show the Nusselt numbers as a function of the Reynolds number for hot water for three selected Prandtl numbers, Pr = 3.0, Pr = 3.9 and Pr = 4.5. The Nusselt numbers were calculated using Equations (29), (36) and (38) derived for six, four and three unknown parameters, respectively, in correlations for the Nusselt number.

A comparison of the Nusselt numbers presented in Tables 4–6 shows that correlations (29) and (36) give similar results, while correlation (38), which contains the same three coefficients on the hot and cold water sides, significantly exceeds the Nusselt numbers obtained assuming six and four unknown parameters.

Similar comparisons of Nusselt number values to those presented in Tables 4–6 for hot water are illustrated in Tables 7–9 for cold water.

Table 4. Selected Nusselt number values for hot water determined using correlations (29), (36) and (38) for Prandtl number Pr = 3.0; correlation (29) was determined assuming six unknown parameters, correlation (36) assuming four unknown parameters, and correlation (38) assuming three parameters identical for hot and cold water; symbol Nu_m denotes the average Nusselt number from the values obtained using Equations (29), (36) and (38).

	Equation (29)	Equation (36)	Equation (38)	
Re_h	$Nu=0.1902Re^{0.6353}Pr^{0.2990}$	$Nu=0.2016Re^{0.6202}Pr^{0.2900}$	$Nu=0.1153Re^{0.7579}Pr^{0.3334}$	Nu_m
50	3.1712	3.1373	3.2281	3.1789
150	6.3730	6.2011	7.4231	6.6657
250	8.8162	8.5125	10.9330	9.4206
350	10.9173	10.4879	14.1091	11.8381
450	12.8072	12.2568	17.0698	14.0446
550	14.5486	13.8813	19.8740	16.1013
650	16.1776	15.3966	22.5567	18.0436
750	17.7172	16.8255	25.1410	19.8946
850	19.1836	18.1837	27.6429	21.6700

Table 5. Selected Nusselt number values for hot water determined using correlations (29), (36) and (38) for Prandtl number Pr = 3.9; correlation (29) was determined assuming six unknown parameters, correlation (36) assuming four unknown parameters, and correlation (38) assuming three parameters identical for hot and cold water; symbol Nu_m denotes the average Nusselt number from the values obtained using Equations (29), (36) and (38).

	Equation (29)	Equation (36)	Equation (38)	
Re_h	$Nu=0.1902Re^{0.6353}Pr^{0.2990}$	$Nu=0.2016Re^{0.6202}Pr^{0.2900}$	$Nu=0.1153Re^{0.7579}Pr^{0.3334}$	Nu_m
50	3.4300	3.3853	3.5232	3.4462
150	6.8930	6.6913	8.1017	7.2287
250	9.5356	9.1855	11.9324	10.2178
350	11.8082	11.3170	15.3989	12.8414
450	13.8524	13.2258	18.6301	15.2361
550	15.7359	14.9786	21.6907	17.4684
650	17.4978	16.6138	24.6187	19.5767
750	19.1631	18.1557	27.4391	21.5860
850	20.7491	19.6212	30.1698	23.5133

Table 6. Selected Nusselt number values for hot water determined using correlations (29), (36) and (38) for Prandtl number Pr = 4.8; correlation (29) was determined assuming six unknown parameters, correlation (36) assuming four unknown parameters, and correlation (38) assuming three parameters identical for hot and cold water; symbol Nu_m denotes the average Nusselt number from the values obtained using Equations (29), (36) and (38).

	Equation (29)	Equation (36)	Equation (38)	
Re_h	$Nu=0.1902Re^{0.6353}Pr^{0.2990}$	$Nu=0.2016Re^{0.6202}Pr^{0.2900}$	$Nu=0.1153Re^{0.7579}Pr^{0.3334}$	Nu_m
50	3.6497	3.5954	3.7757	3.6736
150	7.3345	7.1066	8.6824	7.7078
250	10.1464	9.7556	12.7877	10.8966
350	12.5646	12.0194	16.5026	13.6955
450	14.7397	14.0467	19.9656	16.2506
550	16.7438	15.9083	23.2455	18.6325
650	18.6185	17.6449	26.3833	20.8823
750	20.3905	19.2825	29.4060	23.0263
850	22.0781	20.8390	32.3323	25.0831

Table 7. Selected Nusselt number values for cold water determined using correlations (30), (37) and (39) for Prandtl number Pr = 4.5; correlation (30) was determined assuming six unknown parameters, correlation (37) assuming four unknown parameters, and correlation (39) assuming three parameters identical for hot and cold water; symbol Nu_m denotes the average Nusselt number from the values obtained using Equations (30), (37) and (39).

	Equation (30)	Equation (37)	Equation (39)	
Re_c	$Nu=0.0817Re^{0.8732}Pr^{0.3300}$	$Nu=0.0622Re^{0.9098}Pr^{0.4100}$	$Nu=0.1153Re^{0.7579}Pr^{0.3334}$	Nu_m
60	4.7914	4.7794	4.2430	4.6046
100	7.4848	7.6069	6.2492	7.1136
140	10.0411	10.3313	8.0646	9.4790
180	12.5051	12.9854	9.7569	11.7491
220	14.9000	15.5863	11.3597	13.9487
260	17.2400	18.1447	12.8932	16.0926
300	19.5346	20.6677	14.3703	18.1909
340	21.7906	23.1605	15.8003	20.2505
380	24.0132	25.6268	17.1902	22.2767

Table 8. Selected Nusselt number values for cold water determined using correlations (30), (37) and (39) for Prandtl number Pr = 6.0; correlation (30) was determined assuming six unknown parameters, correlation (37) assuming four unknown parameters, and correlation (39) assuming three parameters identical for hot and cold water; symbol Nu_m denotes the average Nusselt number from the values obtained using Equations (30), (37) and (39).

	Equation (30)	Equation (37)	Equation (39)	
Re_c	$Nu=0.0817Re^{0.8732}Pr^{0.3300}$	$Nu=0.0622Re^{0.9098}Pr^{0.4100}$	$Nu=0.1153Re^{0.7579}Pr^{0.3334}$	Nu_m
60	5.2686	5.3777	4.6701	5.1054
100	8.2302	8.5592	6.8782	7.8892
140	11.0411	11.6246	8.8764	10.5140
180	13.7504	14.6110	10.7390	13.0335
220	16.3838	17.5375	12.5032	15.4749
260	18.9569	20.4162	14.1910	17.8547
300	21.4800	23.2551	15.8168	20.1840
340	23.9607	26.0599	17.3909	22.4705
380	26.4046	28.8350	18.9206	24.7200

Table 9. Selected Nusselt number values for cold water determined using correlations (30), (37) and (39) for Prandtl number Pr = 7.5; correlation (30) was determined assuming six unknown parameters, correlation (37) assuming four unknown parameters, and correlation (39) assuming three parameters identical for hot and cold water; symbol Nu_m denotes the average Nusselt number from the values obtained using Equations (30), (37) and (39).

	Equation (30)	Equation (37)	Equation (39)	
Re_c	$Nu=0.0817Re^{0.8732}Pr^{0.3300}$	$Nu=0.0622Re^{0.9098}Pr^{0.4100}$	$Nu=0.1153Re^{0.7579}Pr^{0.3334}$	Nu_m
60	5.6712	5.8929	5.0308	5.5316
100	8.8592	9.3792	7.4095	8.5493
140	11.8848	12.7383	9.5620	11.3950
180	14.8012	16.0108	11.5685	14.1268
220	17.6358	19.2177	13.4689	16.7742
260	20.4055	22.3722	15.2870	19.3549
300	23.1214	25.4830	17.0384	21.8810
340	25.7917	28.5565	18.7340	24.3607
380	28.4223	31.5975	20.3819	26.8006

In the case of cold water, correlation (39) with the same three coefficients for cold and hot water gives significantly lower Nusselt number values. It can be expected that the overall HTCs for the same Reynolds numbers will be similar regardless of the number of unknown parameters in the Nusselt number correlations. However, it should be emphasised that differences in Nusselt number correlations on the hot and cold water sides lead to different plate temperatures. In the case of high-temperature heat exchangers, the same correlation for cold and hot water may lead to an inaccurate estimate of the wall temperature and incorrect selection of plate material.

The average Nusselt number Nu_m in Figures 4a, 5a, 6a, 7a, 8a and 9a was calculated using the equation

$$\mathrm{Nu}_m(\mathrm{Re}) = \frac{\mathrm{Nu}^{6\mathrm{p}}(\mathrm{Re}) + \mathrm{Nu}^{4\mathrm{p}}(\mathrm{Re}) + \mathrm{Nu}^{3\mathrm{p}}(\mathrm{Re})}{3} \tag{40}$$

where the symbols $\mathrm{Nu}^{6\mathrm{p}}$, $\mathrm{Nu}^{4\mathrm{p}}$ and $\mathrm{Nu}^{3\mathrm{p}}$ denote the Reynolds numbers calculated using correlations containing six, four and three parameters, respectively.

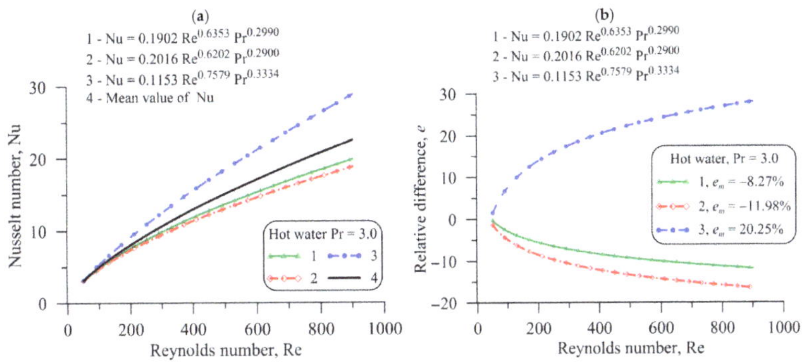

Figure 4. Comparison of Nusselt numbers for Prandtl number Pr = 3.0 calculated using correlations for hot water calculated using the following equations: (29)—curve 1, (36)—curve 2, and (38)—curve 3 (**a**); relative differences e_i between Nusselt number values calculated using Equations (29), (36) and (38), respectively, and the average Nusselt number value for a given Reynolds number (**b**).

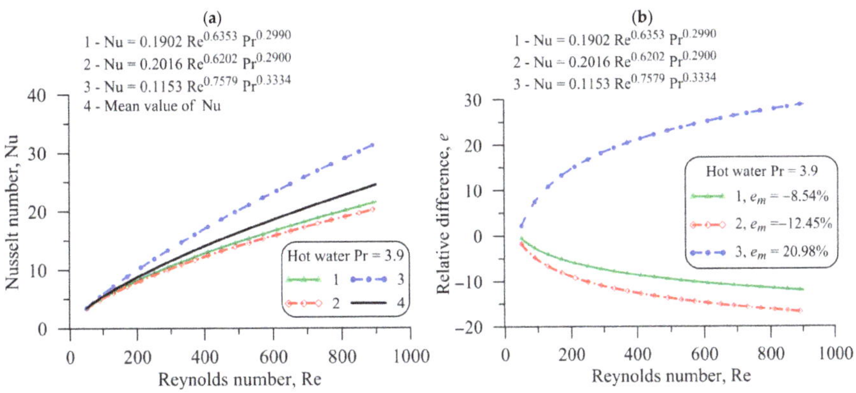

Figure 5. Comparison of Nusselt numbers for Prandtl number Pr = 3.9 calculated using correlations for hot water calculated using the following equations: (29)—curve 1, (36)—curve 2, and (38)—curve 3 (**a**); relative differences e_i between Nusselt number values calculated using Equations (29), (36) and (38), respectively, and the average Nusselt number value for a given Reynolds number (**b**).

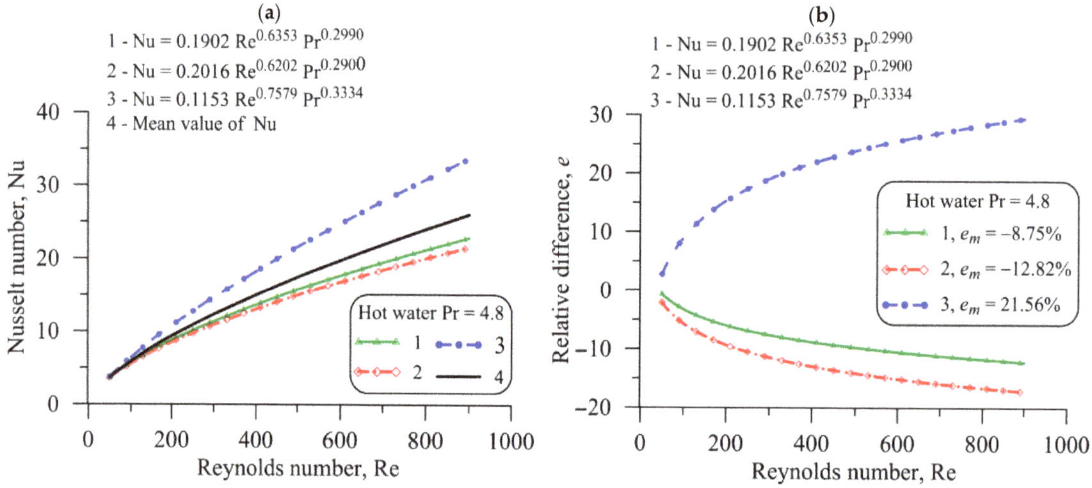

Figure 6. Comparison of Nusselt numbers for Prandtl number Pr = 4.8 calculated using correlations for hot water calculated using the following equations: (29)—curve 1, (36)—curve 2, and (38)—curve 3 (**a**); relative differences e_i between Nusselt number values calculated using Equations (29), (36) and (38), respectively, and the average Nusselt number value for a given Reynolds number (**b**).

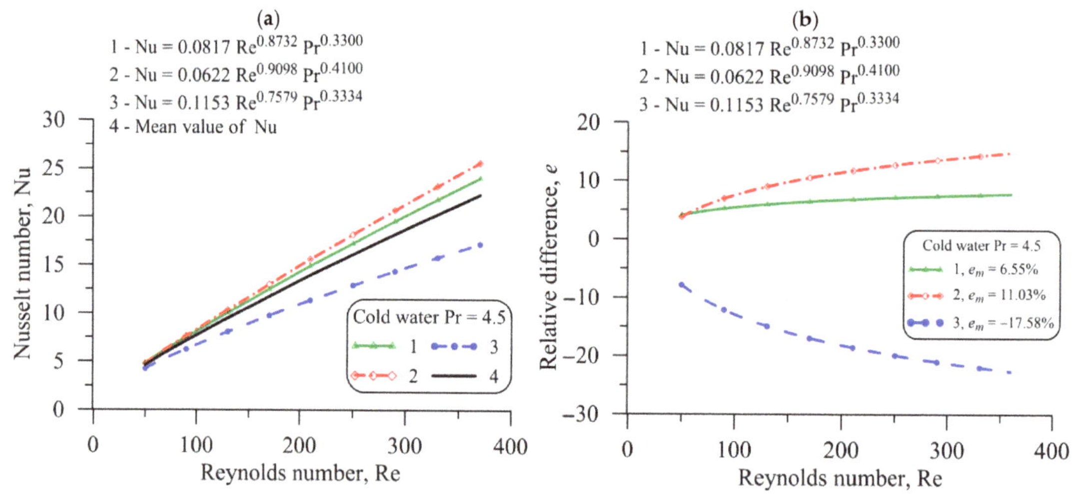

Figure 7. Comparison of Nusselt numbers for Prandtl number Pr = 4.5 calculated using correlations for cold water calculated using the following equations: (30)—curve 1, (37)—curve 2, and (39)—curve 3 (**a**); relative differences e_i between Nusselt number values calculated using Equations (30), (37) and (39), respectively, and the average Nusselt number value for a given Reynolds number (**b**).

The relative differences shown in Figures 4b, 5b, 6b, 7b, 8b and 9b were calculated using the following equation

$$e(\mathrm{Re}) = \frac{\mathrm{Nu}(\mathrm{Re}) - \mathrm{Nu}_m(\mathrm{Re})}{\mathrm{Nu}_m(\mathrm{Re})} \cdot 100\% \tag{41}$$

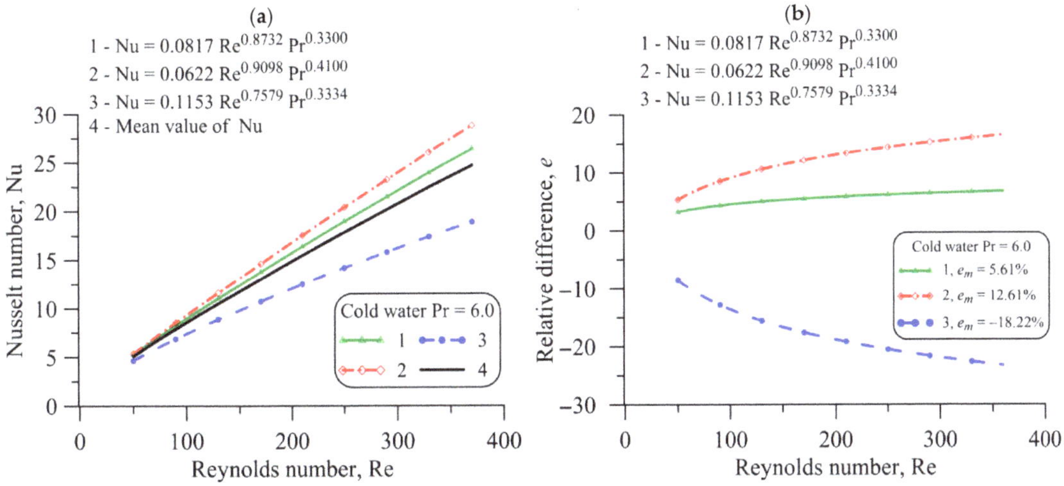

Figure 8. Comparison of Nusselt numbers for Prandtl number Pr = 6.0 calculated using correlations for cold water calculated using the following equations: (30)—curve 1, (37)—curve 2 and (39)—curve 3 (**a**); relative differences e_i between Nusselt number values calculated using Equations (30), (37) and (39), respectively, and the average Nusselt number value for a given Reynolds number (**b**).

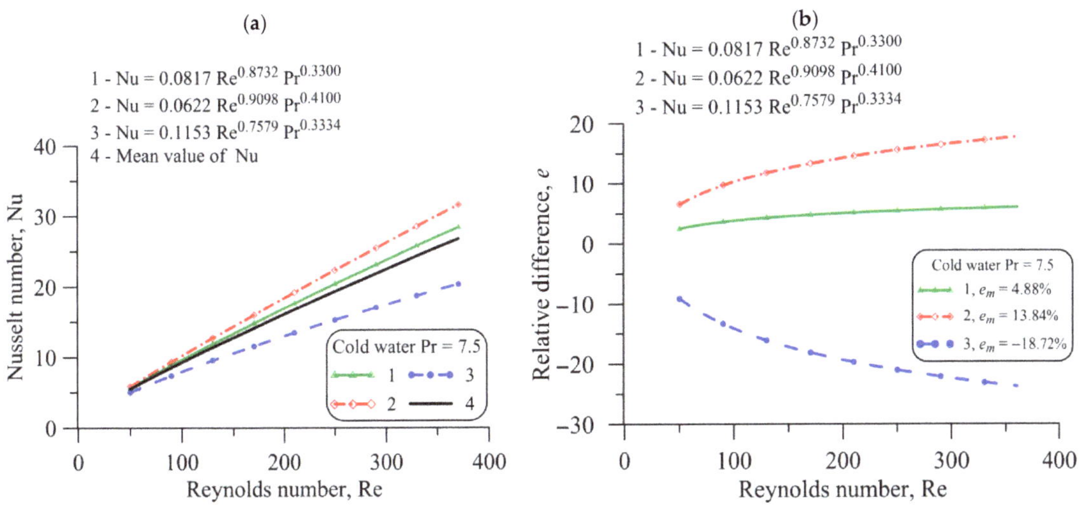

Figure 9. Comparison of Nusselt numbers for Prandtl number Pr = 7.5 calculated using correlations for cold water calculated using the following equations: (30)—curve 1, (37)—curve 2, and (39)—curve 3 (**a**); relative differences e_i between Nusselt number values calculated using Equations (30), (37) and (39), respectively, and the average Nusselt number value for a given Reynolds number (**b**).

The average error value e_m was calculated using the equation

$$e_m = \frac{\sum_{i=1}^{n_f} \mathrm{Nu}(\mathrm{Re}_i)}{n_f} \tag{42}$$

where n_f = 86 is the number of points for hot water and n_f = 33 is the number of points for cold water. The step for calculating the Reynolds number Re_i was equal 10.

The average relative differences e_m between the values Nu (Re) and Nu_m, calculated using Equation (42), are as follows for hot water:

- Pr = 3.0
  −8.27%, −11.98%, and 20.25% in accordance with Equation (29) (six unknown parameters, separate correlations for hot and cold water), Equation (36) (4 unknown parameters, separate correlations for hot and cold water), and Equation (38) (3 unknown parameters, one common correlation for hot and cold water),
- Pr = 3.9
  −8.54%, −12.45%, and 20.98% in accordance with Equation (29) (six unknown parameters, separate correlations for hot and cold water), Equation (36) (4 unknown parameters, separate correlations for hot and cold water), and Equation (38) (3 unknown parameters, one common correlation for hot and cold water),
- Pr = 4.8
  −8.75%, −12.82%, and 21.56% in accordance with Equation (29) (six unknown parameters, separate correlations for hot and cold water), Equation (36) (4 unknown parameters, separate correlations for hot and cold water), and Equation (38) (3 unknown parameters, one common correlation for hot and cold water).

The average relative differences e_m for cold water are as follows:

- Pr = 4.5
  6.55%, 11.03%, and −17.58% in accordance with Equation (30) (six unknown parameters, separate correlations for hot and cold water), Equation (37) (4 unknown parameters, separate correlations for hot and cold water), and Equation (39) (3 unknown parameters, one common correlation for hot and cold water),
- Pr = 6.0
  5.1%, 12.61%, and −18.22% in accordance with Equation (30) (six unknown parameters, separate correlations for hot and cold water), Equation (37) (4 unknown parameters, separate correlations for hot and cold water), and Equation (39) (3 unknown parameters, one common correlation for hot and cold water),
- Pr = 7.5
  4.88%, 13.84%, and −18.72% in accordance with Equation (30) (six unknown parameters, separate correlations for hot and cold water), Equation (37) (4 unknown parameters, separate correlations for hot and cold water), and Equation (39) (3 unknown parameters, one common correlation for hot and cold water).

The analyses of the results presented in Tables 4–8 and Figures 4–9 show that the HTCs on the hot and cold water sides should be calculated using different correlations. Separate correlations for hot and cold water better approximate the experimental data, which are characterised by different ranges of Reynolds and Prandtl number changes for cold and hot water.

It is recommended to determine separate correlations for the Nusselt number on the hot and cold fluid sides in order to better account for the range of changes in the Reynolds and Prandtl numbers on each side. The separate correlations for hot and cold water can be recommended for practical applications because of their better accuracy. They can also be used to calculate the heat transfer resistance from hot to cold water in the heat exchanger under test.

5. Conclusions

Knowledge of HTCs on the hot and cold sides is important not only in design and performance calculations of the heat exchanger, but is also essential for correctly determining the temperature of the plate and, in general, the temperature of the wall separating the hot and cold fluids.

The presented method of simultaneous determination of correlations for the Nusselt number on the hot and cold water sides is characterised by high accuracy. It is competitive with the Wilson method, which is more labour-intensive due to the need for iterative determination of correlations for Nusselt numbers on both sides of the partitions, in this case, plates. The advantage of the proposed method is the possibility of determining the uncertainty of the estimated parameters by determining 95% confidence intervals.

In the paper, three different heat transfer correlations for calculating the Nusselt number in a chevron plate heat exchanger are proposed. In the first correlation, six parameters were determined based on experimental data, four parameters were determined in the second correlation, and three were determined in the third correlation. The final correlation is identical for hot and cold water, while in the case of six and four parameters, separate correlations are used for hot and cold water. The correlations with six or four give similar Nusselt numbers for the same Reynolds and Prandtl numbers.

The accurate correlation with three or two parameters determined on each side of the plate results from different ranges of Reynolds and Prandtl number changes on the hot and cold water sides. The ranges of Reynolds and Prandtl numbers change on the hot water side are as follows: $55.44 \leq \mathrm{Re}_h \leq 852.96$ and $2.95 \leq \mathrm{Pr}_h \leq 4.6$, while on the cold water side, they are different: $62.38 \leq \mathrm{Re}_c \leq 378.89$ and $4.46 \leq \mathrm{Pr}_c \leq 7.82$.

However, in the third correlation, the three common parameters for hot and cold water are used. The analyses carried out in this study show that a single correlation for hot and cold water with three specified parameters does not give good results, as the experimental data for hot and cold water cover different ranges of Reynolds and Prandtl numbers. Since the determined parameters depend to a large extent on the range of changes in the Reynolds and Prandtl numbers, it is difficult to obtain satisfactory accuracy for hot and cold water using a single correlation for both.

It is recommended to determine separate correlations for the Nusselt number on the hot and cold fluid sides in order to better account for the range of changes in the Reynolds and Prandtl numbers on each side. The separate correlations for hot and cold water can be recommended for practical applications because of their accuracy. They can also be used to calculate the heat transfer resistance from hot to cold water in the heat exchanger under test.

6. Future Work

The general method presented in the article for simultaneously determining heat transfer correlations on the hot and cold sides is universal and can be used to determine correlations for Nusselt numbers in various types of heat exchangers. In the future, heat transfer correlations will be determined in coil, shell-and-tube heat exchangers and PFTHEs with round, elliptical and rectangular tubes and various types of plate fins.

The correlations derived in the paper for calculating HTCs for hot and cold water will be used to determine the heat transfer resistance from hot to cold water in plate heat exchangers with clean surfaces without scale deposits. Plate heat exchangers are used in heat substations for domestic hot water preparation and building heating in municipal central heating systems. Water from the municipal water supply is heated by hot water from a district heating network. Cold mains water is often characterised by a high content of mineral salts deposited on the plates' surface in scale. For this reason, plate heat exchangers become fouled and must be cleaned periodically and replaced with new ones after several chemical cleanings. The build-up of limescale on the plate surface is accompanied by a decrease in the overall HTC, which decreases heat flow rate from hot to cold water. In addition, the active cross-sectional area between the plates decreases, which causes an increase in the pressure drop on the heated hot water side. Thermal resistance of scale deposits is the difference between the inverse of the HTC of a fouled heat exchanger and the HTC of a non-fouled heat exchanger with clean plate surfaces.

$$r_f = \frac{1}{U_f} - \frac{1}{U} \tag{43}$$

where r_f—thermal resistance of scale deposits, $(\mathrm{m^2K/W})$; U_f—overall HTC of fouled heat exchanger, $\mathrm{W/(m^2K)}$; U—overall HTC of the clean heat exchanger, given by Equation (14), $\mathrm{W/(m^2K)}$.

The overall HTC U for the heat exchanger with clean plate surfaces is not constant and varies depending on the mass flow of hot and cold water and the temperature of hot and cold water at the inlet to the exchanger. When monitoring the thermal resistance r_f of fouling, the overall HTC U for a clean exchanger is calculated online using the Nusselt number correlation for cold and hot water proposed in the paper. The uncertainty in calculating the overall HTC U for a clean heat exchanger is small, as this coefficient is calculated with high accuracy in the proposed method. Even if the h_h and h_c coefficients are calculated with less accuracy, this does not affect the determined U value. If one of the heat transfer coefficients, e.g., h_h, is too high, then the h_c coefficient must be lower so that the U value remains the same.

The overall HTC of the fouled heat exchanger is determined online using the following equation:

$$U_f = \frac{\dot{Q}}{A \Delta T_{lm}} \tag{44}$$

The symbol $\dot{Q}$ in Equation (44) represents the heat flow rate in the heat exchanger from hot to cold water; ΔT_{lm} is the logarithmic mean temperature difference (LMTD) between hot and cold water and A designates the heat transfer area.

A numerical method for determining Nusselt numbers on the side of the cold and hot water in the clean plate-and-frame heat exchanger was developed based on flow-thermal measurements. The proposed method for determining the thermal resistance of scale deposits will be applied in a computer system to monitor heat substation fouling in large city's district heating network. The online monitoring system for the fouling degree of heat exchangers will monitor several to several thousand heat exchangers in the central heating system. Installation of the system does not require any hardware modifications to the heating system. Unknown parameters in correlations for Nusselt numbers for a clean heat exchanger are determined based on flow and thermal tests of a clean exchanger in a laboratory or based on flow and thermal measurements of a clean heat exchanger installed in a municipal central heating system. Correlations for calculating HTCs are determined once. In the monitoring system, HTCs on the cold and hot water side are calculated using previously developed correlations, and then the overall HTC is calculated using Equation (14). The time required to calculate the overall heat transfer coefficient U and thermal resistance r_f is several to several dozen times shorter than the time step for collecting measurement data in the heat exchanger monitoring system.

Author Contributions: Conceptualization, D.T. and E.Z.; methodology, D.T.; software, J.T., E.Z. and T.C.; validation, T.S., M.J. and J.T.; formal analysis, D.T. and M.M.; investigation, T.S., M.J. and E.Z.; resources, M.M.; data curation, M.M.; writing—original draft preparation, D.T. and E.Z.;

writing—review and editing, T.C.; visualization, M.M.; supervision, J.T. and D.T. All authors have read and agreed to the published version of the manuscript.

Funding: This research received no external funding.

Data Availability Statement: All data are available in the main text. Additional datasets related to this study are available from the corresponding author upon reasonable request.

Conflicts of Interest: The authors declare no conflicts of interest.

Abbreviations

The following abbreviations are used in this manuscript:

CFD	Computational fluid dynamics
HTC	Heat transfer coefficient
IHCP	Inverse heat conduction problem
LMTD	Logarithmic mean temperature difference
NTU	Number of transfer units
PFTHE	Plate-fin and tube heat exchanger
P-NTU	Effectiveness—Number of transfer units
ε-NTU	Effectiveness—Number of transfer units

References

1. Kakaç, S.; Liu, H.; Pramuanjaroenkij, A. *Heat Exchangers. Selection, Rating, and Thermal Design*, 4th ed.; CRC-Taylor & Francis Group: Boca Raton, FL, USA, 2020.
2. Kays, W.M.; London, A.L. *Compact Heat Exchangers*, 3rd ed.; McGraw-Hill: New York, NY, USA, 1998.
3. Wilson, E.E. A basis for rational design of heat transfer apparatus. *Trans. ASME* **1915**, *37*, 47–82. [CrossRef]
4. Sekulić, D.P.; Shah, R.K. *Fundamentals of Heat Exchanger Design*, 2nd ed.; Wiley: Hoboken, NJ, USA, 2023.
5. Taler, D. *Numerical Modelling and Experimental Testing of Heat Exchangers*; Springer Nature: Cham, Switzerland, 2019.
6. Dittus, F.W.; Boelter, L.M.K. Heat transfer in automobile radiators of the tubular type. *Univ. Calif. Publ. Eng.* **1930**, *2*, 443–461, reprinted in *Int. Commun. Heat Mass Transf.* **1985**, *12*, 3–22. [CrossRef]
7. Gnielinski, V. New equations for heat and mass transfer in turbulent tube and channel flow. *Int. Chem. Eng.* **1976**, *16*, 359–368.
8. Taler, D. A new heat transfer correlation for transition and turbulent fluid flow in tubes. *Int. J. Therm. Sci.* **2016**, *108*, 108–122. [CrossRef]
9. Nasrfard, H.; Rahimzadeh, H.; Ahmadpour, A.; Naderan, H. Experimental study of condensation heat transfer for R141b in intermittent flow regime within a smooth horizontal tube. *Exp. Therm. Fluid. Sci.* **2019**, *105*, 109–122. [CrossRef]
10. Fu, Y.; Bian, B.; Liu, Y.; Zhang, L.; Li, M.; Wen, J.; Xu, G. Airside heat transfer analysis using Wilson plot method of three analogous serpentine tube heat exchangers for aero-engine cooling. *Appl. Therm. Eng.* **2024**, *248*, 123238. [CrossRef]
11. Shah, W.; Abbas, A.; Ayub, Z.H.; Ayub, A.H.; Moreira, T.A.; Ribatski, G.; Li, W. Shell side direct expansion evaporation of ammonia on a 3-D structured surface tube bundle with exit superheat effect. *Int. J. Refrig.* **2023**, *147*, 1–9. [CrossRef]
12. Nguyen, D.H.; Kim, T.; Kim, J.M.; Kim, T.; Arkadumnuay, T.; Mahian, O.; Ahn, H.S.; Wongwises, S. Enhancing the vertical downward condensation heat transfer of a plate heat exchanger by electrochemical etching. *Int. J. Heat Mass Transf.* **2024**, *225*, 125277. [CrossRef]
13. Li, L.; Gou, Y.; Min, H.; Gao, N.; Li, Q. Experimental study on the pool boiling heat transfer of R134a outside various enhanced tubes. *Int. J. Heat Mass Transf.* **2024**, *235*, 126140. [CrossRef]
14. Shokouhmand, H.; Salimpour, M.R.; Akhavan-Behabadi, M.A. Experimental investigation of shell and coiled tube heat exchangers using Wilson plots. *Int. Commun. Heat Mass Transf.* **2008**, *35*, 84–92. [CrossRef]
15. Fronk, B.M.; Garimella, S. Condensation of ammonia and high-temperature-glide ammonia/water zeotropic mixtures in minichannels—Part I: Measurements. *Int. J. Heat Mass Transf.* **2016**, *101*, 1343–1356. [CrossRef]
16. Taler, D.; Taler, J.; Trojan, M. Experimental verification of an analytical mathematical model of a round or oval tube two-row car radiator. *Energies* **2020**, *13*, 3399. [CrossRef]
17. Yu, X.Y.; Huang, W.S.; Liu, X.L.; Liu, P.T.; Tang, G.H.; Li, X.L. Thermal-hydraulic performance and optimization for finned-tube heat exchanger in gas wall-hung boilers. *Appl. Therm. Eng.* **2025**, *262*, 125241. [CrossRef]
18. Marcinkowski, M.; Taler, D.; Węglarz, K.; Taler, J. Advancements in analysing air-side heat transfer coefficient on the individual tube rows in finned heat exchangers: Comparative study of three CFD methods. *Energy* **2024**, *307*, 132754. [CrossRef]

19. Zhu, X. Relationship between chevron angle and heat transfer performance of plate heat exchangers. *Case Stud. Therm. Eng.* **2025**, *69*, 106032. [CrossRef]
20. Taler, D. Experimental determination of correlations for average heat transfer coefficients in heat exchangers on both fluid sides. *Heat Mass Transf.* **2013**, *49*, 1125–1139. [CrossRef]
21. Marchetto, D.B.; Marinheiro, M.M.; Netto, A.T.; Furlan, G.; Ribatski, G.; Thome, J.R.; Tibiriçá, C.B. Condensation flow inside tubes: A review of heat transfer coefficient measurement techniques, experimental databases and prediction methods. *Exp. Therm. Fluid. Sci.* **2025**, *160*, 111298. [CrossRef]
22. Thulukkanam, K. *Heat Exchanger Design Handbook*, 2nd ed.; CRC-Taylor & Francis: Boca Raton, FL, USA, 2013.
23. Mills, A.F. *Basic Heat & Mass Transfer*, 2nd ed.; Pearson: New York, NY, USA, 2014.
24. Levenberg, K. A method for the solution of certain non-linear problems in least squares. *Q. Appl. Math.* **1944**, *2*, 164–168. [CrossRef]
25. Marquardt, D.W. Algorithm for least-squares estimation of nonlinear parameters. *J. Soc. Ind. Appl. Math.* **1963**, *11*, 431–441. [CrossRef]
26. Seber, G.A.F.; Wild, C.J. *Nonlinear Regression*; Wiley-Interscience: Hoboken, NJ, USA, 2003.

MDPI AG
Grosspeteranlage 5
4052 Basel
Switzerland
Tel.: +41 61 683 77 34

Energies Editorial Office
E-mail: energies@mdpi.com
www.mdpi.com/journal/energies

www.ingramcontent.com/pod-product-compliance
Lightning Source LLC
Chambersburg PA
CBHW061557220926
51850CB00005B/357
* 9 7 8 3 7 2 5 8 5 9 8 7 0 *